Nursing the Critically Ill Adult

Nursing the Critically Ill Adult

Nancy Meyer Holloway, BSN, MSN
Instructor in Nursing Service
Staff Development
University of California,
San Francisco

Addison-Wesley Publishing Company
Medical/Nursing Division   Menlo Park, California
Reading, Massachusetts • London • Amsterdam
Don Mills, Ontario • Sydney

Sponsoring Editor: James Keating
Production Editor: Pat Franklin
Developmental Editor: Paula Cizmar
Cover Design: Michael A. Rogondino
Book Design: Linda S. Stinchfield
Artist: Jack Tandy

Library of Congress Cataloging in Publication Data

Holloway, Nancy Meyer, 1947–
    Nursing the critically ill adult.

    Bibliography: p.
    Includes index.
    1. Intensive care nursing. I. Title.
RT120.I5H64   610.73'6   78–21153
ISBN 0–201–02948–0
ABCDEFGHIJ–AL–782109

The author and publishers have exerted every effort to ensure that drug selection and dosage set forth in this text are in accord with current recommendations and practice at the time of publication. However, in view of ongoing research, changes in government regulations and the constant flow of information relating to drug therapy and drug reactions, the reader is urged to check the package insert for each drug for any change in indications of dosage and for added warnings and precautions. This is particularly important where the recommended agent is a new and/or infrequently employed drug.

Addison-Wesley Publishing Company
Medical/Nursing Division
2725 Sand Hill Road
Menlo Park, California 94025

Foreword

Of recent years the critical care nurses have, in many ways, been the leaders of clinical nursing. Faced with the burgeoning influx of scientific advances in medicine, surgery, anesthesiology and electronics into the patient setting, these nurses recognized the need for additional information and advanced knowledge. Quick to see the advantages offered to patient care, intensive care nurses sought help from the most visible informed group of experts, the physicians. The doctors who themselves were feeling the threat and push from the technological and scientific developments, and who needed informed, cogent, expert observers, responded with on-site teaching and classes to satisfy the immediate needs of the nurses and the demands of the public. It is therefore of little wonder that current textbooks are primarily based on a medical model and emphasize "how to" rather then "why." By focusing on a single physical system or specialty area, the totality of the patient seen through the development of thoughtful nursing care plans was lost to the immediacy of the moment. This book with its emphasis on a conceptual framework of patient needs, therefore, differs markedly from what is usually offered.

The book presents another difference to existing critical care nursing texts in that the content, the frameworks, the drawings, the sequence and the guidelines have been tested using real nurses, real patients, and a real setting. This gives the material an authenticity that cannot be attained in any other way, and a relevance that is not able to be duplicated.

The book evolved from a portion of a 1975 program in critical care nursing supported by the Nursing Service at the University of California, San Francisco. The program consisted of 5 weeks of didactic experience and 7 weeks of clinical experience in a variety of critical care settings at the university. The students were registered nurses with 1–5 years of general nursing experience, some of whom would take permanent positions in the units and some of whom would form the nucleus of a critical care "float pool". To meet the needs of such a diverse group of learners, the program focused on helping them learn the commonalities in the care of critically ill patients.

The conceptual framework likewise is a pragmatic approach to nursing, developed by a nurse, that concentrates on nursing concerns about patient needs. The commonalities are therefore outgrowths of the essential requirements of individualized patient care. The format of factors, fluids, aeration, nutrition, communication, activity and pain (FANCAP), formally came about to afford students with a simple, easily remembered tool for patient assessment and planning of care. The book appropriately provides a modification of the original mnemonic to afford an expansion of content for the informed or advanced learner. The chapters are, thus, organized around patient needs for fluids, aeration, nutrition, communication, activity and stimulation (FANCAS). In the analysis for patient care, the physical systems are viewed not as entities in themselves but as contributing concerns and strengths to be considered in meeting the patient's vital needs.

Unlike other current texts on critical care nursing, this book presents the concepts of anatomy and physiology not as introductory material to a discussion of disorders, but as integrated content. Principles of anatomy and physiology are interwoven throughout the discussion of assessment techniques, pathophysiology and care. Such a technique promotes relevance, learning, recall, and use of the information in the clinical setting.

To ensure that the learner is able to use the information, each chapter begins with behavioral objectives based on the conceptual framework. The objectives state what the learner should be able to do (rather than know) upon completion of the learning experience. The objectives will help guide learning and assist in judging learner progress and competence as a critical care nurse.

The author's attention to practical application and usefulness is evidenced by inclusion of basic information with solid grounding in significance to clinical nursing. Attainment of basic knowledges and skills is recognized as being an essential prerequisite to advanced subspecialty development. Numerous line drawings and tables which summarize information and relationships further enhance the book's usefulness in the clinical setting where quick reference and clarification are essential. The book, however, is not intended as a comprehensive treatise of in-depth critical care nursing. A bibliography at the end of each chapter provides guidance for further study.

Examples of care plans written by a nurse proficient in critical care are included to: 1) afford review of familiar care problems associated with specific pathophysiological conditions; 2) provide opportunity for discussion; 3) permit argument and dissension with the expert and 4) stimulate thinking and further exploration.

The book contains an appendix on the USCF program. Included are guidelines for establishing a similar program, a possible curriculum and examples of evaluation tools. These are offered as take-off points for: 1) the practitioner as ideas for setting up individualized learning experiences and 2) the educator as adjunct material in course planning or ideas for meeting individual learner needs.

As the originator of FANCAP, I find this book to be one of nursing's real forward steps toward definition of responsibilities, capabilities and direction. The book differs significantly from current texts in its use of a uniquely nursing framework to present tested, pragmatic and practical content. The information offered is basic to critical care and one who wishes to be an expert will profit from careful study, thought and clinical application of the principles and techniques.

In summary, this book will be useful to you if you are . . . an RN beginning your career in critical care nursing . . . an RN already working in critical care who wants to review and strengthen your knowledge base . . . a nursing student needing practical information to gain the most from your clinical experiences . . . a critical care educator in a nursing service staff development department, or . . . a critical care educator in a school of nursing.

June C. Abbey, RN, PhD, FAAN

Preface

Nursing the Critically Ill Adult is meant for you, the R.N. or R.N. student interested in critical care nursing. To gain the most from the material, you should already have completed courses in basic anatomy and physiology. You also should have education and experience in nursing adults with common noncritical pathologies, such as chronic lung disease, and should be proficient in implementing basic nursing skills, such as aseptic technique and administration of medications. You will gain the maximum benefit from the book if you intersperse study of it with periods of clinical practice under the supervision of an experienced critical care nurse.

Acknowledgments   Many people have contributed to the genesis of this book. Over 40 of my colleagues reviewed chapters to ensure their accuracy and relevance. To each of them, I owe a debt I can never repay. Jacqueline Georges, Linda Vanderbout, and Lisa Johnsen devoted hundreds of hours to preparing the manuscript. Paula Cizmar edited and polished the prose, while the artwork of J. P. Tandy and Associates expertly illustrated key points. At Addison-Wesley Publishing Company, Pat Franklin shepherded the book through producton, while Jim Keating oversaw the entire project; each provided both expertise and encouragement at crucial points. Finally, I am indebted to my family for the love which nourished me through the years of work, especially my husband Mike and my small son Jason, whose cries and gurgles provided welcome diversion from the challenging and exciting job of writing this text on critical care nursing.

Nancy Meyer Holloway

Contents

Nursing the Critically Ill Adult

Chapter 1

Introduction

Outline

Nursing process   Assessment/Planning and Implementation/Evaluation

FANCAS

Core concepts and skills

Conclusions

References

Henderson (1966) has written: "The unique function of the nurse is to assist the individual, sick or well, in the performance of those activities contributing to health or its recovery (or to peaceful death) that he would perform unaided if he had the necessary strength, will, or knowledge." As a critical-care nurse, you offer your patients and their families something very special: direct assistance with life-and-death crises. This assistance can be both an awesome responsibility and a tremendously exciting challenge.

Critical-care nursing is the nursing of people undergoing life-threatening physiologic crises. The essence of critical-care nursing is anticipation and early intervention in problems besetting the critically ill. Prediction of patient problems must be based on a sound understanding of anatomy and physiology and astute patient assessment. For this reason, significant portions of this book are devoted to helping you acquire this information. Critical-care nursing also requires adeptness at nursing care planning, intervention, and evaluation. These subjects also are discussed in depth in this book.

In a short time of clinical practice, you can learn the mechanics of critical care—the application of ECG electrodes, manipulation of hemodynamic monitoring lines, and so on. You can become adept at these technical skills,

1

however, without truly comprehending the principles upon which they are based. Without understanding the underlying principles, you may find yourself depending upon physicians' orders and the habitual behavior of other nurses for guidance; crises seem to occur with alarming frequency, and you may become increasingly anxious about your ability to cope with them. Your patients suffer, too, because you are unable to spot problems early and prevent them from reaching crisis proportions. Tired and tense, you may also find you cannot give patients and families the emotional support they desperately need. Slowly, the satisfaction and pride you initially felt as a critical-care nurse evaporates and your nursing becomes just a crisis-oriented, highly stressful job beset with staff shortages, "assembly line" patient care, and too many dying patients. Eventually, "burnt out," you decide critical-care nursing really is not for you and leave the field.

This scenario, replayed many times in critical-care nursing, is one reason for rapid turnover of nursing staff in many critical-care units. It is tragic: the nurse feels she somehow has failed to "measure up" and patients are deprived of an experienced critical-care nurse. Worse, it is a tragedy that could be prevented.

The critical-care nurse must be assisted in evolving a nursing style which both nurtures her and enables her to provide optimum patient care.

Nursing process

The keys to such a nursing style—anticipation, judgment, and creativity—depend upon skillful application of the nursing process in critical-care situations. This process consists of four interdependent phases: assessment, planning, implementation, and evaluation. Andreoli and Thompson (1977) state:

> In order to use the nursing process, nurses must possess intellectual skills for problem-solving, critical thinking, and nursing judgments; interpersonal skills for the ability to communicate, listen, inform, and obtain necessary data in a manner that enhances the individuality of the client as a person; and finally, technical skills to relate methods, procedures, and machines used to bring about specific results or the desired behavioral responses of the client.

Although separated in this book for analysis, the phases of the nursing process interact synergistically in practice.

Assessment

The admitting physician's goal is the diagnosis of medical problems. To this end, he will perform a comprehensive history and physical examination to the extent appropriate to the patient's current status. The health history usually consists of the patient's chief complaint, profile, family history, past health history, history of the present problem, and a review of systems, in which the patient is questioned about the presence and characteristics of symptoms. A detailed physical examination then follows.

Comprehensive nursing assessment of the patient necessitates collection of data from many sources: the health record, your own physical assessment of the patient, interviews with the patient and/or the family, monitoring devices, diagnostic studies, and laboratory tests. When gathering data from these sources, remember that your focus is on the patient's current condition and information with nursing implications. The sections of the book addressing patient assessment present one way to examine these data systematically. By following a logical sequence in assessment, you avoid accidentally overlooking an important source of information about your patient.

Obviously, it is neither expedient nor appropriate to collect all the data presented in these sections for every patient. Within the first 5–10 minutes of admission, you should obtain a brief nursing history and perform a rapid examination guided by the patient's symptomatology. In this rapid assessment, you should seek to identify the patient's major problems, the rapidity with which they are developing, and how well he is compensating for them. You then will be able to determine priorities and initiate any urgent care. More complete assessment can be undertaken once care for the patient's immediate life threats has been instituted.

By developing knowledge and skill in patient assessment, you can enhance your ability to deliver comprehensive, high-quality patient care. You will be better able to detect significant changes early, institute care, and evaluate the results of your actions. You also will be better able to understand the detailed examinations performed by physicians and appreciate the significance of their findings. Finally, you will be able to demonstrate to patients, visitors, and other staff the increasing responsibility nurses are assuming for anticipation, prevention, and early intervention in the myriad disorders that can plague the critically ill.

Planning and implementation

An analogy can be made between a neophyte cook and a neophyte critical-care nurse. When you are learning to cook, a cookbook guides you into selecting the proper ingredients in the proper proportions and informs you what others have found to be the most effective ways to prepare the dish so that it ends up a delight instead of a disaster. As you develop skill in cooking, you begin to experiment, adapting the ingredients and techniques to fit what you have on hand. Eventually, for familiar dishes you may not need the cookbook at all, consulting it only when you prepare a dish you serve infrequently. In fact, you may even become a gourmet cook, inventing your own recipes.

This book describes concepts and techniques used in critical-care nursing. But just as you cannot become a great cook by blind adherence to recipes, you cannot become an excellent critical-care nurse by rote application of concepts; nor can you learn motor skills from written descriptions only. You must care for patients under the guidance of an experienced practitioner who can help you develop the ability to sort through concepts and facts, select the ones pertinent to your patient and practice setting, and synthesize them into a plan of action. Even in seemingly routine situations, you must be alert for special circumstances and adapt your care accordingly. With practice, you may discover that you no longer need this book's guidelines in familiar situations. Instead, you will return to them from time to time to refresh your memory and to guide your care in unfamiliar circumstances.

Evaluation

Evaluation is a crucial phase of the nursing process because it enables you to judge the accuracy of your decisions and actions during the earlier phases. To help you evaluate your assessments, plans, and interventions, each chapter of this book contains a list of patient outcome criteria, that is, the desirable outcomes toward which your care is oriented. These are ideal outcome criteria and you again must use your judgment about their applicability in a given situation.

In addition to the nursing process, two other unifying concepts guided the selection and organization of the body of knowledge in this book: FANCAS and the core approach.

FANCAS

Nursing education long has been patterned upon the traditional "body systems" approach, which evolved from a medical model of patient care. This book departs from that model and instead uses a conceptual approach based on a model developed by a nurse, Dr. June C. Abbey.* In 1963, Dr. Abbey identified six areas of concern to nurses in caring for a patient: fluid balance, aeration, nutrition, communication, activity, and pain. The teaching tool she developed to help nurses remember these concerns carries the mnemonic FANCAP (1976). The model used in this book is an adaptation of FANCAP called FANCAS (Swendsen 1975). In this adaptation, data related to a patient's pain may be recorded under the category to which it most closely relates. The S stands for stimulation.

FANCAS serves as a memory aid to help you discover a patient's problems and project solutions to them. The order of the letters is not significant. The categories deliberately are broad to allow maximum flexibility of the tool in various clinical settings. The definitions and subcategories shown in Table 1-1 are derived from Abbey and Swendsen. Dr. Abbey states that any categorization of a given problem is correct provided it can be supported logically.

Professor, Physiological Nursing Programs, University of Utah, Salt Lake City.

Table 1-1 FANCAS and selected core concepts and skills in critical-care nursing

Letter	Category	Definition	Core concepts	Core skills
F	Fluid balance	Movement of fluids and electrolytes among body compartments	Cardiac anatomy and physiology	Cardiac physical assessment
			Nursing care in arrhythmias	Hemodynamic pressure monitoring
			Nursing care in myocardial failure, infarction, and tamponade	ECG interpretation
				Interpretation of reports of cardiac diagnostic procedures
			Vascular anatomy and physiology	Vascular physical assessment
			Hematopoietic anatomy and physiology	Interpretation of complete blood count and coagulation values
			Nursing care in shock	
			Renal anatomy and physiology	Renal physical assessment
			Nursing care in acute renal failure	Interpretation of urinalysis, BUN, creatinine, and related laboratory tests
			Dialysis	
			Fluid and electrolyte physiology	Fluid and electrolyte physical assessment
			Nursing care in fluid and electrolyte imbalances:	Interpretation of serum osmolality, serum electrolytes, and related laboratory tests
			Fluid excess	
			Fluid deficit	
			Hypo/hypernatremia	
			Hypo/hyperkalemia	
			Hypo/hypercalcemia	
			Hypo/hypermagnesemia	
			Nursing care in therapeutic hypothermia	Use of hypothermia blanket

Table 1-1 (*continued*)

Letter	Category	Definition	Core concepts	Core skills
A	Aeration	Movement of gases to provide energy and eliminate volatile waste products	Respiratory anatomy and physiology Nursing care in acute disorders of aeration: Acute respiratory failure Atelectasis Pulmonary edema Pulmonary embolism Pneumothorax	Aeration physical assessment Interpretation of bedside pulmonary function test reports Interpretation of arterial blood gases Interpretation of chest x-ray reports Nursing skills related to oxygen therapy, chest physiotherapy, artificial airways, tracheal suctioning, mechanical ventilation, and chest drainage
			Acid-base physiology Nursing care in acid-base imbalances: Respiratory acidosis Respiratory alkalosis Metabolic acidosis Metabolic alkalosis	Interpretation of arterial blood gases Interrelationships among blood gases and serum electrolytes
N	Nutrition	Intake, digestion, and absorption of nutrients; removal of solid waste products	Abdominal anatomy and physiology Nursing care in hyperalimentation	Assessment of nutritional status Abdominal assessment Nursing skills related to hyperalimentation

Table 1-1 (*continued*)

Letter	Category	Definition	Core concepts	Core skills
C	Communication	Verbal and nonverbal interchange between person and his environment	Stages of adaptation Crisis intervention Anatomy and physiology of vision, hearing, and speech	Assessment of communication process and content
A	Activity	Expenditure of physical or psychological energy	Physiological effects of bedrest Body image Sensory disturbances Sexuality Nursing care of bedridden patients	Assessment of activity Prevention of detrimental effects of bedrest: range-of-motion exercises, positioning procedures Environmental control
S	Stimulation	Perception, interpretation, and integration of stimuli	Anatomy and physiology of nervous system Nursing care in increased intracranial pressure	Stimulation physical assessment Intracranial pressure monitoring

FANCAS provides a convenient way to distingush aspects of a patient for study. In reality, these aspects are so inextricably intertwined that they mandate a holistic approach to each individual.

Core concepts and skills

The concept of core knowledge and skills implies that there are some common principles and techniques in the care of critically ill patients. These standard elements provide a fruitful approach to mastering the general principles and skills of critical-care nursing, which can be applied to a wide variety of patients. Table 1-1 also lists the core concepts and skills discussed in this book.

Conclusions

Nursing in the past has functioned largely on a perceptual basis, that is, the nurse perceived a problem and then acted upon it. Her behavior often was prescribed by common sense or ritualistic practice. In recent years, the profession increasingly has emphasized an intellectual approach to patient care. With the addition of cognition to perception and action (Doona 1976), nursing is becoming a science as well as an art.

Such an approach is crucial for developing the body of nursing knowledge, but it must be tempered by an awareness of the realities of day-to-day practice in the clinical setting. According to Doona (1976), the dynamic interaction of perceptual and conceptual data is the key to ideal judgment. Tempering your scientific knowledge with judgment will enable you to become a wise critical-care nurse. Add imagination to the mix, and you also will become a creative one.

References

Abbey, J. 1976. FANCAP: a descriptive study of a useful tool for teaching clinical nursing. Unpublished doctoral dissertation. University of California, San Francisco.
Historical development, relevant teaching/learning theory and comparative analysis of FANCAP's use in several schools of nursing.

Andreoli, K., and Thompson, C. 1977. The nature of science in nursing. *Image* 9:32–37.
Thought-provoking discussion of the relationship between science and nursing, concluding that although science exists in nursing, the science of nursing is still embryonic.

Doona, M. 1976. The judgment process in nursing. *Image* 8:27–29.
Importance of judgment in nursing; theory and types of judgment.

Henderson, V. 1966. *The nature of nursing.* New York: Macmillan Publishing Company, Inc.
Philosophical definition of nursing and its development as a profession.

Swendsen, L. 1975. FANCAS: a framework for nursing assessment. University of California School of Nursing, San Francisco.
Definitions of FANCAS categories and classification of patient data.

Chapter 2

Cardiac Assessment

There are numerous cardiac diagnostic techniques. This chapter presents those that you are most likely to encounter in the bedside care of the patient. At the end of this chapter, you will have the theoretical knowledge necessary for beginning skill in (1) physical assessment of your patients, (2) interpretation of cardiac pressure data, (3) ECG analysis, and (4) nursing care related to selected diagnostic procedures.

Outline

History

Physical examination   Inspection / Palpation / Percussion / Auscultation / Hemodynamic monitoring data / Nursing goals / Prevention of complications

Electrocardiogram   ECG recording / ECG interpretation

Diagnostic procedures   Chest roentgenology / Echocardiography / Phonocardiography / Vectorcardiography / Cardiac catheterization

Objectives

- Identify ribs and intercostal spaces by reference to the angle of Louis
- State the location of the cardiac chambers and great vessels in relation to external chest landmarks
- Inspect and palpate the precordium

- Define S_1, S_2, S_3, S_4, and murmur
- Auscultate the precordium
- Compare and contrast the normal pressure curves and values for the atria, ventricles, and great vessels
- Compare and contrast the advantages and disadvantages of a left atrial pressure line, pulmonary artery line, and central venous pressure line
- Assist with the insertion of a hemodynamic monitoring line
- Obtain accurate pressure readings and interpret them
- Identify and prevent potential patient problems related to hemodynamic monitoring lines
- Record a 12-lead ECG
- Place a patient on a cardiac monitor
- Define resting membrane potential, threshold, depolarization, and repolarization
- Explain why the SA node is the usual cardiac pacemaker
- Identify the events represented by the P wave, PR interval, QRS, ST segment, and T wave
- Analyze the ECG for basic arrhythmias
- Briefly describe the technique, diagnostic value, and nursing care related to chest roentgenology, echocardiography, phonocardiography, vectorcardiography, and cardiac catheterization

As noted in the Introduction, the first category in the FANCAS system is that of fluid balance. Fluid balance is a complex process primarily regulated by the interdependent actions of the cardiac, vascular, and renal systems. This chapter focuses on nursing assessment of the cardiac system.

History

An important initial step in assessment is a review of the patient's history to the point at which the nurse is assuming responsibility for his or her care. The purpose of this review is to note data with implications for the planning and delivery of nursing care. Sources of this information include the patient's health record, the nursing Kardex, and the change-of-shift report. Examples of important historical data are factors that precipitate or alleviate chest pain, an allergy to morphine, and death of a family member following a myocardial infarction.

Your review of the patient's history must be supplemented by a "hands on" assessment of current physical status. The following sections discuss in detail the physical examination of the patient.

Physical examination

When examining the patient, remember that physical examination is based on the techniques of inspection, palpation, percussion, and auscultation. These techniques demand the refinement of your senses of sight, touch, and hearing to detect subtle indicators of patient status.

Inspection

Search for noncardiac clues   Nurses sometimes hurry through the phase of general inspection in their eagerness to auscultate the heart and investigate data from mechanical equipment. Developing the skill of inspection, however, can provide you with a great deal of information about your patient.

For instance, does your patient look apprehensive? cyanotic? Is the patient gasping or doubled over in pain? diaphoretic? These signs suggest a calamity, such as myocardial infarction or a large pulmonary embolus, and are hard to miss. Unless you look specifically for more subtle signs, however, you may not notice such clues as cyanosis of the tongue and clubbing of the fingers, both indicative of hypoxemia, or distended neck veins, indicative of right-sided heart failure.

In addition to overall inspection, you can gain valuable information about the patient's cardiac status by examining the peripheral vascular and pulmonary systems. Pertinent techniques for evaluating these systems are presented in Chapters 5 and 9. The remainder of this chapter will focus on cardiac assessment. One convenient format for assessment is shown in Table 2-1.

External chest landmarks   To examine the heart and understand your findings, you must have a clear idea of the cardiac structures and their relationship to external chest markings. These external chest landmarks serve as reference points in describing your cardiac findings.

The heart sits in the mediastinum. It is positioned above the diaphragm and between the lungs. The *precordium* is that portion of the external chest wall which overlies the heart.

When reporting your physical findings, describe their location in relation to the nearest rib or intercostal space (ICS) and imaginary reference line (Figure 2-1).

To locate the intercostal spaces, feel for a bony ridge across the sternum about two inches below the suprasternal notch. This ridge is called the *sternal angle* or *angle of Louis*. It marks the attachment of the second rib and is a handy reference point from which to count the ribs and intercostal spaces. Place your second and third fingers on either side of the ridge and slide them out past the sternal border until you feel a depression under your third finger. This depression is the second intercostal space. Continue numbering the ribs and spaces by palpating downward and laterally in an oblique line. Remember that the ribs

Table 2-1   Cardiac assessment format

1. History _____

2. Physical

    A. Inspection/palpation

    PMI _____

    Precordial movements _____

    B. Auscultation

    Heart sounds

    S_1 _____ S_2 _____

    S_3 _____ S_4 _____

    Murmurs _____

    Rubs _____

3. Diagnostic procedures and laboratory tests

    Cardiac pressures   CVP _____ RA _____ RV _____ LA _____

    LV _____ PA _____ PCWP _____ Aorta _____

    ECG _____

    Chest x-ray _____

    Cardiac cath _____

    Cardiac enzymes _____

    Other _____

4. Other relevant data _____

slope down at about a 45° angle from their attachment to the thoracic spine to their anterior attachment to the costal cartilages.

The imaginary reference lines on the anterior chest are the midsternal and the midclavicular. On the lateral chest, the lines are the anterior and posterior axillary lines—drawn downward from the axillary skin folds—and the midaxillary line.

In some cases, clinical practice under the guidance of an experienced practitioner will be a necessary addition to the theoretical knowledge you gain from this book.

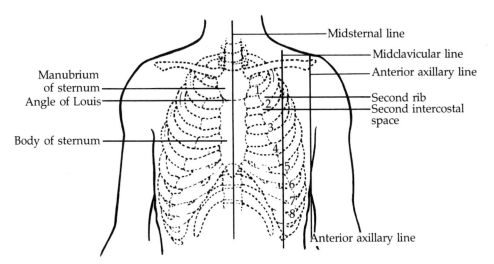

Midsternal line

Midclavicular line

Anterior axillary line

Manubrium of sternum

Angle of Louis

Second rib

Second intercostal space

Body of sternum

Anterior axillary line

Figure 2-1.   Location of angle of Louis, intercostal spaces, and reference lines. Numbers designate intercostal spaces.

The heart is a hollow muscular organ which lies obliquely in the anterior and inferior part of the chest. The sternum and ribs are anterior to the heart, and the esophagus, descending aorta, and the fifth through eighth thoracic vertebrae are posterior. The heart somewhat resembles an inverted triangle, with its narrow apex in the fifth intercostal space at approximately the left midclavicular line (MCL) and its broad base at the level of the attachments of the third ribs to the sternum. About two-thirds of the heart lies to the left of the midsternal line. The apex is more anterior than the base.

The heart consists of a right side and a left side, separated by the septum (Figure 2-2). Each side has an atrium, which receives blood, and a ventricle, which pumps it out. Because of the heart's oblique position in both the frontal and horizontal planes, each chamber is not equidistant from the chest walls (Figure 2-3). The right ventricle (RV) is most anterior, lying directly under the sternum. The left atrium (LA) is most posterior. The right atrium (RA) is on the right side of the heart and the left ventricle (LV) on the left side.

The major blood vessels enter and leave the heart at its base. The superior and inferior venae cavae (SVC and IVC) bring deoxygenated blood to the right atrium. The pulmonary artery (PA) arises from the right ventricle and slants off to the left. It carries deoxygenated blood from the right ventricle to the lungs, and the four pulmonary veins (PV) return oxygenated blood to the left atrium. The aorta (Ao) arises from the left ventricle and slants off to the right. It carries oxygenated blood from the left ventricle to the systemic circulation.

The cardiac valves help control blood flow through the chambers and great vessels. The tricuspid valve (TV) lies between the right atrium and right ventricle, at the attachment of the fifth rib to the right side of the sternum. The mitral

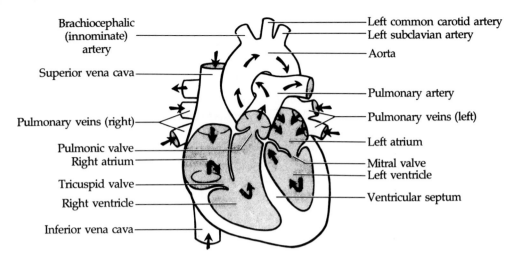

Figure 2-2. Cardiac structures. Arrows show direction of blood flow.

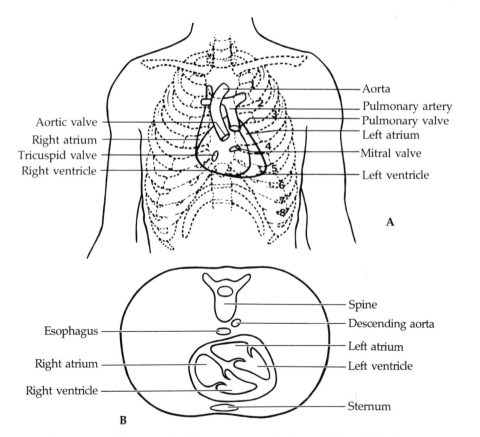

Figure 2-3. Position of cardiac structures. **A,** Frontal plane; **B,** horizontal plane.

valve (MV) lies between the left atrium and left ventricle, at the attachment of the fourth rib to the left side of the sternum. The mitral and tricuspid valves sometimes are called atrioventricular valves. Each is anchored by chordae tendinae to the papillary muscles on its ventricular floor.

The pulmonic valve (PV) lies between the right ventricle and the pulmonary artery. The aortic valve (AV) lies between the left ventricle and aorta. The pulmonic and aortic valves are located under the sternum at approximately the level of the attachments of the third ribs to the sternum. They are not anchored by chordae tendinae, closing instead because blood presses against their cuplike cusps. Because of their shape, the aortic and pulmonic valves sometimes are called semilunar valves.

Because the valves are grouped so closely (Figure 2-4), it is not possible to differentiate them with a stethoscope applied directly over their anatomical locations. Instead, you must listen in the auscultatory areas to which the sounds produced by each valve are best transmitted. In general, these areas are "downstream" from the valve along the path of blood flow through the heart; there are, however, some exceptions.

At present, there are several ways of labeling these favored sites (Figure 2-5). One way is to refer to the nearby valve; another is to refer to the nearby chamber; a third way is to give the general anatomical location; and a fourth is to give the specific anatomical location. Thus, the tricuspid listening area, right ventricular area, and lower left sternal border all describe the same site on the chest wall, that is, the fourth and fifth intercostal spaces to the left of the sternum. The mitral listening area, left ventricular area, and apical area all describe the fifth intercostal space at the midclavicular line. The pulmonic area and upper left sternal border are synonymous with the region of the second and third intercostal spaces to the left of the sternum (remember that the pulmonary artery slants off to the left of the heart). The aortic area and upper right sternal border are

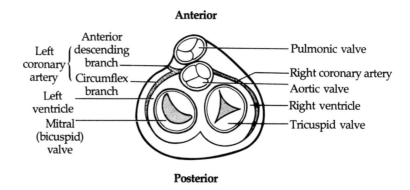

Figure 2-4.   Anatomical grouping of heart valves (viewed from above during diastole, with the atria removed).

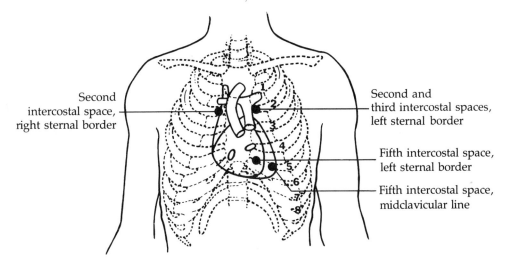

Second intercostal space, right sternal border

Second and third intercostal spaces, left sternal border

Fifth intercostal space, left sternal border

Fifth intercostal space, midclavicular line

Figure 2-5.   Auscultation sites. Second intercostal space at right sternal border is also referred to as aortic area; second and third intercostal spaces at left sternal border are also referred to as pulmonic area; fifth intercostal space at the left sternal border is also referred to as tricuspid area or lower left sternal border; fifth intercostal space at midclavicular line is also referred to as mitral area or apical area.

synonymous with the second intercostal space to the right side of the sternum (the aorta slants off to the right of the heart).

Hurst and Schlant (1974) strongly discourage labeling by valve name. They point out that such terms as mitral area can be misleading because they imply the sounds heard are due only to the nearby valve. This implication is not valid; for example, an aortic ejection click usually is heard best in the so-called mitral area (Hurst and Schlant 1974).

To fix the preceding information in your mind, it is most helpful to study anatomical specimens or a three-dimensional replica of the heart. Comprehension of the relationships between the cardiac structures and the external chest landmarks is crucial to true understanding of the possible sources of phenomena detectable at a particular chest site.

Palpation

Inspection and palpation of the precordial pulsations   Normally, the only pulsation detectable is the apical impulse caused by forward rotation of the heart at the beginning of systole. Palpate with the palm of your hand to locate the point of maximal impulse (PMI). It usually is located about the fifth intercostal space in the left midclavicular line. The normal apical impulse is less than 2–3 cm in diameter and lasts for about a third of systole. In many patients, this impulse is not detectable. If it is, note its location, size, and character. In left ventricular hypertrophy, the impulse is displaced to the left and is larger, longer, and more forceful than normal. Also note any other abnormal precordial movement, such as a systolic parasternal lift (indicative of right ventricular enlargement), extra impulses, or vibrations (thrills).

Percussion

Percussion involves striking the chest and evaluating the resulting vibrations. It is of very limited value in examining the heart and so is not discussed here.

Auscultation

The cardiac cycle and heart sounds   Auscultation allows you to assess the sounds generated by blood flow inside the heart. Before you can understand the data it provides, you must have a thorough understanding of the relationship of the cardiac cycle to the sounds generated by the heart.

The cardiac cycle is that series of events between one ejection of blood from the heart and the next. During the different phases of the cycle, blood rapidly accelerates or decelerates against myocardial structures. These rapid changes in blood flow cause tensing and vibration of valves and other cardiac structures. The vibrations are thought to generate sounds that can be assessed by phonocardiography and auscultation.

The events of the cardiac cycle are diagrammed in Figure 2-6.

The cycle begins with passive filling of the ventricles with blood. At this time, the atrioventricular valves are open, but the semilunar valves are shut. After about two-thirds of the atrial blood has entered the ventricles passively, the atria contract to actively fill the ventricles with the remaining third. At the end of this event, blood is decelerating very rapidly because it is entering against increasing pressure in the ventricles. This rapid deceleration causes the structures of the mitral and tricuspid valves to tense and vibrate just before the valves close. Authorities differ as to whether these vibrations or the actual valve closure produce the first heart sound, known as S_1. The mitral valve usually closes slightly before the tricuspid valve. The closure of the valves signals the onset of ventricular systole.

The ventricles now are closed chambers since both the atrioventricular and semilunar valves are shut. Ventricular contraction begins with a tremendous increase in ventricular pressure, because the blood has no place to go (ventricular isovolumetric contraction).

As ventricular pressure increases, it causes the pulmonic and aortic valves to open. Blood is ejected rapidly into the pulmonary artery and aorta. Toward the end of this phase, the blood decelerates very rapidly due to the increasing

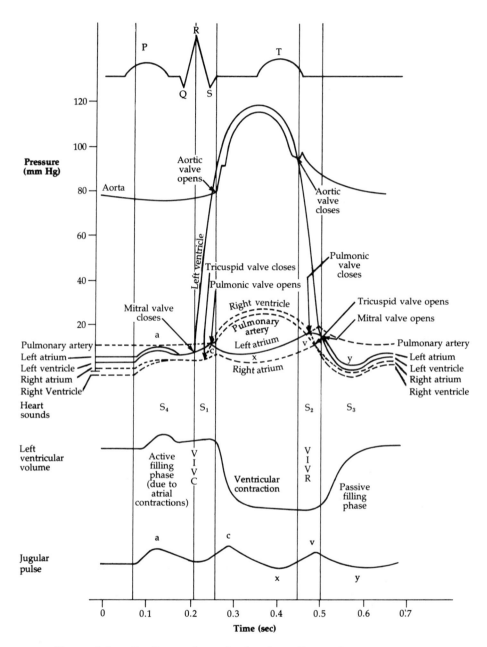

Figure 2-6. Cardiac cycle and related cardiovascular events. *VIVC*, Ventricular isovolumetric contraction; *VIVR*, ventricular isovolumetric relaxation. (Adapted from THE HEART. 3rd ed., J. Hurst, and R. Logue, eds. Copyright © 1974 by McGraw-Hill, Inc. Used with permission of McGraw-Hill Book Company.)

pulmonary arterial and aortic pressures. This deceleration causes the structures of the pulmonic and aortic valves to vibrate just before the valves close, ending ventricular systole. The vibrations and/or valve closures create the second heart sound, S_2. (Normally, the aortic valve closes slightly before the pulmonic, creating two components of S_2. Usually, the aortic component (A_2) is louder and heard all over the precordium, while the softer pulmonic component (P_2) is heard only in the pulmonic area.)

The ventricles now are closed chambers again. As they relax, they cause a decrease in pressure without a change in volume (ventricular isovolumetric relaxation). When the pressure drops sufficiently, the tricuspid and mitral valves open, beginning the ventricular passive filling phase again. The cycle then repeats itself.

From this description, you can tell that S_1 marks the beginning of ventricular systole and S_2 its end. The time between S_2 and the next S_1 marks ventricular diastole. Because systole is usually shorter than diastole, the pause between S_1 and S_2 is shorter than that between S_2 and S_1.

Abnormal heart sounds   Among the abnormalities of S_1 and S_2 that may be detected are increased, decreased, or varying intensity of either sound. It also is possible to detect an abnormal relationship between the components of the second heart sound. As mentioned earlier, A_2 usually occurs before P_2. On inspiration, the split between these sounds widens. Although the exact cause is uncertain, many cardiologists believe that the increased negativity of chest pressure during inspiration causes different amounts of blood to be delivered to and therefore ejected from each ventricle. The negativity may cause pooling of blood in the pulmonary vasculature, so that less blood enters the left ventricle. Because less blood is ejected, the aortic valve closes a little early. At the same time, the increased negativity produces a suction effect on the systemic veins, causing more blood to enter the right side of the heart. Because more blood is ejected from the right ventricle, the pulmonic valve closes a little later than on expiration. As a result of the early A_2 and late P_2, the split between the sounds widens. A number of conditions may cause S_2 to have no variation (a *fixed split*) or reversed (*paradoxical*) split, in which P_2 occurs before A_2 and widens on expiration.

Gallop rhythms result from an extra ventricular sound during diastole, generated by the rapid deceleration of blood as it enters against elevated ventricular pressure. Some gallop rhythms result from an extra sound in early diastole, during the phase of rapid passive ventricular filling. The sound is called S_3 and the rhythm is called a ventricular gallop. An S_3 is normal in children and adults under age 30 years. It is almost always pathologic in adults over 30 years of age. Other gallop rhythms result from an extra sound in late diastole, during the phase of active ventricular filling, which results from atrial contraction. The sound is called S_4 and the rhythm, an atrial gallop. A physiologic S_4 may be heard in infants and small children. It is rarely, if ever, a normal finding in adults.

Table 2-2 presents a classification of abnormal sounds based on the works of Marriott (1967).

A *murmur* is a long series of audible vibrations generated by turbulent blood flow.

A murmur usually results from an obstruction to blood flow, flow into a dilated vessel, a high rate of flow across a normal valve, forward or backward flow across an abnormal valve, or flow through an abnormal arteriovenous communication.

A murmur is identified on the basis of its timing, location, radiation, loudness, pitch, intensity (shape), quality, and response to respiration, position changes, and pharmacologic agents.

Timing in the cardiac cycle may be systolic, diastolic, or continuous. A systolic murmur may be described further as holosystolic (lasting throughout systole) or systolic ejection (midsystolic) murmur. The chest site where the murmur is loudest is its location, while radiation describes its transmission to other chest sites, the neck, or extremities. Loudness is graded on a scale from 1 to 6. A grade 1 murmur can barely be heard; a 2 is faint, but detectable; 3, moderately loud; 4, loud; 5, louder; and 6 is so loud it can be heard with the stethoscope just above but not in contact with the chest wall. Pitch is produced by the number of vibrations per second; high frequency sounds are high-pitched, low frequency ones are low-pitched. The shape of a murmur is described as crescendo (increasing), decrescendo (decreasing), or crescendo-decrescendo (diamond-shaped). The quality depends on the mixture of pitches creating the sound and usually is described as harsh, blowing, rumbling, or musical.

The characteristics of murmurs vary considerably; only the most common are included here (Table 2-3).

The timing of murmurs is easier to understand if you recall the events of the cardiac cycle. For instance, S_1 occurs at the time of mitral and tricuspid valve closure and marks the onset of systole. At this time, the aortic and pulmonic valves still are closed. S_2 is heard at the time of aortic and pulmonic valve closure, marking the end of systole. A holosystolic murmur occurs when blood flows from a chamber with a continuously higher pressure during systole into one with a lower pressure; thus it logically may result from mitral or tricuspid insufficiency or a ventricular septal defect. It usually is high-pitched and blowing, harsh, or musical. The murmur of mitral insufficiency is best heard at the apex, tricuspid insufficiency at the lower left sternal border, and ventricular septal defect at the left sternal border.

Systolic ejection murmurs occur after S_1, the phase of isovolumetric contraction, and the opening of the aortic and pulmonic valves. These murmurs, typical of aortic and pulmonic stenosis, have a crescendo-decrescendo shape due to the blood ejection increase and decrease. They end before their respective component of S_2 (A_2 or P_2) marks the closure of the valve. They usually are harsh and high-pitched. The murmur of aortic stenosis is heard best at the upper right sternal border; it often radiates to the apex and carotid arteries. The pulmonic stenosis murmur is loudest at the upper left sternal border. Systolic ejection

Table 2-2 Abnormal heart sounds*

Sound	Abnormality	Mechanism	Examples
S_1	Louder than normal	1. Valve wide open	Short PR interval, premature beats, tachycardia, mitral or tricuspid stenosis
		2. Prolonged ventricular filling	Left to right shunts
	Softer than normal	1. Valve partly closed	First degree AV block
		2. Valve prematurely closed	Severe hypertension
		3. Normal tensing impossible due to leak	Mitral or tricuspid insufficiency
		4. Damping of sound	Thick chest, pericardial effusion
S_2	Persistent or paradoxical split	1. Asynchronous ventricular activation	
		A. Block of bundle branch	RBBB (persistent split), LBBB (paradoxical split), left ventricular (persistent), right ventricular (paradoxical)
		B. Ectopy	
		2. Prolonged ejection on one side of heart	
		A. Systolic overload	Pulmonary stenosis of hypertension (persistent), aortic stenosis of systemic hypertension (paradoxical)
		B. Diastolic overload	Pulmonary insufficiency (persistent), atrial septal defect (persistent), ventricular septal defect (persistent), aortic insufficiency (paradoxical), patent ductus arteriosus (paradoxical)
		C. Other	Right ventricular failure (persistent), left ventricular failure (paradoxical), myocardial infarction (paradoxical), angina (paradoxical)

Sound	Characteristic	Mechanism	Associated diseases
S_2	Single sound	3. Two outlets for ventricular ejection	Mitral insufficiency (persistent), ventricular septal defect (persistent), tricuspid insufficiency (paradoxical)
		1. One component decreased	Severe aortic or pulmonic stenosis
		2. Aortic valve anterior	Tetralogy of Fallot
		3. Murmur obscuring A_2	Atrial septal defect, patent ductus arteriosus, pulmonic stenosis
S_3	Presence	1. Diastolic overloading of ventricles	Valvular insufficiency, atrial septal defect (RV), left to right shunts (LV), high output states†
		2. Decreased ventricular compliance and/or increased ventricular diastolic pressure	Ventricular failure, ischemic heart disease, constrictive pericarditis, cardiomyopathies
S_4	Presence	1. Systolic overloading of ventricles	Aortic or pulmonic stenosis, hypertension (systemic or pulmonary)
		2. Systolic overloading of right atrium	Tricuspid stenosis
		3. Decreased ventricular compliance and/or increased ventricular diastolic pressure	Mitral insufficiency, ventricular failure, ischemic heart disease, cardiomyopathies
		4. Systemic diseases	Severe anemia, severe infections
		5. First degree AV block	

*Adapted from Marriott, H. 1967. *Differential Diagnosis of Heart Disease*, Oldmar, Fla.: Tampa Tracings.

†Rv = right ventricular overloading; LV = left ventricular overloading.

Table 2-3   Simplified characteristics of murmurs

Type	Timing	Pitch	Quality	Location
Mitral insufficiency	Holosystolic	High	Blowing, harsh, or musical	Apex
Tricuspid insufficiency	Holosystolic	High	Blowing, harsh, or musical	LLSB
Ventricular septal defect	Holosystolic	High	Blowing, harsh, or musical	Left sternal border, 3–4 ICS
Aortic stenosis	Systolic ejection	High	Harsh or musical	URSB
Pulmonic stenosis	Systolic ejection	High	Harsh or musical	ULSB
Aortic insufficiency	Early diastolic	High	Blowing	URSB
Pulmonic insufficiency	Early diastolic	High	Blowing	ULSB
Mitral stenosis	Mid- to late diastolic	Low	Rumbling	Apex
Tricuspid stenosis	Mid- to late diastolic	Low	Rumbling	LLSB

murmurs also occur with flow into a dilated vessel (as in systemic or pulmonary hypertension) or increased flow across the valve (as in aortic or pulmonic insufficiency).

In diastole, the semilunar valves should be closed and the atrioventricular valves open. Early diastolic murmurs logically may result from aortic or pulmonic insufficiency (manifesting itself soon after closure of the valve, which is marked by S_2). They are soft, blowing, high-pitched, decrescendo murmurs. The murmur of pulmonic insufficiency is heard best at the upper left sternal border, that of aortic insufficiency at the upper right sternal border.

Mid- to late diastolic murmurs occur during the phase of rapid ventricular filling as blood rushes across the atrioventricular valves. They are heard in mitral and tricuspid stenosis. They cause low-pitched rumbles. A tricuspid stenosis murmur is appreciated best at the lower left sternal border, that of mitral stenosis at the apex.

Be particularly alert for the sudden appearance of the following murmurs. A new holosystolic murmur along the left sternal border may indicate rupture of the ventricular septum following myocardial infarction, while a new holosystolic murmur at the apex may result from rupture of the papillary muscles, which anchor the mitral valve. These murmurs are rare and are often accompanied by sudden left and right heart failure. In a patient with a suspected aneurysm or descending aortic dissection, the onset of a murmur of aortic insufficiency may herald additional proximal dissection (Schroeder and Daily 1976).

Other sounds that may be heard are opening snaps (due to valve openings), clicks (thought to be due to abnormal valves), sounds of artificial valves, and pericardial friction rubs. This last sound is a scratchy sound that signifies pericardial inflammation; it is discussed in Chapter 4.

Given the scope of this book, it is not possible to do justice to the wealth of information on the causes and characteristics of cardiac sounds. If you wish to know more about them, the annotated bibliography at the end of the chapter will guide your further investigation.

Selection of a stethoscope   A variety of stethoscopes is available in the marketplace. When selecting one for your personal use, it is helpful to know what characteristics are most desirable (Estes 1974).

The eartips should fit snugly without hurting you. Some manufacturers now include various sizes of eartips so that you can select the size that best suits you. Adjust the metal portion of the earpieces so that the long axis of their upper portion is aligned with the external ear canal, and check to see that they stay in this position.

Select an instrument with double tubes to the chestpiece portion rather than Y-shaped tubing; Y-shaped tubing seriously distorts high frequencies. The tubes should be about 10 to 12 inches long; longer tubing diminishes the clarity of sounds.

The stethoscope should have two chestpieces connected by a valve that you can switch easily. The flat diaphragm enhances your ability to hear high-frequency vibrations by filtering out low-frequency ones. The bell (preferably trumpet shaped rather than a low dome) is used for low-frequency sounds.

Techniques of auscultation   There are many systems for listening to cardiac sounds; this is one useful method. Have the patient lie down. If the patient stands or sits, many low frequency sounds such as diastolic filling sounds or murmurs will diminish or disappear because of orthostatic pooling.

First, create as quiet an environment as possible: turn off the television if one is present; ask visitors or staff to be quiet; and so on.

Start with the diaphragm. Press it against the chest firmly enough to leave a ring on the skin when you later remove it. Inch the diaphragm along the chest, progressing from the apex to the left lower sternal border, left upper sternal border, and finally the right upper sternal border. Repeat the process with the bell, but press it on the skin just enough to seal the edges. To keep both the diaphragm and bell from moving on the skin and creating distracting noises, keep the finger tips holding the chestpiece in contact with the chest.

Unless you use both chestpieces, you will miss some cardiac sounds. The diaphragm, best for detecting high-pitched sounds and murmurs, enables you to hear clearly S_1, S_2, and murmurs of valvular regurgitation. The bell, best for low-pitched sounds and murmurs, allows you to hear clearly S_3, S_4, and diastolic rumbles from the mitral and tricuspid valves.

As you auscultate the precordium, make the following observations:

1. What is the relationship between S_1 and S_2? Identify S_1 by listening to the heart while you palpate the carotid pulse. S_1 coincides with or slightly precedes the carotid pulse. To understand this fact, remember that S_1 represents the vibrations at the time of mitral and tricuspid closure. Closure of these valves is followed by ventricular systole, which causes the aortic (and therefore carotid) pulse.

Although S_1 may be heard all over the precordium, normally it is louder than S_2 at the apex and softer than S_2 at the base. Try to identify whether S_1 is louder or softer than normal or is variable.

2. After you identify S_1 and S_2, listen at the left upper sternal area to hear the split of S_2. You can identify which component is A_2 by comparing the sounds you hear at the pulmonic area to the sound you hear at the aortic area. After you have identified the components, listen while observing the patient's respiration to identify whether the sounds widen normally, paradoxically, or not at all.

3. Next characterize any abnormal sounds. Do they occur during systole or diastole? In which areas do you hear them best? Can you hear them better with the bell or with the diaphragm? Are they continuous or discrete? Do you hear them best with the patient supine or in another position?

Skill at auscultation takes considerable practice under the guidance of a knowledgeable practitioner. It helps to listen to audiotapes of heart sounds and to begin practicing with patients whose heart rates are under 70 beats per minute. Although you may be unable to diagnose abnormal sounds, your ability to identify their presence and to describe them will assist you in detecting changes in the patient's condition; alert a more experienced nurse or a physician to the need for further assessment.

Hemodynamic monitoring data

The cardiac cycle and pressure waves   As blood flows from chamber to chamber, as valves open and close, and as the myocardium contracts and relaxes, pressures are generated in various parts of the heart. These pressures may be measured and, in some cases, seen and felt as pulsations.

This section again will look at the cardiac cycle, concentrating not on heart sounds this time but instead on pressures. Refer back to Figure 2-6.

The atrial curve consists of three ascending and two descending waves. The *a wave* is produced by atrial contraction. The *c wave* may result from bulging of the valves into the atria during ventricular contraction. The c wave may also result from the impact of the carotid arterial pulse on the nearby jugular vein. The *x descent* occurs as atrial pressure drops during atrial diastole. It is possible that the onset of ventricular contraction contributes to this descent by tugging downward on the atrioventricular valves. The *v wave* occurs as the atria fill and their pressure increases. The *y descent* shows the rapid drop in atrial pressure after the atrioventricular valves open and the rapid, passive ventricular filling phase ensues.

These waves can be seen on tracings recorded by catheters in the right or left atrium. The left atrial tracing also can be seen in recordings from a catheter in the pulmonary artery, after it has been positioned to record pressures in the pulmonary capillary bed. The right atrial pressure waves can be seen and palpated in the neck as the jugular venous pulse. Increased neck vein pressure also can be seen as neck vein distention. The technique for estimating distention is discussed in Chapter 5.

The ventricular curve demonstrates a gradually increasing pressure during ventricular filling, with a small bulge at the time of atrial contraction. After the atrioventricular valves close, the pressure increases sharply during systole until it causes the semilunar valves to open. Then the pressure drops rapidly, until the semilunar valves close and diastole begins.

The arterial wave form is seen in tracings from both the pulmonary artery and the major systemic arteries. After the semilunar valves open, the wave form shows a rapid upstroke during ventricular ejection. The more gradual downstroke is interrupted by the dicrotic notch, which indicates closure of the semilunar valves. The pulmonary arterial wave form is detectable only with a catheter in the pulmonary artery. The systemic arterial wave form is seen on recordings from an arterial catheter and palpated as the arterial pulse. Noninvasive evaluation of the arterial pulse also is discussed in Chapter 5.

Although the wave configurations are similar for the right- and left-sided chambers, the *pressures* at which the waves occur differ, as discussed in the following section.

Pressure measurements   Cardiovascular pressures can be measured and monitored through catheters whose tips are placed in the atria, pulmonary artery, or systemic arteries (Figure 2-7).

The most important cardiac pressure is that of the left ventricle because it is a major determinant of systemic perfusion. The pressure in the left ventricle just before systole is called the *left ventricular end diastolic pressure (LVEDP)*. This pressure reflects the compliance of the left ventricle, that is, its ability to receive blood from the left atrium during diastole. When left ventricular compliance decreases, the LVEDP rises. Myocardial infarction and left ventricular failure are two examples of conditions in which left ventricular compliance decreases. Direct monitoring of LVEDP would be very helpful in detecting changes in the patient's condition and in guiding optimal fluid therapy in shock. Unfortunately, left ventricular pressure cannot be monitored at the bedside owing to the high potential for thromboembolization directly to the brain or other vital organs.

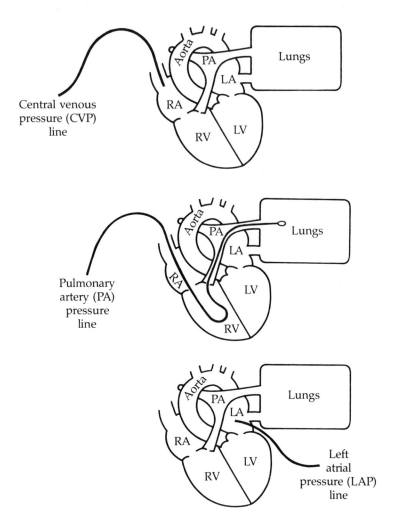

Figure 2-7.   Location of hemodynamic monitoring catheter tips. *RA,* Right atrium; *RV,* right ventricle; *LA,* left atrium; *LV,* left ventricle; *PA,* pulmonary artery.

In the presence of a normal mitral valve, LVEDP is reflected by *left atrial pressure (LAP)*. Left atrial pressure can be monitored at the bedside, but a LAP line can be dangerous because it provides a direct path for air or clots to enter the left ventricle and become systemic emboli.

In the person with a normal mitral valve and normal lungs, the LVEDP also is reflected by the pressure in the pulmonary capillary bed and the pressure in the pulmonary artery at the end of diastole. This latter pressure sometimes is referred to as the *pulmonary artery end diastolic pressure (PAEDP)*.

The pulmonary capillary and pulmonary arterial pressures can be monitored at the bedside with a balloon-tipped catheter placed in the pulmonary artery. With the balloon deflated, one can measure pulmonary artery systolic, diastolic, and mean pressures with the catheter. When the balloon is inflated, it wedges the catheter in a small distal branch of the pulmonary artery. The pressure that is recorded is that reflected back from the left atrium through the pulmonary capillary bed. This pressure sometimes is called the *pulmonary capillary wedge pressure (PCWP)*.

The least sensitive indicator of left ventricular pressure is the *central venous pressure (CVP)*. It is monitored at the bedside through a catheter whose tip is located at the juncture of the superior vena cava and right atrium, or through one lumen of the balloon-tipped pulmonary artery catheter that opens in the same location. The CVP reflects the pressure in the right atrium and systemic veins. It is affected primarily by changes in right-sided heart pressures and only secondarily by changes in left-sided pressures, so the CVP may be the last cardiac pressure to reflect increased LVEDP. Moreover, because the CVP can be affected by pulmonary disease, pulmonic or tricuspid stenosis, and other right atrial or ventricular abnormalities, an elevated CVP is not necessarily an accurate indication of an elevated LVEDP. The CVP line is safer than the LAP and PA lines. It is used to measure venous pressure, estimate blood volume, obtain venous blood samples, and administer fluids and some medications. It may also be used to monitor the patient in heart failure when PA monitoring is unavailable.

Systemic arterial pressure can be monitored indirectly with a sphygmomanometer or directly through a catheter (arterial line) placed into a major systemic artery. For a discussion of the variables affecting systemic arterial pressure, see Chapter 5.

Values for normal resting cardiac pressures vary from institution to institution. Schroeder and Daily (1976) give the following as normal values in millimeters of mercury (mm Hg):

- Superior vena caval or right atrial pressure is 2–6 mean
- Right ventricular pressure is 20–30 systolic and 0–5 diastolic
- Pulmonary artery pressure is 20–30 systolic, 10–20 diastolic, and 10–15 mean
- Pulmonary capillary wedge pressure is 4–12 mean
- Left atrial pressure is 4–12 mean
- Left ventricular pressure is 100–140 systolic and 60–80 diastolic; left ventricular end diastolic pressure is 5–12
- Aortic pressure is 100–140 systolic, 60–80 diastolic, and 70–90 mean

Uses of hemodynamic lines   Hemodynamic lines have several uses. They enable you to sample venous and arterial blood without repeated vascular punctures. They provide a way to monitor arterial wave forms, which can provide clues to patient status. The combination of pulmonary arterial and systemic arterial lines can be used to calculate cardiac output. Most importantly, these lines enable you to monitor directly various cardiac pressures. Interpretation of these pressures can guide you and the physician in planning and evaluating therapy in shock, fluid overload or deficit, cardiac failure, and other conditions.

Insertion   The LAP line is placed in the atrium during cardiac surgery and brought out through the chest wall. The other lines can be inserted at the bedside by a physician. They may be inserted percutaneously or via cutdown. The CVP line usually is inserted in the antecubital or subclavian vein. The pulmonary artery (PA) line is inserted in any large vein and floated into the right atrium. The balloon is inflated, and normal blood flow then carries the tip into the pulmonary artery. The arterial line usually is placed in the radial, brachial, or femoral artery.

The nurse has three primary responsibilities related to insertion of a hemodynamic line.

Preparing the patient and family   Prior to insertion, whenever possible, explain to the patient and immediate family how the procedure will help in the patient's care. Tell the patient what sensations to expect. Reassure the patient that you will be observing and that you should be told promptly of any discomfort. Consult with the physician before giving an analgesic or sedative since such drugs can alter baseline pressure measurements. Obtain baseline vital signs. Mark on the patient's chest the reference point for measurements. This point usually is on the lateral chest wall, midway between the anterior and posterior chest. It is important to mark it so that readings are taken at a consistent level. If they are not, variations in readings may be attributed to changes in the patient's condition when they actually result from changes in the recording technique.

Preparing the equipment   Monitoring equipment usually consists of a specific type and size of catheter, a device to measure pressures, a flush solution and related tubing, and a carpenter's level. Insertion equipment includes local anesthetic, skin preparatory solution, sterile gloves, dressing supplies, and a cutdown tray if indicated.

The measuring device may be a water manometer or a pressure transducer and oscilloscope. The water manometer (Figure 2-8) is suitable for low pressures (under 40 cm of water), when it is not necessary to see the wave forms. It commonly is used for CVP and LAP measurement. A transducer (Figure 2-9) is an instrument that converts pressure waves to electrical energy, which then can be displayed on an oscilloscope. It usually is used for pressures too high for the water manometer or in situations where depiction of the wave form is useful, such as with pulmonary or systemic arterial pressures.

Flush systems consist of a solution (such as heparinized 5% dextrose in water) and a method of irrigating the line. The least desirable irrigation method

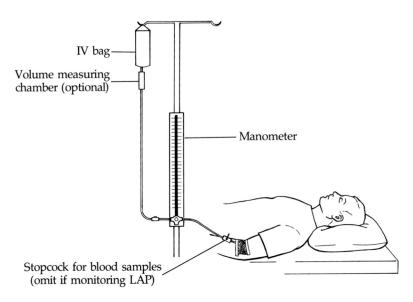

Figure 2-8. Pressure monitoring with manometer.

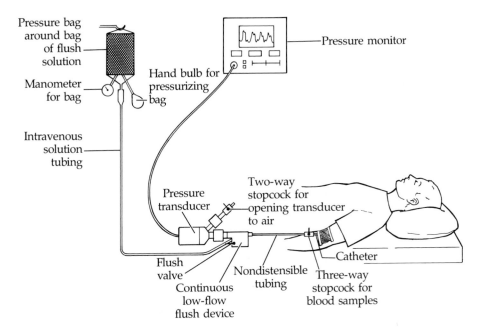

Figure 2-9. Pressure monitoring with transducer. Pressure transducer and continuous flush device enlarged to show detail.

is a syringe inserted in a stopcock port because of the potential for infection and excessively high flushing pressures. The most desirable method is a continuous low-flow flush device, which is a closed system that infuses solution at a constant slow rate. When you want a rapid flush, you can pull the "tail" on the device and flush the system without breaking sterility.

Details of the equipment and set-up procedure vary from unit to unit. In general, before the procedure begins, connect the equipment (except for the catheter itself) together sterilely and securely. Flush air out of the system. If you are using a transducer, balance and calibrate it according to the manufacturer's directions. Label the system with tags at several points: the solution bag or bottle, the tubing near the rate control clamp, and the tubing near stopcocks or medication ports. Critically ill patients often have several hemodynamic and fluid infusion lines. When they are unlabeled, it is easy to confuse them and accidentally alter the flow rate or inject medication into the wrong line.

Assisting and observing   To assist the physician, act as the unsterile person to pour prep solution, hold the bottle of local anesthetic, and open the catheter package. As the line is inserted, observe the patient for pain and cardiopulmonary distress. As soon as blood drips out the end of the catheter, connect it to the system. The physician will dress the site of insertion while you obtain the initial measurement.

Nursing goals

Hemodynamic lines have several potential problems so there are multiple nursing goals in securing and utilizing the data they provide.

Obtaining accurate measurements   Each time you measure the pressure, follow these steps:

1. Place the patient in the baseline position, that is, the position in which all readings are taken. The usual position is supine with the bed flat. If necessary for a particular patient, the head of the bed may be elevated, but it should be placed at the same degree of elevation for each reading. If the patient is on a ventilator, you may leave it connected during the reading. Be sure to note "on ventilator" when you record the pressure.

2. Check the level of the measuring device. Use a carpenter's level to make sure the "O" on the manometer or the diaphragm of the transducer is level with the reference mark on the patient's chest.

3. Look for and remove any air bubbles in the line or transducer; they can cause a damped, distorted reading or failure to get any reading.

4. Check the patency of the line by observing on the oscilloscope the normal wave form transmitted by the transducer, observing fluctuations in the manometer when it is opened, or aspirating blood from the line.

5. Measure the pressures. If you are using a manometer, you will be able to

measure only mean pressure. Turn the stopcock on the manometer so that fluid flows from the fluid source into the manometer. Let the manometer fill several centimeters above the expected reading but do not let the upper end of the manometer become contaminated with fluid.

Turn the stopcock to open the line between the manometer and the patient. The fluid level should fall and fluctuate with respirations. The average level of the fluid represents the reading. After noting the value, turn the stopcock so that the fluid again can flow from the fluid source to the patient.

If you are using a transducer, you will be able to measure systolic, diastolic, and mean pressures. You can obtain these pressures for the pulmonary or systemic artery by placing the switch on the pressure monitor on the appropriate settings. To measure pulmonary capillary pressure, place the switch on "mean." Inflate the balloon with no more than the specified amount of air for that size catheter. Insert the air until the characteristic PCWP wave form (with its a, c, and v waves) appears on the oscilloscope. To keep the balloon inflated while you read the pressure from the monitor, hold the syringe in place or use the lever on the catheter's end to lock the air in place. After taking the reading, be sure to remove the syringe or release the lock so the balloon can deflate.

There are other nursing actions to maintain accurate pressure measurements:

1. To ensure that the catheter is positioned properly, immobilize the extremity.

2. Prevent kinking of the tubing. You will not only increase the accuracy of pressure readings but will also protect your patient from fluctuating dosages of any drugs being administered through the line.

3. To ascertain whether the tip is in the correct location, obtain a chest x-ray after insertion of all except the systemic arterial line.

4. At least every eight hours, balance and calibrate the transducer according to the manufacturer's recommended procedure.

5. If you are using a systemic arterial line, compare its measurement to the blood pressure obtained with a sphygmomanometer at least every eight hours. Remember that many factors can give you discrepancies between the cuff BP and arterial line. Among the most common are wrong cuff size, arrhythmias, peripheral vasoconstriction or vasospasm, and unbalanced or uncalibrated equipment.

Analyzing the pressures critically   There are several principles to remember in interpreting pressure data:

1. Compare the values obtained at this time to the patient's normal values rather than an arbitrary standard. If the patient has undergone cardiac catheterization within the past few months, pressures obtained at that time may be used as baselines. If not, you must predict general values on the basis of your knowledge of the so-called normal values and your patient's pathology. For example, you would expect the patient with a narrowed mitral valve to have an elevated

LAP. The patient with chronic obstructive lung disease probably would have both high PA pressures and CVP.

2. Single readings are not as significant as the trend of values.

3. Consider the pressures in relation to each other. If one pressure is measured with a manometer and another with a transducer, you may want to convert them to the same scale. To convert millimeters of mercury (Hg) to centimeters of water, multiply by 1.34. Remember that abnormal values are not always due to primary pathology of the monitored chamber. For example, an elevated CVP in association with normal or low PA pressures suggests that the cause lies between these two sites, that is, with the pulmonary valve, right ventricle, or tricuspid valve. In contrast, an elevated CVP in conjunction with elevated PA pressures suggests that the cause is pulmonary disease, left-sided heart disease, or fluid overload.

4. Remember that a normal value does not necessarily indicate an absence of pathology. For instance, a patient may have a normal LAP but be intensely vasoconstricted due to hypovolemia.

Observing the wave forms periodically   If the patient is being monitored with a transducer, wave forms should be periodically observed. The CVP, LAP, and PCWP will display the characteristic atrial wave forms discussed earlier in this chapter. The PA and arterial line will display the arterial wave forms already presented. Changes in wave forms can be clues to malposition of the catheter tip, obstructions in the line, or changes in the patient's clinical state. Frequently, a PA catheter will float and wedge itself spontaneously. Unless you are alert to the change in wave form, the patient might suffer a pulmonary infarction. The loss of the dicrotic notch in an arterial line most commonly indicates damping and a need to flush the line; it might, however, suggest the development of aortic insufficiency.

Prevention of complications

Anticipate and prevent complications by taking the appropriate nursing measures. The following complications may occur with any line.

Infection   Maintain scrupulous sterile technique. Observe the insertion site for signs of inflammation every eight hours. Clean the site and change the dressing at least daily. Check the patient's temperature at least once every eight hours and call unexplained elevations to the physician's attention.

Discomfort   Position the limb comfortably. Do gentle range of motion exercises distal to the site three times a day. Palpate pulses and note skin color and temperature distal to the site, to detect developing ischemia. If the patient is alert, teach him to tell you promptly about any pain or abnormal sensations in the extremity.

Thrombosis   Utilize a continuous low-flow flush system whenever possible. Flush lines after blood samples are drawn, including flushing the stopcock port from which the sample was obtained. Also flush promptly if the tracing becomes damped (that is, the amplitude of the wave forms decreases).

Emboli   If you are unable to aspirate blood or infuse fluid, the line may be clotted. Do not attempt to clear the line by a forceful manual flush because you may cause a thrombus to embolize.

There are several ways to prevent air emboli. Be sure that air is flushed from the line before initial use. During insertion of the CVP or PA line in the subclavian vein or jugular vein, place the patient's head below the level of the thorax. If you spot air bubbles in the line, remove them with a needle and syringe or disconnect the line and let it bleed back. Whenever it is necessary to open the transducer to air (as in balancing it or removing blood that has leaked into the dome), first turn the stopcock off to the patient.

The PA line presents another source of potential air emboli from breakage of the balloon used to obtain the PCWP. Prevent breakage by inserting no more air than appropriate for the specific size catheter, by releasing the air after the reading, and by aspirating before injecting air for subsequent readings. You should feel a slight resistance to inflation of the balloon. If the balloon breaks, you will know because the air will enter with minimal resistance, no wedge tracing will appear, and blood may leak out of the balloon lumen. If you suspect breakage, turn the lumen off to the patient and notify the physician. The small amount of air in the balloon is not dangerous, but repeated injections of air by well-meaning misinformed staff can be unsafe.

Hemorrhage   Secure connections by taping them together or taping them to a tongue blade. After blood samples are drawn and the stopcock port is flushed, close it so the patient will not exsanguinate.

When a line is removed, ensure hemostasis by exerting pressure over the insertion site until bleeding stops. For an arterial line, you usually must maintain firm pressure uninterrupted for at least 5 minutes. Dress the sites until healing occurs. During the first 15 minutes after removal, check frequently for hemorrhage or hematoma formation.

Drug toxicity   Do not give any drugs via the PA or LAP lines. When giving drugs via the CVP line, dilute them according to the manufacturer's and physician's recommendations, and administer them at the recommended rate. For the arterial line, give only drugs specifically intended for intraarterial use, such as some chemotherapy agents.

Fluid overload   Fluids commonly are administered only via the CVP or peripheral venous lines. On these lines, use measuring chambers and small-drop infusion sets. Do not infuse fluids via the PA, LAP, or arterial lines other than the small amounts necessary to keep the lines patent. When recording fluid balance at the end of the nursing shift, include the amount used to keep the lines patent.

In addition to the above problems common to all monitoring lines, anticipate and prevent problems associated with specific lines.

Ventricular arrhythmias   Ventricular arrhythmias can be caused by displacement of the CVP or PA catheters into the right ventricle. In the case of the PA catheter, this displacement will cause a change in the contour of the wave form, from the typical PA tracing to a right ventricular tracing. This problem again emphasizes the need to keep an eye on the wave forms displayed on the oscilloscope. Notify the physician and inflate the balloon to see if it will float back up into the pulmonary artery. If it does not, the physician will need to reposition the catheter. A displaced CVP catheter also requires repositioning. After repositioning, get a new chest x-ray to verify catheter placement.

Pulmonary infarction   Pulmonary infarction may result if the PA catheter balloon is left inflated or if the deflated balloon spontaneously wedges itself in the capillary bed. Adhere to the safety precautions described under the problem of air embolization. You may be able to dislodge a spontaneously wedged catheter by having the patient cough or turn. If these measures are unsuccessful, notify the physician promptly.

Pneumothorax   Pneumothorax may occur during insertion of the CVP or PA line into the subclavian or jugular vein. The reason for this complication is that the apex of the lung extends above the clavicle. Since it is in close proximity to these veins, it may be punctured accidentally during insertion. For information on the recognition and treatment of pneumothorax, see Chapter 10.

Electrocardiogram

Contraction of the cardiac chambers is provoked by an electrical stimulus. The initiation and propagation of this stimulus can be recorded on an electrocardiogram (ECG).

The transmission of the electrical current is detected by sensors placed on the skin. These sensors are called *electrodes*. The electrodes view the activity in only one plane (frontal or transverse) at a time.

ECG recording

To prepare the patient, explain the purpose of the procedure and tell him that although it will not hurt, he must remain still for the duration. It is unnecessary to restrict diet or activity prior to the ECG.

The routine 12-lead ECG usually is obtained by a technician. In an emergency, such as severe chest pain, you should be able to record a 12-lead ECG yourself.

Leads   The standard electrocardiogram consists of six limb leads and six precordial leads, each of which has a slightly different orientation toward the heart. The limb leads are I, II, III, AVR, AVL, and AVF. They look at the heart in the frontal plane. The six precordial leads are V_1 through V_6. They give a horizontal view of cardiac activity.

To obtain the frontal leads, electrodes are placed on the arms and legs. The right leg electrode serves as a ground. The ECG machine determines the polarity of each remaining electrode for each lead. Leads I, II, and III are called standard limb leads (Figure 2-10). In lead I, the machine reads the right arm (RA) electrode as negative and the left arm (LA) electrode as positive. In lead II, it reads the RA electrode as negative and the left leg (LL) as positive. In lead III, it reads the LA as negative and the LL as positive. Each of these leads measures the difference in potential between two electrodes, each of whose actual potential is unknown (Andreoli et al 1975). The standard limb leads therefore are called bipolar leads.

In contrast, the remaining limb leads and the precordial leads are unipolar leads, that is, they measure the actual potential under one electrode. The explanation for measuring actual potential is based on Einthoven's law, which states that at any given instant, the algebraic sum of the potentials of leads I, II, and III is zero. Therefore, if the electrodes from which these leads are recorded are connected to a common terminal, its potential is zero. This common electrode is called the *neutral* or *indifferent electrode.* If this electrode is connected to one pole of a galvanometer, an electrode connected to the galvanometer's other pole will record the true potential under itself. This electrode is called the *exploring electrode.*

Leads I, II, and III form an equilateral triangle, whose apices are the right arm, left arm, and left leg electrodes. These electrodes are considered to be electrically equidistant from the heart, which is at zero potential. Because a unipolar lead records the difference between the common electrode at zero

Figure 2-10.   Standard limb leads. The three dotted lines represent the leads as recorded and are labeled to show the direction of current from negative to positive poles. The solid lines represent the shifting of these axes (without altering their direction) so that they intersect at the zero point, the heart. The solid lines are labeled at their positive poles.

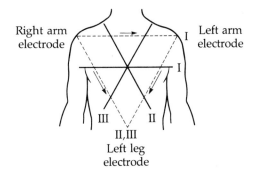

Right arm electrode   Left arm electrode

I

I

III   II

II,III

Left leg electrode

potential and the exploring electrode, it measures the difference between the center of the heart and the exploring electrode also.

For the augmented limb leads (AVR, AVL, and AVF), the limb electrodes are left in the same positions as for the standard limb leads (Figure 2-11). The machine then reads one electrode as positive and combines the remaining two electrodes to create the neutral electrode. For example, to record AVR, the right arm electrode is read as positive and the left arm and left leg electrodes are joined to form the neutral electrode. Originally, the right arm, left arm, and left leg electrode all were summed to form the neutral electrode, so that in VR, for example, the right arm electrode was both the exploring electrode and part of the neutral electrode. This technique created a very low potential for the exploring electrode. When the exploring electrode is not also connected to the neutral terminal, an augmented voltage is obtained and the resulting lead is called an augmented lead (Schamroth 1971). Each augmented lead measures the difference in potential between the center of the heart and the limb wearing the positive electrode. The three standard limb leads and the three augmented limb leads intersect at the heart forming a hexaxial reference system (Figure 2-12).

The remaining six leads (V_1 through V_6) also are unipolar leads (Figure 2-13). A separate exploring electrode is placed at different positions on the precordium, and the indifferent electrode is created by combining the right arm, left arm, and left leg electrodes.

The twelve leads intersect at the heart, thus providing 12 views of the heart, six frontal and six horizontal.

12-lead ECG recording technique   A photograph of the control panel of a typical machine is included in Figure 2-14. To obtain a 12-lead ECG, follow these steps:

1. Place the ECG machine on the patient's left side whenever possible. When you work from that side, you decrease the chance of artifact in the recording because you do not need to drape the cable over the patient's chest or abdomen. Plug the machine in and turn it on.

2. Place the electrodes on the limbs. They are labeled with the initials of the appropriate limb. Expose the arms and legs. Since the machine will record

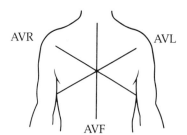

Figure 2-11.   Augmented limb leads. Leads are labeled at their positive poles.

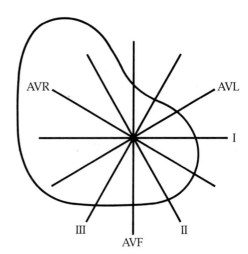

Figure 2-12. ECG views of the heart, frontal plane (hexaxial reference system). Leads are labeled at their positive poles.

muscle activity and introduce artifact into the recording, place the electrodes anywhere on the limbs over areas of minimal muscle.

Before applying an electrode, put a small dab of electrode jelly on it or put an alcohol wipe on the skin. Secure the electrode with the rubber strap just firmly enough to keep the electrode from sliding.

3. Check that the sensitivity button is on its standard setting of 1 millivolt (mv) and that the paper speed switch is on its standard setting of 25 millimeters (mm) per second.

4. Turn the selector knob to "run." Look to see whether the line being recorded is centered on the paper. If it is not, use the position knob to center it. Avoid touching the stylus (writing arm) itself as it is very delicate and also very hot. Check the standardization by quickly tapping the "standard" button. The stylus should record a narrow deflection that is the height of two of the large boxes on the recording paper. (If it is inaccurate, run the ECG anyway, and notify the

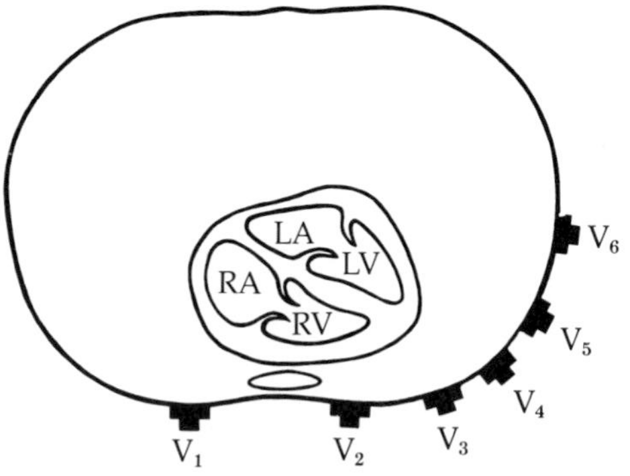

Figure 2-13. ECG views of the heart, horizontal plane (precordial leads). *RA,* Right atrium; *RV,* right ventricle; *LA,* left atrium; *LV,* left ventricle.

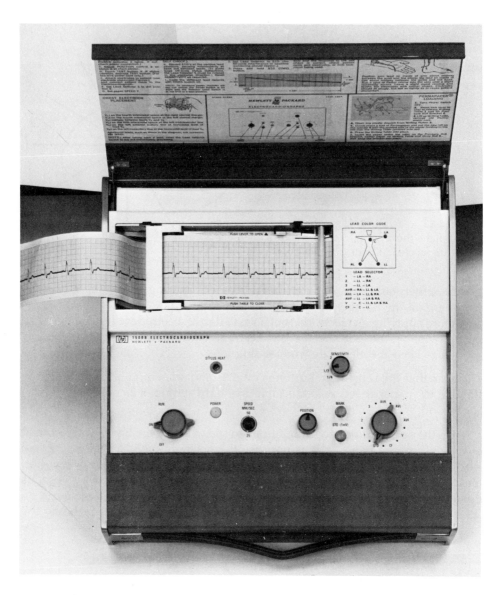

Figure 2-14. ECG machine. (Courtesy Hewlett-Packard Company.)

person responsible for maintaining the machine after the emergency is over.) Turn the switch back to "on." Write the patient's name, date, and time on the recording paper.

5. Record the limb leads by turning the switch to "run" and the selector knob to I, II, III, AVR, AVL, and AVF in sequence. At the start of each lead, write the

name of the lead or use the automatic marker on the machine. Also record a standardization mark by pressing the standard button so that the mark falls on the baseline (flat line between the deflections being recorded). Record six to eight electrical complexes unless the rhythm is irregular; in that case, record about 12–16. The knob usually has dots indicating stop positions between each lead to facilitate marking.

6. Place the selector knob on the stop after AVF. Locate the electrode positions for the chest leads by palpating the patient's precordium as described earlier in the chapter. Figure 2-15 diagrams the positions.

The fourth intercostal space at the right sternal border is the location of the first precordial lead, V_1. Mark the location with a pen. Directly across the sternum, at the fourth intercostal space at the left sternal border, mark the site of V_2. Next locate V_4 by palpating down to the next (fifth) intercostal space and over to the midclavicular line, which is imaginary. Mark this site and then make a mark midway between V_2 and V_4; this site is V_3. Next, imagine a horizontal line drawn

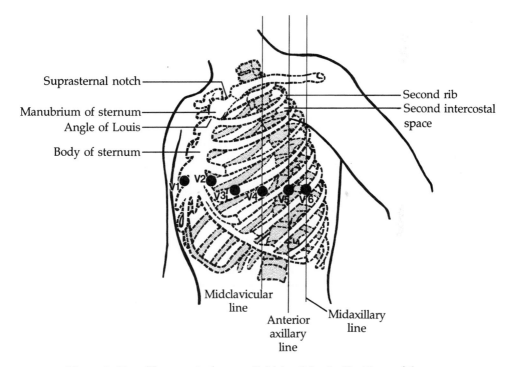

Figure 2-15.   Placement of precordial (chest) leads. Positions of the precordial electrode: V_1, Fourth intercostal space at right sternal border; V_2, fourth intercostal space at left sternal border; V_3, midway between V_2 and V_4; V_4, fifth intercostal space at midclavicular line; V_5, directly lateral to V_4 at anterior axillary line; V_6, directly lateral to V_5 at midaxillary line.

from V_4 intersecting an imaginary vertical line drawn down from the anterior axillary skin fold; this is V_5. V_6 is also on the horizontal line emanating from V_4, at its intersection with the midaxillary line. Note that while V_5 and V_6 are on a horizontal line drawn from V_4 they are not necessarily in the same intercostal space because the ribs slant downward as they come from the thoracic spine to the sternum.

7. Place a small dab of electrode jelly on each chest lead site. Squeeze the suction cup and place it on the V_1 site. Turn the selector knob to "V" and record the lead as you did with the limb leads. Turn the knob to a stop position and remove the cup. Squeeze it and place it at V_2. Turn the knob to "V" again to record the rhythm. Continue through the remaining chest leads.

8. When done, turn the machine off. Remove the electrodes and wipe the jelly off the patient's chest and the electrodes. Since wiping the jelly off usually wipes the electrode position marks off too, use a pen or felt-tip marker to remark electrode positions if serial ECGs are anticipated.

Problems   You may encounter several problems while doing the ECG. The most common are wandering baseline, thickened baseline, muscle artifact, and excessively large deflections in one or more leads. Figure 2-16 shows examples of these problems.

When the baseline does not remain centered but instead moves up and down on the paper, it is said to be wandering. Wandering baseline is due to respiratory movement and is more common in the chest leads. Do not attempt to counter this by moving the position knob continually. Instead, ask the patient to hold his/her breath briefly while the lead is recorded.

The baseline may appear thickened due to poor electrode contact or electrical interference with the machine. If you are using alcohol swabs under the electrodes, try repositioning them; if contact is still poor, remove them and use the jelly instead. Reposition the electrodes over more bony areas and make sure the straps are tight enough to hold them securely. With 60-cycle interference, you may be able actually to see 60 tiny peaks per second in the baseline. If the patient's bed is electric, unplug it. Also check for broken electrode wires or cable. Ground other electrical equipment in the immediate vicinity.

Muscle artifact appears as random narrow deflections in the tracing. Make sure the patient is in a comfortable position and is warm. Position the electrodes over less muscular areas. Large deflections in one or more leads will cause the tracing to appear as though the upper part of the deflections were cut off. If this occurs, proceed to the next lead and continue taking the ECG on the standard sensitivity. Then reset the sensitivity on "1/2" or "1/4" and take the lead(s) you had to skip.

Bedside cardiac monitoring   Modifications of the standard 12 leads are used for routine cardiac monitoring at the bedside. Specifics of monitors vary from

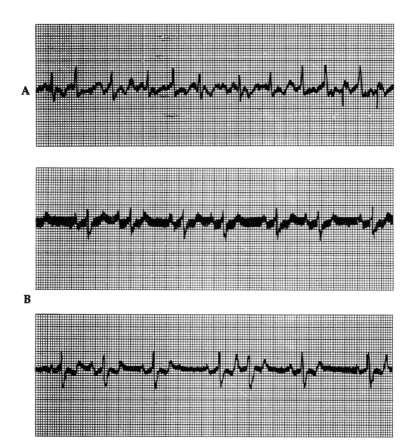

Figure 2-16.   ECG artifacts. **A**, Muscle movement; **B**, 60-cycle interference.

manufacturer to manufacturer. The following general guidelines will help you work with a variety of models.

The bedside monitor consists of a monitor console, a patient cable, and electrode wires that can be connected to disposable electrodes. The console contains an oscilloscope screen to display the tracing and various buttons and switches to obtain the tracing. In most units, the bedside monitors also are connected to displays at the nurses' desk.

When you are notified of an admission, turn the monitor on with the power switch to let it warm up. Connect electrodes to the electrode wires. Connect the electrode wires to the patient cable and plug the cable into the monitor itself. Check that the following switches are on their standard settings. The sweep speed switch controls the rate at which the beam traverses the screen; its usual setting is 25 mm per second. The filter switch controls the amount of external interference in the tracing. It has two settings, "diagnostic" and "monitor." The usual setting for routine monitoring is "monitor" because it filters out most of the muscle artifact.

When the patient arrives, take these steps:

1. Explain to the patient why and how you will monitor cardiac rhythm. The following is a sample explanation:

> Mr. Johnson, have you ever been in a CCU before? No? Well, while you are here, we will observe your heart rhythm constantly so that we can help you immediately if you have any problems. This machine, called a monitor, will help us to observe your rhythm, even if we are not standing here at your bedside. I will attach it to you by placing these adhesive disks on your chest after I clean the skin with alcohol and shave small areas of your chest. This cable will connect the disks to the monitor, and I will pin it on your gown to reduce tugging on it.
>
> The monitor has alarms on it to let us know right away if you have any difficulty. Unfortunately, the alarms can be fooled when you move your chest muscles a lot. The alarm sounds like this when it goes off (demonstrate the alarm). When you hear it, remember that it may be due just to movement. We'll still come into your room to check you, though, unless we can observe the screen at the nurse's desk and see that it's just momentary movement.
>
> I'll tell your family about this monitor, too. Do you have any questions about it?

Of course, depending on the patient's condition, you may need to modify or delay this explanation. In many cases, however, you can explain the monitor and simultaneously connect the patient to it.

2. Prepare the electrode sites. If they are hairy, shave them. Rub the skin briskly with an alcohol sponge (let the shaved patient know that the alcohol may sting). Allow the sites to dry.

The electrodes currently being used by most hospitals are silver-silver chloride. They are centered in an adhesive disk, with a depression in the center containing electrode gel. Peel the electrodes off their backing without touching the gel or the adhesive surface.

3. Position the electrodes according to the lead you wish to monitor. The most common routine monitoring leads are lead 2 and MCL_1. Lead 2 provides the same view of cardiac activity as standard lead II; the difference is that lead 2 electrodes are placed on the chest while lead II electrodes are placed on the limbs. Lead 2, however, is not the ideal lead for visualizing atrial activity or ventricular activity. A superior lead is the right chest lead, V_1, because it clearly records the sequence of ventricular depolarization. It thus facilitates differentia-

tion of right from left premature ventricular beats; right from left bundle branch block; and premature left ventricular beats from premature right bundle aberrant beats. Unfortunately, routine monitoring in this lead is mechanically inconvenient since it requires four limb electrodes plus a precordial electrode. MCL_1 is a lead developed by Marriott (1970) to overcome the diagnostic disadvantages of lead 2 and the mechanical disadvantages of lead V_1. The designation MCL does not stand for "modified chest lead" as is commonly believed. CL was a lead in use before V leads, the C standing for chest and the L for the placement of the indifferent electrode on the left arm. The numbers after the L designated various chest positions, with CL_1 corresponding to the current V_1, and CL_6 to V_6. In this modification, the indifferent electrode is placed on the chest instead of the left arm (Marriott 1972).

Most companies mark their electrodes in one or more of three ways: a color code, initials, or electrical polarity symbols ($+$, $-$, and ground). If the monitor does *not* contain a lead, initials and polarity symbols are based upon lead I, so that the negative electrode is labeled RA, the positive electrode is labeled LA, and the ground electrode is labeled LL. Color codes may vary among manufacturers.

Most monitors today use a three-wire electrode system. Placements of the electrodes will vary depending upon the lead you want to monitor and whether your monitor has a lead selector switch. Figure 2-17 illustrates the most common situations you may encounter when placing electrodes.

- Placement for limb leads when the monitor has a selector switch.

  Put the negative (RA) electrode anywhere on the right upper chest. Place the positive (LA) electrode anywhere on the upper left chest. A useful upper chest location is just under the clavicle in the midclavicular line, because of minimal muscle there. Place the ground (LL) electrode anywhere on the lower left chest. The best place is over the sixth or seventh intercostal space in the anterior axillary line, because this position will not interfere with the interpretation of chest x-rays or pick up diaphragmatic movement.

  Set the selector switch for whichever lead you desire (1, 2, 3, AVR, AVL, or AVF). The machine automatically will change the polarity of the electrodes according to the lead you select.

- Placement for limb leads, when the monitor does not have a selector switch.

  If there is no selector switch, you must place the electrodes in the locations determined by the lead you want to monitor. If you wish to monitor lead 2, for instance, place the negative electrode on the upper right chest and the positive electrode on the lower left chest. The reference electrode may go either on the upper left or lower right chest.

- Placement for MCL, when the monitor has a selector switch.

  Similarly, the placement for monitoring MCL_1 or MCL_6 varies according to the presence or absence of a lead selector switch. If a selector switch is present, position the electrodes as follows.

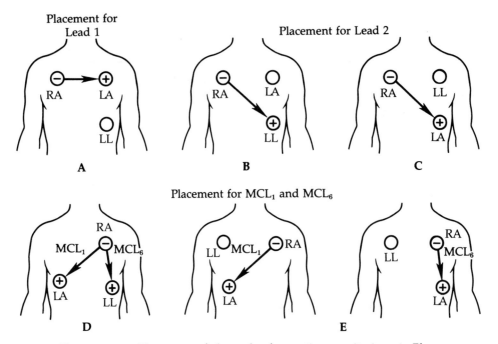

Figure 2-17.   Placement of electrodes for routine monitoring. **A,** Place electrode marked ⊖ or RA under right clavicle, electrode marked ⊕ or LA under left clavicle and electrode marked ground or LL at sixth or seventh intercostal space in anterior axillary line. If monitor has lead selector switch, place it on lead 1. **B, C,** If monitor has a lead selector switch, place electrodes as in lead 1 and set switch on lead 2. **C,** If monitor does not have a lead selector switch, place electrode marked ⊖ or RA under right clavicle, electrode marked ⊕ or LA in 6th or 7th intercostal space in anterior axillary line, and electrode marked ground or LL under left clavicle. **D,** If monitor has a lead selector switch, place electrode marked ⊖ or RA under left clavicle, electrode marked ⊕ or LA in V_1 position, and electrode marked ground or LL in V_6 position. Then switch selector to lead 1 position to obtain MCL_1 and lead 2 position to obtain MCL_6. **E,** If monitor does not have a lead selector switch, place negative (RA) electrode under left clavicle, ground (LL) electrode under right clavicle, and positive (LA) electrode in V_1 position (for MCL_1) or V_6 position (for MCL_6).

Place the negative (RA) electrode on the upper left chest. Place the positive (LA) electrode in V_1 position (fourth intercostal space at the right sternal border). Place the ground (LL) electrode in the V_6 position (at the intersection of a horizontal line from V_4 and the midaxillary line). Now, place the selector switch on the lead 1 position to monitor MCL_1; switch to the lead 2 position to monitor MCL_6.

- Placement for MCL when the monitor does not have a lead selector switch.

To monitor MCL_1, place the negative electrode on the upper left chest, the positive electrode in the V_1 position, and the ground electrode on the upper right chest. To monitor MCL_6, place the negative electrode on the upper left chest, the positive electrode in the V_6 position, and the ground on the upper right chest.

4. After placing the electrodes and setting the selector knob (if there is one), observe the ECG pattern on the screen. Adjust the position of the baseline with the position knob. If the complexes are not tall enough to be counted by the machine's rate meter, increase them with the sensitivity knob. (This knob sometimes is labeled "gain" or "size.")

5. Next note the rate being displayed on the rate meter. Set the rate alarms according to the limits at which you want to be alerted. For the patient with a satisfactory rate, these limits usually are ±20 beats from the patient's normal rate. For patients with abnormally slow or fast rates, you may wish to narrow the limits to deviations of 10 beats per minute in the abnormal direction. For example, for a patient with a heart rate of 60, you might place the low-rate alarm at 50 and the high-rate alarm at 90.

6. Trigger a printout of the rhythm by pressing the appropriate button or switch on the monitor. Analyze the rhythm and mount it in the patient's chart along with your admission nursing assessment.

When caring for a monitored patient, you should know the following items: the lead being monitored, the normal appearance of the patient's rhythm in that lead, the alarm settings, the sounds of the different alarms, the technique for triggering a printout at the bedside and the central console, and whether the monitor has a memory, that is, whether it records the last few seconds of cardiac activity before you trigger the printout.

Routine monitoring shares with the 12-lead ECG the problems of thickened baseline (due to dry electrodes or 60-cycle interference) and muscle artifact. To cope with these problems, review the section on 12-lead ECGs presented earlier in this chapter.

ECG interpretation

ECG analysis is most meaningful when you comprehend the relationship between the electrical forces in the heart and the recording obtained at the chest surface.

Membrane potentials and the ECG   All heart cells have a membrane potential, which is simply a difference in electrical charge across a semipermeable cell membrane. There are two types of potentials: the *resting membrane potential*

(RMP), and the *action potential*, which has two stages, depolarization and re-polarization. These potentials and their relationship to ionic movement are depicted in Figure 2-18, which diagrams the potentials for a ventricular cell.

Membrane potentials are affected by both the permeability of the cell membrane to sodium (Na+) and potassium (K+) ions and the rate at which these ions pass across the membrane. In the resting state, no electrical activity is occurring. This stage is represented by an isoelectric line and is called phase 4. In the resting state, the cell membrane is less permeable to sodium than to potassium. Sodium and potassium each establishes its own equilibrium across the cell membrane. Relatively more sodium is outside than inside the cell. Relatively more potassium is inside than outside the cell. Although the cell contains many positively charged potassium ions and fewer positively charged sodium ions, these positive charges are exceeded by negatively charged ions, primarily proteins and phosphates. As a result, the cell is polarized with more negative charges inside and more positive charges outside.

When a sufficient stimulus occurs, membrane permeability changes. This stimulus may be electrical, chemical (as in hypoxia), or mechanical (as in chamber dilatation). If the stimulation is strong enough, the membrane will reach a certain point at which its potential changes significantly. This point is

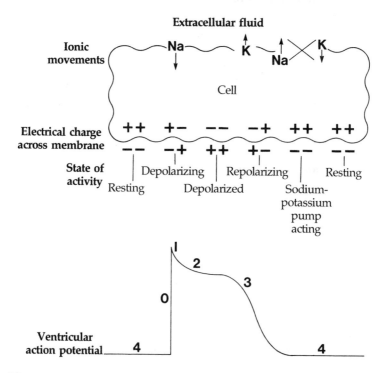

Figure 2-18.   Ionic movements related to ventricular action potential.

called the *threshold*. If the membrane reaches threshold, an action potential occurs on an all or none basis—that is, either the whole membrane changes its potential or none of it does. The action potential results from the movement of ions into and out of the cell according to the membrane's permeability for each ion and the gradient of each ion across the cell membrane.

When stimulation occurs and threshold potential is reached, the membrane becomes much more permeable to sodium. It allows such a large amount of sodium ions to rush into the cell, carrying their positive charges with them, that the inside of the cell rapidly becomes positive. Due to an electrochemical gradient, potassium moves out of the cell. Because the cell now is more positive inside than outside (the reversal of the polarized state), this process is called *depolarization*. On the action potential diagram, it is seen as a rapid upstroke (phase 0).

After depolarization occurs, a series of further ionic movements restores the ionic balance to normal. A short rapid drop in positivity immediately after the upstroke causes a spike on the action potential diagram (phase 1). *Repolarization* then slows down to almost zero rate for a short while, creating a plateau (phase 2). As repolarization continues, it accelerates again (phase 3). The details of repolarization are unclear, but it is thought that sodium permeability decreases and potassium permeability increases. As potassium diffuses out of the cell, the potential becomes progressively more negative until it returns to resting potential, phase 4. Although the overall balance of positive versus negative charges is restored, the distribution of most of the sodium and potassium is the reverse of what it was in the original polarized state. Using energy, the sodium-potassium pump in the cell membrane transports sodium out of the cell and potassium back in to restore the correct balance. This restoration does not disrupt the phase 4 baseline.

Conduction system   Changes in membrane potential spread more rapidly along the heart's conduction system than through other cardiac cells. Figure 2-19 shows the major components of the conduction system. They are not nerves but rather specialized muscle tissue. Normally, impulses arise in the sinoatrial (SA) node at the juncture of the right atrium and superior vena cava. From the sinus node, they spread across the atria and over preferential pathways to the atrioventricular (AV) node and left atrium. The preferential pathways to the AV node are the anterior, middle, and posterior internodal bundles. Bachmann's bundle, a branch of the anterior internodal bundle, is the preferential pathway to the left atrium. The AV node is located just to the right of the base of the interatrial septum and above the tricuspid valve. The impulses next travel to the bundle of His, which extends leftward from the AV node into the upper membranous part of the interventricular septum. (The AV node and bundle of His sometimes are referred to as the AV junction.) The bundle of His, also called the common bundle, splits into right and left bundle branches that travel down the muscular interventricular septum. The left bundle branch has two major divisions to the

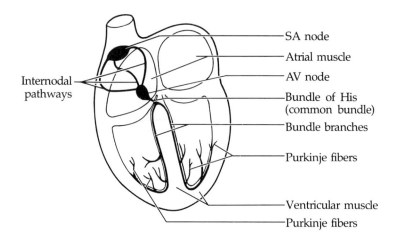

Figure 2-19.   Cardiac conduction system.

left ventricle, the anterior-superior branch and the posterior-inferior branch. The bundle branches split into the terminal part of the conduction system, the network of Purkinje fibers, which spreads the impulses from the endocardium to the epicardium.

Cells in the conduction system have different transmembrane potentials from cells outside the system (Figure 2-20). The most important difference relates to the resting phase. The phase 4 of cells outside the system is stable; they must wait for a stimulus to depolarize them. In contrast, the resting phase of cells inside the system shows a gentle positive slope. These cells are able to reach threshold potential spontaneously, thus depolarizing themselves. This property of spontaneous diastolic depolarization is called *automaticity.* These cells also have the property of *rhythmicity,* that is, they can depolarize themselves rhythmically.

Because cells in the conduction system can depolarize themselves, they can function as pacemakers to depolarize the rest of the heart. Pacemaker cells are of two types, dominant and latent. Although latent pacemakers exhibit diastolic depolarization, they usually become excited by an impulse transmitted from higher up in the system before they reach threshold spontaneously. A latent pacemaker may become a dominant pacemaker if it speeds up, a higher

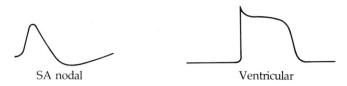

Figure 2-20.   SA nodal versus ventricular action potentials.

pacemaker slows down, or impulses from a higher pacemaker become blocked. Normally, the SA node is the dominant pacemaker because it can depolarize itself faster than the other potential pacemakers, 60–100 times a minute. If it slows down, fails, or becomes blocked, the next pacemaker to take over is the AV junction, at 40–60 beats per minute. If the Purkinje fibers are not depolarized by the SA node or AV junction, they will depolarize spontaneously at 20–40 beats per minute.

Impulse formation and propagation are affected by many stimuli discussed elsewhere in the text. The nervous control of the heart is presented in detail in Chapter 15. Briefly, sympathetic nerves (from the cervical and upper thoracic sympathetic ganglion chain) innervate the SA node, AV node, and ventricles. When sympathetic stimulation is increased, impulses are formed and conducted more quickly, and the ventricles contract more forcefully.

Parasympathetic control is provided by the vagus nerves from the medulla. Parasympathetic fibers innervate the SA and AV nodes, but not the ventricles. When parasympathetic stimulation is increased, impulses are formed and conducted more slowly.

Refer to Chapters 5–7 for detailed discussion of vascular dynamics and hormonal and chemical influences on cardiac impulses. The blood supply to the conduction system is discussed in detail in the myocardial infarction section of Chapter 4.

Vectors and the ECG   To interpret an ECG, you must have a clear mental picture of the relationship between the 12 leads and the heart's position in the frontal and transverse planes. If you are unclear, review the previous sections of this chapter dealing with those topics before proceeding with the following sections of ECG analysis.

At a given point in time, numerous cardiac cells' individual membrane potential changes interact to form an electrical force. This force, called a *vector*, has both direction and magnitude. It can be recorded by an ECG electrode on the chest surface.

It is important to recognize that the ECG records only the heart's electrical activity, not its mechanical activity (which follows electrical activation). It thus can record depolarization and repolarization, but not chamber contraction and relaxation nor valvular motion.

The ECG is able to record the relatively large vectors of the atria and ventricles, but not the smaller vectors of individual parts of the conduction system. Whenever it is unable to detect electrical activity, it records a straight line, called the *baseline* or *isoelectric line*. When it detects a vector, it records a deflection from the baseline.

The direction and magnitude of the deflection depend on (a) the distance between the the force's starting point and the lead, and (b) the relation between the force's direction and the lead's axis, the imaginary line between the poles of the lead (Figure 2-21). If the force's direction is toward the lead's positive pole, a

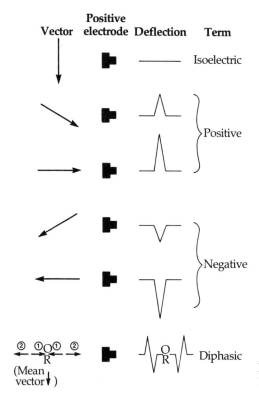

| | Positive | | |
| Vector | electrode | Deflection | Term |

Figure 2-21. Vectors and associated ECG deflections.

positive deflection is recorded. If it is directed away from the positive pole, a negative deflection is recorded. The more parallel the force is to the lead, the larger the recorded deflection; the more perpendicular, the smaller the deflection. If the force and lead are completely perpendicular to each other, no deflection is recorded. When the positive and negative forces are equal, a diphasic deflection is recorded. In this case, the mean vector is perpendicular.

By convention, the deflections are labeled with the letters P through U (Figure 2-22). Atrial depolarization (*not* atrial contraction) produces the P wave. Ventricular depolarization causes the QRS complex. Ventricular repolarization is seen as the T wave.

Intervals including or between these deflections are labeled as follows. The PR interval is from the start of atrial depolarization (the P wave) to start of ventricular depolarization (the QRS). It represents the length of time for an impulse to depolarize the atria and travel through the AV junction, bundle of His, and bundle branches. The ST segment is the interval between the end of ventricular depolarization (QRS) and the T wave. The end of the S wave and start of the ST segment sometimes is referred to as the J point. The QT interval is the duration of ventricular depolarization and repolarization.

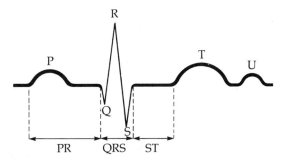

Figure 2-22.   ECG deflections and intervals.

P and T waves are called that whether they are positive, negative, or diphasic (part positive, part negative). In contrast, the letters used to label the QRS complex vary with the polarity and sequence of the deflections. *QRS complex* is a generic term applied to any ventricular depolarization; combinations of these letters are used to designate specific ventricular configurations (Figure 2-23). The first negative deflection after the P wave is called a Q wave. The first positive deflection after the P wave is called an R wave. The first negative deflection after the R wave is called an S wave. If the QRS complex consists of only one negative wave, it is called a QS configuration. Other variations include the notched R, when the negative deflection after the R wave does not reach the baseline, and

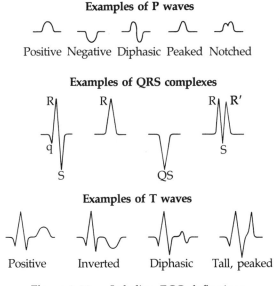

Figure 2-23.   Labeling ECG deflections.

the RSR', when it does. The relative size of the ventricular deflections can be indicated by using small letters for small waves and capital letters for large ones.

The QRST complex corresponds approximately to the phases of the ventricular action potential described earlier (Figure 2-24). The QRS complex reflects ventricular depolarization and the rapid start of repolarization (phases 0 and 1). The ST segment represents phase 2, the plateau in repolarization. During phases 0, 1, and 2, the myocardial cells cannot respond to another impulse. This is called the *absolute refractory period*. During phase 3, later repolarization, the cell may respond to an impulse. This period, the *relative refractory period*, corresponds with the T wave (Estes 1974). During the first part of the relative refractory period, a stimulus must be stronger than usual to evoke a response. During the later part of the period, however, there is a temporary increase in excitability, known as the supernormal period. During it, a weaker than normal impulse can provoke a response. The relative refractory period includes a vulnerable period during which another stimulus can cause repetitive depolarization. The vulnerable period corresponds with the 0.04 seconds before the crest of the T wave (Ritota 1975). The flat baseline between complexes corresponds to phase 4, during which excitability is normal.

These facts are clinically significant. For example, a premature atrial beat falling during the ventricles' absolute refractory period cannot cause them to

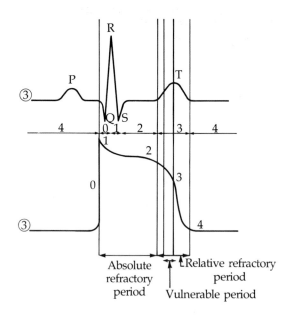

Figure 2-24.   Ventricular action potential phases correlated with ECG deflections.

depolarize. A premature ventricular beat occurring during the 0.04 seconds before the crest of the T wave (R-on-T phenomenon), however, can provoke lethal ventricular tachycardia or ventricular fibrillation. For this reason, you must keep an eagle eye on the distance between T waves and premature ventricular beats!

Frontal plane vectors can be plotted on the hexaxial reference system (Figure 2-25). This reference system is formed by the intersection of the six frontal leads, which divide the frontal plane into 30° units. By convention, all degrees in the upper half of the figure are negative and all those in the lower half are positive.

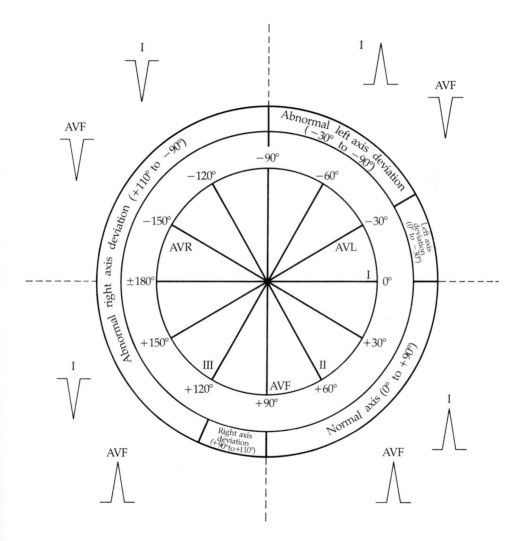

Figure 2-25. Hexaxial reference figure for determination of mean frontal QRS vector.

This convention is unrelated to the positive and negative poles of a lead. For example, AVL's positive pole is at −30°, while AVR's negative pole is at +30°.

The hexaxial reference system is divided into quadrants by leads I and AVF. Lead I divides the body into superior and inferior parts and lead AVF, into right and left sides. By examining deflections in those leads, you can determine the quadrant of the reference figure into which the vector falls and the direction of the vector in the heart.

For instance, suppose you found a patient's QRS complex to be positive in both leads I and AVF. You could refer to Figure 2-25 and note that the quadrant in which both of these leads have positive QRSs is the quadrant of normal axis. Alternatively, you could reason out the axis. If the QRS is positive in lead I, the electrical activity must be traveling toward the positive pole of lead I, that is, the left side of the body. If it is positive in lead AVF, it must also be traveling toward AVF's positive pole, that is, the foot. Thus, the vector is leftward and inferior.

It is possible to locate the vector more precisely. Find the lead which contains a transitional complex, a diphasic complex that is as much positive as negative. As explained earlier, a deflection is diphasic in the lead most perpendicular to a vector, so the vector must be almost perpendicular to the lead you are examining. It also must be almost parallel to the lead at right angles to the lead containing the transitional complex. For example, if the transitional complex were in lead III, you would know that the vector was almost perpendicular to lead III and almost parallel to lead AVR. You still would not know in which direction the vector was traveling, though. To determine that, you would look at the complex in AVR. If it were negative, the vector must be traveling toward AVR's negative pole. You would look on the hexaxial figure and note that AVR's negative pole is at +30°, so your patient's mean frontal QRS axis would be approximately +30°.

If no lead contains a transitional complex, find the one which contains the largest deflection. A deflection is largest in the lead which most closely parallels the vector. Next, determine whether the vector is traveling toward or away from the positive pole of that lead by noting whether the deflection in the lead is positive or negative.

Horizontal plane vectors also can be plotted on a precordial reference figure formed by the six precordial leads. Note the lead which contains a transitional complex, draw the vector perpendicular to that lead, and identify its direction by observing which V leads contain positive complexes.

Although you may not actually plot vectors, it is extremely important to understand the vector concept for two reasons: axis normality or deviation is determined by vector analysis, and comprehension of normal vectors will help you to spot whether a given deflection is normal for the lead in which it appears.

The most important vectors are the mean frontal P, QRS, and T vectors and the initial QRS vector. The mean frontal P, QRS, and T vectors of the normal electrocardiogram lie within the quadrant bounded by the positive sides of leads I and AVF (0° to +90°). This signifies that the mean direction of atrial depolarization, ventricular depolarization, and ventricular repolarization is leftward and inferior. Since this is the normal direction, the person is said to have a normal axis. If the vectors fall outside the quadrant, axis deviation is present. Axis deviation can result from different positions of the heart within the chest cavity, cardiac disease (such as hypertrophy or conduction disturbances), or disease of other chest organs which alters their ability to conduct electrical impulses.

A mean QRS vector between $+90°$ and $-90°$ indicates right axis deviation. That within the range of $+90°$ to $+110°$ may be normal. Right axis deviation from $+110°$ to $-90°$ is abnormal and usually results from right ventricular hypertrophy or right bundle branch block. A mean QRS vector between $0°$ and $-90°$ represents left axis deviation. The range from $0°$ to $-30°$ may be normal. Abnormal left axis deviation ($-30°$ to $-90°$) suggests left ventricular hypertrophy or left bundle branch block.

The next section discusses the P, QRS, and T wave vectors and the ECG complexes they produce. The vectors are shown diagramatically in Figure 2-26. Figure 2-27 is example of a normal 12-lead ECG and associated patterns of depolarization.

The P wave represents right atrial depolarization followed by left atrial depolarization. Sinus P waves usually are rounded and symmetrical, with a maximum width of 0.10 seconds and maximum amplitude of 2.5 mm (Ritota 1975). The normal mean frontal P wave axis is about $+60°$ (Estes 1974). Looking on the hexaxial reference figure, you can see that the leads closest to this vector are II and AVR, with the vector moving toward the positive pole of lead II and away from the positive pole of AVR. You can anticipate, then, that in normal sinus rhythm, II and AVR are the leads which will best display atrial activity, and the P wave will be positive in II and negative in AVR. The P wave normally is positive in the remaining limb and precordial leads. Occasionally, however, the normal P wave is negative, flat, or diphasic in III, AVL, V_1 and V_2.

Following atrial depolarization, an isoelectric line is recorded as the impulse travels through the AV node, the bundle of His, and bundle branches. The

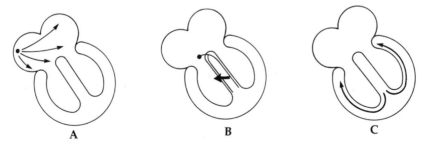

Figure 2-26.   Sequence of depolarization. **A,** Atrial depolarization, P wave vector is anterior, inferior, and leftward; **B,** septal depolarization, initial QRS vector is anterior, either inferior or superior, and rightward; **C,** free ventricular wall depolarization, mean QRS vector is posterior, inferior, and leftward.

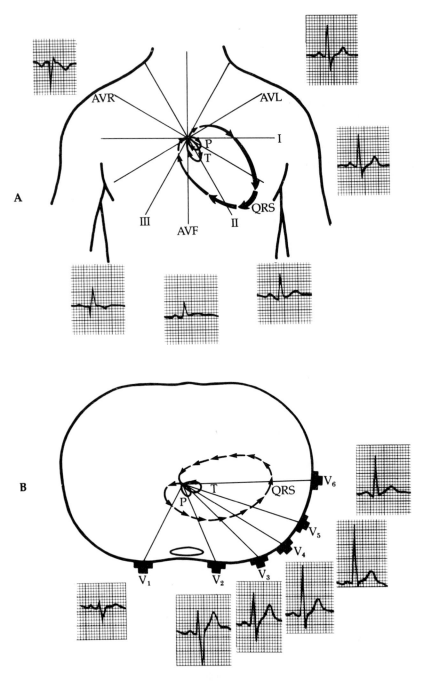

Figure 2-27.   Normal patterns of depolarization and related deflections on 12-lead ECG. **A,** Frontal plane; **B,** horizontal plane.

interval from the start of the P wave to the end of this isoelectric line (that is, to the start of the QRS) is known as the PR or PQ interval. Its normal value is constant and within 0.12–0.20 seconds.

Atrial repolarization usually is not recorded because it is obscured by ventricular depolarization.

The following information on QRS and T vectors is drawn primarily from Estes (1974).

The QRS complex represents ventricular depolarization. The frontal plane QRS axis varies with age. It is about +60°–+90° in the young adult and moves leftward (more horizontally) with increasing age.

Ventricular depolarization normally starts on the left side of the interventricular septum and initially moves to the right across the septum and anteriorly to the tip of the right ventricle. This anterior direction of the mean initial QRS vector causes initial positive waves (R waves) in the earlier precordial leads. This initial QRS vector also moves either inferiorly or superiorly. The inferior orientation is more common in the person with a more horizontal mean QRS vector. It produces small negative deflections (normal Q waves) in leads I and AVL for this person. The superior orientation is more common in the person with a vertical mean QRS vector. It produces normal Q waves in leads II, III and AVF for this person. These normal Q waves represent septal depolarization.

In addition to the patient's axis and lead in which Q waves are seen, normal Q waves are defined by width and depth. These criteria vary with leads, but in general a Q wave is abnormal if it (1) appears in a lead where it was not present earlier, (2) is more than 0.04 seconds wide, (3) is greater than ¼ the height of the R wave, or (4) accompanies a left bundle branch block in leads I, AVL, AVF, V_4, V_5 or V_6 (Ritota 1975). The reason for the latter criterion is that left bundle branch block usually causes the loss of normal Q waves in leads oriented toward the left ventricle, so the appearance of even a small Q wave in these leads usually indicates an infarction in addition to the bundle branch block.

Depolarization next spreads through the right and left free ventricular walls, from endocardium to epicardium. Because the muscle mass of the left ventricle is larger than that of the right ventricle, the ECG reflects primarily left ventricular vectors, which are oriented leftward and inferiorly. They progress from the initial anterior orientation toward a strongly posterior orientation, because the bulk of the left ventricle is posterior.

The posterior base of the ventricles is the last area depolarized. This vector is posterior, superior, and rightward.

The changing QRS vectors are reflected in the ECG. They cause increasingly positive waves (R waves) in leads towards whose positive poles they are traveling and increasingly negative waves (S waves) in leads away from whose positive poles they are traveling. Thus, lead II normally is characterized by a small Q wave (of septal depolarization) and large R wave. AVR displays a normal deep, wide QS wave, while V_1 normally is characterized by either a large wide Q wave or a small R wave and large S wave. The R wave becomes progressively larger and the S wave progressively smaller from V_1 to V_6. The normal duration of the QRS complex is 0.06–0.12 seconds.

The ST segment is isoelectric because early ventricular repolarization is very slow. The ST segment should be level with the PR interval line. Abnormal elevation is 1mm or more above the line and abnormal depression 1mm or more below it. ST segment deviations may indicate myocardial ischemia, injury, and infarction and are discussed in greater detail in Chapter 4.

The T wave represents ventricular repolarization and is evaluated by vector, size, and shape.

The mean frontal T wave axis normally is within 50° of the QRS axis and is related to the direction of the QRS axis. It usually lies to the left of the QRS axis if the QRS axis is more vertical and to the right of the QRS axis if the QRS axis is more horizontal. Normally, then, the T wave is positive when the QRS is predominantly positive and negative when the QRS is negative. If the T wave's polarity is opposite to the QRSs, the T wave is called inverted. Thus, an inverted T wave could be negative (with a positive QRS) *or* positive (with a negative QRS). The common assumption that a negative T wave always is inverted is a misconception.

The T wave usually is rounded and symmetrical. A T wave above 13mm tall in a precordial lead is abnormally high or deep and may be seen in ischemia and left ventricular hypertrophy (Ritota 1975). Tall, narrow, peaked T waves are seen in hyperkalemia. Giant inverted T waves commonly appear with myocardial infarction and ventricular premature beats.

Sometimes, a slow wave is recorded after the T wave. This U wave is poorly understood but may represent the very end of ventricular repolarization.

Analyzing the ECG   Train yourself to use a systematic approach to ECG analysis so that you do not overlook important data. The exact sequence is not as important as your consistency in using it. The following approach integrates analyses of vectors and the timing of cardiac events. It requires the use of a measuring device called *calipers*.

1. Note ventricular regularity and measure ventricular rate. The rate can be determined in relation to the measurements on the ECG paper (Figure 2-28). By convention, horizontal measurements represent time (vertical measurements represent electrical voltage). At the standard recording rate of 25 mm/sec, each small box measured horizontally equals 0.04 seconds. By remembering this value, you can figure out that each large box (five small boxes) equals 0.20 seconds, and 30 large boxes equal 6 seconds.

If the rhythm is regular, there are several ways to calculate rate. Since 300 boxes equal one minute, you can count the number of large boxes between the same point on two consecutive R waves and divide into 300. This method is accurate only if each of the R waves falls on the edge of a big box. Since 1500 small boxes also equal one minute, another way is to count the number of small boxes between two consecutive R waves and divide into 1500.

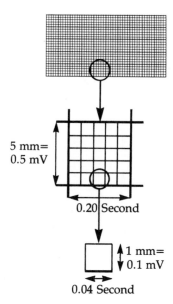

5 mm=
0.5 mV

0.20 Second

1 mm=
0.1 mV

0.04 Second

Figure 2-28. Time and voltage measurements on ECG paper (when recording speed 25 mm/sec).

A third method is that recommended by Dubin (1974) (Figure 2-29):

A. *Find a deflection occurring on a heavy black line.* For instance, to calculate ventricular rate, look for a QRS on a heavy black line. Use the distance between it and the same point on the next QRS to calculate the rate. If there is no QRS falling exactly on a heavy line, measure the distance between two QRSs with your calipers by placing one caliper point on the first QRS and the other on the same point on the next QRS. Without changing the relative position of the points, lift the calipers to the edge of the strip and place the first point on a heavy line. Then count to the second caliper point to determine the rate.

B. *Count out the rates represented by each heavy black line until you reach the ones closest to the second caliper point.* The rates represented by each heavy line are shown in the figure and may be memorized easily. You can see that the rate of the strip in the figure lies between 60 and 75.

(A deflection occurring on each heavy line is occurring at a frequency of 1 per 0.2 seconds, or 300 per minute. One occurring every other black line equals a frequency of 1 per 0.4 seconds, or 150 per minute. The remaining rates were calculated in a similar fashion.)

C. *To pinpoint the rate, know the values represented by the small black lines.* Although they are not as easy to remember, frequent practice with them will make them second nature. The precise ventricular rate of the strip in the figure is 65.

These smaller rate divisions also were determined logically, by dividing frequencies into 300. For example, the rate 125 was obtained by adding 0.4

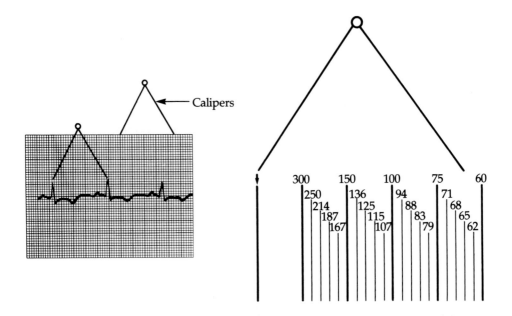

Figure 2-29.   Rapid rate calculation for regular rhythms. (From Dubin, D., 1974. *Rapid Interpretation of EKGs.* 3rd ed. Tampa, Florida: COVER Publishing Company. Used with permission of Dale Dubin, M.D., and C.O.V.E.R. Publishing Company.)

seconds (the frequency of the next highest heavy line) to the 0.08 seconds (the frequency represented by two additional small boxes), and dividing the sum 0.48 into 60 to get 125 beats per minute.

If the rate is irregular, you can get an estimate by counting the number of R waves in a 6 second (30 large boxes) strip and multiplying it by 10.

2. Note atrial regularity and measure the atrial rate. Use the above methods, but calculate the distance between the same point on two consecutive P waves.

3. Examine the P waves to identify the source of atrial activity. What is their contour, width, and amplitude? Do all the Ps resemble each other? Do they occur before, during or after the QRS? Is their polarity normal for the lead you are examining?

4. Measure the PR interval to evaluate conduction through the atria, AV junction, and bundle of His. To do this, measure from the onset of the P wave to the onset of the first ventricular deflection (it may not always be an R wave). Multiply the number of small boxes between these points by 0.04 seconds to get the measurement. Is the measurement normal, shortened, or prolonged? Is the PR interval constant, irregular with a consistent pattern, or completely irregular?

5. Examine the QRS to analyze the length and sequence of ventricular depolarization. Measure from the onset of the first ventricular deflection from the baseline to the end of the last ventricular deflection, that is, the return to the baseline. (If the demarcation between the baseline and the deflections is not clear, the onset and termination of the QRS may be difficult to detect. Sometimes, you will be able to see the change from a thick deflection, caused by slow electrical activity, to a thinner line resulting from the faster ventricular depolarization.) Multiply the number of small boxes by 0.04 seconds to get the measurement. Is the patient's value normal or prolonged? Is it constant, variable with a consistent pattern, or completely variable?

Examine the QRS deflections to assess the direction of ventricular depolarization. Are the deflections appropriate to the lead? If a Q wave is present, is its presence normal for that patient and lead? Is the appearance of the QRS similar for all complexes?

6. Examine the ST segment and T wave to evaluate ventricular repolarization. Is the ST segment normal (isoelectric and level with the flat part of the PR interval), elevated above the baseline, or depressed? Is the T wave normal or abnormal?

In summary, the normal ECG has the following characteristics. The impulse originates in the SA node at a rate of 60–100 beats a minute. It produces a P wave which is symmetrical, rounded, and precedes ventricular activity. It travels across the atria, AV node, and the bundle of His in 0.12–0.20 seconds. It produces a QRS complex that lasts 0.06–0.12 seconds. The complex is followed by an isoelectric ST segment and a T wave that is symmetrical, rounded, and of the same polarity as the QRS. The vectors of the P wave, QRS complex, and T wave are appropriate for the lead being examined.

This chapter has dealt with the mechanics of obtaining and examining the ECG. Identification, prevention, and treatment of arrhythmias and conduction defects are complex and so important that they are discussed separately in Chapter 3.

Diagnostic procedures

A wide variety of procedures is available to the physician in diagnosing cardiac disorders. Although you will not perform them yourself, you should read the reports and understand their significance. The diagnostic maneuvers reviewed here are chest roentgenology, echocardiography, phonocardiography, vectorcardiography, and cardiac catheterization. Interpretation of serum enzymes will be discussed in Chapter 4.

Chest roentgenology

This diagnostic technique utilizes an x-ray beam directed through the patient's chest to expose film placed against the opposite chest wall.

The differing densities of chest structures allow differing amounts of radiation to pass through the thorax and strike the exposed film. As a result, it is possible to differentiate on the developed film the shadows cast by the various structures. Air, which is the most radiolucent, appears black. Fat appears dark gray. Water appears light gray. Bone, which is the most radiopaque, appears white. The following descriptions of radiographic findings are based on Weens and Gay (1974) and Sanderson (1972).

Because of the anatomical positions of the chambers, individual ones are seen best on different projections. These projections are obtained by placing the chest in various positions in relation to the x-ray beam and film. In the preferred method, the patient stands, takes a deep breath and holds it while the film is taken with a beam six feet away.

In the posteroanterior view (PA view), the film is placed against the anterior chest, so the beam travels from the back to the front of the thorax. The lateral view positions the film against the right or left lateral chest wall. The right or left anterior oblique view positions the plate against the right or left chest so the beam traverses the thorax obliquely from the opposite portion of the posterolateral chest wall.

Figure 2-30 shows the cardiac structures visible in the different projections.

Since critically ill patients cannot tolerate being transported to the x-ray department and positioned upright, the films most commonly seen in the critical care unit are portable chest films. The patient is supine or sometimes the thorax is elevated. The x-ray beam traverses the chest from about two feet away, in an anteroposterior (AP) projection. Due to these variations in technique, the cardiac structures have a different size and shape on the AP view than on the PA view. Although the AP view is more distorted than the PA view, it nonetheless provides useful information in patient care. For example, it can indicate whether an endotracheal tube is positioned properly and whether there is a collection of air or blood in the pleural space.

In analyzing the cardiac significance of chest films, the interpreter considers heart size, signs of chamber enlargement, calcifications of myocardial structures, and evidence of altered pulmonary blood flow.

Cardiac size may be determined in several ways; the most useful methods compare the size of the heart with the size of the patient. A description of the techniques for calculating the heart's transverse diameter, frontal area, or volume is contained in Weens and Gay (1974). The calculated measurements then are compared against tables of normal values.

In addition to knowing whether the whole heart is enlarged, it is useful to know whether a specific chamber is enlarged. Individual chambers will display signs visible in different projections.

Enlargement of the right atrium will cause bulging of the right heart border on the PA view and the anterior border on the left anterior oblique (LAO) view. Bulging of these borders may be difficult to attribute to right atrial enlargement, since the chamber often is displaced by enlargement of other chambers.

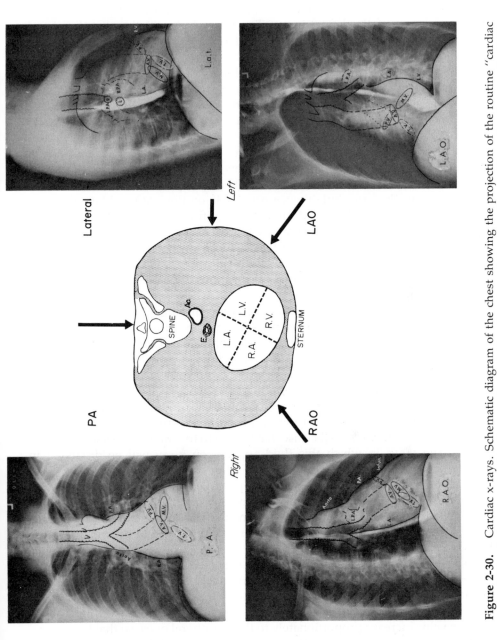

Figure 2-30. Cardiac x-rays. Schematic diagram of the chest showing the projection of the routine "cardiac series." The dark arrows in this diagram indicate the direction of the x-ray beam. (From Sanderson, R., 1972. *The Cardiac Patient.* Philadelphia: W. B. Saunders Company. Used with permission of Richard G. Sanderson, M.D., and W. B. Saunders Company.)

Enlargement of the right ventricle will produce an anterior superior bulge on the oblique and lateral views. Little change is visible on the PA projection.

Enlargement of the left atrium will cause a bulge of the posterior heart border, thereby producing esophageal displacement. The patient may be asked to swallow barium so the esophagus may be seen clearly. The displacement is seen best in the lateral and right anterior oblique (RAO) views.

Left atrial enlargement may also cause an elevated left bronchus, because the chamber is situated just below the juncture of the trachea and bronchi. This displacement is visible on PA and LAO projections, as a widening of the bifurcation of the trachea.

Enlargement of the left ventricle produces alterations in the left, inferior and posterior cardiac borders. On the PA view, the left border becomes more rounded and is displaced more to the left. The apex projects below the level of the diaphragm. Posterior bulging is most visible on the LAO and lateral views.

Calcifications of cardiac structures are significant clues in diagnosing the type of cardiac disease. They appear as white areas, because they have the same density as bone. Calcifications of valves, almost always the mitral and aortic, may appear as partial or complete rings. Calcifications of chamber walls appear as curved densities. Coronary arterial calcifications appear as small flecks, often in parallel lines.

Cardiac abnormalities often create alterations in pulmonary blood pressures or blood flow. Elevated pulmonary pressure may be arterial, venous, or both. Venous hypertension results when the pulmonary veins cannot empty normally into the left atrium. Initially, the veins emptying closest to the left atrium will dilate.

As the condition progresses, the superior veins will dilate significantly, while the inferior veins remain normal or constrict, producing an antler pattern of hilar shadows, often seen in mitral stenosis. As pressure continues to increase, fluid will move from the vascular system to the lung tissue itself, creating edema. The ways in which this fluid appears on x-ray will be discussed in Chapter 9.

Pulmonary arterial hypertension causes marked dilatation of the main pulmonary artery and the right and left pulmonary arteries, down to smaller arteries called segmental arteries. These segmental arteries remain normal or constrict so that the ratio of the size of the central to peripheral pulmonary artery branches exceeds the normal 5:1.

Normal pulmonary blood flow is equal to systemic blood flow. An increased or decreased ratio of systemic to pulmonary blood flow, such as occurs in congenital heart disease, will produce characteristic x-ray findings. When pulmonary blood flow exceeds about twice the systemic flow, both the central arteries and the veins increase proportionately to the peripheral ones, so that the normal ratio between central and peripheral vessels remains. When pulmonary flow decreases, the arteries and veins appear smaller and the lung is more radiolucent than normal.

Echocardiography

In this procedure, ultrasonic waves are beamed into the heart and their echoes are recorded. It is the only noninvasive procedure for following the mechanical activity of intracardiac structures. The procedure usually is performed by a physician or specially trained technician.

The patient is positioned supine or on his left side. A transducer is placed in various positions on his chest, avoiding the lungs and bones. Common locations are the left sternal border at the fourth intercostal space, the right sternal border, and the suprasternal notch. The transducer emits sound waves, which bounce back from the interfaces of dissimilar materials, such as blood and muscle. By aiming the transducer in different directions, the operator picks up echoes from different cardiac structures. Correct positioning of the transducer beam is difficult and time consuming, so the procedure usually takes 30–60 minutes. Figure 2-31 shows an example of a position to record the mitral valve.

When the beam encounters a boundary between substances with different acoustic properties (such as cardiac muscle and blood), a portion of it is reflected. The returning sounds (echoes) are recorded on a strip chart or on an oscilloscope, which is photographed. The acoustic characteristics of the substances determine the intensity of the echo. Blood is recorded as a black (echo-free) space, while tissue appears white. The length of time before the echo returns indicates the structure's distance from the transducer. By comparing the echocardiogram to a simultaneously-recorded electrocardiogram, the physician can interpret the timing of various mechanical events.

Among the conditions that can be diagnosed from an echocardiogram are disorders of mitral or aortic valve motion, left atrial tumors, pericardial effusion,

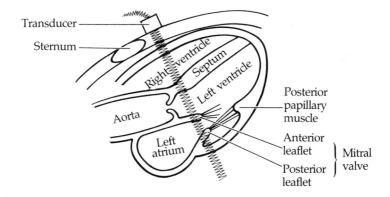

Figure 2-31. Echocardiography. With the transducer directed as shown, the echocardiogram will record echoes from the chest wall, right ventricular wall, ventricular septum, anterior and posterior leaflets of the mitral valve, and posterior left ventricular wall.

septal defects, and aortic aneurysms. In addition, it is possible to calculate chamber sizes and blood volumes, including cardiac output.

There are no complications of echocardiography. Post-procedure nursing care involves resuming previous interventions, including providing emotional support as the patient tries to cope with his concern about an impending or confirmed diagnosis.

Phonocardiography

This noninvasive diagnostic maneuver uses a microphone to pick up the sounds of blood flow and transmits them to a screen, which is photographed. An electrocardiogram is recorded simultaneously to help the physician interpret the tracing.

Patient preparation involves a brief explanation of its value in diagnosing his disorder and a description of the technique. Although it is unnecessary to restrict diet or activity before this procedure, it is essential that the patient remain still and quiet during it. Let the patient know that it will not hurt and the sound waves will not damage his heart.

The test should be done in a quiet room. Electrodes are placed on the chest for the ECG. A microphone is strapped on the chest, at the apex and/or base of the heart. When the base phonocardiogram is done, the microphone is placed on the left sternal border in the second intercostal space so that A_2 and P_2 changes with respiration can be recorded. Recordings are taken in the upright, supine, and left lateral oblique positions. A physician listens with a stethoscope to be sure the phonocardiogram is recording the sounds accurately.

Figure 2-32 is a diagram of a phonocardiogram. The recording is evaluated for timing, amplitude, duration, and frequency of sounds. Among the phenomena recorded are variations in the intensity of heart sounds, paradoxical splitting, gallop sounds, and murmurs. The visual representation of auditory phenomena is useful in diagnosing valvular disorders and other anatomical defects.

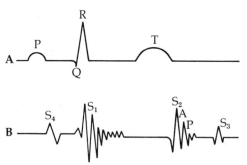

Figure 2-32. Phonocardiogram. **A,** ECG; **B,** apex phonocardiogram.

The test is of limited value in patients with tremors, chronic obstructive lung disease, or obesity. Misplacement of transducers and inexperience in interpretation may make the tracing difficult to analyze.

There are no complications of this procedure. Post-procedure nursing care is the same as that for echocardiography.

Vectorcardiography

Vectorcardiography is the noninvasive process of simultaneously plotting electrical voltage according to two perpendicular leads. As cardiac electrical activity occurs, it causes many simultaneous electrical forces originating from the same point in the heart. These electrical forces, which possess both duration and magnitude, are known as vectors. The recording thus can display the spatial orientation, direction, magnitude, and sequence of electrical activity in the heart.

It is possible that vectorcardiography is not available in your institution since it is a relatively new technique. If it is available, and your patient is scheduled for a vectorcardiogram (VCG), explain its purpose and technique. You do not need to restrict activity or diet before this procedure.

The patient will be taken to a special laboratory. Electrodes will be placed on his thorax and connected to an oscilloscope, which can be photographed. Electrode placement is not standardized yet. Different systems place the electrodes in different locations to obtain the equivalent of an anteroposterior lead, a horizontal lead, and a vertical lead.

On paper, a vector can be drawn as an arrow. The head of the arrow will indicate the direction of the force, and the length of the arrow will indicate its magnitude. Paper, however, is two-dimensional in nature, while cardiac electrical activity is three-dimensional. If you imagine the tips of the arrows as dots, you can conceive of a three-dimensional loop of dots representing cardiac electrical activity.

This three-dimensional loop can be detected by the VCG electrodes and projected onto a two-dimensional surface, an oscilloscope. Figure 2-23 is a diagram of vectorcardiographic loops. Also see Figure 2-27 for ECG deflections correlated with vector loops.

A light beam on the oscilloscope will record a line, indicating a continuous set of dots. The beam is interrupted periodically, which results in a series of tear-shaped dashes. The blunt end of the tear indicates direction and its length can be used to determine duration.

Usually three projections are recorded—frontal, transverse, and sagittal. Depending on which two leads are being recorded, the appearance of the same three-dimensional loop will vary in different projections.

Interpretation of the loops is difficult. In general, the interpreter examines the atrial and ventricular loops for spatial orientation, appearance, relationship to each other, and timing in correlation with the ECG.

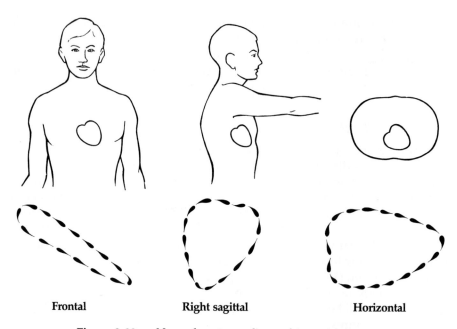

Frontal   Right sagittal   Horizontal

Figure 2-33.   Normal vectorcardiographic projections.

Because of its time scale, the ECG is best for measuring intervals and identifying arrhythmias. Both the ECG and the VCG are useful in diagnosing conduction defects within the ventricles, hypertrophy of the left ventricle, and most
infarcts. The VCG is superior for diagnosing hypertrophy of the right ventricle
and smaller or complicated infarcts, particularly those on the dorsal surface of
the heart.

There are no complications of vectorcardiography. Post-procedure nursing
care consists of resuming previous care and continuing emotional support.

Cardiac catherization

Cathererization is an invasive diagnostic procedure to study anatomical and
mechanical aspects of cardiac function. It is used to evaluate the patient with
atypical chest pain or inadequate response to medical therapy, to identify
anatomical lesions and associated conditions in order to plan drug or surgical
therapy, and to evaluate postoperative hemodynamic status.

The only absolute contraindication to catheterization is the patient's failure
to give informed consent to the procedure. Among the relative contraindications
are infection, acute myocardial infarction, and ventricular irritability.

Patient preparation   Collaborate with the physician and catheterization laboratory staff in emotionally preparing the patient and the family. Before the

patient goes to the procedure, they should have a clear idea of its benefits and risks, pre- and post-procedure care, and the steps of the procedure. In discussing the steps, focus on the sensations the patient may expect, and ways to interact effectively with the team.

Among the sensations the patient may experience are stinging as the local anesthetic is injected, the sense of pressure as the catheter is inserted or advanced, palpitations as the catheter is positioned in the heart, and intense warmth, a headache, and nausea as the dye is injected. These sensations are unpleasant but last only a minute or two. Let the patient know that in the room there will be many personnel in surgical dress. He should tell any of them if he experiences discomfort or does not understand what is being done.

Catheterization is a frightening experience to many patients. Assisting the patient to verbalize and cope with his fears not only will contribute to his equanimity during the procedure but also may reduce the likelihood of such complications as catecholamine-induced arrhythmias and vasovagal reaction (hypotension and bradycardia resulting from massive discharge by the autonomic nervous system).

Physical preparation includes several steps. Blood is drawn for coagulation studies. If the patient is on anticoagulants, they may be discontinued several hours before the procedure. The patient usually is not permitted anything by mouth (except oral medications) for eight hours prior to the procedure. Prophylactic antibiotics may be administered. Catheter insertion sites are scrubbed and shaved. The patient usually is premedicated with atropine (to prevent bradycardia) and diazepam. Glasses or dentures may be worn to the laboratory. The latter will be necessary if a Fick output will be done.

In the laboratory, preparation consists of the application of ECG electrodes, insertion of an arterial line, skin preparation, and draping with sterile sheets. The patient will be positioned supine on a narrow cradle which can be tilted sideways to facilitate various x-ray projections, since the procedure is performed under image-intensification fluoroscopy with television monitoring and videotape playback.

Catheterization procedures   The catheterization proceeds according to a protocol determined individually for each patient. The approach to the vascular system may be percutaneous (favored for femoral vessels) or by cutdown (favored for the brachial artery or basilic vein). Among the factors that influence the choice of site are the presence of obesity or peripheral vascular disease.

Catheterization of the right heart is achieved from the basilic or femoral vein most commonly. The left side of the heart may be catheterized via a retrograde arterial approach across the aortic valve, via a trans-septal puncture from the right atrium across the fossa ovalis, or via direct puncture through the chest wall.

Generally, the right heart is catheterized first. The catheter is left in place while the left heart is catheterized. Once that catheter is positioned, the peripheral arterial, left ventricular, and pulmonary capillary pressures are measured simultaneously.

Data recorded   During the catheterization the pressures are measured and the pressure waveforms are recorded for further study (see pages 26–29).

Oxygen contents and saturations are measured at several sites. These can be studied to determine the presence of shunts (abnormal blood flows within the heart). The usual oxygen saturation on the right side of the heart is 75% while on the left it is about 95%. Oxygen content varies from 14–15 volumes percent on the right side of the heart to 19 volumes percent on the left. An abnormal increase in oxygen content or saturation is called a *step-up* and is a clue to the presence of a shunt. For instance, an abnormally high oxygen content or saturation in the right atrium suggests that better oxygenated blood is mixing with venous blood in the right atrium. Among the conditions that might cause this finding are a defect in the atrial septum or a pulmonary vein returning to the right atrium instead of the left.

Cardiac output also is calculated. Cardiac output is the amount of blood pumped out by the heart each minute. It is a product of the heart rate and stroke volume, which is the amount of blood pumped out with each ventricular contraction. During catheterization, the cardiac output usually is measured both at rest and after exercise with a hand-grip or bicycle wheel mounted at the end of the table.

Cardiac output can be calculated in several ways. The most common is the Fick method. It is based on the theory that the amount of oxygen the body consumes equals that used by the tissues times the blood flow to the lungs. Oxygen consumption is measured by occluding the nose, having the patient breathe in a known concentration of oxygen, and analyzing the concentration in the air he expires. The amount of oxygen used by the tissues is measured by taking simultaneous arterial and mixed venous blood samples, and subtracting the venous oxygen content from the arterial. The values then can be entered into the Fick equation:

$$\frac{\text{Oxygen consumption (ml/min)} \times 100}{\text{Arteriovenous oxygen content difference (ml/100 ml blood)}} = \text{Cardiac output (ml/min)}$$

Cardiac output also may be calculated by the indicator dilution technique. In the catheterization laboratory, the indicator commonly used is a dye. A known amount of dye is injected centrally and its concentration is measured continuously at a peripheral arterial site. A dye-dilution curve is recorded, and the cardiac output can be calculated by computing the area under the curve.

A variation on the indicator dilution technique is the use of temperature as an indicator. A known amount of solution, at a known temperature, is injected centrally. A catheter with a temperature-sensitive tip continuously measures the temperature of the blood at a more distal point. A thermodilution curve is obtained and cardiac output is calculated from it. This thermodilution technique is used most commonly at the bedside. The catheter used has an opening in the right atrium, through which the indicator may be injected, and a thermistor in the pulmonary artery.

The value obtained for cardiac output is more meaningful when related to the patient's size, specifically his body surface area. The resulting value is the cardiac index; its normal range is 2.8–4.2 L per minute per square meter of body surface (2.8–4.2 L/min/m²).

Similarly, the volume pumped out with each stroke is more meaningful when related to the patient's size. The normal stroke index is 30–65 ml/beat/m².

The volume of blood in each chamber also can be measured. From the left ventricular volumes at end-systole and end-diastole, it is possible to calculate the ejection fraction. This value indicates the percentage of ventricular diastolic volume that the ventricle is able to eject. To maintain an effective cardiac output, the ejection fraction usually must be at least 0.60.

Myocardial metabolites such as lactate can be measured to evaluate oxygen supply to the myocardium.

Valve orifice areas can be calculated. Normal valve areas are 5–6 cm² for the mitral and 2.5–3.5 cm² for the aortic valve. The gradients (pressure differentials) across the valves also can be determined.

Vascular resistance also can be calculated. Normal total systemic vascular resistance is 770–1500 dynes-sec-cm⁻⁵; usual total pulmonary vascular resistance is 100–300 dynes-sec-cm⁻⁵.

Contrast media may be injected to opacify various cardiac structures. The general term for this procedure is *angiography*. *Ventriculography* is the injection of dye into the left ventricle to assess its contractility. *Aortography* is the use of contrast media to examine the function of the aorta and aortic valve. *Coronary arteriography* is the injection of dye into the coronary arteries to assess their patency. These studies are filmed for further analysis.

At the completion of the catheterization (which may last from two to four hours), the catheters are removed. The vessels may be stripped proximally and distally to remove clots. If a cutdown was performed, the vessel is sutured. The site is covered with an antibiotic ointment and an occlusive dressing is applied. Since it is difficult to apply an occlusive dressing at the groin, a sandbag may be placed over the dressing at the femoral site.

Complications   Among the complications that may occur during catheterization are cardiac arrest, acute myocardial infarction, arrhythmias, vasovagal reaction, anaphylactic shock, dye injection into the myocardium or pericardium, emboli to the lungs or brain, and sudden fluid shift due to the hypertonicity of contrast media.

After the catheterization, potential complications include thromboemboli; hemorrhage or hematoma; and hypotension because excretion of the hypertonic dye causes an osmotic diuresis. The patient usually is on bedrest until the next day and on intravenous fluids until his oral intake equals his fluid output. When the patient first returns from catheterization, check his temperature, perfusion distal to the insertion sites, hemostasis at the sites, blood pressure, and intake and output. Usually, you should make these checks, excepting temperature, every 15 minutes until the patient is stabilized and then gradually decrease frequency of the checks for the first 24 hours. Transient diminution of the arterial pulse is common but any pulse decrease should be reported promptly to the physician because it may signal impending arterial occlusion. If you are unable to monitor the patient constantly at the bedside, be sure to teach him and his family to alert you to any coolness, numbness, or paresthesias distal to the incision sites. Protect the healing of the site by not inflating a blood pressure cuff on that extremity, and by teaching the patient to keep it straight and not put his weight on it for the first eight hours or so.

A sound understanding of the above information will reinforce your comprehension of cardiac anatomy and physiology. In addition, your knowledge of the normal values will help you understand catheterization reports on your patients and use them to predict nursing problems. For instance, you might note that your patient had extremely high left atrial and pulmonary arterial pressures. This knowledge would alert you that your patient was at high risk for developing pulmonary edema; you then would know to monitor the patient closely for the onset of signs and symptoms, and take such preventive measures as close attention to fluid balance.

References

Andreoli, K., Fowkes, V., Zipes, D., and Wallace, A. 1975. *Comprehensive cardiac care.* 3rd ed. St. Louis: C. V. Mosby Company.
Outstanding reference on the care of the cardiac medical patient, covering anatomy and physiology, coronary artery disease, physical assessment, arrhythmias, and treatment.

Dubin, D. 1974. *Rapid interpretation of EKG's.* 3rd ed. Tampa: COVER Publishing Company.
Introductory text with information clearly presented in programmed instruction format.

Estes, E. 1974. Electrocardiography and vectorcardiography. In *The heart.* 3rd ed., eds. J. Hurst and R. Logue, pp. 297–313. New York: McGraw-Hill Books, Inc.
Highly detailed information on assumptions underlying these diagnostic techniques; ECG analysis; atrial ECG; ventricular ECG; criteria for diagnosis of hypertrophy and conduction disturbances; and ECG signs of myocardial infarction.

Grossman, W., ed. 1974. *Cardiac catheterization and angiography.* Philadelphia: Lea and Febiger.
Essential reading if you frequently work with catheterized patients. Clear and logical presentation of major concepts, principles, and technical details.

Hurst, J., and Schlant, R. 1974. Auscultation of the heart. In *The heart,* 3rd ed., eds. J. Hurst and R. Logue, pp. 215–281. New York: McGraw-Hill Books, Inc.
Principles of auscultation; advice on choosing a stethoscope; descriptions of normal and abnormal cardiac sounds.

Marriott, H. 1967. *Differential diagnosis of heart disease.* Oldsmar, Florida: Tampa Tracings. *Collection of tables and diagrams (from Marriott's* Bedside diagnosis of heart disease*) covering physical signs of heart disease, valvular disease, congenital heart disease, arrhythmias, and miscellaneous topics related to cardiac disease.*

_____ 1970. Constant monitoring for cardiac dysrhythmias and blocks. *Modern Concepts of Cardiovascular Disease.* 39: 103–108.
Advantages of MCL $_1$, illustrated with several ECG strips.

_____ 1972. *Workshop in electrocardiography.* Oldsmar, Florida: Tampa Tracings. *Conversational text based on Marriott's popular ECG workshops; includes numerous slide reproductions and dialogue with audience.*

Ritota, M. 1975. *A basic approach to the electrocardiogram.* Newark, New Jersey: M.E.D.S. Corporation.
Criteria for normality and abnormality of each component of the ECG.

Sanderson, R., ed., 1972. *The cardiac patient.* Philadelphia: W. B. Saunders Publishing Company.
Brief overview of various diagnostic techniques in Chapter 5.

Schroeder, J., and Daily, E. 1976. *Techniques in bedside hemodynamic monitoring.* St. Louis: C. V. Mosby Company.
Descriptions by cardiologists and cardiovascular nurse specialists of continuous bedside hemodynamic monitoring techniques and related patient care.

Weens, H., and Gay, B. 1974. Routine radiologic examination of the heart. In *The heart,* 3rd. ed., eds. J. Hurst and R. Logue, pp. 323–337. New York: McGraw-Hill Books, Inc.
Interpretation of radiographic findings; numerous illustrative x-rays.

Supplemental Reading

Franch, R. 1974. Cardiac catheterization. In *The heart.* 3rd ed., eds. J. Hurst and R. Logue, pp. 354–376. New York: McGraw-Hill Books, Inc.
Detailed presentation with numerous x-rays, diagrams, and formulae for data analysis.

Hoechst Pharmaceuticals. 1972. *Directions in cardiovascular medicine. Book 4: Cardiac catheterization.* Rev. ed. Somerville, New Jersey.

Hoechst Pharmaceuticals. 1972. *Directions in cardiovascular medicine. Book 5: Clinical vectorcardiography.* Rev. ed. Somerville, New Jersey.
Simplified but clearly presented, with many diagrams.

Silverman, M., and Schlant, R. 1974. Anatomy of the cardiovascular system. In *The heart.* 3rd ed., eds. J. Hurst and R. Logue, pp. 20–34. New York: McGraw-Hill Books, Inc. *Detailed information on cardiac structures.*

Sones, F. 1974. Coronary cinearteriography. In *The heart.* 3rd ed., eds. J. Hurst and R. Logue, pp. 377–385. New York: McGraw-Hill Books, Inc. *Authoritative presentation of various techniques of coronary cinearteriography.*

Chapter 3

Arrhythmias and Conduction Defects

The previous chapter showed you the mechanics of analyzing the ECG. This chapter will assist you in recognizing and responding appropriately to the arrhythmias and conduction defects you are most likely to encounter.

Outline

Assessment   Risk conditions / Arrhythmia detection / Significance of the arrhythmia

Planning and implementation of care   General principles governing treatment / Therapeutic procedures

Outcome evaluation

Objectives

- Anticipate and prevent arrhythmias
- Recognize these arrhythmias: sinus bradycardia, tachycardia, arrhythmia, arrest; atrial tachycardia, flutter, fibrillation; junctional rhythm, accelerated rhythm, tachycardia; supraventricular tachycardia, wandering pacemaker; ventricular rhythm, accelerated rhythm, tachycardia, fibrillation, asystole
- Recognize these conduction defects: first degree atrioventricular (AV) block; second degree AV blocks (Mobitz I, Mobitz II, advanced); third degree AV block; bundle branch blocks
- Recognize AV dissociation
- Recognize premature beats: atrial, junctional, ventricular; ectopy vs. aberration; capture; fusion

- Evaluate the arrhythmia's significance in relation to cardiac output and prognosis
- State the indications, technique, and nursing responsibilities for common treatment modalities: cardiopulmonary resuscitation; pharmacologic agents; vagal stimulation; cardioversion and defibrillation; and artificial pacemakers
- State desirable outcome criteria for the patient with an arrhythmia

Assessment

Critically ill patients are subject to a wide variety of arrhythmias which range from inconsequential to lethal. Since the inception of ECG monitoring, nurses have assumed increasing responsibility for accurate recognition and rapid termination of life-threatening arrhythmias. Remember that the monitor is but a tool in patient care. Focus on the patient, not just the monitor!

Risk conditions

Learn to anticipate and prevent arrhythmias by recognizing the conditions which increase the patient's risk of developing an arrhythmia. The risk conditions are numerous: major categories include myocardial hypoxia, electrolyte imbalances, catecholamine stimulation, vagal stimulation, and trauma or structural interruption of the conduction system. Myocardial hypoxia can result from systemic hypoxia, anemia, inadequate coronary artery filling time (for example in severe tachycardia), insufficient coronary artery perfusion pressure (for example in shock), or coronary artery disease. In some cases, the patient with coronary artery disease may have an oxygen supply that is sufficient at rest or for minimal exertion, and may only develop myocardial hypoxia when myocardial workload increases (such as in tachycardia) because oxygen demand exceeds oxygen supply. Local areas of myocardial hypoxia may be present in myocardial infarction.

Electrolyte imbalances, particularly those of potassium, may contribute to arrhythmias. These imbalances are discussed in Chapter 6.

Catecholamine stimulation, which predisposes toward tachyarrhythmias and premature beats, may occur in hypotension, hypertension, emotional excitement, increased muscular work, and administration of some drugs, such as vasoconstrictor agents. Vagal stimulation, which contributes to bradyarrhythmias and heart block, may occur with digitalis intoxication, Valsalva maneuvers, or tracheal stimulation. A Valsalva maneuver is a forced expiration against a closed glottis; it often occurs when a patient is moving about in bed or moving his bowels. Tracheal stimulation resulting in bradycardia or heart block may occur during tracheal suctioning, intubation, or vomiting.

Other factors which may provoke arrhythmias are trauma to the conduction system (such as during cardiac surgery), structural defects (such as a ventricular septal defect), myocarditis, and stretching of myocardial fibers due to volume overload.

Whenever possible, prevent conditions of risk. One of the key goals of critical care nursing is to develop the skill of taking preventive measures to avoid complications whenever possible. The following nursing measures are examples of ways to assist in preventing arrhythmias.

- Reduce catecholamine stimulation, which can produce tachycardias and premature beats. Minimize the patient's anxiety and pain and avoid hypotension. Promote physical and emotional rest.
- Avoid vagal stimulation, which can produce bradycardia and blocks. Take the following actions:
  1. Monitor patients on digitalis to detect digitalis intoxication promptly.
  2. Teach the patient to avoid Valsalva maneuvers. Also consult the physician about using stool softeners to reduce straining during bowel movements.
  3. When suctioning the trachea, watch the cardiac monitor for the onset of bradycardia and observe recommended time limits for suctioning. (The trachea is innervated with vagal fibers.)
- Avoid or alleviate fluid and electrolyte imbalances. Follow the care plans listed in the chapter on fluid and electrolyte imbalances.

Arrhythmia detection

To improve your ability to spot arrhythmias promptly, develop good arrhythmia detection habits. Monitor the cardiac rhythm constantly with an oscilloscope. Observe the scope for changes in rate, rhythm, P wave, PR interval, QRS duration and configuration, ST segment, and T wave. Analyze the rhythm strip and mount in the patient's record every 1–8 hours depending on the stability of his condition. When significant changes occur, document with a rhythm strip or 12-lead ECG. Read the 12-lead ECG reports (or the ECGs themselves) to keep informed about the progression of ECG changes. Auscultate the apical pulse for rate and regularity.

Common arrhythmias and conduction defects   Rhythms traditionally have been classified on the basis of their origin and their underlying mechanisms. The origin of an arrhythmia may be the sinus node, atria, AV junction, or ventricles. Mechanisms usually are grouped into disturbances of impulse formation (rate or origin) and disturbances of impulse conduction (blocks). Definitions of disturbances of impulse formation follow.

A *bradycardia* is any rhythm with a regular ventricular rate under 60 beats per minute (bpm).

A *tachycardia* is any rhythm with a regular ventricular rate over 100 bpm. Not all interpreters use this terminology. For instance, a spontaneous ventricular rhythm usually has a rate between 20 and 40 bpm. If the rate exceeds 40, some interpreters call it ventricular tachycardia; similarly, a junctional rhythm over 60 bpm may be called a junctional tachycardia. You can see how confusing this usage is, since "tachycardia" used this way can refer to a ventricular rate above 40, 60, or 100 bpm. For clarity, restrict the term tachycardia to rates over 100. Rates less than 100 bpm, but above normal for their sources, are best called accelerated.

Flutter is a regular rhythm, more rapid than tachycardia, with a sawtoothed appearance. The term usually is applied only to an atrial arrhythmia, although an occasional author calls ventricular tachycardia with this contour, ventricular flutter.

Fibrillation refers to chaotic depolarization. It produces an irregular, wavy baseline in which complexes cannot be distinguished clearly.

The disturbances of impulse formation are named by combining their source with their mechanism, for example *sinus bradycardia*. To enable you to compare and contrast the basic sinus, atrial, junctional, and ventricular rhythms, their characteristics are presented in tabular form and illustrated with ECG strips. Tables 3-1, 3-2, and 3-3 present sinus, atrial, and junctional arrhythmias. Table 3-4 presents supraventricular rhythms. A supraventricular rhythm is one which arises above the ventricles but whose source cannot be identified clearly as sinus, atrial, or junctional. Table 3-5 presents ventricular arrhythmias.

Disturbances of impulse conduction also may occur. These are called *blocks* and are subdivided into sinus, atrioventricular (AV), bundle branch, and hemi-blocks (block of a subdivision of the left bundle branch). AV blocks and bundle branch blocks are the most common and are presented in this chapter. Readers interested in learning about sinus block and hemiblocks should consult the supplemental reading list at the end of the chapter.

A block may be superimposed on any disturbance of the cardiac rhythm; thus, a patient might have an atrial tachycardia with AV block or a normal sinus rhythm with bundle branch block. Labeling of atrioventricular blocks can be confusing. To label an AV block, count the number of P waves per QRS. For example, if a rhythm had two P waves for each QRS, it would be described as a 2:1 block. Occasionally, an atrial wave may be obscured by the QRS deflections. To detect a hidden wave, use your ECG calipers to measure the P–P interval on visible waves. If the distance between the P waves just before and just after a QRS is twice the measured P–P interval, you can deduce that a P wave is being obscured by the QRS.

Atrioventricular blocks are shown in Table 3-6.

Table 3-7 presents an example of *atrioventricular dissociation*. AV dissociation is not a primary arrhythmia. Instead, it is a term that says the atria and ventricles are beating independently, that is, dissociated. Because it is not a primary ar-rhythmia, whenever you use the term you also must state the primary rhythms causing atrial and ventricular beating, for example AV dissociation with sinus bradycardia and ventricular rhythm. AV dissociation may occur in three different ways. If the primary pacemaker slows, a rhythm may escape from a lower site. An example is the sinus bradycardia and ventricular rhythm mentioned above. AV dissociation also may occur if the primary pacemaker discharges at a normal rate, but an ectopic pacemaker accelerates. An example of this category is sinus rhythm and ventricular tachycardia. The third way that AV dissociation may occur is if impulses from the primary pacemaker become completely blocked (third degree AV block). This type of dissociation is detected easily if the atrial rate is greater than the ventricular. If the ventricular rate is greater than the atrial, however, you cannot say just from the ECG strip that a third degree block is present, although it is possible that a third degree block occurred and was followed by acceleration of a rhythm from a junctional or ventricular focus. In order to diagnose the cause of the dissociation in this case, the physician will attempt to accelerate the rhythm driving the atria to see whether a block is in fact present.

In the first two types of dissociation, AV conduction is normal. Occasionally, then, when a P wave is far enough away from a QRS, it may be conducted to the ventricles, thus capturing (depolarizing) them. Such a beat is called a *capture* beat. It occurs because the impulse reaches the ventricles at a time when they can respond, that is, when they are not already refractory from the impulses otherwise driving them. Capture beats are shown in Table 3-7.

Bundle branch blocks are a type of conduction disturbance in which the right or left bundle branch fails to conduct impulses. To understand the ECG patterns which result from bundle branch blocks, it is helpful to understand the relationship between the sequence of ventricular activation and the corresponding ECG deflections (Table 3-8). Normally, ventricular depolarization occurs in two major steps. Septal depolarization proceeds from left to right, followed by free ventricular wall depolarization. The right ventricle depolarizes from left to right; simultaneously, the left ventricle depolarizes from right to left. Because left ventricular muscle mass exceeds that of the right ventricle, the ECG normally reflects primarily left ventricular depolarization. This normal sequence of ventricular depolarization can be seen clearly in ECG recordings from V_1, an electrode over the right ventricle, and V_6, an electrode over the left ventricle. The wave of septal depolarization travels toward V_1 (which records a small positive or R wave) and away from V_6 (which records a small negative or Q wave). The wave of free ventricular wall depolarization travels in the opposite direction—away from V_1 (which records a large negative or S wave) and toward V_6 (which records a large positive or R wave). As a result, normal bundle branch conduction produces an rS pattern in V_1 and a qR pattern in V_6.

When the right bundle branch is blocked, right ventricular stimulation is delayed. Septal depolarization proceeds normally, from left to right. The ventricles, however, no longer depolarize simultaneously; instead the left ventricle depolarizes before the right ventricle. Left ventricular depolarization proceeds

Text continued on p. 92

Table 3-1   Sinus rhythms

| Regularity and rate | | P waves | AV Conduction | | QRS |
Ventricular	Atrial		P:QRS ratio	PR Interval	
Normal sinus rhythm					
Regular, 60–100	Same as ventricular	Symmetrical, rounded	1:1	0.12–0.20 sec	0.06–0.12 sec

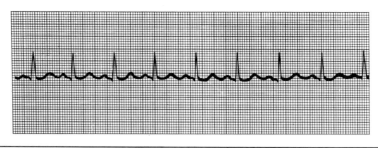

Sinus bradycardia					
Regular, below 60	Same	Same	Same	Same	Same

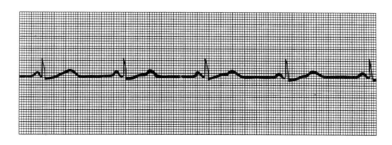

Sinus tachycardia					
Regular, above 100 (usually up to 180)	Same	Same	Same	Same	Same

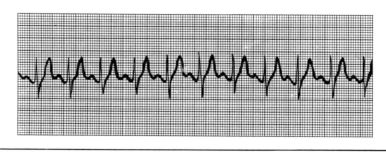

(continued)

Comments	Causes	Significance	Treatment
	Normal heart	Normal rhythm	None
	Normal heart; athletic heart; sleep; vagal stimulation; myocardial infarction; increased intracranial pressure	Significance depends on rate; if moderate, allows for increased ventricular filling and decreased myocardial oxygen demand. If too slow, inadequate cardiac output	None if asymptomatic; if symptomatic, atropine, isoproterenol, artificial pacemaker
	Normal heart; tea, coffee, tobacco, alcohol; physical or emotional stress; inflammatory heart disease; coronary artery disease	Usually not significant except in patient with heart disease; then may cause angina, infarction, congestive heart failure, shock	If asymptomatic, none; if symptomatic, treatment of cause

(continued)

Table 3-1   Sinus rhythms *(continued)*

Regularity and rate		P waves	AV Conduction		QRS
Ventricular	Atrial		P:QRS ratio	PR Interval	
Sinus arrhythmia					
Irregular, 60–100	Same	Same	Same	Same	Same

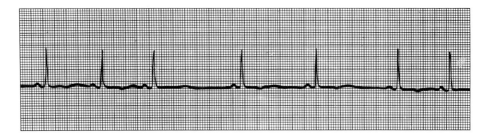

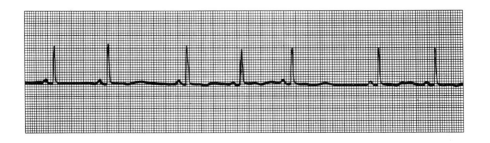

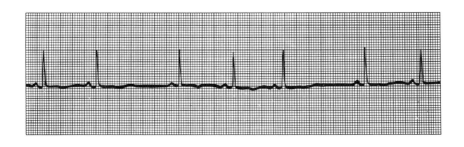

(continued)

Comments	Causes	Significance	Treatment
Rate increases with inspiration, decreases with expiration, in cyclical fashion	Normal heart (variation in sympathetic and parasympathetic stimulation during respiration)	Normal variant	None

(continued)

Table 3-1   Sinus rhythms *(continued)*

| Regularity and rate | | P waves | AV Conduction | | QRS |
Ventricular	Atrial		P:QRS ratio	PR Interval	
Sinus arrest					
Regular but with occasional absence of entire PQRST complex; any rate	Same	Same	Same	Same	Same

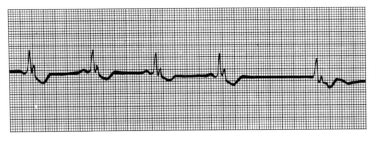

Table 3-2   Atrial rhythms

| Regularity and rate | | P waves | AV Conduction | | QRS |
Ventricular	Atrial		P:QRS ratio	PR Interval	
Paroxysmal atrial tachycardia					
Regular, 150–250	Same as ventricular	Contour slightly different from sinus P waves	1:1	Normal	Normal

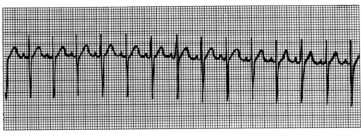

(continued)

Comments	Causes	Significance	Treatment
Cycle containing missed beat is not a multiple of the basic sinus cycle	Failure of sinus node owing to infarction, increased vagal tone, fibrosis, digitalis toxicity	May be transient or prolonged; if transient, no significance. If prolonged, patient develops asystole unless escape rhythm occurs.	If prolonged, atropine, isoproterenol, or artificial pacemaker

Comments	Causes	Significance	Treatment
Onset and termination sudden	Normal heart; stimulation from coffee, tea, tobacco; coronary artery disease; hyperthyroidism; rheumatic heart disease	May produce heart failure, shock, angina, dizziness	Depends upon patient's tolerance, cause, and history of previous attacks; rest, sedation, vagal stimulation, cardioversion, right atrial pacing, propranalol

(continued)

Table 3-2   Atrial rhythms *(continued)*

Regularity and rate		P waves	AV Conduction		QRS
Ventricular	Atrial		P:QRS ratio	PR Interval	
Atrial tachycardia with block					
Regular if block is constant, ir-regular if block is variable; any rate	Regular, 150–250. If block is constant, atrial rate is multiple of ventric-ular rate	Same as above	More than 1:1	Normal on conducted beats	Normal

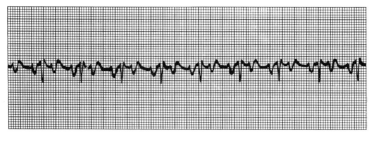

Atrial tachycardia with 2:1 block

Atrial flutter					
Regular or irregular depending upon constancy of block; any rate	Regular, 200–350. If block is constant, atrial rate is multiple of ventric-ular rate.	Sawtooth	More than 1:1. Usually constant even block— 2:1, 4:1, etc.	Normal on conducted beats	Normal

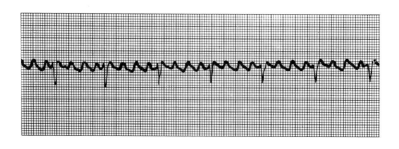

(continued)

Comments	Causes	Significance	Treatment
Block is physiologic owing to arrival of some atrial impulses at AV node during its refractory period	Coronary artery disease; digitalis intoxication	Symptoms depend upon ventricular rate	If asymptomatic, observation; if digitalis is cause: discontinuation of drug, administration of potassium chloride; if digitalis not cause, digitalis to slow ventricular rate
Same comment as atrial tachycardia with block	Normal heart; heart disease	Carotid sinus massage increases degree of block temporarily but does not terminate arrhythmia	Cardioversion digitalis quinidine propranolol

(continued)

Table 3-2   Atrial rhythms *(continued)*

Regularity and rate		P waves	AV Conduction		QRS
Ventricular	Atrial		P:QRS ratio	PR Interval	
Atrial fibrillation					
Irregular, rate varies	Unmeasurable	Chaotic (fine or coarse) fibrillatory (f) waves, seen as wavy baseline	Very variable; numerous f waves per QRS	Variable	Normal

Table 3-3   Junctional rhythms

Regularity and rate		P waves	AV Conduction		QRS
Ventricular	Atrial		P:QRS ratio	PR Interval	
Junctional rhythm					
Regular, 40–60	0 or same as ventricular	Absent; before QRS and inverted; during QRS; or after QRS	0 or 1:1	If present, less than 0.12 seconds	Normal

(continued)

Comments	Causes	Significance	Treatment
	Normal heart; mitral stenosis; thyrotoxicosis; pericarditis; coronary artery disease; hypertensive heart disease	No effective atrial contraction; predisposes to pulmonary or systemic thromboemboli (about one-third of patients develop)	Cardioversion digitalis quinidine

Comments	Causes	Significance	Treatment
If P waves are present, junctional stimulus has been conducted retrograde to atria	Failure of sinus node	Protects patient from asystole	Treatment of failure of sinus node; atropine, isoproterenol to increase junctional rate; or artificial pacemaker

(continued)

Table 3-3   Junctional rhythms *(continued)*

| Regularity and rate | | P waves | AV Conduction | | QRS |
Ventricular	Atrial		P:QRS ratio	PR Interval	
Accelerated junctional rhythm					
Regular, 60–100	0 or same as ventricular	Same as above	0 or 1:1	Same	Same

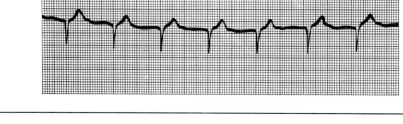

Junctional tachycardia					
Regular, over 100	0 or same as ventricular	Same	Same	Same	Same

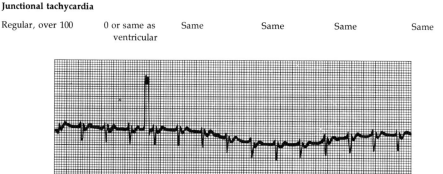

normally, from right to left. Because the right bundle branch cannot conduct the impulse to the right ventricle, right ventricular depolarization occurs via spread of the impulse from the left ventricle. This spread occurs slowly because the impulse travels outside the conduction system; as a result, the QRS measures greater than 0.12 seconds. Although the length of right ventricular depolarization is prolonged, the direction remains the same, left to right. The three steps of ventricular depolarization are reflected in the ECG. Instead of the normal rS, a V_1 electrode records a triphasic (rSR') deflection: a small positive wave of septal depolarization, a large negative wave of free left ventricular wall depolarization, and a large positive wave of free right ventricular wall depolarization. The V_6 electrode also records a triphasic deflection, but it is a qRS; the q wave reflects

Comments	Causes	Significance	Treatment
Same	Same	Same; in addition, produces near normal cardiac output	Treatment of cause

Nonparoxysmal junctional tachycardia:

Comments	Causes	Significance	Treatment
Same; if onset and termination sudden, called paroxysmal junctional tachycardia	Myocardial infarction, myocarditis, post-cardiotomy, digitalis intoxication	Depends upon patient's tolerance; usually stops spontaneously if tolerated well	If asymptomatic, treatment of cause; if symptomatic, discontinuation of digitalis, cardioversion, digitalis (if not cause)

Paroxysmal junctional tachycardia: see paroxysmal atrial tachycardia

septal depolarization, the R wave reflects left free ventricular wall depolarization, and a wide S wave reflects the slow free right ventricular wall depolarization. Due to abnormal ventricular repolarization, the T wave which follows a right bundle branch block is inverted.

When the left bundle branch is blocked, the pattern of depolarization is disrupted to a greater extent. Septal depolarization no longer proceeds from left to right; its direction is reversed. The right ventricle depolarizes next, in its normal direction (left to right). Left ventricular stimulation is delayed and occurs via spread of the impulse from the right ventricle, again outside the conduction system. The left ventricle therefore depolarizes last, but in the abnormal direction, right to left. The ECG patterns again reflect the ventricular activity clearly.

Table 3-4   Miscellaneous supraventricular rhythms

Regularity and rate		P waves	AV Conduction		QRS
Ventricular	Atrial		P:QRS ratio	PR Interval	
Wandering pacemaker					
Slightly irregular, any rate	Same as ventricular	Variable: sinus, atrial and/or junctional	1:1	Variable	Normal

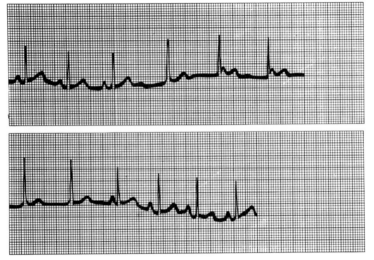

Wandering pacemaker (continuous strip)

Supraventricular tachycardia

Regular, over 100	←————————Not detectable————————→				Normal

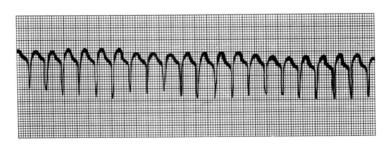

(continued)

Comments	Causes	Significance	Treatment
	Normal heart; athletic heart; heart disease	Several pacemakers are tending to fire at similar rates, so pacemaker site "wanders" from SA node to atria and/or AV junction; only one site is dominant at a given moment	Rarely necessary; atropine or isoproterenol
	See sinus, atrial and junctional tachycardia	Global term indicating rhythm originating above ventricles but whose source cannot be identified (because P waves are not clearly visible)	Differentiation requires additional maneuvers such as carotid sinus massage, study of a waves in jugular venous pulse, and assessment of S_1 intensity and S_2 splitting

(continued)

Table 3-4   Miscellaneous supraventricular rhythms

Regularity and rate		P waves	AV Conduction		QRS
Ventricular	Atrial		P:QRS ratio	PR Interval	
Supraventricular tachycardia with aberration					
Regular, over 100	←——————————Not detectable——————————→				Wide RBBB or LBBB pattern

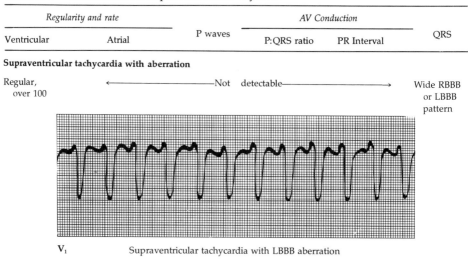

V₁   Supraventricular tachycardia with LBBB aberration

V_1 records a small negative wave of septal depolarization, sometimes a small positive wave of right ventricular depolarization, and a large negative wave of free left ventricular wall depolarization. These deflections usually are seen as a monophasic QS wave, sometimes with a small positive notch. The V_6 electrode records a small positive wave, sometimes a small negative wave, and a large

Table 3-5   Ventricular rhythms

Regularity and rate		P waves	AV Conduction		QRS
Ventricular	Atrial		P:QRS ratio	PR Interval	
Ventricular rhythm					
Regular, 20–40	Absent, or if present, unrelated to ventricular activity				Greater than 0.12 seconds

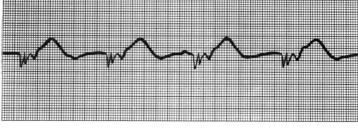

(continued)

Comments	Causes	Significance	Treatment
	See sinus, atrial and junctional tachycardia	As in sinus, atrial and junctional tachy-cardia; temporarily abnormal conduction through bundle branches because supraventricular impulses fall when one branch still refractory; easily confused with ventricular tachycardia	As above

positive wave, resulting in a wide, monophasic R wave, occasionally with a small negative notch. The T wave usually is inverted, due to abnormal ventricular repolarization.

Because the initial forces in the right bundle branch block are not changed, ECG signs of myocardial infarction can be detected on the patient's ECG. In

Text continued on p. 106

Comments	Causes	Significance	Treatment
	Failure of higher pacemakers or complete AV block	Escape rhythm	Atropine, isoproterenol, artificial pacemaker

(continued)

Table 3-5   Ventricular rhythms (*continued*)

Regularity and rate		P waves	AV Conduction		QRS
Ventricular	Atrial		P:QRS ratio	PR Interval	

Accelerated ventricular rhythm

Regular, 40–100	Absent, or if present, unrelated to ventricular activity				Greater than 0.12 seconds

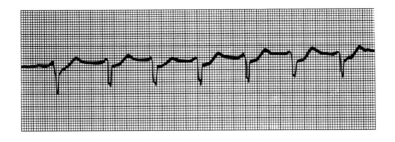

Ventricular tachycardia

Regular, above 100	Absent, or if present, unrelated to ventricular activity				Greater than 0.12 seconds

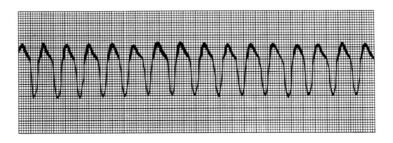

Ventricular fibrillation

0	Absent, or if present, unrelated to ventricular activity				None

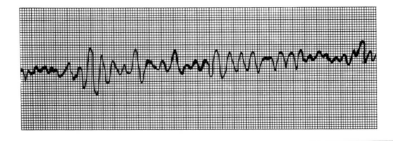

(continued)

Comments	Causes	Significance	Treatment
	Acute myocardial infarction; digitalis intoxication	Ectopic ventricular pacemaker accelerates to rate approximating normal sinus rhythm.	Close observation; treatment of cause; rarely, atropine or lidocaine
	Acute myocardial infarction; coronary artery disease; premature ventricular beat (R on T phenomenon)	Ominous as may progress to ventricular fibrillation; symptoms depend on underlying heart disease, rate, and duration of VT; may cause angina, cardiac failure, shock	If hemodynamic decompensation, immediate counter-shocks; if no decom-pensation, lidocaine bolus IV followed by lidocaine infusion
Chaotic depolarization produces grossly irregular, bizarre ECG deflections	Acute myocardial infarction; coronary artery disease; electrical shock; premature ventricular beat (R on T phenomenon); dying heart	Lethal within 4–6 minutes; symptoms include loss of con-sciousness, pulse, heart sounds and respirations; seizures; absent blood pressure	Immediate defibrillation followed by cardiopulmonary resuscitation

(continued)

Table 3-5 Ventricular rhythms *(continued)*

Regularity and rate		P waves	AV Conduction		QRS
Ventricular	Atrial		P:QRS ratio	PR Interval	
Ventricular asystole					
0	Absent, or if present, unrelated to ventricular activity				None

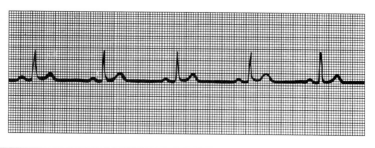

Ventricular standstill

Table 3-6 Atrioventricular blocks

Regularity and rate		P waves	AV Conduction		QRS
Ventricular	Atrial		P:QRS ratio	PR Interval	
First degree AV block					
Regular, any rate	Same as ventricular	Sinus or atrial	1:1	Constant but greater than 0.20 seconds	Normal

(continued)

Comments	Causes	Significance	Treatment
In illustration, deflections are P waves	Acute myocardial infarction; coronary artery disease; complete heart block; dying heart	Same as ventricular fibrillation	Immediate cardiopulmonary resuscitation

Comments	Causes	Significance	Treatment
All impulses are conducted through AV node but slower than usual	Normal heart; coronary artery disease; digitalis intoxication; conduction system fibrosis; myocarditis; cardiac surgery	Relatively benign; may progress to second or third degree blocks	None necessary

(continued)

Table 3-6   Atrioventricular blocks (*continued*)

Regularity and rate		P waves	AV Conduction		QRS
Ventricular	Atrial		P:QRS ratio	PR Interval	

Second degree AV blocks: (1) Mobitz I (Wenckebach I)

Irregular but consistent pattern, any rate	Regular, faster than ventricular	Sinus or atrial	1:1 except for nonconducted P wave	Lengthens progressively until one P wave not conducted; cycle then repeats itself	Normal

Mobitz I second degree AV block

(2) Mobitz II (Wenckebach II)

Irregular but with no consistent pattern, any rate	Regular, faster than ventricular	Sinus or atrial	1:1 except for nonconducted P wave	Constant on conducted beats, 0.12–0.20 seconds	Normal

Mobitz II second degree AV block

(*continued*)

Comments	Causes	Significance	Treatment
In second degree blocks, some impulses are not conducted; in Mobitz I, impulses are delayed progressively until one reaches AV node while it is absolutely refractory, so it cannot conduct that impulse	Same as first degree block	Relatively benign: does not diminish cardiac output, usually transient, does not usually progress to greater degree of block	Usually, none necessary; if symptomatic, atropine; discontinue digitalis if cause
Impulses are conducted normally until one is suddenly blocked	Same as first degree block except not digitalis intoxication	More ominous than Mobitz I; often precedes sudden complete heart block	Atropine, isoproterenol, prophylactic artificial pacemaker

(continued)

Table 3-6   Atrioventricular blocks *(continued)*

| Regularity and rate | | P waves | AV Conduction | | QRS |
Ventricular	Atrial		P:QRS ratio	PR Interval	
		(3) Advanced (high grade)			
Regular or irregular, depending upon constancy of block	Regular, faster than ventricular	Sinus or atrial	More than 1:1	Constant on conducted beats, 0.12–0.20 seconds	Normal

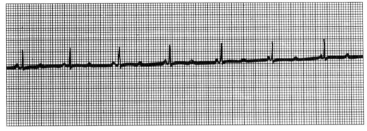

Advanced second degree AV block

Third degree (complete) AV block

Absent or regular	Regular, faster than ventricular	Sinus or atrial	0; no relationship between Ps and QRSs	Appears variable but P waves actually not conducted	Absent, normal or wide, depending on presence and source of escape rhythm

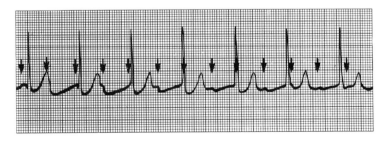

Comments	Causes	Significance	Treatment
Many impulses not conducted; block may be constant or variable; illustration shows 2:1 block	Same as first degree block	Block often physiologic (high atrial rate causes some impulses to reach AV node while it is refractory; block protects ventricles from excessive stimulation); if block severe, inadequate cardiac output	If asymptomatic, treatment of atrial arrhythmia; if ventricular rate too slow, atropine
No impulses conducted through AV node; Ps and QRSs must be far enough apart that conduction could occur if block was not present; in illustration, arrows point to P waves	Same as first degree block	If no escape rhythm, patient dies	Isoproterenol; artificial pacemaker

Table 3-7   AV dissociation

Regularity and rate		P waves	AV Conduction		QRS	Comments
Ventricular	Atrial		P:QRS ratio	PR Interval		
Regular unless capture beats present, any rate	Regular, any rate	Unrelated to QRS	Unrelated	Appears variable but Ps actually not con- ducted	Normal or wide, de- pending on source of escape rhythm	In illustration, strips are non- continuous; arrows mark P waves

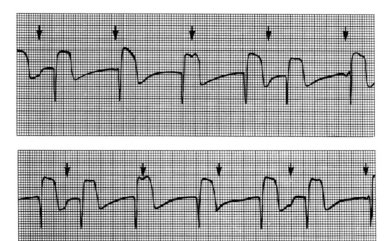

Analysis of strip

Dominant rhythm:	Ventricular rate = 57, Atrial rate = 47; QRS = 0.08; P waves unrelated to QRS complexes
Early beats:	QRS = 0.08; each beat preceded by a P wave; constant relationship between P and QRS (PR = 0.28); in these beats, the P wave *is* conducted to and depolarizes the ventricles
Diagnosis:	AV dissociation (sinus bradycardia and junctional rhythm) with frequent capture beats

contrast, left bundle branch block does alter the initial forces; when myocardial infarction occurs in the patient with left bundle branch block, its characteristic ECG signs often are obscured.

Funny looking beats   Often when you examine an ECG strip you will notice "funny looking beats". These usually are *ectopic beats* (an ectopic beat is one which arises outside the sinus node). Because ectopic beats vary in significance, it is important to use a logical method to analyze a "funny looking beat". A good method of analysis is:

1. Determine whether a beat is early or late by comparing the interval between it and the preceding beat to an R–R interval of the dominant rhythm. If it is late, it is an *escape beat.*

   Escape beats occur when the dominant pacemaker fails to fire and depolarize slower sites of impulse formation. They appear "late", that is, after the next-expected dominant beat. If the funny looking beat is an escape beat, you can identify it further as an escape junctional or escape ventricular beat by looking for a P wave and measuring the QRS. If it is early (occurs before the next-expected dominant beat), it is a *premature beat.* Supraventricular premature beats may be blocked, conducted normally, or conducted aberrantly. This last term means the beat is conducted down the bundle branches, although abnormally. *Aberration* is a transient conduction abnormality, which occurs because the premature impulse reaches the bundle branches before they are fully repolarized. Since the bundle branches have unequal refractory periods, a premature impulse may find one branch still refractory (usually the right). The impulse still can travel the conduction pathway, but in a temporarily abnormal manner. A premature supraventricular beat with aberration somewhat resembles a ventricular premature beat at first glance. It is important to differentiate them because their significance and treatment differ. Continue to follow a logical, consistent approach to analyzing the beat.

2. Measure the QRS duration. A normal duration means the beat's origin is supraventricular. A wide QRS (when the dominant QRS is normal) can mean either a supraventricular beat with aberration or a ventricular beat.

3. Look for a P wave related to the premature beat. Its presence strongly suggests the beat is supraventricular.

4. Analyze the pause after the premature beat. To do this, compare the interval consisting of two dominant cycles to the interval between the two dominant beats surrounding the premature beat. (See Figure 3-1). If the interval containing the premature beat is shorter than the interval containing two dominant cycles, the pause is called noncompensatory. It occurs because the premature impulse has depolarized the SA node, causing it, and therefore the ventricles, to pause. If the interval containing the premature beat is equal to or longer than twice the dominant cycle, the pause is called *compensatory.* It occurs because the impulse has not depolarized the SA node but has made the ventricles refractory to the next sinus impulse. That is, the SA node does not pause but the ventricles do—until the second sinus impulse after the premature beat, which arrives at a time when they can respond.

5. Compare the coupling intervals. The *couple* is the premature beat and the dominant beat immediately preceding it. Compare the interval between these R

Table 3-8   Bundle branch blocks

Regularity and rate		P waves	AV Conduction		QRS
Ventricular	Atrial		P:QRS ratio	PR Interval	
Normal conduction					
Regular or irregular, any rate, depending upon basic rhythm		Sinus or atrial	Normal or abnormal, depending on basic rhythm		0.06–0.12 seconds V₁: rS V₆: qR

Normal sequence

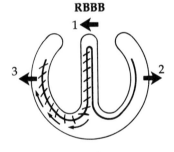
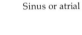
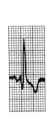
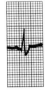

V₁   V₆

Regularity and rate		P waves	AV Conduction		QRS
Right bundle branch block					
Regular or irregular, any rate, depending upon basic rhythm		Sinus or atrial	Normal or abnormal, depending on basic rhythm		Greater than 0.12 seconds V₁: triphasic rSR' V₆: triphasic QSR, with wide S wave

RBBB

Left bundle branch block					
Same as above		Same as above	Same as above		Greater than 0.12 seconds V₁: monophasic QS V₆: monophasic wide R wave

LBBB

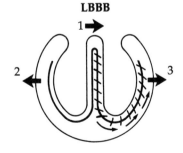
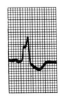
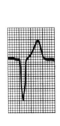

Comments	Causes	Significance	Treatment
Not a bundle branch block; included for comparison	Normal heart	Normal conduction	None necessary
	Normal heart; coronary artery disease	Does not affect cardiac output	None necessary, unless accompanied by block of one division of left bundle branch; in that case, prophylactic artificial pacemaker
	Normal heart; coronary artery disease; valvular heart disease; hypertension	More serious than right bundle branch block because results from more serious disorders and often accompanied by cardiomegaly	None

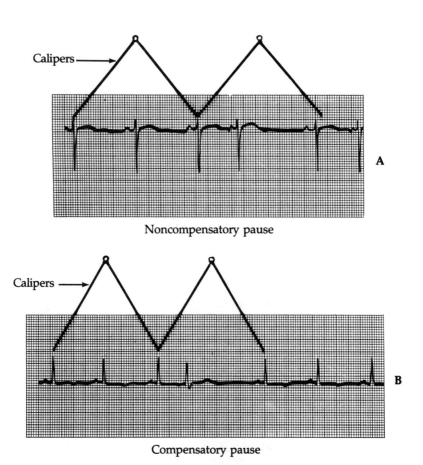

Figure 3-1.   Noncompensatory versus compensatory pauses. To determine whether the pause following a premature beat is noncompensatory or compensatory, use your calipers to measure an interval consisting of two dominant cycles. Then, without changing the relative position of the caliper points, place the left point on the R wave preceding the premature beat. **A,** If another dominant QRS falls *before* the right point, the two cycles surrounding the premature beat are less than two dominant cycles; that is, the pause is *noncompensatory.* **B,** If the dominant QRS falls on or after the right caliper point, the cycles surrounding the premature beat are equal to or longer than the dominant cycles; that is, the pause is *compensatory.*

waves to that of other couples in the strip. Constant (fixed) coupling is a characteristic of ventricular premature beats.

6. Compare the R–R interval immediately preceding the premature beat to others in the dominant rhythm. A sudden lengthening just before the premature beat predisposes to aberration. The reason for this is that the refractory period of

the bundle branches depends on the length of the preceding R–R interval—when the interval is long, the refractory period is long.

7. Examine the pattern of QRS deflections compared to the dominant QRS and to other premature beats:

A. Initial deflections similar to those of dominant beats suggest the impulse is traveling the usual conduction system, that is, it is supraventricular.

B. A pattern of deflections similar to that of other premature beats suggests that you probably are seeing a premature beat from the same source.

C. A bundle branch block (BBB) pattern may indicate supraventricular aberration or ventricular ectopy.

Aberration produces a BBB pattern when the early impulse reaches the ventricles while one bundle branch is still refractory. Since the refractory period of the right bundle branch usually is longer than that of the left bundle branch, aberration usually appears as a right BBB configuration.

Ventricular ectopy also may cause a BBB pattern. You will remember that in BBB, the impulse must spread cell to cell from the normally stimulated ventricle to the blocked one. Since a ventricular premature beat arises outside the conduction system, it also spreads cell to cell to the other ventricle. For this reason, a premature beat from the left ventricle may form the same QRS configuration as a right BBB, while a right ventricular premature beat may simulate a left BBB.

Certain QRS configurations are more likely to represent ectopy than others. Marriott's clues to whether a QRS is ectopic or aberrant (1972) are presented in Figure 3-2.

Premature beats may be classified in many ways in addition to the designations ectopic or aberrant. When classified by site of origin, they are identified as atrial, junctional, or ventricular. Another classification refers to the number of foci (sites) from which they arise, beats from one site being called unifocal and those from more than one site being called multifocal. These and other characteristics of premature beats are summarized and illustrated in Tables 3-9 and 3-10.

Differentiation of general ECG patterns   So far, rhythms have been grouped primarily according to site of origin. As you learned them, you undoubtedly noticed that different specific rhythms may have a similar general effect on the ECG. For instance, tachycardias from several sites have the same effect of a rapid, regular rhythm. When you first scan an ECG strip, it is the overall pattern that catches your eye, so your first impression is that of a tachycardia, bradycardia, and so on. Then, you proceed to differentiate the rhythms that could cause that effect. Marriott has elaborated on this concept by originating an immensely useful list that identifies the specific rhythms which cause a similar general ECG pattern. Those causes that are discussed in this book are given in Table 3-11.

Manifestation		Favors	Odds
RSR' variant in V$_1$ or MCL$_1$		Aberration	10:1
qRs in V$_6$ or MCL$_6$		Aberration	20:1
R or qR in V$_1$ or MCL$_1$ with taller left "rabbit ear"		LV ectopy	10:1
R or qR in V$_1$ or MCL$_1$ with taller right "rabbit ear"		Neither	—
QS in V$_6$ or MCL$_6$		LV ectopy	20:1
rS in V$_6$ or MCL$_6$(NO q)		LV ectopy	7:3
LBBB pattern with wide r in V$_1$ or MCL$_1$		RV ectopy	10:1

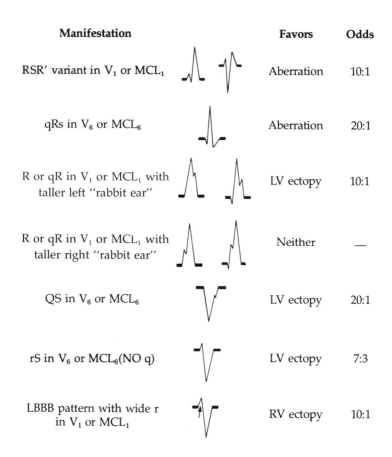

Figure 3-2.   Ventricular aberration versus ectopy: morphologic clues. (From Marriott, H. 1972. *Workshop in Electrocardiography.* Oldsmar, Fla.: Tampa Tracings.)

Significance of the arrhythmia

Effect on cardiac output   Cardiac output equals the heart rate times stroke volume. Normal sinus rhythm is the optimal rhythm because it provides enough time for the atrial and ventricular filling, proper coordination of valve openings and closings, and coronary artery filling during diastole. The coordination of AV valve movements is important because it permits the active phase of ventricular filling. During this phase, atrial contraction contributes about 30% of atrial volume to ventricular filling volume (and therefore to cardiac output). Patients with poor myocardial reserve are particularly dependent upon this mechanism to maintain cardiac output. When it is lost (as in sudden atrial fibrillation), the resulting drop in cardiac output may produce signs of shock.

Bradycardia decreases cardiac output if its onset is sudden. If its onset is gradual, a compensatory increase in stroke volume may occur to maintain a normal cardiac output.

Tachycardia increases cardiac output up to the point at which it infringes seriously on ventricular filling time. At that rate (which varies from patient to patient), cardiac output drops. The patient's ability to tolerate a tachycardia depends not on its source but on its rate, the heart size, and additional insults (such as systemic hypoxia).

Tendency to become more serious   An arrhythmia may progress to more serious arrhythmias. It is good nursing practice to watch for such a tendency, and take appropriate measures when changes occur. Following are examples of some possible progressions to more serious problems.

Tachycardia predisposes to the development of faster rhythms by decreasing coronary artery filling time at the same time it increases myocardial oxygen demand. The resulting myocardial hypoxia alters the resting membrane potential of cardiac cells, enhancing the likelihood of spontaneous depolarization.

Premature beats indicate cellular irritability. They predispose toward rapid, repetitive depolarization, that is, tachycardia, flutter, and fibrillation.

Bradycardia encourages beats to escape from lower sites of impulse formation. It does so by failing to depolarize these sites and by decreasing coronary artery perfusion pressure. These escape beats may accelerate and become the dominant rhythm.

Lower degrees of block may progress to more complete blocks.

Planning and implementation of care

Treat serious arrhythmias promptly. Selection of the treatment modality is the prerogative of the physician. Since some arrhythmias require immediate treatment and consultation with a physician may be delayed, many units have standing medical orders to guide the nurses and protect them legally. Find out the policies for your unit.

General principles governing treatment

The general principles governing treatment instituted by the nurse under standing medical orders are as follows:

1. Do not initiate treatment of an arrhythmia if the patient is stable hemodynamically and if the rhythm is unlikely to worsen.

2. Immediately treat life-threatening arrhythmias causing pulselessness: ventricular asystole, ventricular fibrillation, and sometimes ventricular tachycardia. The techniques will be discussed later in detail.

Text continued on p. 123

Table 3-9   Premature beats

QRS Duration	P wave	PR Interval	Pause	Coupling	QRS Deflections
Atrial premature beat (APB)					
Normal	Atrial	Normal	Usually noncompensatory	Variable	Same as dominant QRS

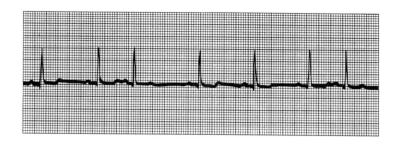

Blocked or nonconducted APB					
Absent	Atrial	Absent	Usually noncompensatory	Variable	Absent

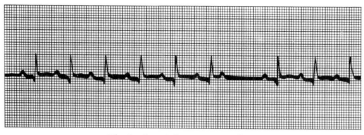

Blocked atrial premature beat

(continued)

Comments	Cause	Significance	Treatment
	Normal heart; coffee, tobacco, alcohol stimulation; stress; myocarditis; myocardial ischemia	Ectopic atrial focus; usually benign but may precede atrial tachycardia, flutter or fibrillation	Usually, none necessary; if very frequent, treatment of cause; sedation; digitalis
Same	Same	Same	Same as APB

(continued)

Table 3-9   Premature beats *(continued)*

QRS Duration	P wave	PR Interval	Pause	Coupling	QRS Deflections
Aberrantly conducted APB					
Wide	Atrial	Normal	Usually noncom-pensatory	Variable	Usually, initial deflection same as dominant QRS; usually, right bundle branch block pattern

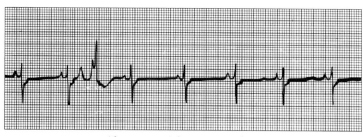

Aberrant atrial premature beat

Junctional premature beat (JPB)					
Normal	Absent; before, during, or after QRS	Absent or less than 0.12 seconds	Usually noncom-pensatory	Variable	Same as dominant QRS

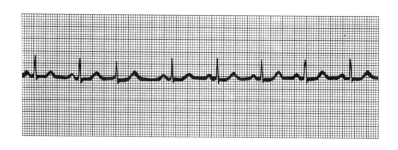

(continued)

Comments	Cause	Significance	Treatment
Prolonged preceding R-R interval may be present	Same	Same	Same as APB
	Same as APB	Ectopic junctional focus; usually insignificant but may precede junctional tachycardia	Same as APB

(continued)

Table 3-9   Premature beats *(continued)*

QRS Duration	P wave	PR Interval	Pause	Coupling	QRS Deflections
Aberrantly conducted JPB					
Wide	Absent; before, during or after QRS	Absent or less than 0.12 seconds	Usually noncompensatory	Variable	Usually, initial deflection same as dominant; usually, right bundle branch block pattern

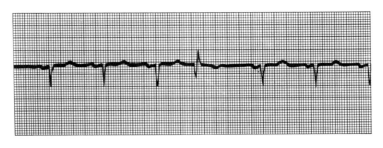

QRS Duration	P wave	PR Interval	Pause	Coupling	QRS Deflections
Ventricular premature beat (VPB)					
Wide	Unrelated	Absent	Usually compensatory	Depends upon type	Bizarre; initial deflection usually opposite to dominant QRS

QRS Duration	P wave	PR Interval	Pause	Coupling	QRS Deflections
Fusion beat					
Intermediate between dominant and ectopic durations	Yes	Normal or no more than 0.06–0.08 seconds less than dominant beat	Variable	Constant	Intermediate between dominant and ectopic contours

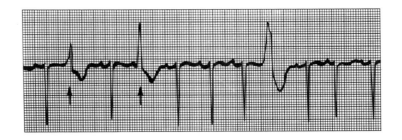

Comments	Cause	Significance	Treatment
Prolonged preceding R–R interval may by present	Same	Same	Same
Followed by large inverted T wave; numerous sub-categories shown in Table 3–10	Normal heart; myocardial ischemia or infarction; electrolyte imbalances; others as in APB	Ectopic ventricular focus; may progress to ventricular tachy-cardia or fibrillation, especially if more than 3 in a row, more than 6 per minute, multi-focal, or falling on or near preceding T wave	None if infrequent; if frequent, lidocaine bolus IV followed by lidocaine infusion; quinidine; procainamide; treatment of cause
	As in other premature beats	Simultaneous de-polarization of atria or ventricles by one normal and one ectopic focus (normal sinus beat and artificial pacemaker; normal sinus beat and APB; or supra-ventricular beat and VPB)	None necessary

Table 3-10 Subcategories of VPBs

Characteristics	*Examples*

Unifocal VPB

Fixed coupling, constant QRS contour

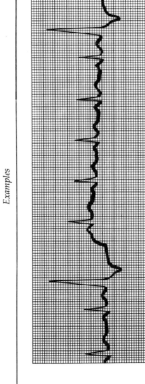

Multifocal VPB

Variable coupling, variable QRS contour

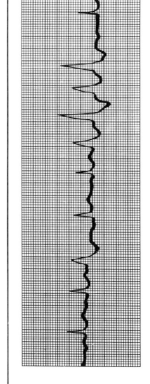

Interpolated VPB

No pause, "sandwiched" between dominant beats

Left ventricular VPB

Right bundle branch block pattern or primarily positive deflection in leads oriented toward right ventricle

Right ventricular VPB

Left bundle branch block pattern or
primarily positive deflection in leads
oriented toward left ventricle

Isolated VPB

Occurring infrequently

Bigeminy (ventricular)

VPB alternating with dominant beat

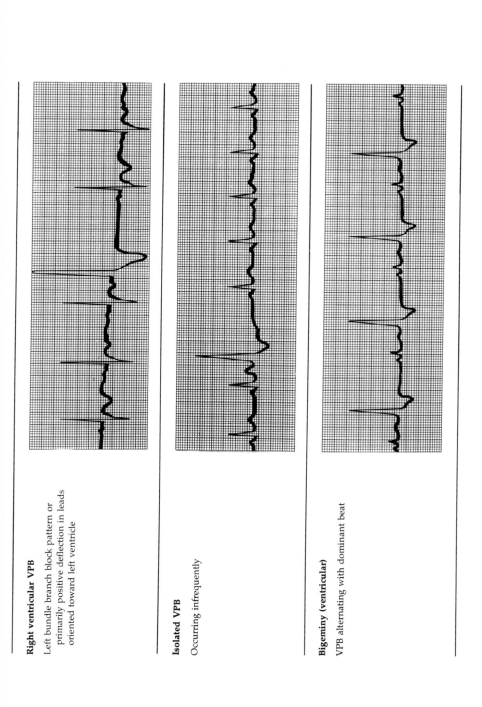

Table 3-11 Specific causes of general ECG patterns*†

General pattern	Possible specific causes
Regular rhythm, normal rate	Normal sinus rhythm Accelerated junctional rhythm Accelerated ventricular rhythm Sinus tachycardia with 2:1 block Atrial flutter with 4:1 block AV dissociation : atrial fibrillation and accelerated escape rhythm
Bradycardia	Sinus bradycardia Junctional rhythm Ventricular rhythm Second degree AV block with high-grade degree of block Third degree AV block with escape rhythm
Tachycardia	Sinus tachycardia Atrial tachycardia Junctional tachycardia Ventricular tachycardia
Pauses	Nonconducted atrial premature beat Second degree AV block (type I or II)
Premature beats	Atrial premature beat Junctional premature beat Ventricular premature beat Capture beat
Bigeminy	Premature beats coupled to a sinus, junctional, or ventricular beat Atrial flutter with alternating 4:1 and 2:1 conduction 3:2 AV block
Groups of beats	Premature beat occurring every third beat Two premature beats coupled to a sinus, atrial, or ventricular beat Premature beat in atrial fibrillation Grouping in atrial fibrillation Grouping in ventricular tachycardia 4:3 AV block
Chaos	Atrial fibrillation Atrial flutter with varying AV block Wandering pacemaker Multifocal atrial tachycardia Multifocal premature beats Mixed arrhythmias Ventricular fibrillation

*Adapted from Marriott, H. 1972. *Workshop in Electrocardiography;* and 1967. *Differential Diagnosis of Heart Disease.* Oldsmar, Fla.: Tampa Tracings.

†Table limited to those patterns and causes presented in this text.

3. Promptly terminate tachyarrhythmias that are causing hemodynamic deterioration or are likely to accelerate.

For atrial tachycardia, flutter, or fibrillation with rapid ventricular response, apply vagal stimulation to increase the degree of block or cardiovert at 10–50 joules. If unrelieved, consult with the physician about the use of digitalis, quinidine, diphenylhydantoin, or atrial pacing.

For ventricular tachycardia causing pulselessness, defibrillate instantly. For ventricular tachycardia not causing pulselessness, give lidocaine 50–100 mg as an IV bolus followed by an infusion of 1–4 mg per minute. If unsuccessful, consult the physician about using diphenylhydantoin or propranalol. Recurrent or persistent ventricular tachycardia may warrant atrial pacing, cardiac catheterization, myocardial revascularization, or cardiac sympathectomy.

4. Immediately suppress premature beats if they are dangerous. Supraventricular beats rarely are; keep the physician informed of their presence and follow his or her therapeutic plan. If premature ventricular beats are more than six per minute, more than three in a row, multifocal, or falling on or near the T wave, administer an IV bolus of 50–100 mg lidocaine and start an infusion.

5. Promptly relieve bradycardia causing hemodynamic deterioration. For sinus bradycardia and AV blocks, give 0.5 mg atropine as an IV bolus. If unsuccessful, contact the physician about the use of isoproterenol or artificial pacing.

Therapeutic procedures

Develop your knowledge and skill with therapeutic procedures. An understanding of the commonly used treatment methods will enhance your ability to implement the therapeutic plan, evaluate its effectiveness, and protect the patient from harmful side effects.

Cardiopulmonary resuscitation (CPR)   When a respiratory and/or cardiac arrest occurs, you must respond quickly and effectively. Standards for resuscitation have been developed by the American Heart Association and National Academy of Sciences-National Research Council (1974).

These standards cover a wide variety of settings. The recommendations fall into several categories: the adult, child, and infant arrest; arrest in a person on a cardiac monitor; unmonitored arrest; and airway obstruction. Although the resuscitation techniques are the same, their sequencing differs with the circumstances in which the arrest occurs. The sequences for all but pediatric arrests and airway obstruction are integrated in Figure 3-3.

The recommendations presented here are only those most likely to be useful to you in your work setting: the ones pertinent to the adult patient in a critical care unit. To develop competence in their application, you must practice them on a manikin under the supervision of a competent instructor. It is recommended strongly that you achieve certification as a Basic CPR Provider by attending a course offered by the American Heart Association or American Red

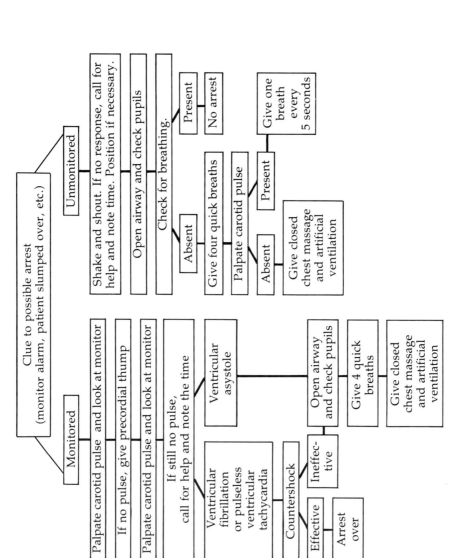

Figure 3-3. Decision tree: adult arrest.

Cross. Because the recommendations are refined frequently, you also must keep yourself informed of revisions.

Monitored cardiopulmonary arrest: one person rescue.

Since almost every patient in a critical care unit is on a cardiac monitor, the initial sign that the patient has had a cardiopulmonary arrest often is the audible monitor alarm. In these circumstances, you are alerted immediately to the possibility of arrest and are able to begin CPR at once. You therefore follow the recommended sequence for a monitored arrest situation.

1. Because a monitor alarm may be set off by a number of arrhythmias as well as faulty machinery, patient movement, and loose leads, first establish that the patient has arrested. Simultaneously palpate the carotid pulse for 5–10 seconds and look at the monitor. There are three rhythms which can cause an absent pulse: ventricular asystole, ventricular fibrillation, and ventricular tachycardia (the latter does not always cause pulselessness).

2. Thump the sternum once with the fleshy part of your fist, from about 8–10 inches above the chest (1–2 seconds). This thump generates a small electrical stimulus, which may be effective in interrupting ventricular tachycardia or fibrillation, or in initiating a heart beat during asystole.

3. Again palpate the carotid pulse and look at the cardiac monitor. If the arrest continues, call for help and note the time.

4. If the rhythm is ventricular tachycardia or fibrillation, countershock immediately. If the countershock is ineffective or if the rhythm is asystole, institute cardiopulmonary resuscitation.

5. Open the airway (1–2 seconds). Remove the pillow if one is present. Put one hand on the forehead, the other under the neck, and tilt the head back so the chin is in a line with the earlobes (Figure 3-4). As you do so, check the pupils. Because dilated pupils may be caused by drugs or by other conditions, they are an unreliable sign of hypoxia unless you know the patient's history and therapy at that time. Reactive pupils are a good baseline against which to evaluate later the efficacy of resuscitation.

6. Start mouth-to-mouth resuscitation. Keep your hand in contact with the forehead and pinch the nose shut. Seal the patient's mouth with your mouth and deliver four quick breaths in 3–5 seconds. In between these breaths, remove your mouth only enough to let the air escape partially; do not let the lungs deflate completely. Deliver about 800 ml per breath. Assess the effectiveness of ventilation by feeling resistance as the lungs inflate, feeling your lungs empty, and watching the chest rise.

7. If you are unable to ventilate the patient, an airway obstruction is present. Recheck the head tilt and try again (4–7 seconds). If you still cannot ventilate the

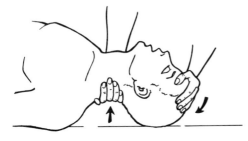

Figure 3-4. Opening the airway: head tilt. Hyperextend the head by lifting up with the hand under the neck and pressing down with the hand on the forehead, until the chin is in line with the earlobes.

patient, attempt to dislodge an airway obstruction through a combination of back blows, manual thrusts, and finger probes. Roll the patient toward you and support him/her against your thighs with one hand. With the heel of the other hand, give four rapid blows between the shoulder blades. Next, roll the person on his/her back and give four rapid manual thrusts, either chest thrusts or abdominal thrusts. To deliver a chest thrust, position your hands as for closed chest cardiac massage (described below) and thrust downward. To deliver an abdominal thrust, place the heel of one hand between the lower sternum and navel; place your other hand on top of the first and thrust upward into the abdomen. In neither case should you put your hands over the xiphoid process, as thrusting over it significantly increases the risk of rupture or laceration of internal organs. Finally, probe the mouth to detect any foreign body dislodged by the back blows and thrusts. Turn the head away from you, unless the patient has a neck injury. In that case, raise the arm opposite you and roll the head and shoulders as a unit so the head ends up supported on the arm. Open the mouth; one way is with the crossed-finger technique. To use it, cross your thumb and index finger. Place them in the upper corner of the mouth and pry open the mouth (Figure 3-5). While holding it open, use the index and third fingers of your other hand to reach back to the pharynx and sweep out the mouth. Roll the head back in position, tilt it, and again try to ventilate. If you still cannot ventilate, continue attempts to open the airway and ventilate the patient until medical

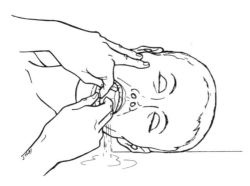

Figure 3-5. Removing obstructions in the mouth. Open the mouth by inserting your crossed thumb and index finger in the upper corner of the mouth and crossing them further. Scoop out the pharynx and mouth with the second and third fingers of your other hand.

help arrives. As the patient becomes unconscious, the muscles will relax and the positive pressure may force some air around the obstruction.

8. Once ventilation has been established, position yourself rapidly but accurately to give closed chest cardiac massage. Climb on the bed and kneel next to the patient's chest. Using whichever hand is closer to the patient's feet, slide your third finger along the costal margin to the costal angle. Place the index finger on the sternum, touching the third finger. Place the heel of the other hand on the sternum next to the index finger (Figure 3-6). Place the heel of the first hand directly over the heel of the other and interlock your fingers to keep them off the chest. Lean forward over the patient so your shoulders are directly over the sternum.

9. Massage the chest 60 times a minute. Keep your elbows straight and press vertically 1½ to 2 inches. Then release the pressure completely while keeping your hands in contact with the sternum.

Count out loud to maintain the correct ratio of 15 compressions to two ventilations. The Heart Association recommends you count: "one and two and three and four and five, one and two and three and four and ten, one and two and three and four and fifteen," compressing on each number. Tilt the head, give two full breaths without letting the lungs deflate completely in between, reposition your hands, and resume compressing. When performing CPR by yourself, deliver 4 cycles per minute (15 seconds per cycle) to give 60 compressions and 8 ventilations per minute. Note that the rate of compression must be 80/min, because you lose time while ventilating the patient. Stop briefly after the first minute and then every 5 minutes to check for the return of spontaneous pulse and respirations.

Unmonitored arrest: one person rescue.

Sometimes, you may encounter an arrest in an unmonitored person, such as a visitor, or coronary care patient just before transfer to a general floor.

1. Shake the patient's shoulder vigorously and loudly call his name. Failure to respond establishes that the patient is unconscious, not just asleep. Call for help and note the time.

2. Position him for possible resuscitation: roll him on his back if necessary and remove any head pillows.

3. Open his airway and check his pupils as described previously. Occasionally, opening the airway will be enough to make him resume breathing if he has stopped.

4. Check for breathing (3–5 seconds). Place your ear within an inch of his mouth and look at his chest. If he is not breathing (respiratory arrest), quick action may prevent the arrest from degenerating into a cardiopulmonary arrest. Give four

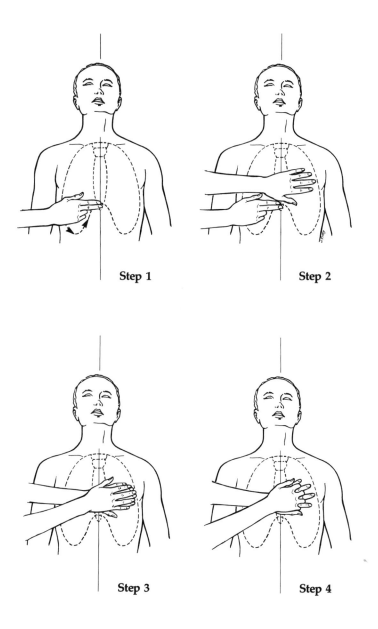

Figure 3-6.   Hand placement for external cardiac compression. **Step 1.**
Place third finger (of hand closest to patient's feet) in costal angle and
second finger directly next to it on sternum. **Step 2.** Place heel of other
hand on sternum so that it touches the tip of the second finger. **Step 3.**
Place heel of first hand over heel of hand on sternum. **Step 4.** Raise
fingers off the chest and interlock them.

quick breaths. Then give one breath every 5 seconds (12 times a minute). An alternative to mouth to mouth resuscitation is ventilation with a self-inflating bag, mask, and 100% oxygen. To hold the mask in place, hook your third, fourth, and fifth fingers under the chin. Press down on the mask with your thumb and second finger to make a tight seal (Figure 3-7). If the airway is obstructed, follow the sequence of back blows, manual thrusts, and finger probes (described earlier) until it is clear or until an emergency endotracheal intubation or tracheotomy is performed.

5. Palpate the carotid pulse for 5–10 seconds. If it is absent (cardiac arrest), give closed chest cardiac massage as described earlier.

Since the differences between the monitored and unmonitored sequences may be confusing, a handy way to remember them is in terms of priorities:

- monitored arrest: circulation, airway, breathing (C, A, B)
- unmonitored arrest: airway, breathing, circulation (A, B, C)

Two person rescue.

So far, we have been discussing what to do if you are alone. More commonly, other health care personnel will be nearby and assist you.

While the first person (to discover the arrest) initiates CPR as described above, the second person should do the following:

1. Page the cardiac arrest team.
2. Bring the defibrillator to the bedside. Countershock the patient, if he needs countershocking and it has not yet been done.
3. Bring the emergency cart to the bedside.
4. Place the cardiac arrest board under the patient's back.
5. Suction the airway if vomit or secretions are present.

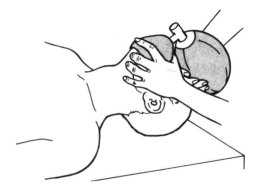

Figure 3-7. Ventilating with a bag and mask. Use your last three fingers to hyperextend the head and lift the mandible. Use your thumb and index finger to press the mask on the patient's face. Squeeze the bag with your other hand.

6. Bag ventilate the patient with 100% oxygen. Begin squeezing the bag on the fifth upstroke, interposing the breaths between compressions so there is no pause in the chest massage. To maintain the correct ratio of five compressions to one ventilation, the compressor should count "one one-thousand, two one-thousand, three one-thousand, four one-thousand, five one-thousand". In two-person CPR, deliver 12 cycles per minute (5 seconds per cycle), for a total of 60 compressions and 12 ventilations per minute. In between breaths, the ventilator should check for a palpable carotid pulse coinciding with compressions, reactive pupils, and the return of spontaneous breathing.

By the time you have established CPR, a physician should be on the scene. Assist him or her to intubate the patient, establish a peripheral venous line if none is available, and administer emergency medications. The most common ones for immediate use are summarized in Table 3-12.

Drugs   Various drugs are used in the treatment of arrythmias and conduction defects. Knowledge of the effects of pharmaceuticals is essential in providing astute nursing care.

Atropine blocks the transmission of parasympathetic impulses from the vagus nerve. It does so by competing with acetylcholine (the usual parasympathetic chemical mediator) for receptor sites. Because the vagus inhibits impulse initiation by the SA or AV node and impulse conduction through the AV junction, blocking the vagus causes improved impulse initiation and conduction. Since the ventricles lack parasympathetic innervation, atropine does not improve ventricular contractility. The usual dose for a sinus bradycardia, junctional rhythm, or AV block is a 0.5–1.0 mg IV bolus. After you give it, observe the patient for the minor side effects of dry mouth, blurred vision, and flushed dry skin. If they occur, reassure the patient they are drug-induced and temporary; ease them by such nursing measures as lemon and glycerin mouth swabs. Also observe for the major side effects of a paradoxical decrease in heart rate, myocardial ischemia resulting from the therapeutic effect of increased heart rate, decreased urinary tone leading to urinary retention, decreased gastrointestinal tone producing constipation, and the precipitation of acute glaucoma. If these occur, consult with the physician about discontinuing the drug.

Isoproterenol (Isuprel) is a sympathomimetic. Because it stimulates only the beta adrenergic receptors in the heart and blood vessels, it increases the heart rate and contractility and causes peripheral vasodilatation, leading to decreased venous return to the heart. For these reasons, it is suitable for the patient with hypotension and an expanded blood volume (as in congestive heart failure). It usually is given as an intravenous infusion titrated to the patient's blood pressure. Prepare the infusion by adding 1 mg (5ml) of the 1:5000 preparation to 250 ml of 5% dextrose in water. This dilution is equivalent to 4 μg per ml. Use a measuring chamber, microdrop administration set, and controlled-volume infusor. The usual dose is 1–4 μg (15–60 microdrops) per minute. Toxic effects are most common in the first 15 minutes; observe closely for tachycardia, ventricular irritability, and hypotension.

Digitalis and its derivatives have two major therapeutic effects: increased myocardial contractility and decreased AV conduction. It is thought that digitalis inhibits the sodium/potassium pump, allowing more sodium inside the cell and more potassium outside it than normal. The sodium then is exchanged for calcium, which increases the binding of actin and myosin (Kones and Benninger 1975), thereby improving contractility.

Digitalis decreases AV conduction by decreasing conduction speed and increasing the refractoriness of the AV junction. These effects are due to both decreased sympathetic stimulation and increased vagal stimulation. Digitalis is used primarily for atrial arrhythmias and for shock caused by decreased myocardial contractility. The therapeutic dose varies considerably with the specific preparation, age, electrolyte status, and renal and hepatic function. When rapid digitalization is desired, the preparations most commonly used are Digoxin (Lanoxin) 0.5–1.0 mg or Lanatoside C (Cedilanid) 1 mg IV bolus.

When a patient is on digitalis, the ECG will show characteristic changes. Therapeutic doses produce a sagging, depressed ST segment, prolonged PR interval, and shortened QT interval. Toxic doses produce a wide variety of atrial and ventricular arrhythmias due to increased automaticity or decreased AV conduction. The tendency toward increased automaticity is increased in the presence of serum hypokalemia, probably because that condition worsens the depletion of intracellular potassium. Frequently seen rhythms include paroxysmal atrial tachycardia (PAT) with block, and ventricular bigeminy. Decreased AV conduction may produce bradycardia, complete heart block, or asystole.

In addition to monitoring the ECG, note such toxic signs as nausea and vomiting, headache, and disturbed color vision. These signs may be minimal or absent with the more purified preparations. Also watch for underdigitalization, which may occur especially in the patient treated for atrial arrhythmias. In this case, only enough digitalis may be present to produce increased vagal stimulation of the AV junction and a normal ventricular rate at rest. Exercise or emotional excitement may produce increased sympathetic and decreased parasympathetic stimulation, resulting in 1:1 conduction of the rapid atrial impulses and a sudden drop in cardiac output. This problem is treated by increasing the dose to achieve both digitalis' vagal and extravagal effects.

Quinidine, procainamide (Pronestyl), and *propranalol (Inderal)* decrease AV conduction, intraventricular conduction, and automaticity. They are suitable for most atrial and ventricular arrhythmias and are often combined to manage complex arrhythmias such as recurrent PAT.

Quinidine rarely is given IV due to the dangers of hypotension and myocardial depression. The usual dose is 200–400 mg 4–6 times daily, orally or intramuscularly.

Therapeutic doses of quinidine produce a widened QRS, a prolonged QT interval, and a wide, notched, low, or inverted T wave. Toxic doses produce a

Table 3-12   Drugs used in cardiac arrest: Adult doses

Drug	Indications	Availability	Mixing directions
Atropine	Bradycardia	1 ml vial = 1 mg	None
Calcium chloride	Asystole ↓ Myocardial contractility	10 ml ampule = 1 gm = 14 mEq	None
Sodium bicarbonate	Acidosis	50 ml preloaded syringe	None
Epinephrine (Adrenalin)	Asystole	10 ml preloaded syringe = 1 mg 1 ml ampule = 1 mg (1 mEq/ml)	As is = 1:10,000 dilution Dilute 1 ampule with 9 ml saline = 10 ml of 1:10,000
Isoproterenol (Isuprel)	↓ Cardiac output	5 ml ampule (1:5000) = 1 mg (0.2 mg/ml)	Dilute 1 ampule in 250 ml D_5W. Use microdrop administration set.
Dopamine (Intropin)	↓ Cardiac output	5 ml ampule = 200 mg (40 mg/ml)	Dilute 1 ampule in 250 ml D_5W. Use microdrop administration set.
Lidocaine (bolus)	Ventricular tachycardia Premature ventricular beats	5 ml preloaded syringe (2%)	None
Lidocaine (infusion)	Ventricular tachycardia Premature ventricular beats	25 ml vial (4%) = 1.0 gm (40 mg/ml)	Dilute 1 vial in 250 ml D_5W. Use microdrop administration set.

Important: Preparations and intravenous administration sets differ among manufacturers. Always check the label of the drug and administration set you use for specific information.

QRS widened more than 25% from its predrug value. The decreased AV conduction may cause heart block, intraventricular conduction defects, or asystole. The decreased automaticity may cause slowing of atrial impulses to the point where they are conducted 1:1 through the AV junction, producing tachycardia. The decreased contractility may provoke a drop in cardiac output or worsen congestive heart failure. Also observe for gastrointestinal distress, visual disturbances, and ringing in the ears—signs of quinidine toxicity.

Final concentration	Usual dose	Administration
1 mg/ml	1.0 mg (0.02 mg/kg)	IV push
100 mg/ml; 1.4 mEq/ml	1.0 gm (20 mg/kg)	IV push
1 mEq/ml	50 mEq (2 mEq/kg)	IV push q 5–10 min Depends on arterial blood gases
0.1 mg/ml 0.1 mEq/ml	1 mg Always use as 1:10,000 solution	Intracardiac or IV push
4 µg/ml	1–4 µg/min (.01 µg/kg/min) initially then titrate to desired response	1 µg/min = 15 gtts/min 2 µg/min = 30 gtts/min 3 µg/min = 45 gtts/min 4 µg/min = 60 gtts/min
800 µg/ml	2–5 µg/kg/min initally then titrate to desired response	200 µg/min = 15 gtts/min 400 µg/min = 30 gtts/min 600 µg/min = 45 gtts/min 800 µg/min = 60 gtts/min
20 mg/ml	100 mg (1–2 mg/kg)	IV push
4 mg/ml	1–4 mg/min (20 µg/kg/min)	1 mg/min = 15 gtts/min 2 mg/min = 30 gtts/min 3 mg/min = 45 gtts/min 4 mg/min = 60 gtts/min

Used with permission of Donald Kishi, Pharm D., Associate Clinical Professor, University of California School of Pharmacy, San Francisco.

Procainamide hydrochloride (Pronestyl hydrochloride) usually is given as a loading dose of 0.5–1 gm followed by 500 mg 4–6 times a day or 50–100 mg IV followed by an intravenous infusion of 1–5 mg/min. Monitor for the same toxic signs as with quinidine and for signs of lupus erythematosis, as a lupuslike syndrome has been reported.

Propranalol hydrochloride (Inderal) is a beta blocker with effects similar to quinidine. The usual dose is 0.5 mg IV over 2–3 minutes, or up to 80 mg four times daily, orally. It is particularly prone to depressing myocardial contractility and thus may precipitate or worsen congestive heart failure. It also can precipitate bronchial asthma and mask the signs of hypoglycemia.

Diphenylhydantoin (Dilantin) is used for both atrial and ventricular arrhythmias. It is valuable especially in the treatment of digitalis-induced arrhythmias. It may be administered as an IV bolus of 100 mg over 3–5 minutes or 100 mg p.o. q.i.d. Observe for nausea and vomiting, hypotension, and cardiac arrest (the latter two if given rapidly IV).

Lidocaine (Xylocaine) is used to decrease ventricular irritability. The preparation used is different from that used for nerve blocks; the antiarrhythmic preparation contains no epinephrine or preservative. Lidocaine may be given 200 mg IM. More commonly, it is administered as an IV bolus of 25–100 mg over 1–2 minutes. This dose may be repeated to a total of 300 mg over 30–60 minutes. Since the effects of the bolus last about 15 minutes, it usually is followed by an infusion of 1–4 mg/min. Prepare it by pouring solution out of a 250 ml bag or bottle of 5% dextrose in water until the 225 ml mark. Add 1 gm of the drug, which is supplied as 1 gm in 25 ml. This dilution will equal 4 mg/ml. Use a measuring chamber, microdrop administration set, and mechanical controlled-volume infusor to maintain the desired rate of 1–4 mg (15–60 microdrops) per minute.

Monitor the patient closely for hypotension, increased ventricular irritability, and central nervous system stimulation or depression seen as twitching, seizures, or drowsiness.

Vagal stimulation   Vagal stimulation is used to terminate PAT and to increase AV block in other rapid atrial rhythms.

There are several ways to produce vagal stimulation. The blood pressure in the carotid sinus can be increased; the carotid baroreceptors then will cause reflex slowing of the heart rate via vagal stimulation. This effect can be provoked by telling the patient to hold his breath and bear down (the Valsalva maneuver), massaging the carotid sinus on one side of the neck, or administering vasopressors to cause transient hypertension. Vagal stimulation also can be achieved by delaying the breakdown of the vagal neurotransmitter, acetylcholine. The neuromuscular blocking agent used most frequently is edrophonium chloride (Tensilon), 10 mg IV bolus.

Defibrillation and cardioversion   A direct current electrial countershock may be successful in terminating both atrial and ventricular tachyarrhythmias. Cardioversion and defibrillation are similar in that each involves a countershock which depolarizes all the cells simultaneously, thereby allowing the sinus node to resume its dominance. They differ in that cardioversion uses a lower wattage and requires synchronization of the shock with the R wave. Synchronization is necessary so that the shock will not fall during the vulnerable period of repolarization and therefore cause repetitive depolarization. Cardioversion usually is not an emergency procedure; defibrillation is. Cardioversion usually is performed by a physician, defibrillation by the nurse if no physician is immediately available.

To defibrillate a patient follow these steps:

1. Plug the defibrillator in to a source of direct electrical current (unless it operates on batteries).

2. Place a thin layer of electrode jelly over the surface of each paddle.

3. Select the highest energy level. The number of joules will vary depending on whether the machine delivers a high peak wave form or trapezoidal wave form. The high peak wave form scale goes up to 400 joules. This wave form causes a tonic muscular response (the patient "jumps") and is thought to cause more myocardial damage than the trapezoidal type. The trapezoidal wave form scale goes up to 250–300 joules. This energy delivery does not cause the familiar "jump" response to defibrillation.

4. Turn the machine on.

5. Place the paddles on the chest—one on the upper right chest and the other at the apex of the heart.

6. Warn others to stand clear of the patient and bed. Make sure you yourself are clear.

7. Depress the paddle buttons simultaneously.

8. Observe the ECG. If it is necessary to repeat defibrillation, repeat steps 4–7.

To cardiovert a patient, follow these guidelines:

1. Collaborate with the physician to explain to the patient and family the value and technique of the procedure.

2. If ordered by the physician, administer prophylactic quinidine and/or atropine, restrict food and fluids for 6 hours, and stop administration of digitalis for up to 24 hours before the procedure. Both cardioversion and defibrillation are contraindicated in the digitalized patient, because they may provoke refractory ventricular tachycardia.

3. Place one electrode under the patient's back and the other over the apex.

4. Assist the physician to anesthetize the person with diazepam or thiopental sodium. These drugs are given as a slow IV bolus until the patient loses consciousness.

5. Charge the machine to the ordered energy level, being sure to turn on the R wave synchronizer. Discharge it when cued by the physician.

Post-cardioversion or post-defibrillation, monitor the ECG, blood pressure, and neuromuscular activity. Transient arrhythmias such as APBs, JPBs, VPBs, and sinus bradycardia are common; so is transient hypotension. The patient may throw thromboemboli during the procedure, especially if it was done for atrial fibrillation.

Pacemakers   To effectively nurse a patient with a pacemaker, you must know the reason for insertion, characteristics of the pacemaker and electrode catheter, method of insertion, and appearance of paced and spontaneous beats.

An artificial pacemaker may be inserted prophylactically or therapeutically. Artificial pacing is used for symptomatic bradycardia unresponsive to drugs, second or third degree AV block, bilateral bundle branch block, and refractory ventricular arrhythmias (to overdrive the ventricles, thereby suppressing ectopic sites).

Pacemakers are classified according to their synchronization with the patient's spontaneous beats, to the chamber sensed, and to the chamber paced. The *asynchronous (fixed-rate)* pacemaker delivers a stimulus regardless of the patient's spontaneous cardiac activity. The *synchronous (demand)* pacemaker senses spontaneous activity and either inhibits the artificial stimulus or triggers its delivery while the ventricles are refractory. The *chamber sensed* may be either the atrium or ventricle. The *chamber paced* may be the atrium, ventricle, or both. Many combinations of these characteristics are available commercially. The most popular external pulse generator is the demand ventricular QRS-inhibited pacemaker.

The pacing catheter itself is either unipolar or bipolar. The unipolar catheter has its solitary pole on the catheter tip; the end of the catheter fits into the generator's negative terminal. To create a ground, a wire suture is placed in the skin and attached to the positive terminal on the generator. The bipolar catheter has both poles at the internal tip of the catheter and two wires at the external end which fit into the matching terminals on the generator.

A pacemaker may be temporary or permanent. Temporary pacemaker electrodes can be inserted through a transvenous, transthoracic, or direct epicardial approach.

In the transthoracic approach, the physician inserts a special needle through the fifth or sixth intercostal space to the left of the sternum, into the right ventricle. The pacing catheter is passed through the needle, which is then removed, and the electrode is connected to the external power source. This method is rapid but not suitable for prophylactic use or long-term pacing. Complications include possible hemopericardium and coronary artery laceration.

During cardiac surgery, temporary electrodes may be sutured directly to the epicardium and be brought out through the chest wall. If pacing becomes necessary, the terminals can be connected quickly to the power source. When pacing is no longer necessary, a pull on the wire will break the epicardial sutures so the electrodes can be pulled out.

A permanent pacemaker usually is inserted under fluoroscopy in the cardiac catheterization laboratory.The catheter is inserted under local anesthesia into the external jugular or subclavian vein and positioned in the right ventricle. The pulse generator is implanted in the anterior chest or abdomen. The generator has a set rate and amperage. If necessary, they can be adjusted after implantation with a special needle.

The most common method of temporary pacing is the transvenous. The system consists of a transvenous catheter electrode and an external pulse generator. The catheter usually is inserted in a cardiac catherization laboratory under fluoroscopy. In an emergency, the catheter may be inserted at the bedside by a physician. To assist with bedside insertion, take the following steps:

1. Prepare the patient. If the patient's condition allows time, help the physician in explaining the procedure. An operative permit should be signed and the patient sedated if necessary. An IV should be started, if the patient is without one.

2. Bring to the bedside a cutdown tray, gloves, skin prep solution, local anesthetic, sterile catheter, pulse generator, sterile alligator clamp and wire, topical antibiotic, dressing supplies, and portable fluoroscopy unit or 12-lead ECG machine. Also have a bolus of lidocaine, a defibrillator, and other emergency equipment readily available.

3. The physician will select the brachial, external jugular, subclavian, or femoral vein and cleanse the skin. The catheter can be introduced percutaneously if the subclavian or femoral vein is used. If the brachial or external jugular vein is used, a cutdown must be performed. If the subclavian site is to be used, position the patient flat or lower the head to minimize the risk of air embolism by creating positive venous pressure so air will not be sucked into the vein.

4. Act as the unsterile person to assist while the skin is cleansed and anesthetized and the catheter is passed.

5. Ideally, the physician will position the catheter under fluoroscopy. If a portable unit is unavailable, he or she will attach a sterile alligator clamp to the catheter and pass you the end of the wire. Attach it to the precordial lead of the ECG machine. While the catheter is advanced, keep the physician informed of changes in the P wave, QRS, and ST segment. When it reaches the right atrium, the P and QRS will be about the same height. As the catheter enters the right ventricle, the QRS amplitude will increase significantly. When the tip touches the endocardium, the ST segment will elevate. The physician will try to wedge the tip in the trabeculae of the right ventricle. He or she will then suture the catheter to the skin and dress the site.

6. If a bipolar catheter is used, connect one of its wires to the positive terminal of the pulse generator and the opposite wire to the negative terminal. If a unipolar catheter is used, connect its wire to the negative terminal and the skin suture to the positive terminal.

7. The external pulse generator (see Figure 3-8) contains an on/off switch, a sensitivity setting to indicate what voltage the generator should interpret as a spontaneous QRS, a milliamperage (MA) dial to determine how much voltage the pacemaker discharges, a rate setting, a pacing indicator such as a light or moving line, and, in some cases, a test indicator for battery function. Turn the

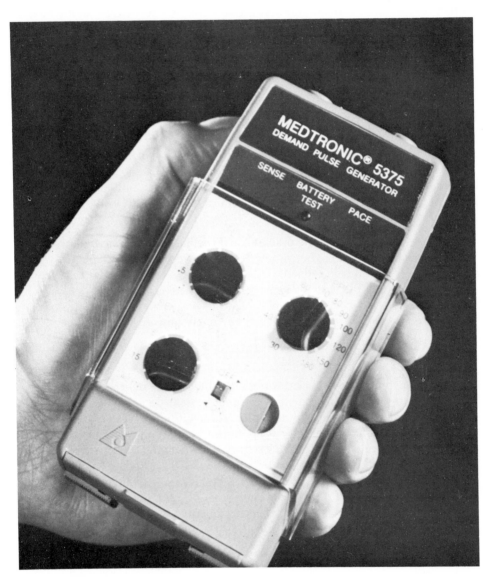

Figure 3-8. External pacemaker. (Courtesy Medtronic, Inc., Minneapolis, Minnesota.)

pacemaker on and set the dials as ordered by the physician. Start with the MA dial at its lowest setting. Increase it until the ECG shows that each pacing spike is capturing (being followed by a QRS). The level at which this occurs is the threshold. Increase the MA setting to twice threshold to allow for variations in discharge voltage and for fibrosis around the catheter tip.

The sensitivity dial determines the pacemaker's response to spontaneous cardiac activity. At greatest sensitivity, it will interpret any amount of voltage as a ventricular depolarization. At least sensitivity, it will ignore all cardiac voltage and will pace at a fixed rate. The usual setting is at a 12 o'clock position, where only a fairly large voltage will be read as a ventricular depolarization.

Set the rate at the number ordered by the physician. It should be at least ± 5 to 10 beats from the patient's spontaneous rate.

After pacemaker insertion, the nursing goals are maintenance of electrical safety, prevention of complications, maintenance of pacemaker effectiveness, and education of the patient:

1. Provide electrical safety. Elimination of electrical hazards is essential because the pacing catheter provides a direct pathway for electricity to reach the heart and induce ventricular fibrillation. All electrical equipment should have three-prong plugs; the third prong connects the instrument to the hospital ground. Never use "cheater" adaptors to connect a three-prong plug and a two-hole electrical outlet. Disconnect from the patient any electrical equipment not currently in use. Connect all other electrical equipment in contact with the patient to a common receptacle. Insulate the pacemaker terminals and exposed electrodes with a rubber glove. Also wear rubber gloves whenever you work with the terminals.

2. Detect potential complications related to insertion. These are most significant with the subclavian site; pneumothorax, hemothorax, air embolism, and injury to the brachial plexus may occur. Local hematoma and infection are possible with all methods. Check the insertion site for inflammation and the patient's temperature for elevation at least once every eight hours. Clean the skin and apply a dry sterile dressing daily.

3. Maintain pacemaker effectiveness. The patient with a temporary or new permanent pacemaker should receive continuous ECG monitoring. Periodically, analyze a rhythm strip, noting in particular these characteristics:

- The appearance of the spike in relation to the P wave and QRS. In atrial pacing, it should be before the P wave; in ventricular, before the QRS, that is, after the P wave (if one is present). In a QRS inhibited pacemaker, no spike should be visible during a spontaneous beat. In a QRS triggered model, a spike should be visible during a spontaneous beat.
- The polarity and amplitude of the spike.

- The appearance of the paced QRS. The appearance will vary depending upon the type of pacemaker. With a right ventricular pacemaker, the paced QRS should be wide, have a left BBB appearance in V_1 and V_6, and a deep S wave in II, III, and AVF.
- Whether the pacemaker rate calculated from the ECG matches the set rate. If the patient has spontaneous beats and a demand temporary pacemaker, simply increase the MA until capture occurs; run a rhythm strip and return the MA to its original setting. If the pacemaker is permanent, hold a magnet over the generator to inactivate the sensing mechanism while you run a strip.
- Whether the paced beats are synchronized with spontaneous beats. If a demand pacemaker is used, a paced beat should occur only when a spontaneous beat fails to appear on time. Fusion beats are common (Figure 3-9).

Also check the pacemaker threshold at least once every 8 hours. To do this, turn the MA dial down to the point at which each spike is capturing. Note the reading and reset the dial at two to three times threshold.

Use the aforementioned observations to detect problems promptly and take appropriate action. Some possible problems are described in the following paragraphs and shown in Figure 3-9.

Failure to pace is indicated by absent pacemaker spikes, bradycardia, and signs of decreased cardiac output. There are numerous possible causes. Check the generator to make sure it is on and the dials are on the correct settings. Make sure the sensitivity dial is on the correct setting; it may have been dislodged to the position where it reads even P waves as QRSs. Also check the rate setting. Check the connections to make certain they are secure. The pacemaker components may have failed. To prevent this, each day use a voltmeter to check the battery voltage of any pacemaker in use. (Once a week, also check the voltage of stored batteries.) If the patient's pacemaker is not pacing, change the battery or whole generator. If none of these interventions works, the cause may be a fractured electrode. You can prevent this by limiting tension on the cable. If you suspect a fractured electrode, notify the physician because it will need replacement.

Failure of the pacing impulse to capture the ventricles is shown by spikes not followed closely by paced ventricular complexes; bradycardia; and decreased cardiac output. This problem usually is caused by catheter displacement. To ensure correct placement, obtain a chest x-ray and 12-lead ECG after bedside insertion. To prevent displacement, minimize movement at the insertion site. Should the pacemaker fail to capture, the catheter may be floating free in the right ventricle; if so, you may see ECG signs of ventricular irritability. Attempt to reposition it by moving the patient's arm or turning him on his side. The catheter may have moved into the right atrium; in this case, the spike will be followed by a P wave instead of a QRS. The catheter may have perforated the septum; the QRS then will manifest a RBBB pattern, being primarily positive in the right chest leads and negative in the left, and ventricular irritability may occur. If you

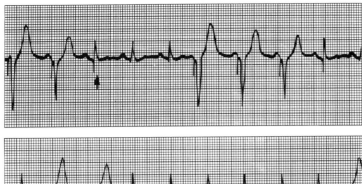

Demand ventricular pacemaker
(Continuous strip; arrows point to fusion beats)

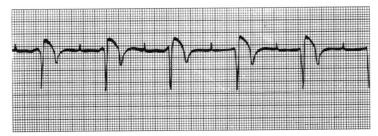

Failure to sense

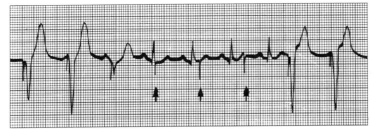

Failure to capture

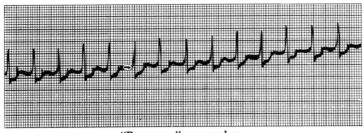

"Runaway" pacemaker
(rate is 150)

Figure 3-9. Pacemaker rhythms.

are unable to reposition a floating catheter or if you suspect migration to the atrium or left ventricle, notify the physician to reposition the catheter.

Another possibility is that the MA setting may be inadequate due to fibrosis at the tip, infection, or potassium imbalance. Increase the MA until a new threshold is reached; then again set the MA dial two to three times threshold. Notify the physician of the increase in threshold.

Failure to sense (competition) is indicated by pacemaker spikes occurring when they should not. This problem may occur due to catheter malposition; try the measures suggested above. It also may result from too low a sensitivity setting; try adjusting the setting. If failure to sense continues and if the spontaneous rhythm is adequate, turn the pacemaker off. If not, leave it on and notify the physician. Competition rarely causes ventricular fibrillation, but be prepared in case it does occur.

A pacing rate change of more than 10 beats from the set rate indicates failure of the pacemaker components. Change the battery or the whole pulse generator.

Other rarer problems include hiccoughs due to phrenic stimulation by the pacing stimulus, pericardial tamponade due to myocardial perforation, and thromboemboli at the catheter tip.

4. Teach the patient and family about the pacemaker. If the patient has a temporary pacemaker, briefly explain to him and his family how it works to aid his heart. Assess their current knowledge and clarify misconceptions. Review cardiac anatomy and emphasize how the pacemaker will relieve the symptoms which hospitalized him. If the patient has a permanent pacemaker, teach him and his family more extensively about it. Teach him and a family member how to check his pulse daily. Stress the need for medical follow-up and the signs of pacemaker failure (rate change greater than ± 10 beats, dyspnea, persistent dizziness, and fluid retention). Explain the need for a battery change every 18–24 months; the change will necessitate aoout three days' hospitalization and local anesthesia. Warn him about the electrical hazards of high voltage areas, microwave ovens, and car ignition systems. He may use other electrical devices providing he does not become dizzy. Encourage specific physical activities, but not to the point of fatigue. Make sure he has a pacemaker warranty card and knows to carry it at all times. For additional insight into the lives of patients with pacemakers, see the supplemental reading list.

Outcome evaluation

Evaluate the patient's progress according to the following outcome criteria. Ideally, the arrhythmic episode will be terminated owing to suitable medical procedure and the patient will develop a normal sinus rhythm. The ideal may not occur, however, particularly in the critically ill patient with pre-existing heart disease. Realistic outcome criteria in the absence of normal sinus rhythm are spontaneous, drug-controlled, or artifically paced rhythms with the following characteristics:

- Ventricular rate 60–100 beats per minute
- Ventricular rate adequate to perfuse core organs and periphery, as manifested by alert mental state; absence of angina; urinary output WNL for patient; warm, pink, dry skin; peripheral pulses bilaterally equal and of normal volume for patient
- Infrequent atrial or junctional premature beats, if any
- Six or fewer ventricular premature beats per minute
- No more than three VPBs in a row
- No multifocal VPBs
- No VPBs falling on or near T waves
- If on maintenance antiarrhythmic medication or permanent pacing, the patient should show no major toxic effects or complications from the therapy. The patient and one family member should be able to state accurately: (a) the reason for and importance of the therapy; (b) necessary administration details such as dosage; (c) precautions to take; (d) complications to watch for; (e) what to do if complications occur; (f) time and locations of follow-up appointments. If unable to meet the preceding criteria, the patient should be referred to a public health nurse for continued supervision. The patient either should verbalize an ability to afford continued care or should be referred to Social Service for financial assistance.

References

American Heart Association and National Academy of Sciences-National Research Council. 1974. Standards for cardiopulmonary resuscitation and emergency cardiac care. *JAMA* 227:833–868.
Essential reading. Specific standards for basic and advanced life support.

Kones, R., and Benninger, G. 1975. Digitalis therapy after acute myocardial infarction. *Heart Lung* 4:99–103.
Mechanism of action and effect on oxygen consumption.

Marriott, H. 1967. *Differential diagnosis of heart disease.* Oldsmar, Florida: Tampa Tracings.
Tables and diagrams on physical signs of heart disease, differential characteristics of types of heart diseases, arrhythmias, and miscellaneous information related to cardiac disorders.

Marriott, H. 1972. *Workshop in electrocardiography.* Oldsmar, Florida: Tampa Tracings.
Conversational text based on author's ECG workshops; topics include arrhythmia analysis, blocks, AV dissociation, and causes of various rhythms.

Supplemental reading

Arrhythmias

Andreoli, K., Hunn, V., Zipes, P., and Wallace, A. 1975. *Comprehensive cardiac care.* 3rd ed. St. Louis: C. V. Mosby Company.
Popular nursing text which includes patient assessment, arrhythmias, and treatment modalities.

Dubin, D. 1974. *Rapid interpretations of EKGs.* 3rd ed. Tampa, Florida: COVER Publishing Company.
Programmed text on interpretation which enhances comprehension of basic concepts through its logical approach.

Fisch, C. 1974. Electrophysiologic basis of clinical arrhythmias. *Heart Lung* 3:51–56.
Transmembrane action potential, automaticity, refractoriness, and re-entry explained and diagrammed.

Marriott, H. 1977. *Practical electrocardiography.* 6th ed. Baltimore: Williams & Wilkins.
One of the classics, progressing from basic concepts to complex arrhythmias.

Ritota, M. 1975. *A basic approach to the electrocardiogram.* Newark: MEDS Corp.
Interesting approach which focuses on P wave, QRS complex, and other components of the ECG, defining limits of normality and abnormalities of each.

Schamroth, L. 1971. *An introduction to electrocardiography.* 4th ed. Oxford: Blackwell Scientific.
Another classic text covering the basic principles and arrhythmias.

Segal, I. and Schamroth, L. 1973. The basic forms of reciprocal rhythms. *Heart Lung* 2:732–735.
Explanations, diagrams, and ECGs illustrating reciprocal rhythms.

Zipes, D. 1974. Modern nomenclature of a.v. dissociation. *Heart Lung* 3:284–287.
Review of mechanisms which produce dissociation.

Pacemakers

Barold, S. 1973. Modern concepts of cardiac pacing. *Heart Lung* 2:238–252.
Comprehensive presentation, including hysteresis, unipolar and bipolar electrograms, and ECG patterns with different types of pacemakers.

Cortes, T. 1974. Pacemakers today. *Nursing* 4(2):22–29.
Review of principles, types, and nursing care.

Preston, T., and Yates, J. 1973. Management of stimulation and sensing problems in temporary cardiac pacing. *Heart Lung* 2:533–538.
Advice on coping with stimulation and sensing difficulties.

Rios, J., and Hurwitz, L. 1974. A simplified logical approach to the evaluation of temporary pacemaker malfunction. *Heart Lung* 3:624–625.
Decision trees to guide problem-solving.

Other therapeutic measures

Kleiger, R., and Wolff, G. 1973. Indications and contraindications for cardioversion for arrhythmias. *Heart Lung* 2:552–560.
History, technique, and results of cardioversion.

Noble, R. 1974. An approach to supraventricular tachycardias. *Heart Lung* 3:64–77.
Significance of these arrhythmias, clinical approach, and specific therapies for each.

Zipes, D., and Nicoll, A. 1974. Therapeutic approach to the patient with a hard-to-control ventricular arrhythmia. *Heart Lung* 3:57–63.
Therapeutic maneuvers for refractory ventricular arrhythmias.

Chapter 4

Cardiac Failure, Infarction, and Tamponade

In addition to arrhythmias, the critically ill patient is at high risk of developing cardiac failure, acute myocardial infarction, or cardiac tamponade. This chapter will help you recognize these disorders and understand the nursing and medical measures used to treat such problems.

Outline

CARDIAC FAILURE

Assessment   Risk conditions/Signs and symptoms

Planning and implementation of care   Nursing measures/Outcome evaluation

ACUTE MYOCARDIAL INFARCTION

Assessment   Risk conditions/Signs and symptoms

Planning and implementation of care   Pain alleviation/Complications/ Outcome evaluation

ACUTE CARDIAC TAMPONADE

Assessment   Risk conditions/Signs and symptoms

Planning and implementation of care   Nursing measures/Outcome evaluation

Objectives

- Define ventricular failure
- Define preload, contractility, and afterload

- State at least two conditions which can alter each factor and produce ventricular failure
- Identify actions you can take to reduce the likelihood of failure
- Recognize the signs and symptoms of right and left ventricular failure
- Identify at least eight nursing or medical measures to treat failure
- Recognize potential complications and initiate the nursing measures to prevent such problems
- Evaluate the patient's progress according to outcome criteria
- List the risk factors for acute myocardial infarction
- Reduce the risk of infarction when caring for patients
- Recognize the common signs and symptoms of infarction
- Define transmural and subendocardial infarction
- Name the three coronary arteries and the structures each supplies
- Analyze the ECG for indicators of ischemia, injury, and infarction
- Identify the leads which will show the clearest indication of anterior infarct, lateral infarct, inferior infarct, and posterior infarct
- List some causes of ST–T changes and QRS changes other than infarction
- Evaluate serum enzymes for characteristic changes in acute MI
- Take measures to relieve the effects of the infarct
- Take steps to alleviate or prevent complications of infarction
- Evaluate the acute myocardial infarction patient's recovery according to outcome criteria
- Define cardiac tamponade
- Recognize factors which increase risk of tamponade
- Identify signs and symptoms of tamponade
- Assist with pericardiocentesis
- Evaluate the tamponade patient's progress according to outcome criteria

CARDIAC FAILURE

Cardiac failure may be defined as an inability of the heart to meet the body's metabolic demands. In cardiac failure, cardiac output *per se* may be low, normal, or high.

Cardiac output is equal to the product of heart rate and stroke volume. *Stroke volume* in turn depends upon myocardial preload, afterload, and contractility. *Preload* refers to the length of ventricular fibers at the end of diastole. It is directly dependent upon the volume of blood in the ventricle; as the volume increases, preload—and therefore stroke volume—increases (Frank-Starling mechanism). This compensatory mechanism for regulating stroke volume will fail if the ventricular volume load becomes excessive. *Afterload* is the resistance against which the ventricle ejects its volume.

Contractility is a complex process initiated by cellular depolarization. Although the exact mechanism by which electrical energy converts to mechanical energy awaits further study, one widely held theory follows in simplified form (James and Sherf 1974, Anthony and Kolthoff 1975).

The myocardial cell (myocardial fiber) is composed of bundles of very fine fibers called myofibrils. Each myofibril consists of small contractile units called sarcomeres. Each sarcomere in turn consists of two kinds of contractile proteins, actin and myosin. The thick myosin filaments partially overlap the thin actin filaments, causing an electron micrograph to record lines of varying density. A diagrammatic representation of a myocardial fiber is shown in Figure 4-1. The sarcomere is bounded at each end by a Z band, to which the actin filaments are attached. The actin filaments extend part way in toward the center of the sarcomere. The myosin filaments alternate with the actin filaments but are not attached to the Z band. The overlapping of thick filaments and thin filaments is seen as the A band. In its center, the absence of the thin filaments is seen as the H band. The area where only actin filaments are seen is the I band.

Myosin filaments contain projections called cross-bridges, which jut out toward the actin filaments. When the fibers are at rest, myosin and actin filaments do not touch each other because another protein (troponin) blocks the attachment of cross-bridges to the actin. The myocardial fiber also contains many mitochondria, which serve as the cell's primary energy source.

The last important component of the myocardial fiber is a complex network of tubules and sacs which surround the myofibrils. This system plays an important role in electrical impulse conduction and excitation-contraction coupling. In

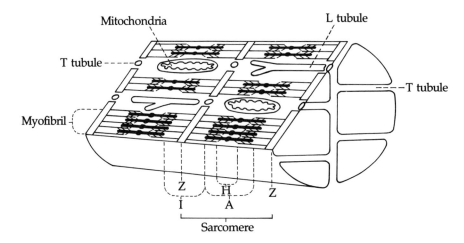

Figure 4-1. Diagrammatic representation of myocardial fiber.

between sarcomeres in the transverse direction is a system of tubules called T tubules. A T tubule is an invagination of the cell membrane; therefore, it communicates with the extracellular fluid.

In between myofibrils in the longitudinal direction is another system of tubules called L tubules. The end of the L tubule is dilated, forming a sac where calcium is stored. The T and L tubules are not in direct contact with each other. When an electrical impulse occurs, it is spread from the outer membrane of the fiber into the fibril along the T tubules. The spread of the impulse into the L tubules causes the release of calcium ions from the sac, and they spread along the L tubules. The calcium ions bind with the troponin, inactivating it. Myosin's cross-bridges then can link up with the actin. This interaction pulls the actin in toward the center, so the filaments slide along each other (Figure 4-2). Using the energy source adenosine triphosphate (ATP), the bridges break and reform several times, each time pulling the actin in closer. When this process occurs in many fibers, it causes the muscle to contract. The efficiency of this mechanism is optimal within only a narrow range of myofibril stretch. When the ventricles are distended excessively, the fibers are pulled too far apart to permit effective coupling of the cross-bridges, and failure ensues.

The right or left ventricle may fail independently, or left ventricular failure may lead to right ventricular failure. At times, the left ventricle may fail so severely that the patient goes into shock. Shock is such an important consideration in the critically ill that it is discussed separately in Chapter 5.

Assessment

Risk conditions

Risk conditions for cardiac failure can be grouped conveniently into five categories: increased metabolic demands, impediments to filling, increased preload, decreased contractility, and increased afterload.

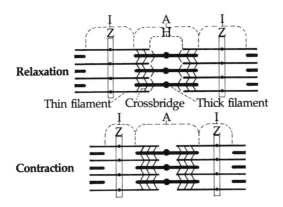

Figure 4-2.   Sarcomere in relaxation and contraction.

With increased metabolic demand, cardiac output is high but still insufficient for the body's needs. This high-output failure may be seen in fever, anemia, hyperthyroidism, or severe physical or emotional stress.

Filling impediments limit the amount of blood that can enter the ventricles. Examples are cardiac tamponade, tricuspid or mitral stenosis, and restrictive cardiac diseases. Severe tachycardia, while not an actual physical impediment, also limits cardiac output by sharply decreasing ventricular diastolic filling time.

With increased preload, the ventricles are unable to contract with maximum efficiency because the excessive end-diastolic volume disrupts the optimal relationship between cardiac fiber length and force of contraction. Valvular regurgitation, intracardiac shunts, severe bradycardia, fluid overload, and dysfunction or rupture of chordae tendinae are examples of conditions which cause increased preload.

Decreased contractility directly decreases cardiac output. Contractility may be impaired by depressant drugs such as propranolol, myocardial ischemia, myocarditis, cardiomyopathy, a decrease in the area of functional myocardium (such as in myocardial infarction, ventricular aneurysm, or ventricular dyskinesis), or ventricular fibrillation or asystole.

Increased afterload can precipitate failure when the heart becomes unable to expel blood efficiently against the increased resistance. Increased right ventricular afterload occurs with pulmonary hypertension and massive pulmonary embolism; increased left ventricular afterload occurs with systemic hypertension.

When you can identify risk factors, you can take steps to reduce them. For example, follow the measures to prevent and/or relieve pulmonary embolism (Chapter 10), arrhythmias (Chapter 3), myocardial infarction, and cardiac tamponade. Also observe the patient for other risk states and call them to the physician's attention.

Signs and symptoms

Signs and symptoms of cardiac failure vary depending upon the ventricle involved and the acuteness of the process. Slow onset allows time for the ventricle to hypertrophy, thus compensating somewhat for the increased volume load.

Right ventricular failure   When the right ventricle is unable to pump out blood adequately, blood inexorably backs up into the right atrium and then into the systemic veins. Right ventricular failure thus produces increases in right ventricular pressure, right atrial pressure, and systemic venous pressure. The elevated right ventricular pressure causes the following manifestations:

- S_3 and sometimes S_4 due to filling against an already distended ventricle
- Pansystolic murmur at the lower left sternal border owing to stretching of the tricuspid ring (relative tricuspid insufficiency)
- Increased myocardial oxygen consumption

The increased right atrial pressure may produce atrial fibrillation or other atrial arrhythmias. Elevated venous pressure causes the following signs and symptoms:

- Increased CVP reading
- Distended jugular veins
- Prominent jugular venous pulsations
- Liver engorgement and tenderness
- Positive hepatojugular reflux (momentary pressure over the liver produces increased jugular venous distention)
- Dependent edema
- Ascites due to fluid accumulation in the peritoneal space
- Decreased appetite, nausea, or vomiting due to pressure on the stomach and bowel from venous engorgement of abdominal vessels
- Increased arterial-venous O_2 difference

Because right ventricular output is decreased, the patient also may show signs of hypoxia, such as cyanosis or dyspnea.

Left ventricular failure   In left ventricular failure, the left ventricle is unable to pump out blood into the systemic circulation efficiently. Initially, the right ventricle is unaffected and continues to pump blood into the pulmonary circuit. Left ventricular failure thus causes increases in left ventricular pressure, left atrial pressure, and pulmonary pressures. The left ventricular pressure elevation produces the following manifestations:

- S_3 and sometimes S_4
- Increased myocardial oxygen consumption
- Pansystolic murmur at the apex caused by relative mitral insufficiency

Atrial fibrillation or other atrial arrhythmias may result from left atrial distention.

Elevated pulmonary pressures cause transudation of fluid into the pulmonary interstitium and alveoli, reflected by the following signs and symptoms:

- Rales or wheezing
- Dyspnea (This may appear as dyspnea on exertion, dyspnea at rest, orthopnea, or paroxysmal nocturnal dyspnea.)
- Pulmonary edema
- Cyanosis
- Hyperventilation and respiratory alkalosis

Because left ventricular output is decreased, the patient also may manifest:

- Dizziness or syncope, because of decreased cardiac output to the brain
- Fatigue, because of diminished oxygenation of skeletal muscles and loss of cardiac reserve
- Metabolic (lactic) acidosis, because of insufficient oxygen for normal cellular aerobic metabolism
- Generalized edema
- Pulsus alternans (alternating volume of arterial pulse), for which the exact cause is unknown. One explanation is that the ventricle does not empty fully with the first contraction. The resulting increase in volume provokes a stronger contraction for the next beat (according to the Frank-Starling mechanism) emptying the ventricle more completely. As a result, the end-diastolic volume for the third beat resembles the first, and the cycle repeats itself.

If left ventricular failure is severe enough, blood will back up from the pulmonary vessels into the right side of the heart. In that case, signs and symptoms of right heart failure also will be present.

Planning and implementation of care

Nursing measures

Various nursing measures can be taken to relieve the increased myocardial workload, hypoxia, and other effects of failure.

Decreasing the preload   The preload can be decreased by taking the following actions. Position the patient with the trunk elevated and the extremities dependent. Place the patient on intake and output recording. Weigh him or her daily. Minimize the volume of intravenous infusions and give them slowly. Use a volume measuring chamber to measure accurately and protect against accidental wide-open infusion due to changes in the position of the needle or arm. Administer diuretics as the physician orders. Utilize rotating tourniquets if deemed necessary by the doctor. If the patient is in pulmonary edema, follow the measures outlined in Chapter 10. Relieve bradycardia if present. Place the patient on a low sodium diet.

Improving myocardial contractility   Medicate the patient with digitalis preparations, if ordered by the physician. Digitalis is useful only if diminished contractility is the cause of failure. It therefore would not be prescribed if the cause were aortic stenosis or restrictive pericarditis, for example. See Chapter 3 for related nursing care. Correct any electrolyte imbalances, especially hypokalemia or hypocalcemia (see Chapter 6), and any acid-base imbalances (see Chapter 11). Consult the physician about discontinuing propranolol if the patient is on it. In certain cases, the patient may benefit from surgical procedures such as myocardial revascularization or aneurysmectomy.

Minimizing myocardial workload   Place the patient on bedrest or cardiac chair rest. Reduce emotional stress by maintaining a calm, optimistic atmosphere and relieving anxiety (see Chapter 13). When the acute episode is past, assist the patient in examining ways to modify his or her lifestyle to minimize cardiac workload.

Relieving hypoxia   Minimize the work of breathing by restricting physical activity and maintaining pulmonary hygiene. Administer supplemental oxygen as ordered by the physician.

Additional nursing measures   Improve cardiac filling, for example by treating tachycardia or cardiac tamponade. Reduce afterload: assist the physician in treating systemic or pulmonary hypertension, aortic or pulmonic stenosis, or pulmonary embolism.

Prevention of complications   Ventricular failure carries with it the possible complications of excessive diuresis, arrhythmias, and pulmonary embolism. Preventive nursing measures will help to avoid these complications.

Avoid the hazards of excessive diuresis. During diuresis, monitor blood pressure, pulse rate and volume, cerebral status, muscular strength, weight, and intake and output. Alert the physician to the development of hypotension, tachycardia, thready pulse, confusion, weakness, precipitous weight loss, and net fluid loss in excess of the amount expected.

Monitor serum potassium levels. Most diuretics cause potassium wasting, which is especially dangerous in the digitalized patient.

Refer back to Chapter 3 for ways to prevent, recognize, and relieve arrhythmias.

Methods of minimizing the risk of pulmonary embolism are presented in Chapter 10.

Outcome evaluation

Evaluate the patient's progress and the effect of therapeutic measures according to these outcome criteria:

- Arterial blood pressure within normal limits for the patient
- When thorax elevated 45°, jugular venous distention and hepatojugular reflux absent; normal jugular venous pulsations

- Heart rate and rhythm normal for the patient; preferably normal sinus rhythm
- No edema, ascites, or liver enlargement or tenderness
- Lungs clear to auscultation
- Blood gases within normal limits for patient
- No dyspnea, orthopnea, or cyanosis

ACUTE MYOCARDIAL INFARCTION

Because of the prevalence of coronary atherosclerosis in the general population and because of the stresses imposed by being critically ill, your patients have a significant risk of developing an acute myocardial infarction (MI).

Assessment

Risk conditions

Be alert for factors associated with an increased risk of MI. Among those implicated by epidemiologic studies are these:

- middle or old age
- male sex
- female sex after menopause
- elevated serum cholesterol or triglycerides
- hypertension
- manifestations of coronary atherosclerotic heart disease before the age of 50 in patient's parents or siblings
- cigarette smoking
- diet high in calories, sugar, salt, cholesterol, total fat, and/or saturated fat
- diabetes, fasting blood sugar over 120 mg/100 ml, abnormal glucose tolerance test
- sedentary lifestyle
- constant emotional tension

In the patient with suspected or confirmed coronary artery disease, the additional following factors are associated with an increased risk of infarction:

- previous infarction
- any factor reducing coronary arterial perfusion or oxygenation (for example, systemic hypoxia, hypotension)

- any factor increasing ventricular workload (for example, physical stress, emotional stress, hypertension, aortic stenosis)

Decrease the risk factors whenever possible. Following are some examples of ways to decrease coronary risk factors.

Educate patients, their families, and the general public about the risk factors and ways to reduce them. (For specific recommendations, consult the most recent literature from the American Heart Association.)

Administer antihypertensive or antilipidemic drugs if prescribed by the physician. Maintain adequate systemic oxygenation and coronary arterial perfusion. Reduce physical stress by limiting ambulation and self-care during acute ischemic attacks. Reduce emotional stress (see Chapter 13).

Signs and symptoms

Be alert to the various signs and symptoms of acute myocardial infarction.

Note the characteristics of pain. Acute infarction pain is usually substernal. The patient may describe it as crushing, "like a weight on my chest," and when asked to localize it will place a clenched fist on his sternum. Frequently, the pain will radiate down the left arm, down both arms, or up into the neck. Less common sites of pain for which you should be alert are the jaw, back, and abdomen. Typically, the pain is constant and unrelieved by rest or by sublingual nitroglycerin (1 tablet q 5 min x 3).

Observe for increased sympathetic stimulation. Most patients develop increased sympathetic stimulation during an infarct. This stimulation produces tachycardia, slight hypertension, diaphoresis and clammy skin, and nausea or vomiting. Some patients suffer cardiovascular depression, possibly due to reflexes from the ischemic area. These people display bradycardia and hypotension.

Check for additional findings. On auscultation, you may hear an S_3, S_4, or paradoxically split S_2 due to decreased left ventricular compliance. The patient usually is short of breath. Blood gases show a metabolic acidosis (due to inadequate tissue perfusion) and respiratory alkalosis (due to hyperventilation). Severe apprehension is common.

Causes and indications   Infarctions may occur for a variety of reasons; the exact cause may be difficult for the physician to diagnose. Most commonly, it is thought to occur as a result of occlusion of a coronary artery. In the past, thrombosis was believed to cause all infarctions. This concept has been proved erroneous. Although thrombosis precedes most infarctions, other causes have been identified. The occlusion may be due to atheromatous narrowing, spasm of the artery, or embolization of thrombi, fatty plaques, air or calcium. In some cases, the infarct may result not from occlusion but from a great disparity between myocardial oxygen demand and coronary arterial supply.

Types of infarcts   There are two major types of infarcts: subendocardial and transmural. The *transmural* involves all the layers of the heart. An estimated 40% of MIs are transmural; of these, about 90% are due to arterial occlusion. In contrast, the *subendocardial* infarct involves only the subendocardium, that is, not the innermost (endocardial) or outermost (epicardial) layers. Some experts believe 60% of MIs are subendocardial. Others contend that all MIs begin subendocardially and that transmural infarcts result from extension of the infarct. Infarcts limited to the subendocardium probably result not from arterial occlusion but rather from microemboli or a disparity between oxygen demand and supply. The subendocardium is particularly vulnerable to infarction because of a combination of factors. Because it has the longest myofibrils in the heart, its O_2 need is greatest. Since coronary arteries lie on the epicardium, the epicardium is oxygenated better than the endocardium. As a result, at the same time the subendocardium needs more O_2 than other cardiac cells, the blood perfusing it has the lowest PO_2 in the heart. In addition, during systole the high pressure in the subendocardium and the wringing effect of contraction preclude perfusion of the subendocardium. Once subendocardial injury has occurred, it is particularly likely to progress to infarction and extension. The swelling of damaged cells and clotting combine to compress surrounding subendocardium, endocardium, and epicardium. These factors also increase coronary arterial resistance, which creates a further decrease in flow both to the injured area and to the areas distal to it.

Coronary blood supply   Since many infarcts are due to arterial occlusion, it is helpful to understand the distribution of the coronary blood supply (Figure 4-3). The heart is supplied by three coronary arteries: the right and two branches of the left main coronary artery (the anterior descending and the circumflex coronary arteries). The right and left main coronary artery arise from sinuses of Valsalva, recesses located on the aorta just above the aortic valve. They lie on the epicardial surface and send small branches into the endocardium.

The right coronary artery courses along the anterior groove or sulcus between the right atrium and ventricle, giving off a branch (the marginal artery) to the apex. It continues along the posterior atrioventricular groove and in some cases descends along the posterior groove in between the ventricles, creating the posterior descending artery. In its course, the right coronary artery supplies the right atrium, right ventricle, posterior third of the septum, and the inferior (diaphragmatic) and posterior left ventricle.

The left main coronary artery soon splits into its two branches. The left anterior descending (LAD) coronary artery passes behind the pulmonary artery and travels down the anterior interventricular groove. In its course, it supplies the anterior two thirds of the septum and the anterior and apical portions of the left ventricle.

The left circumflex (LCX) coronary artery traverses the left atrioventricular groove from anterior to posterior. It sometimes ends as a descending artery

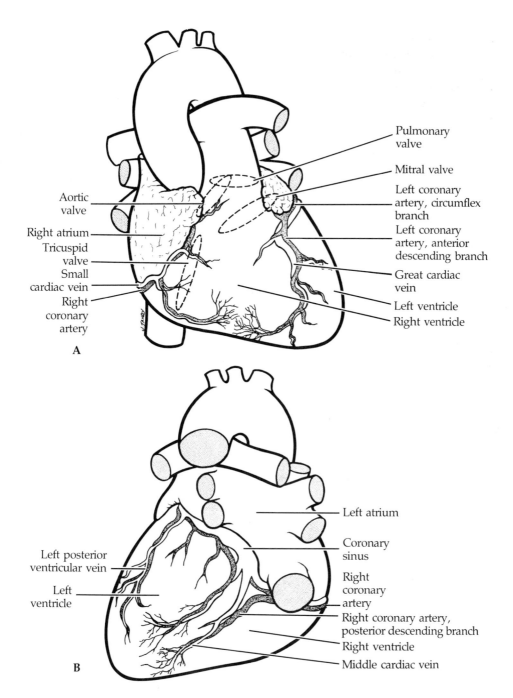

Figure 4-3.   Coronary blood vessels. **A,** Anterior view; **B,** posterior view.

along the posterior left ventricle. The LCX nourishes the left atrium, lateral and posterior left ventricle, and in some cases the inferior left ventricle.

All three coronary arteries supply parts of the conduction system. The SA node is nourished by the right coronary artery in about 55% of the population, and the circumflex artery in 45%. The internodal tracts are supplied by the right coronary artery. The AV node is supplied by the right coronary artery (90%) or circumflex artery (10%). The bundle of His is fed by the right coronary artery or left anterior descending coronary artery.

ECG indicators of infarction   Knowledge of the arterial blood supply will help you to understand the ECG signs of the infarction and predict specific patient problems which may occur.

If you suspect an infarct, obtain immediate medical help while you record a 12-lead ECG. If an infarct is diagnosed, obtain further recordings each of the next three days and thereafter as determined by the physician. Follow the serial 12-lead ECGs for the location and resolution of the infarct.

Myocardial ischemia, injury and infarction usually produce characteristic changes on the ECG (Figure 4-4). These changes are detectable in leads whose positive poles overlie the involved area (indicative leads), as well as in leads whose positive poles overlie the opposite side of the heart (reciprocal leads). Ischemia impairs repolarization and therefore inverts the T wave. Injury to the myocardium prevents cells from becoming fully polarized; it therefore alters the ST segment. Indicative leads will show ST elevation, reciprocal leads ST depression. Infarction produces absence of electrical activity, creating in effect an "electrical window." Leads whose positive poles are closest to this window look "through" it, recording electrical activity on the other side of the heart. Imagine a V_6 electrode, whose positive pole overlies the lateral left ventricle. You will recall that this lead normally displays a large R wave; it does not record right ventricular depolarization because that is obscured by the large positive wave of left ventricular depolarization. When the lateral left ventricle infarcts, its cells no longer transmit current, so no R wave is recorded. Without the positive wave coming toward it, the electrode is free to record electrical activity on the other side of the heart. Because this current is moving away from it, the electrode records a significant negative deflection, that is, a Q wave. Now consider a V_1 electrode, whose positive pole is opposite the infarct. It normally records a small R wave of septal depolarization. Then it records a large S wave, because the combined effect of right and left ventricular depolarization causes a current moving away from it. When the lateral left ventricle infarcts, V_1 will record an initial R wave as it usually does. Now, however, there are no negative left ventricular forces to oppose right ventricular depolarization. V_1 therefore continues to inscribe a positive wave, producing a large R wave. Since the zone of infarction is surrounded by a zone of injury, which in turn is enclosed by a zone of ischemia, signs of all three zones often are visible on the ECG of the patient with a fresh infarct.

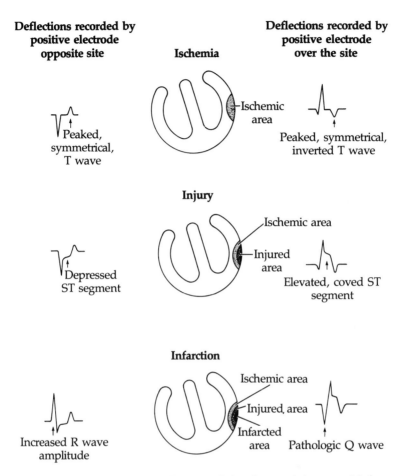

Figure 4-4. ECG patterns of myocardial ischemia, injury, and infarction. Note that as damage progresses, signs are superimposed on earlier changes. For example, the pattern of infarction includes the pathologic Q wave (produced by the infarcted area), an elevated ST segment (from the surrounding injured area), and an inverted T wave (from the surrounding ischemic area).

The location of the infarct may be determined by noting in which leads the characteristic changes appear (Figure 4-5). The positive poles of leads I, AVL, and V_4–V_6 overlie the lateral LV wall. The lateral and inferior walls are opposite each other anatomically. When indicative changes occur in I, AVL, and V_4–V_6, reciprocal changes occur in II, III, and AVF, and vice versa.

The positive poles of chest leads V_2 and V_3 overlie or "look at" the anterior left ventricular wall. Although the anterior and posterior LV walls are opposite anatomically, the 12-lead ECG contains no leads whose positive poles overlie the

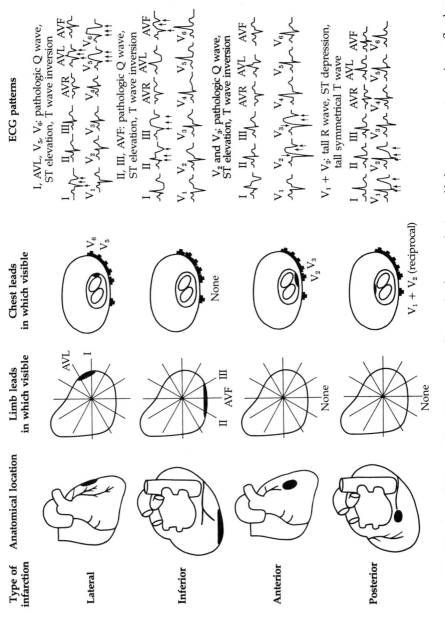

Figure 4-5. Localization of infarcts. *Lateral infarct* usually results from occlusion of left coronary artery, circumflex branch . *Inferior infarct* usually is due to occlusion of right coronary artery, posterior descending branch. *Anterior infarct* usually results from occlusion of left coronary artery, anterior descending branch. *Posterior infarct* usually is due to occlusion of right coronary artery.

posterior wall. If an anterior infarction occurs, indicative changes are seen in leads V_2 and V_3, but there are no leads which display reciprocal changes. If a posterior infarction occurs, there are no leads which demonstrate indicative changes, but V_1 and V_2 may show reciprocal changes. For this reason, it is difficult to diagnose a posterior infarct from a 12-lead ECG; other techniques such as vectorcardiography are more informative.

These ECG changes can be used to identify the acuteness of an infarct (Figure 4-6). An acute infarct is characterized by large ST deviations. After a few days, the ST segment becomes isoelectric. The T waves develop a coved appearance for a few weeks. After 8–12 weeks, the signs of a chronic or old infarct are apparent. The ST segment and T wave are normal, but the significant Q waves and the loss of R wave progression remain.

When examining the ECG for signs of ischemia, injury, and infarction, it is important to remember that changes in the T wave, ST segment, and QRS can be caused by conditions other than myocardial infarction. ST–T changes are nonspecific; tachycardia, hyperventilation, cerebral disorders, electrolyte imbalances, pericarditis, pulmonary embolism, and digitalis administration are common causes. QRS alterations also may result from left ventricular hypertrophy, pulmonary embolism, and complicated congenital heart defects, to name a few. These facts emphasize the importance of evaluating the ECG only in conjunction with other patient data.

Evaluation of serum enzymes   When cells are damaged, they release enzymes into the interstitial fluid and thence into the serum. After a myocardial infarction, different enzymes reach peak serum levels at different times. Serial determinations of serum levels of selected enzymes thus can be a valuable adjunct to the history and physical in evaluating the presence and degree of myocardial infarction. The information contained in this section is drawn primarily from Galen (1975). As with other laboratory tests, the normal values vary among institutions and authorities. The values and time intervals included in Table 4-1 are guidelines which you should evaluate for applicability in your clinical setting. Both the trends of values and the amounts of increases are significant.

According to Galen, enzyme tests vary in terms of their sensitivity, specificity, and predictive value. *Sensitivity* is a measure of frequency of positive test results in patients who have a certain disease (true positives); if most patients with that disease have positive test results, the test is said to be highly sensitive for that disease. *Specificity* is a measure of the frequency of negative results in patients who do not have the disease (true negatives); if most patients without the disease do *not* have positive test results, the test is said to be highly specific for that disorder.

So far, two aspects of cardiac enzyme tests have been considered: whether all patients with the disease have positive results (sensitivity) and whether all patients without the disease have negative results (specificity). A third, vital con-

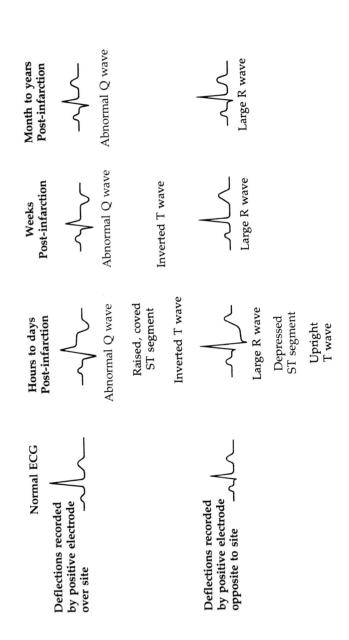

Figure 4-6. Evolutionary changes in myocardial infarction.

Table 4-1 Characteristic serum enzyme changes in acute myocardial infarction

Enzyme	Normal value	Onset	Elevation†		Duration
			Peak time		
CPK	2–83 IU/L (male)* 2–49 IU/L (female)*	4–8 hrs	24 hr		4–5 days
CPK₂ (CPK-MB)	0	4–8 hrs	24 hr		3 days
SGOT	7–26 IU/L*	8–12 hrs	24 hr		4–5 days
LDH	52–149 IU/L*	12–24 hrs	72 hr		10 days
$LDH_1 : LDH_2$	$LDH_1 < LDH_2$ ($LDH_1 = 17–32\%$, $LDH_2 = 23–36\%$)	$LDH_1 > LDH_2$ or LDH_1 almost = LDH_2, with both substantially elevated: 12–24 hrs.	—		Variable; for most patients, less than 7 days
HBD	50–250 IU/L	12–24 hrs	72 hrs		10 days

*Data from Clinical Laboratories, University of California, San Francisco, 1978.
†Data from Galen.

sideration is whether all patients with positive results have the disease, or whether there are false positives, that is, what is the test's *predictive value*? The probability that a person with a positive test result has the disease varies with the prevalence of the disease; the greater the disease's prevalence, the more likely is a person with the positive result to have the disease.

An ideal test for diagnosing a disease would have high sensitivity, specificity, and predictive value. Unfortunately, there is currently no ideal test for identifying myocardial infarction. Instead, the results of several tests must be interpreted in conjunction with each other. The enzyme tests in current use are CPK, CPK isoenzymes, SGOT, LDH, LDH isoenzymes, and HBD.

Creatine phosphokinase (CPK) is found in the brain, the myocardium, and skeletal muscle. A normal CPK level is 2–83 international units per liter (IU/L) for males and 2–49 IU/L for females. In myocardial infarction, CPK begins to increase after 4–8 hours and peaks at 5–10 times normal by 24 hours. The elevation lasts 4–5 days. Galen states that CPK is 96% sensitive, 65% specific, and 75% predictive when used to rule out myocardial infarction in coronary care unit patients on the first day following the onset of chest pain. As such, it is highly sensitive but relatively nonspecific and 25% of its positive results will be false positives.

In addition to an elevated CPK value, myocardial infarction causes significant changes in the levels of CPK isoenzymes. (*Isoenzymes* are alternate molecular structures of an enzyme. Isoenzyme specificity is significantly greater than total enzyme specificity.)

Three CPK isoenzymes have been identified: the brain (CPK-BB or CPK_1), cardiac (CPK-MB or CPK_2), and skeletal muscle (CPK-MM or CPK_3) fractions. A normal CPK serum isoenzyme profile shows 100% of CPK from skeletal muscle and none from the heart or brain, that is, $CPK_3 = 100\%$. CPK elevations occur in cardiac disorders (tachycardia, angina, infarction), skeletal muscle injury (vigorous exercise, intramuscular injections, trauma, major surgery), and neurological disorders (stroke, convulsions, head injuries). Being able to distinguish the source of CPK elevations as skeletal, cardiac, or cerebral obviously is of great diagnostic value. In the heart, up to 40% of CPK is of the cardiac variety and the remainder is skeletal. In acute myocardial infarction, both the skeletal muscle and cardiac levels show increases.

The serum cardiac fraction begins to rise 4–8 hours after the onset of chest pain, peaks at 24 hours, and lasts up to 72 hours. The skeletal muscle fraction remains increased for four or five days. As a result, CPK isoenzyme levels after the third postinfarction day will not enable you to distinguish CPK elevations due to cardiac injury from those due to skeletal muscle injury. Cardiac fraction elevations occur in all myocardial infarction patients within the first 48 hours. Although they also are found in a few other disorders (such as some muscular dystrophies), these diseases are distinguished easily from acute myocardial infarction by their histories and clinical signs.

Serum glutamic oxaloacetic transaminase (SGOT) is found widely in cardiac, renal, hepatic, pulmonary, pancreatic, and skeletal muscle tissue and in red blood cells. The normal SGOT is 7–26 IU/L. SGOT begins to rise 8–12 hours post infarct, reaching 2–3 times normal by 24 hours. The value remains elevated for 4–5 days.

Conditions in which the SGOT is elevated fall into the broad groups of cardiac, skeletal muscle, pulmonary, and hepatic disorders. For example, SGOT elevations may be seen in myocardial infarction, prolonged tachycardia, and congestive heart failure with hepatic congestion; skeletal muscle injury and neuromuscular disorders; pulmonary embolism; and cholecystitis and hepatitis. Moreover, many drugs elevate the SGOT because of hepatoxicity; among those identified are narcotics, analgesics, antibiotics, and steroids. Galen places SGOT's sensitivity at 83%, specificity at 80%, and predictive value at 80% when used to rule out MI in CCU patients on the first day following chest pain onset. He asserts that although SGOT determinations have been popular in the past evaluation of the borderline MI patient, they are unnecessary in current cardiac enzyme analyses because of their relative lack of sensitivity and specificity.

Lactic dehydrogenase (LDH) is present in almost all tissues, with the largest amounts in the liver, skeletal muscle, and heart. The normal serum level is 52–149 IU/L. LDH has five isoenzymes, labeled according to the speed with which they migrate toward the anode in an electrophoretic field. Each isoenzyme is found in a variety of tissues. The normal LDH isoenzyme values are: LDH_1, 17–32%; LDH_2, 23–36%; LDH_3, 20–32%; LDH_4, 4–15%; and LDH_5, 5–18% (UCSF 1978). The relationship between fractions is very important in evaluating LDH isoenzyme results. Normally, LDH_2 is the largest percentage, followed in decreasing order by LDH_1, LDH_3, LDH_4, and LDH_5. The heart contains primarily LDH_1, with a slightly lesser amount of LDH_2 and decreasing amounts of LDH_3, LDH_4, and LDH_5. Liver and skeletal muscle tissue have the opposite pattern, that is, no LDH_1 and increasing amounts of the isoenzymes up to LDH_5. Since LDH is so widely distributed in the body, LDH elevations occur in numerous conditions, including pulmonary embolism, liver disease, renal infarction, and neoplastic conditions. For this reason, an LDH elevation by itself would not enable you to say with certainty that it resulted from myocardial injury, but LDH isoenzymes would help to pinpoint the source. An elevated LDH_5, for instance, points to skeletal muscle or hepatic damage rather than cardiac damage.

Following an infarct, the LDH level begins to rise within 12–24 hours, peaks at 2–3 times normal by the third day, and persists for up to 10 days. Galen reports LDH determination sensitivity of 87%, specificity of 88%, and predictive value of 90% in ruling out MI in CCU patients on the third day following the onset of chest pain.

In addition to an LDH elevation, the LDH isoenzyme profile often changes. As mentioned above, the heart normally contains slightly more LDH_2 than LDH_1. An LDH_1 greater than LDH_2 is called a "flipped LDH" pattern. Eighty percent of acute myocardial infarction patients show this pattern within 48 hours post infarct. Although other conditions (such as renal infarction) can cause the flipped LDH profile, they are rarer and readily differentiated from acute MI.

Alpha-hydroxybutyrate dehydrogenase (HBD) is not an enzyme per se. Instead, it expresses the activity of a sub-unit of LDH on alpha-hydroxybutyric acid. The normal value is 50–250 IU/L. Not suprisingly, HBD shows the same pattern of sensitivity, specificity, predictive value, and elevation postinfarction as LDH. Elevations also occur in liver disease, skeletal muscle injury, neoplasms, muscular dystrophy, and some anemias. Galen believes it is not specific enough to be included routinely in cardiac enzyme studies.

To summarize, the trend in cardiac enzyme determinations is away from the panel of CPK, SGOT, LDH and HBD, popular in the past. SGOT and HBD levels are not specific enough for myocardial infarction to warrant their routine determination. In contrast, CPK and LDH are highly sensitive. Ideally, CPK and LDH levels are determined on admission and at 24 and 48 hours. Although LDH is more specific for MI than CPK, both can be elevated by other conditions. If CPK and LDH levels are elevated, Galen recommends combining the highly sensitive CPK isoenzyme analysis with the highly specific LDH isoenzyme determinations. If the CPK cardiac fraction is not elevated, no myocardial infarction has occurred. An elevated CPK cardiac fraction and flipped LDH indicates that a myocardial infarction definitely has occurred. An elevated CPK cardiac fraction without a flipped LDH may or may not indicate an MI.

In addition to acute myocardial infarction, isoenzyme analysis can provide clues that confirm the presence of other disorders common in acute MI patients. LDH_5 can be monitored to evaluate hepatic damage following infarction or congestive heart failure. LDH_2 and LDH_3 elevate with lung injury. The patient with acute chest pain, an elevated LDH_2 and LDH_3, normal LDH_1: LDH_2 ratio, and normal CPK (MB) probably has suffered a pulmonary rather than myocardial infarction.

Because red blood cells contain SGOT, LDH, and HBD, hemolysis can distort significantly these tests' value in diagnosing MI. When collecting blood samples for enzyme determination, perform the venipuncture as nontraumatically as possible, avoid shaking the container, and promptly send the specimen to the laboratory. Also remember to draw the samples on time and note on the laboratory slip the date and time of drawing; when possible, also note the date and time of the suspected MI. These actions will help to ensure that results are arranged chronologically and peak elevations are detected.

The use of CPK and LDH isoenzyme determinations is limited at present because they are expensive and time-consuming. Hopefully, faster and less expensive methods of determination will be developed because these isoenzymes provide significantly better assistance to the physician and nurse in detecting the presence and progress of acute myocardial infarction.

Additional diagnostic measures   Other laboratory tests and chest x-rays are nonspecific. However, nuclear medicine scans offer a promising method of locating the site of infarction and following serial changes. A tagged isotope such as thallium or rubidium, when injected intravenously, will localize in healthy tissue. A scanning machine can then record a scan of myocardial perfusion. It will fail to localize in regions with diminished flow, altered membrane permeability, or altered cellular metabolism; therefore ischemic, injured, or infarcted tissue will show up as a "cold" spot. (With a large, old infarct, it may be difficult to delineate current ischemic areas.)

The infarct itself can be imaged with a technetium pyrophosphate isotope injected intravenously. This isotope has an affinity for calcium in the mitochondria of new infarcts (1–8 days). It localizes there and appears as a "hot" spot on the scan done 1–2 hours post injection. In the patient with a first myocardial infarction, superimposition of the perfusion scan (with thallium or rubidium localized in healthy tissue) and infarct image (with pyrophosphate localized in infarcted tissue) theoretically could reveal the area of ischemic tissue between them. Other techniques under development include studies of left ventricular wall motion and left ventricular volume.

These nuclear medicine scans are noninvasive and can be performed at the bedside. In contrast to such diagnostic measures as catheterization, they may be repeated up to 15 times a day. Although still in the developmental stage, they offer promise for a significant advance in patient care.

Planning and implementation of care

Pain alleviation

Pain, both physical and psychological, is almost an invariable result of an infarct. To relieve physical pain, administer intravenous morphine sulfate or meperidine hydrochloride as prescribed by the physician. Administer oxygen to relieve myocardial hypoxia.

Also try to relieve psychological pain. Provide as calm and optimistic an atmosphere as possible. Briefly explain to the patient and family what is being done and why. Accompany the family to the bedside as soon as emergency care is completed. When the patient is stable, begin a teaching and rehabilitation program.

Complications

The most frequent complications of an infarct are extension, harmful arrhythmias, congestive heart failure, cardiogenic shock, pericarditis, thromboemboli, and psychogenic invalidism. Prophylactic nursing measures often can prevent potential complications.

Extension   Minimizing the extension of the infarct is an important therapeutic goal. Take measures to protect the ischemic myocardium surrounding the infarct.

The following are means of decreasing the myocardial workload:

1. Provide physical rest in a bed or cardiac chair, and assist the patient with eating, bathing, and toileting. Whenever possible, avoid the supine position; the increased venous return from the legs significantly increases myocardial workload. Fowler's position not only reduces venous return but also facilitates ventilation, by lessening the pressure of abdominal contents on the diaphragm and by promoting drainage of the upper lobes. It also enhances the patient's ability to see his environment and interact with others.

2. Administer stool softeners on the physician's order.

3. Place the patient on an easily-digested diet. Avoid the stimulants of caffeine and extremely hot or cold food.

4. Control hypertension by administering pharmacologic agents as prescribed by the physician.

5. Sedate the patient with diazepam, if ordered by the physician, both to relieve anxiety and to promote rest.

Take the following steps to improve myocardial oxygenation:

1. Administer oxygen (see Chapter 10). Start it without waiting for a physician's authorization if the patient becomes severely dyspneic, develops tachycardia, or displays signs of cyanosis, shock, or congestive heart failure.

2. Prohibit smoking. In addition to smoking being hazardous around oxygen, nicotine has several undesirable physiologic effects. It increases heart rate and stroke volume, thereby increasing myocardial workload. Although the accompanying increase in cardiac output and blood pressure causes increased coronary blood flow, the patient with compromised coronary arterial circulation will be unable to increase myocardial perfusion proportionately to his increased need for it. Moreover, the carbon monoxide produced tends to elevate the carboxyhemoglobin level. Less oxygen then can be carried by hemoglobin (the oxyhemoglobin dissociation curve shifts to the left), so less oxygen is available for release to the myocardium.

3. Improve myocardial oxygenation by administering nitrites and nitrates as ordered by the physician. The mechanism(s) by which they act are controversial. These are believed by various authors to be dilatation of the coronary arteries, dilatation of the peripheral vascular system (thus reducing preload and afterload), and/or altered myocardial metabolism. Sublingual nitroglycerin can be taken at the first sign of ischemia to forestall an anginal attack. Longer-acting preparations such as isosorbide dinitrate (Isordil) are used prophylactically. Remember that flushing, headache, and nausea are frequent and harmless, though annoying, side effects.

Arrythmias   Monitor the patient for arrhythmias. Ventricular premature beats and ventricular tachycardia are common. Ventricular fibrillation may occur without warning. In addition to watching for these rhythms, be alert for those associated with particular types of infarcts. Since the right coronary artery supplies the SA node in 55% of patients and the AV node in 90%, an inferior infarct often produces ischemia or necrosis of those sites. Bradyarrhythmias are common; sinus bradycardia, sinus or atrial rhythms with AV block, or escape junctional or ventricular rhythms may occur. Among the AV blocks, Mobitz I often is seen, resulting from AV junctional ischemia.

The circumflex coronary artery nourishes the SA node in 45% of patients and the AV node in 10%. In these patients, a lateral infarct may produce the same arrhythmias as above.

The left anterior descending coronary artery supplies the anterior third of the septum. When an anterior infarct occurs, septal ischemia or necrosis may produce third degree AV block, bundle branch block, or Mobitz II second degree AV block (due to transient bilateral bundle branch block).

For advice on preventing, recognizing, and treating arrhythmias, see Chapter 3.

Congestive heart failure and/or cardiogenic shock   Observe closely for signs of congestive heart failure and/or cardiogenic shock. Both of these conditions are common post infarct, particularly when more than a third of the left ventricle has been destroyed by the current or previous infarcts. These conditions are discussed separately, heart failure in an earlier section of this chapter and shock in Chapter 5.

In the patient with an acute MI, several potential complications increase his susceptibility to failure or shock. The left ventricular papillary muscles may become ischemic or infarcted. Papillary muscle ischemia presents as congestive heart failure with an apical pansystolic or systolic ejection murmur. Papillary infarction, which is uncommon, presents as sudden, severe congestive heart failure and shock. Because the right coronary artery usually supplies the posteromedial papillary muscle, this muscle is the one likely to dysfunction in an inferior infarct. Occasionally the circumflex artery also supplies this muscle, so the posteromedial papillary muscle may fail in a lateral infarct. The circumflex coronary artery nourishes the anterolateral papillary muscle, so it is the one involved in a lateral infarct.

In addition to papillary muscle dysfunction or rupture, shock and failure may occur if the ventricular septum or free ventricular wall ruptures. Septal rupture is a danger with an anterior infarct. It is most likely to occur in the first week. It produces a pansystolic murmur loudest at the lower left sternal border and a systolic thrill at the same location. Rupture of the free ventricular wall may result from a lateral infarct. The reported incidence is 5–10%. It is most likely to occur in the first two weeks and is associated with excessive effort or hypertension. The massive bleeding into the pericardium which results tamponades the heart and rapidly causes death.

Pericarditis   Be alert for the development of pericarditis. Sudden, severe chest pain worsened by deep breathing, and a pericardial friction rub suggest the patient has developed pericarditis, estimated to occur in 15% of acute MIs. The rub may be apparent in systole and/or diastole. It may have three components, due to heart movement during atrial systole, ventricular systole, and ventricular diastole. It sounds scratchy, often varies with respiration, and may be transient. You are most likely to hear it from the second to seventh day. Since the pain mimics infarction, a 12-lead ECG often is useful to differentiate the two conditions. Pericarditis is displayed as ST elevation in the limb and precordial leads without reciprocal depression in opposite leads and without significant Q waves.

Thromboemboli   Lessen the risk of thromboemboli. Thrombi may form due to stasis resulting from bedrest, congestive heart failure, or arrhythmias; or from clotting at the site of damaged myocardium. For these reasons, many physicians routinely prescribe anticoagulants. Others prescribe them only if the patient has an extensive infarct or a history of congestive heart failure or thromboemboli. See Chapter 10 for nursing care related to thromboemboli.

Psychogenic invalidism   Assist the patient and family to recover psychologically from the infarct. Chronic psychogenic invalidism is a tragic result of infarction, particularly when it occurs because of inadequate teaching or counseling by those caring for the patient. Although some excellent myocardial rehabilitation programs exist across the nation, many hospitals do not yet have them. Too many nurses make haphazard, poorly informed attempts to assist psychological recovery. Worse yet, some nurses display no responsibility for rehabilitation, leaving it up to the physician. If the physician and nurse are too busy, poorly informed, or unaware of the patient's and family's concerns, the patient's return to a satisfying lifestyle may be thwarted permanently. See Chapter 14 for specific details of myocardial infarction rehabilitation programs.

Outcome evaluation

Evaluate the patient's progress and the effects of your nursing interventions according to these outcome criteria:

- Heart rate and rhythm normal for patient
- Cardiac output adequate, as manifested by: BP within patient's normal limits; alert, oriented state; absence of refractory angina or serious arrhythmias; urinary output above 60 ml/hr; warm, dry skin; peripheral pulses WNL

- Realistic plans made by patient and family for return to a satisfying lifestyle after discharge

ACUTE CARDIAC TAMPONADE

The heart is surrounded by the pericardial sac, which fits loosely around it and protects it against friction. The sac attaches to the great vessels but not to the heart itself. Silverman and Schlant (1974) make an analogy between the heart with its pericardial sac and a fist invaginated into a partially filled balloon. The inner layer of the sac (the part in direct contact with the heart) is the visceral pericardium or epicardium. The outer layer, the parietal pericardium, is fibrous. Both layers are lined with serous tissue. The space between the layers, the pericardial space, normally contains only 10–20 ml of pericardial fluid.

Cardiac tamponade results when increased intrapericardial pressure interferes with diastolic filling of the heart. The pressure may rise because of a space occupying lesion, such as a tumor, or more commonly because of bleeding into the pericardial sac.

Assessment

Risk conditions

Certain conditions increase the likelihood of tamponade. Be on the alert for these conditions:

- Pericarditis, especially in an anticoagulated patient
- Cardiac trauma, penetrating or nonpenetrating, such as: cardiac surgery, cardiac biopsy, perforation of a transvenous pacing wire, myocardial infarction
- Rupture of heart or great vessels

Prevent or alleviate high-risk conditions whenever possible. For instance: consult with the physician about discontinuing anticoagulants when a patient develops pericarditis; maintain the patency of mediastinal chest tubes postcardiotomy and decrease cardiac workload for the patient with a recent myocardial infarction.

Signs and symptoms

Recognize the signs of developing tamponade. They vary with the amount of fluid and the rapidity of its accumulation.

Observe for signs of restricted venous return to the heart. These include distended neck veins, liver enlargement, elevated CVP readings, and/or dyspnea. A paradoxical arterial pulse (pulsus paradoxicus) is an important finding in tamponade as well as in certain other cardiac disorders. Its etiology and assessment technique are presented in Chapter 5.

Observe for signs of decreased cardiac output. Especially watch for a falling systolic blood pressure, muffled heart sounds (sometimes), poorly palpable apical pulse, and tachycardia.

Follow the results of diagnostic procedures. The ECG may be normal or show nonspecific signs of pericarditis. Alternating voltage (electrical alternans) of all P, QRS, and T deflections is thought to be diagnostic of tamponade; however, it is an infrequent finding. The echocardiogram will show an echo-free zone. The chest x-ray usually shows a widened mediastinum.

Planning and implementation of care

Nursing measures

Assisting with pericardiocentesis   If the symptoms are progressing rapidly, obtain *immediate* medical help and prepare for a pericardial tap (pericardiocentesis).Following are the steps to take in assisting with pericardiocentesis:

1. Elevate the patient's thorax about 60°.

2. Monitor the cardiac rhythm, CVP, and BP before and during the procedure. Have an emergency cart and defibrillator nearby. Accidental laceration of a coronary artery or the myocardium can cause shock and death.

3. Obtain a pericardiocentesis tray, sterile gloves, prep solution, and ECG machine and sterile "alligator" clips and wires. Act as the unsterile person to unwrap the tray and add to it the alligator clips and wire. The physician will connect the clips to the sterile needle and pass you the end of the wire. Connect it to the precordial lead wire of the ECG machine.

4. The physician will insert the needle at the cardiac apex or in the angle between the left costal margin and the xiphoid. As he or she does so, watch the pattern on the ECG machine and say immediately when the PR segment or ST segment elevates. These elevations indicate the needle has reached the myocardium, producing a local current of injury. They therefore warn the physician to withdraw the needle a few millimeters to avoid myocardial laceration.

5. After the fluid is aspirated, the physician will withdraw the needle and apply pressure on the site.

6. Send the aspirated fluid for diagnostic studies ordered by the physician.

Other measures.   Collaborate with the physician to treat the cause of tamponade. For example, administer antibiotics if the cause is bacterial pericarditis.

Continue monitoring the patient for recurrent tamponade. Repeated tamponade may necessitate surgical opening of the pericardium.

Outcome evaluation

Use these outcome criteria to evaluate the patient's progress:

- Heart rate and rhythm normal for patient
- Cardiac output sufficient, as evidenced by arterial blood pressure, mental status, urinary output, peripheral pulses, skin temperature and color normal for patient
- Heart sounds as loud and palpated apical pulse as strong as before the tamponade

References

Anthony, C., and Kolthoff, N. 1975. *Textbook of anatomy and physiology.* 9th ed. St. Louis: C.V. Mosby Company.
Anatomy and physiology of body, including myocardial cells.

Galen, R. 1975. The enzyme diagnosis of myocardial infarction. *Prog. Human Path.* 6:141–155.
Detailed information on cardiac enzymes and isoenzymes. Highly recommended for in-depth study.

University of California Hospitals, San Francisco. 1978. Clinical laboratory values. University of California, San Francisco.

James, T., and Sherf, L. 1974. Ultrastructure of the myocardium. In *The heart.* 3rd ed., eds. J. Hurst and R. Logue, pp. 63–79. New York:McGraw-Hill Books, Inc.
Myocardial cells, subcellular components, sliding filament theory of contractility.

Silverman, M., and Schlant, R. 1974. Anatomy of the cardiovascular system. In *The heart.* 3rd ed., eds. J. Hurst and R. Logue, pp. 20–35. New York:McGraw-Hill Books, Inc.

Supplemental Reading

Ventricular failure

Hurst, J., and Spann, J. 1974. Etiology and clinical recognition of heart failure. In *The heart.* 3rd ed., eds. J. Hurst and R. Logue, pp. 987–1003. New York: McGraw-Hill Books, Inc.
Thorough discussion of signs, symptoms and syndromes.

_____. 1974. Treatment of heart failure. In *The heart*. 3rd ed., eds. J. Hurst and R. Logue, pp. 464–491. New York: McGraw-Hill Books, Inc.
Detailed information on digitalis preparations and diuretics; recommended therapeutic approaches to slight, moderate, and severe failure.

Schlant, R. 1974. Altered physiology of the cardiovascular system in heart failure. In *The heart*. 3rd ed., eds. J. Hurst and R. Logue, pp. 416–433. New York: McGraw-Hill Books, Inc.
Mechanisms of failure, hemodynamic effects, physiologic adjustments.

Tuttle, E. 1974. Hormonal factors in congestive heart failure. In *The heart*. 3rd ed., eds. J. Hurst and R. Logue, pp. 432–437. New York: McGraw-Hill Books, Inc.
Causes of sodium and water retention in failure.

Acute myocardial infarction

Apps, M., and Tinker, J. 1978. The measurement and control of myocardial infarct size. *Intens. Care Med.* 4:21–27.
Estimation of infarct size by chemical, electrocardiographic, and radioisotopic methods; interventions to reduce infarct size.

Cassem, N., and Hackett, T. 1973. Psychological rehabilitation of myocardial infarction patients in the acute phase. *Heart Lung* 2:382–388.
Essential reading if you work with patients with infarcts. Advice on when, how much, and what types of exercise to institute during the acute phase.

Denzler, T., Fuller, E., and Eliot, R. 1974. Angina pectoris and myocardial infarction in the presence of patent coronary arteries: a review. *Heart Lung* 3:646–653.
Nine theories about this puzzling condition, including small artery disease, sympathomimetic hyperfunction, and studies supporting the contention that infarction causes thrombosis rather than vice versa.

DiGirolamo, M., and Schlant, R. 1974. Etiology of coronary atherosclerosis. In *The heart*. 3rd ed., eds. J. Hurst and R. Logue, pp. 987–1003. New York: McGraw-Hill Books, Inc.
Risk factors, including types of hyperlipoproteinemias, theories about genesis of atherosclerosis.

Doyle, J. 1974. Tobacco and the cardiovascular system. In *The heart*. 3rd ed., eds. J. Hurst and R. Logue, pp. 1536–1567. New York: McGraw-Hill Books, Inc.
Review of literature pertaining to tobacco's physiological effects.

Eliot, R., and Edwards, J. 1974. Pathology of coronary atherosclerosis and its complications. In *The heart*. 3rd ed., eds. J. Hurst and R. Logue, pp. 1003–1017. New York: McGraw-Hill Books, Inc.
Processes, clinical syndromes, complications. Numerous photographs of pathologic specimens.

Houser, D. 1976. What to do first when a patient complains of chest pain. *Nursing 76* November: 54–56.
Differentiation of myocardial infarction pain from that of angina, pericarditis, pleuropulmonary disease, esophageal-gastric pathology, musculoskeletal disease, and psychosomatic origin.

Hurst, J., and Logue, R. 1974. The clinical recognition and medical management of coronary atherosclerotic heart disease. In *The heart*. 3rd ed., eds. J. Hurst and R. Logue, pp. 1038–1132. New York: McGraw-Hill Books, Inc.
Diagnostic measures (including interpretation of cardiac enzymes), management of hyperlipidemias and other risk factors, prognosis, differential diagnosis of infarction, management of clinical syndromes.

Netter, F. 1969. *The CIBA collection of medical illustrations, Volume 5: the heart.* New York: Colorpress Publishing Company.
Numerous elegant illustrations useful for study and teaching. See particularly pp. 63–64 on localization of infarcts, pp. 212–222 on arteriosclerotic heart disease, and pp. 238–244 on myocardial revascularization surgery.

Romhilt, D., and Fowler, N. 1973. Physical signs in acute myocardial infarction. *Heart Lung.* 2:74–80.
Includes brief discussion of the late complications of MI: Dressler's syndrome, aneurysm, and shoulder-hand syndrome.

Scalzi, C. 1973. Nursing management of behavioral responses following an acute myocardial infarction. *Heart Lung* 2:62–69.
Behavioral responses to anxiety, denial, depression, and sexual concerns. Recommends what to teach patients about sexual activity after MI.

Schlant, R. 1974. Altered cardiovascular physiology of coronary atherosclerotic heart disease. In *The heart*. 3rd ed., eds. J. Hurst and R. Logue, pp. 1017–1037. New York: McGraw-Hill Books, Inc.
Physiologic mechanisms in angina, infarction, and its complications; cardiac reflexes in infarction.

Wolf, P., Lohr, T., Hoffman, S., Mersch, J., and Hudak, C. 1973. Assessment skills for the nurse. In *Critical care nursing,* eds. C. Hudak, B. Gallo, and T. Lohr, pp. 113–119. Philadelphia: Lippincott.
Cardiac enzyme interpretation.

Chapter 5

Vascular Assessment and Shock

Although separated in this text for purposes of clarity, cardiac and vascular dynamics are so closely interwoven that an understanding of one is incomplete without the other. Cardiac assessment, disorders, and nursing care are discussed in detail in Chapters 2–4. Chapter 2 in particular includes information related to invasive cardiovascular monitoring techniques, such as pulmonary arterial and central venous pressure lines. This chapter will focus primarily on noninvasive assessment of the peripheral vascular system and on nursing care for patients in shock.

Outline

Vascular system assessment   Physical examination / Laboratory tests

Shock   Risk conditions / Early signs of shock / Later effects of shock / Treatment of shock / Prevention or relief of complications / Outcome evaluation

Objectives

- Recognize signs of vascular disease detectable on inspection of the skin
- List the chief factors affecting arterial pressure—cardiac output, stroke volume, heart rate, and peripheral resistance—and the nature of the relationships between the variables

- Differentiate among the inherent, nervous, and humoral controls of the circulation
- Describe the key points about the sympathetic vasoconstrictor system
- Identify the location of the primary baroreceptors and explain their influence on arterial pressure
- Explain the effect of chemoreceptors on arterial pressure
- Identify the role of the central nervous system ischemic response in the control of blood pressure
- Identify the major blood control mechanisms operating within various periods of time following an arterial pressure drop
- Check the palpatory and auscultatory blood pressures
- Recognize the auscultatory gap and identify its significance
- Estimate the pulse pressure and mean arterial pressure
- Check for paradoxical pulse; state its possible significance
- Evaluate the peripheral arterial pulses
- Examine the neck veins to evaluate venous pressure
- State the causes of the a, c, v, x, and y components of the jugular venous pulse
- Palpate the skin for temperature, tenderness, and edema
- Check for Homan's sign and identify its significance
- Describe the factors affecting capillary diffusion
- Identify the mechanisms by which edema can develop
- Interpret laboratory tests of hematopoietic function and clotting
- Evaluate the CBC and reticulocyte count
- Interpret the blood coagulation values
- Describe the steps involved in reaching hemostasis after a blood vessel rupture
- Plan and implement measures to prevent shock
- Recognize early and late signs of shock
- Identify the type of shock and take appropriate emergency measures
- Define the purpose of a fluid challenge
- Differentiate among pharmacologic agents that are alpha stimulators, beta stimulators, and vasodilators
- Calculate the number of micrograms per minute when using a microdrop intravenous administration set
- Prevent or treat complications of shock: respiratory failure, renal failure, paralytic ileus, acute myocardial infarction, DIC, and cardiopulmonary arrest
- Evaluate the patient's progress using outcome criteria

Vascular system assessment

The *vascular system* consists of arteries, small arteries (called arterioles), capillaries, small veins (called venules), veins, venous reservoirs, and the structures which control them. Approximately 15% of the blood volume is contained in arteries, 5% in capillaries, and 64% in veins yielding a total of 84%. The remainder is contained in the heart (7%) and pulmonary vessels (9%) (Guyton 1976).

Assessment of the vascular system includes evaluation of arterial and venous pressures and pulses, cell counts, and coagulation tests. Such assessment enables you to determine the adequacy of central and peripheral perfusion and blood coagulation. A convenient format for vascular assessment is shown in Table 5-1.

As with examination of any system, it is helpful to obtain a history and description of relevant symptoms. Particularly note the presence of such signs as abnormal sensations or coldness of the extremities, muscular pain provoked by exercise (intermittent claudication), and pain at rest.

Physical examination

Inspection   Inspect the skin for color, trophic changes, and signs of bleeding. Color abnormalities may include pallor, mottling, cyanosis, or rubor (redness produced by reactive hyperemia when a severely ischemic limb is allowed to become dependent). Trophic changes, which result from prolonged tissue malnourishment, include thickened nails, hairlessness, shiny taut skin, or skin ulcers. Signs of bleeding include frank bleeding, hematomas, bruises, and petechiae (small, round red spots indicating an increased tendency to bleed). Also note the presence of varicose veins.

In the remainder of the vascular examination, blend palpation and auscultation to assess vascular dynamics. (Percussion is not helpful in evaluating this system.)

Blood pressure measurement   The measurement of blood pressure is of vital importance in patient assessment because it is a prime indicator of the adequacy of organ perfusion. To interpret the measurements you obtain, it is necessary to comprehend the factors which affect blood pressure and their interrelationships. These are presented graphically in Figure 5-1 and discussed in detail in the paragraphs that follow.

The factors which affect blood pressure and their interrelationships are extremely complex and involve feedback mechanisms at many levels. The explanations presented here are simplified and are based primarily upon the works of Guyton (1976), Schlant (1974), and Anthony and Kolthoff (1975). For more sophisticated explanations, consult the original works or other anatomy and physiology sources.

Table 5-1   Vascular assessment format

1. History _____

2. Physical

   A. Inspection/palpation

      Skin: color _____ temperature _____

         trophic changes _____

         vascular lesions _____

         tenderness _____

         edema _____

      Neck veins _____

      Arterial pulses

         carotid _____ brachial _____ radial _____

         femoral _____ popliteal _____

         dorsalis pedis _____ posterior tibial _____

   B. Auscultation

      BP _____

      Bruits _____

3. Diagnostic procedures and laboratory tests

   A. CBC: RBC _____ Hgb _____ Hct _____

          WBC _____ Differential _____

   B. Clotting time _____ PT _____ PTT _____

   C. Other _____   _____

4. Other relevant data _____

The interrelationships among flow, pressure, and resistance in blood vessels with laminar flow are expressed in Poiseuille's law. This law states that fluid flow equals the difference in pressure from one end of the vessel to the other divided by the resistance to flow. Expressed mathematically, the equation is as follows, where Q = flow, Δ = change, P = pressure, R = resistance.

$$Q = \frac{\Delta P}{R}$$

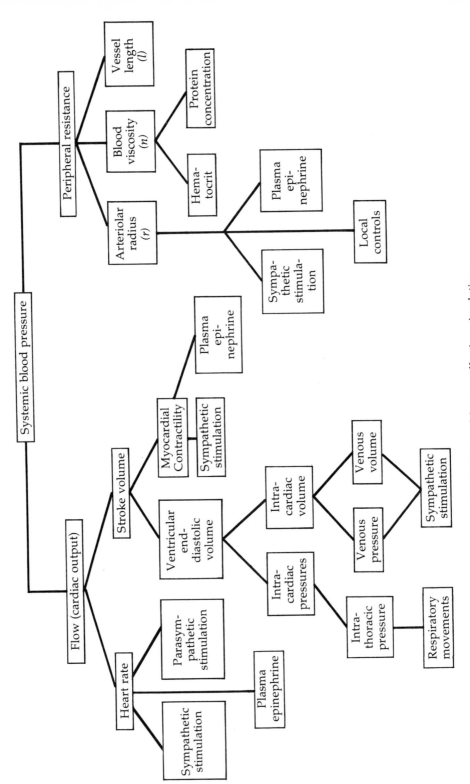

Figure 5-1 Multiplicity of factors affecting circulation

Transposing the terms of the equation results in the recognition that the change in pressure equals flow times resistance, or

$$\Delta P = Q \times R$$

In the clinical setting, we use this relationship to understand the ways in which blood pressure is affected by fluid flow and resistance.

When this equation is applied to the total body circulation, it is apparent that the arterial blood pressure varies directly with cardiac output (which is the total fluid flow) and also varies directly with peripheral resistance. The total blood flow is the cardiac output, which averages about 5 liters per minute. It equals the amount of blood the left ventricle ejects with each beat (the stroke volume) times the number of beats per minute (the heart rate). Both stroke volume and heart rate are related directly to arterial blood pressure. The stroke volume is determined by the ventricular volume at the end of diastole and by the ventricular contractility. These factors in turn are influenced by the venous return to the heart and by nervous and hormonal stimulation. The heart rate, the other chief determinant of cardiac output, responds primarily to nervous and hormonal stimuli.

Peripheral resistance is affected chiefly by blood vessel length, blood vessel radius, and blood viscosity. Stated mathematically in Poiseuille's law,

$$R = \frac{8nl}{\pi r^4}$$

where R = resistance, n = viscosity, l = length, and r = radius of the vessel. Blood vessel length and blood viscosity are related directly to peripheral resistance and therefore to arterial pressure. Changes in blood vessel length are much less important than changes in viscosity. As blood viscosity increases (for example, due to an increased hematocrit or serum protein level), peripheral resistance also tends to increase and so does arterial pressure. In contrast, blood vessel radius and peripheral resistance are related inversely—as the radius increases, resistance decreases, and, because of the direct relationship between resistance and pressure, arterial pressure also tends to decrease. Because resistance is related inversely to the fourth power of the radius, even small changes in arteriolar radius can have a profound effect on arterial pressure. As explained in greater detail later, the chief determinants of arteriolar radius are nervous stimulation, hormonal stimulation, and local tissue needs.

Intrinsic control of the circulation   The multiple factors controlling the circulation can be grouped into intrinsic, nervous, and humoral controls (Guyton 1976). To a large degree, the vascular system is capable of functioning without outside control. The inherent mechanisms that enable it to do so are termed *intrinsic controls*. The most important intrinsic control is local control of blood flow in response to tissue demands. The following description of local control is based upon Guyton. Blood flows into capillary beds through arterioles, which have a continuous muscular coat and can exert up to about half of the total peripheral vascular resistance. From arterioles, blood next flows into meta-arterioles, which are surrounded intermittently by smooth muscle fibers. At the point where meta-arterioles give rise to capillaries, a smooth muscle fiber called the *precapillary sphincter* surrounds the blood vessel. These sphincters act in two ways. In each, the individual sphincter either is completely open or closed at a given time. In some tissues, the meta-arterioles and precapillary sphincters also display intermittent contraction and relaxation, called *vasomotion*. Because of this phenomenon, blood spurts intermittently into the capillaries. If many capillaries are present, vasomotion does not occur. Instead, some of the sphincters remain open while others remain closed.

Each tissue can control its own blood flow by altering sphincter activity to influence the frequency and duration of the vasomotor cycle or the number of open precapillary sphincters. The most important regulators of tissue blood flow are oxygen need and/or carbon dioxide (CO_2) accumulation. When the tissue oxygen concentration drops and/or CO_2 level rises (the latter particularly important in the brain), the proportion of dilated precapillary sphincters increases substantially; vasomotion occurs more frequently; and the duration of blood flow during vasomotion lengthens. These acute responses normally serve to restore tissue oxygen and/or carbon dioxide concentration toward normal. Other factors which may alter local flow, such as histamine, are under investigation. In tissues which suffer a prolonged but moderate oxygen deficit, flow also is increased by dilatation of already existing bypass channels (collateral vessels) plus increases in the number and size of new blood vessels, which are laid down continuously in tissues.

Guyton stresses that it is the tissues themselves which control cardiac output, not the heart, because it is they that control peripheral vascular resistance and venous return to the heart.

The two other intrinsic controls of major importance are the Frank-Starling mechanism and the relationship between arterial pressure and urinary output. The Frank-Starling mechanism enables the heart automatically to adjust its pumping to the volume of venous blood it receives. Within physiologic limits, therefore, an increased venous return causes an increased ventricular end-diastolic volume. The resulting stretching of the fibers causes them to contract more forcefully, thereby ejecting an increased cardiac output. Similarly, a decreased venous return results in a decreased cardiac output.

The relationship between arterial pressure and urinary output also provides an automatic circulatory control: as arterial pressure increases, pressure in the kidney's afferent arterioles rises, glomerular filtration increases, and more fluid is excreted, thus tending to return pressure toward normal. The effectiveness of this mechanism can be judged by Guyton's statement that at an arterial pressure of 100 mm Hg, the kidneys excrete about 1 ml of urine each minute, while at a pressure of 200 mm Hg, they excrete about 6 ml/min. This pressure/urine volume relationship also applies as pressure drops; the kidneys conserve volume until at a pressure of about 60 mm Hg, urine output is nil.

Nervous control of the circulation   Nervous control of the circulation is mediated via complex pathways, most of which are part of the autonomic nervous system. Parasympathetic control of the vascular system is relatively unimportant, affecting arterial pressure only through its ability to slow the heart rate. In contrast, sympathetic stimuli are very important.

The sympathetic vasodilator system is believed to be important primarily in increasing blood flow to skeletal muscles during exercise. Impulses probably travel from the motor cortex to the anterior hypothalamus, through the midbrain, and down the cord to sympathetic nerves innervating the blood vessels of the involved muscles (Guyton 1976). These nerves secrete a transmitter, which produces vasodilatation and therefore increased flow to the exercising muscles.

The most important nervous regulator of the circulation is the sympathetic vasoconstrictor system which operates through the vasomotor center. The "vasomotor center" is thought to be located in the lower pons and upper medulla. From this center, impulses pass through the spinal cord to vasoconstrictor fibers, which innervate arteries and veins. These fibers secrete norepinephrine, which acts directly on the smooth muscle of blood vessels to cause constriction.

The vasomotor center controls circulation chiefly by altering the degree of blood vessel vasoconstriction. The lateral parts of the center constantly discharge stimuli which keep the blood vessels partially contracted (vasomotor tone).

When stimulated to raise arterial pressure, the lateral portions of the vasomotor center increase sympathetic stimuli. This stimulation can increase arterial pressure in a number of ways. It constricts the veins and venous reservoirs, diminishing their capacity and thereby increasing blood volume. It accelerates the heart rate. By increasing constriction of the arteries and arterioles, it raises peripheral resistance. The center can also send impulses to the adrenal medullae, provoking secretion of epinephrine and norepinephrine which are carried in the bloodstream and reinforce vasoconstriction. All these mechanisms raise arterial pressure.

When stimulated to lower arterial pressure, the medial portion of the vasomotor center inhibits the center's release of sympathetic stimuli, thereby inhibiting vasoconstriction and decreasing the effects described in the paragraph above. The medial portion of the center also sends parasympathetic impulses via the vagus nerve to the heart, slowing its rate.

Numerous stimuli affect the vasomotor center. Higher nervous centers located throughout the cerebral cortex, diencephalon, midbrain, and pons can produce excitation or inhibition of the vasomotor center. This fact explains why motor activity, emotional responses, and the "fight or flight" response to stress are accompanied by circulatory changes. More important than the higher controls for day to day regulation, however, are the vasomotor reflexes provoked by baroreceptors, chemoreceptors and central nervous system (CNS) ischemia. The following information about these reflexes is derived from Guyton. Within the physiologic range of blood pressure (approximately 60–180 mm Hg), baroreceptors are the major regulators. *Baroreceptors* (pressoreceptors) sense changes in pressure. The most important ones are contained in the aortic arch and in the carotid sinuses, which are located in the internal carotid arteries just above the bifurcation of the internal and external carotid arteries. When blood pressure drops, they transmit a decreased number of impulses to the vasomotor center. (Impulses from the aortic baroreceptors traverse the vagus nerve to the medulla. Those from the carotid baroreceptors travel along the carotid sinus nerve [Hering's nerve] to the glossopharyngeal nerve to the medulla.) The center responds by increasing vasoconstriction, increasing the heart rate, and increasing myocardial contractility. Baroreceptor response starts within minutes of a pressure change and can correct about two-thirds of the fall in pressure.

If pressure falls to within 40–80 mm Hg, chemoreceptors come into play. Chemoreceptors respond primarily to changes in O_2 concentration and, to a lesser extent, CO_2 concentration and pH of arterial blood. The most important are located in the aortic and carotid bodies (in the aortic arch and carotid bifurcations). They send impulses along the same paths as baroreceptors. An oxygen deficit causes increased chemoreceptor activity and excitation of the vasomotor center.

As pressure continues to fall below 50 mm Hg, the very powerful CNS ischemic response is triggered. Although the exact mechanism is uncertain, it is thought that the drop in pressure allows CO_2 to accumulate in the central nervous system, producing intense stimulation of the vasomotor center. An example of a CNS ischemic response is the Cushing reflex. It occurs when an extreme elevation in cerebrospinal fluid pressure cuts off the blood supply to the brain.

If these mechanisms are ineffective in restoring an adequate arterial pressure, neuronal cells become inactive; the pressure falls to about 40 mm Hg because all tonic vasoconstrictor activity is lost.

The vasomotor reflexes act within seconds but are effective only temporarily (hours to days) because baroreceptors adapt to the new pressure level, the circulatory system adapts to the sympathetic stimuli, and local controls override the sympathetic response. Longer-range restoration of blood pressure is provided by an extracellular fluid shift and by the kidneys.

Within a few minutes of a blood pressure drop, fluid begins shifting from the interstitial compartment to the capillaries. This mechanism is about twice as effective as the baroreceptors in returning pressure toward normal, but it acts much more slowly. Finally, within hours to one day, renal regulatory mechanisms (particularly diminished glomerular filtration, renin, and aldosterone) come into play to conserve volume and restore pressure toward normal.

Humoral control of the circulation   Humoral regulation of the circulation, the least significant of the three types, is mediated mostly through the actions of aldosterone, norepinephrine and epinephrine, and the renin-angiotensin cycle.

Aldosterone, secreted by the adrenal cortex in response to decreased blood volume, causes increased renal reabsorption of sodium and water, thus returning blood volume to normal. (Also see Chapters 6 and 7 for information on aldosterone.) As mentioned earlier, norepinephrine release from sympathetic vasoconstrictor nerves plays an important role in nervous control of the circulation. Norepinephrine can also be secreted by the adrenal medullae in response to sympathetic stimuli from the vasomotor center, as can epinephrine. Norepinephrine causes vasoconstriction in almost all blood vessels. Epinephrine, however, causes some blood vessels to constrict and others to dilate. Adrenal medullary release of epinephrine and norepinephrine probably is unimportant in the normal control of blood pressure and significant only when the organism is stressed severely (Schlant 1974). Angiotensin is produced by an interplay of several chemicals in the renin-angiotensin mechanism. (It too is discussed in greater detail in Chapter 7.) When blood pressure drops below physiologic levels, the kidney secretes renin. Renin activates a series of reactions which finally produce angiotensin, a stimulator of aldosterone release and a powerful arteriolar vasoconstrictor. Histamine already has been mentioned as a controller of local arteriolar dilatation. The unclear roles of other chemicals, such as serotonin and bradykinin, remain a promising area for further investigation in the understanding of vascular dynamics.

Technique of blood pressure measurement   When measuring the blood pressure noninvasively, it is essential to adhere to certain guidelines. These criteria often are overlooked in practice, resulting in the hasty recording of inaccurate pressures.

The following are guidelines for accurate pressure measurement:

1. Use a sphygmomanometer cuff with a bladder that is 20% wider than the limb diameter and long enough to go halfway around the limb. Too small a cuff produces a falsely high BP, and too large a cuff a falsely low one. Usually, a cuff 12–14 cm wide is appropriate for the arm and one 18–20 cm wide is appropriate for the thigh of an average adult.

2. Identify the palpatory and auscultatory pressures. Place the limb so that the artery you will use is at the level of the heart, and palpate the arterial pulse. Center the bladder over the artery and wrap the cuff snugly. While palpating the pulse again, inflate the cuff to about 30 mm above the point at which the pulse disappears. Then lower the pressure 2–3 mm per second, until you detect the pulse again. This point is the palpatory systolic pressure, and its importance will be explained shortly. Next, center the stethoscope over the artery and reinflate the cuff to about 30 mm above the palpatory systolic level. Auscultate the artery while you lower the pressure about 3 mm/second, noting the changes in arterial sounds (Korotkoff sounds).

There are five phases of Korotkoff sounds, caused by the vibrations of turbulent flow in the partially compressed artery. The following descriptions are based on Nutter and Paulk (1974). Phase I occurs when the cuff pressure reaches the peak systolic pressure in the artery and is characterized by clear tapping sounds of increasing intensity. In Phases II and III, the sounds take on a murmuring quality. Phase III sounds are more intense than Phase II sounds because of the increased volume of blood flowing through the artery. In Phase IV, the slowing blood flow causes the sounds to muffle suddenly and take on a blowing quality. They then gradually decrease in intensity to Phase V, where they disappear because the compression no longer is sufficient to cause turbulent flow. Phase V may never be reached in high flow states such as fever, anemia, or thyrotoxicosis.

Phase I is recorded as the systolic level. Since there is controversy over whether Phase IV or V represents the diastolic pressure, either follow the prevailing recording practice at your institution or record both levels, for example "130/85/75".

In severely hypertensive patients, the sounds may completely disappear for an interval below the true systolic pressure. If you fail to establish the systolic pressure by palpation, and instead follow the common practice of inflating the cuff only a short interval above the appearance of sounds, the point at which you stop inflation may well fall within this auscultatory gap. The first sounds you hear on deflation then will be the bottom of the auscultatory gap, rather than the true systolic pressure. Another source of error is to raise the cuff pressure high enough to hear the true systolic pressure but release the pressure when sounds disappear; in the person with an auscultatory gap, you will be misled into interpreting the point at which sounds disappear as the diastolic level. Obviously, hasty checking may underestimate seriously the true systolic reading or overestimate the real diastolic reading. For this reason, it is wise to develop the habits of checking the systolic level by palpation before auscultating the blood pressure and continuing to auscultate until the cuff pressure is 0, particularly in patients you suspect are hypertensive. Record an auscultatory gap in this manner: "280/140 with an auscultatory gap from 250 to 220".

If you are unable to hear the pressure, deflate the cuff completely and wait two minutes before rechecking. Failure to observe this caveat causes venous congestion, which falsely elevates the diastolic BP. Venous congestion also may decrease the intensity of Phase I or II sounds so much that they may not be heard: the recorded systolic pressure then will be falsely low (Nutter and Paulk 1974).

Particularly on initial evaluation, check the pressure in both arms. A difference of up to 10 mm Hg is normal. An increased difference is seen in dissection of the aorta and some congenital diseases.

3. Calculate the pulse pressure and mean arterial pressure. The pulse pressure is the difference between the systolic and diastolic readings. Pulse pressure depends upon stroke volume, the rate of ventricular ejection, peripheral resistance, and vessel distensibility (Nutter and Paulk 1974). Increased pulse pres-

sure is seen as a normal variant or in conditions which increase stroke volume (for example, circulatory overload or anxiety), decrease peripheral vascular resistance (fever), or decrease arterial distensibility (aging, hypertension). Decreased pulse pressure is usually not seen in normal subjects. Conditions which can cause it are decreased stroke volume (for example, shock, heart failure, hypovolemia), increased peripheral vascular resistance (shock, hypovolemia, vasoconstrictor drugs), or obstructions to ventricular ejection (mitral insufficiency, aortic stenosis).

The mean arterial blood pressure averages out cycle-to-cycle variations in BP and therefore is the average pressure under which blood flow to the tissues occurs. A true mean BP can be obtained electrically via an intra-arterial line. To approximate the mean for patients without intra-arterial lines, add one-third the pulse pressure to the diastolic pressure; for a pressure of 120/80, the mean BP is 93 mm Hg. (Note that this value is not an arithmetic mean, which would result from adding the systolic and diastolic values and dividing by 2. Because diastole is longer than systole, the mean BP is closer to the diastolic reading.)

4. Check for a paradoxical pulse if you suspect cardiac tamponade. Inspiration normally makes intrathoracic pressure more negative causing pulmonary vessels to expand and causing blood to pool in the vessels. The resulting decrease in venous return to the left side of the heart causes cardiac output to decrease and systolic arterial pressure to drop. (Although inspiration also causes increased venous return from the body to the right side of the heart, by the time this blood traverses the pulmonary circuit, inspiration is almost over.)

In conditions which increase the disparity between inspiratory pressure changes in the heart and pulmonary vessels, an exaggerated drop in systolic arterial pressure may occur. For instance, conditions which restrict cardiac expansion cause relatively greater pressure drop in the pulmonary vessels than in the heart (Fowler 1974) so more blood pools in the pulmonary vessels and the systolic arterial pressure shows a greater decline than normal. Examples are cardiac tamponade and constrictive pericarditis. Severe obstructive lung disease also causes an exaggerated response, because the increased fluctuations in pulmonary pressures are transmitted to the heart and great vessels. The exaggerated systolic arterial pressure response to inspiration is known as a paradoxical pulse, although the name is poor because the response is merely an accentuation of the normal response rather than a paradox (a reversal of the normal situation). A paradoxical pulse often must be detected by blood pressure auscultation rather than palpation.

To check for a paradoxical pulse, inflate the cuff above the known systolic level. As you deflate it very slowly, note the level at which you first detect sounds. At first, sounds will be audible only on expiration. Continue lowering the pressure and note the level at which you hear sounds on both inspiration and expiration. A difference of less than 10 mm Hg between the two points indicates a normal BP response to inspiration. A greater difference indicates a paradoxical pulse. If its other causes are ruled out, this finding can be particularly valuable in confirming the presence of cardiac tamponade and the trend of readings useful in evaluating its progression.

Evaluation of peripheral arterial pulses   The locations of the clinically most important pulses are presented in Figure 5-2. The pulses of leg arteries sometimes can be difficult to locate. To find the popliteal artery, flex the patient's knee slightly and feel behind the knee with the fingertips of both hands. The dorsalis pedis pulse is congenitally absent or nonpalpable in 5–12% of the population (Gifford, Dewolfe, and Young 1974).

When evaluating peripheral pulses, compare them bilaterally for rate, rhythm, volume, and contour. Describe pulse volume as absent, small (weak), normal, or large (bounding). The pulse volume depends upon many of the same factors as arterial pressure (stroke volume, peripheral resistance, etc.) as well as characteristics of the vessel and its distance from the heart.

The contour of the pulse refers to the shape of its wave form. Normally, the contour of the arterial pulse changes from the aorta to the periphery (Figure 5-3), because of changes in vessel elasticity, damping of some parts of the pulse, distortion by reflected waves, and other factors. The following descriptions are based on Hurst and Schlant (1974) and the American Heart Association (1972).

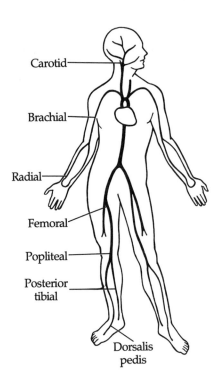

Carotid

Brachial

Radial

Femoral

Popliteal

Posterior tibial

Dorsalis pedis

Figure 5-2.   Primary arterial pulses.

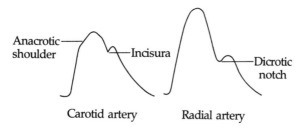

Figure 5-3.   Central versus peripheral pulse contours.

The pulse in the aorta or carotid artery is characterized by a rapid upstroke with a slight pause (anacrotic shoulder) just before the peak pressure. The peak of the wave is rounded. It is followed by a slight downstroke, a sharp downstroke (the incisura) produced by aortic valve closure, a slight rise, and then a gradual downstroke until the next beat. As the wave moves out toward the periphery, the upstroke becomes steeper and the pause on the upstroke disappears. The systolic pressure becomes higher and the peak becomes sharper. The incisura becomes smoother and is replaced by the dicrotic notch, which occurs later and at a lower pressure than the incisura. The diastolic and mean pressures become lower. Although visible on pulse recordings, the anacrotic shoulder, incisura, and dicrotic notch normally are not palpable.

Selected abnormalities of the arterial pulse are presented in Figure 5-4.

Particularly on initial evaluation, it also is helpful to auscultate the major arteries. Auscultation normally reveals no bruits, although systolic abdominal bruits occur normally in about 25% of young people (Schroeder and Daily 1976). In partially occluded vessels (primarily the carotid or femoral arteries), bruits indicate turbulent blood flow secondary to atherosclerosis or other pathology.

Examination of neck veins   As part of the patient examination, examine the neck veins. There are two purposes for this procedure: to evaluate venous pressure noninvasively and to study the waves of the venous pulse.

The venous system is a low-pressure, low-resistance system. Because it is so distensible, it can easily accommodate an increase in blood volume. Since it responds to a lesser degree of sympathetic stimulation than arteries and arterioles, the venous system easily shifts blood into the circulating blood volume when the need arises.

Venous reservoirs exist in all parts of the body except the heart, brain, and skeletal muscles (Anthony and Kolthoff 1975). The most important are those in the abdominal organs, particularly the liver and spleen, and in the skin.

Among the factors affecting venous return to the heart are venous pressure (in turn affected by blood volume, venous distensibility, gravity, and right atrial pressure), venous valves, sympathetic stimulation, the contraction of skeletal and abdominal muscles, and intrathoracic pressure changes occurring during respiration.

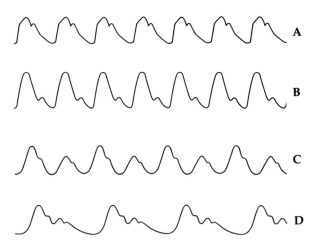

Figure 5-4.   Abnormal arterial pulses. **A,** Normal. **B,** Large, bounding (water hammer) pulse. Characterized by rapid rise, sharp crest, rapid fall. Seen in hyperkinetic states (anxiety, fever, anemia, exercise), rapid arterial runoff (aortic regurgitation), sometimes in atherosclerosis and hypertension. **C,** Pulsus alternans. Regular alternation of pulse amplitude, due to alternation of left ventricular end-diastolic volume and contractility; seen in left ventricular failure. **D,** Bigeminal pulse. Irregular alternation of pulse amplitude, most often due to premature ventricular beats coupled to normal beats. Premature beats have small volume, normal beats larger volume due to prolonged diastolic filling after premature beats.

In contrast to arteries, venous flow from capillaries is nonpulsatile; however, pressure changes resulting from atrial and ventricular filling are transmitted to the neck veins and can be appreciated as pulsations.

Following are procedures for evaluating venous pressure and pulse by examining the neck veins:

1. Estimate the venous pressure as normal or increased. To evaluate the venous pressure and pulse, first identify the neck veins, preferably the internal jugular veins. Elevate the head of the bed slightly if you anticipate a relatively normal venous pressure or approximately 45° if you suspect an elevated pressure, as in congestive heart failure. Place a small pillow under the neck to relax the neck muscles. Turn the head slightly away from you.

Shine a light tangentially across the neck. Identify the carotid artery, external jugular vein, and internal jugular vein (Figure 5-5). The inexperienced examiner easily may confuse the carotid artery with the jugular veins, particularly the internal jugular, which is located very close to it. To distinguish them, keep these points in mind. The carotid pulse is palpable, with a single strong rapid

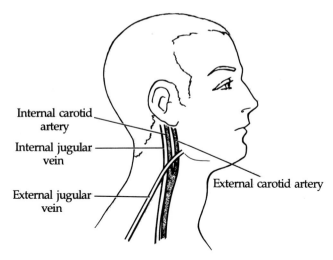

Figure 5-5.   Relationship of carotid arteries and jugular veins.

upstroke. It is unaffected by respiration and cannot be obliterated easily by pressure. The external jugular vein is superficial. Because the external jugular's valves usually interfere with the transmission of right atrial pressure, the internal jugular vein (especially the right one), is preferred for evaluation of venous dynamics (Hurst and Schlant 1974). It lies deep, under the sternocleidomastoid muscle. Its pulsations usually are not palpable, instead being seen in movements of the overlying tissue. Bates (1974) suggests looking for the internal jugular venous pulsations "in the suprasternal notch, between the attachments of the sternomastoid on the sternum and clavicle, or just posterior to the sternomastoid." In contrast to the arterial pulse, the venous pulse consists of two or three slower, smaller upstrokes (the a, c, and v waves discussed in a later section). The level of pulsation descends with inspiration and rises with expiration. The pulsations are obliterated easily by pressure on the vessel just above the clavicle.

Vary the degree of elevation of the head of the bed until you can see the maximum pulsations of the upper level of the fluid column in the internal or external jugular veins. Then make the following observations:

A. Note the degree of elevation of the head of the bed.

B. Measure the vertical distance between the top of the fluid column and the angle of Louis.

C. Note whether the level decreases on inspiration and increases on expiration.

D. Apply pressure on the vein just above the clavicle; the vein will distend. Release the pressure suddenly and note whether the vein immediately empties to its previous level.

E. Perform a *hepatojugular reflux (HJR)* test. Ask the patient to breathe normally. Press the right upper quadrant of the abdomen firmly for 30 seconds, while you observe the neck veins. This maneuver increases venous return from the abdomen to the heart. If this test increases venous distention one centimeter or less, venous pressure is normal. An increase of more than 1 cm (positive HJR) indicates increased venous pressure, such as in right heart failure or constrictive pericarditis. This test is invalid if the patient holds his breath or bears down during it.

F. Repeat the examination on the other side of the neck. To summarize, the signs of normal venous pressure are neck veins that are visible at 0° elevation, less than 3 cm distention at 30° elevation, a fluid level that falls on inspiration and rises on expiration, a rapid return to the previous level upon release of occlusive pressure on the vein, and negative hepatojugular reflux test.

Increased venous pressure is indicated by distention of more than 3 cm above the sternal angle, and a positive hepatojugular reflux. Severely increased pressure appears as a parodoxical rise in the level of distention during inspiration (Kussmaul's sign) or distention of the entire vein (no visible top of the fluid column) even at 90° elevation.

2. Examination of waves of the venous pulse. As mentioned in Chapter 2, the venous pulse consists of three positive waves and two descents, which are related to pressure changes during the cardiac cycle (Figure 5-6). When the right atrium contracts, forcing blood into the right ventricle during the end of diastole, the slight rise in atrial pressure produces the *a wave.* Tricuspid valve closure and atrial diastole cause a drop in pressure, known as the *x descent.* It is interrupted by the *c wave,* which occurs as a result of bulging of the tricuspid valve during ventricular systole and/or a neck vein reflection of the nearby carotid pulse.

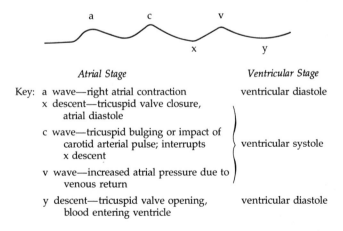

	Atrial Stage	*Ventricular Stage*
Key:	a wave—right atrial contraction	ventricular diastole
	x descent—tricuspid valve closure, atrial diastole	
	c wave—tricuspid bulging or impact of carotid arterial pulse; interrupts x descent	ventricular systole
	v wave—increased atrial pressure due to venous return	
	y descent—tricuspid valve opening, blood entering ventricle	ventricular diastole

Figure 5-6.   Venous pulse waves.

During the last part of ventricular systole, venous return raises the atrial pressure and produces the *v wave*. The opening of the tricuspid valve and rush of blood into the ventricle create a drop in atrial pressure, the *y descent*. The cycle then repeats itself.

To identify the individual waves, look at the venous pulse while you either palpate the carotid artery on the other side of the neck or auscultate the heart. The a wave just precedes S_1 and the carotid upstroke. The c wave usually cannot be seen. The v wave coincides with S_2.

A variety of abnormal venous pulses may be seen and related logically to the conditions that produce them. In atrial fibrillation, for example, effective atrial contraction does not occur, and no a wave is seen. Large, regular a waves indicate resistance to atrial emptying into the right ventricle, as in tricuspid stenosis or pulmonary hypertension. Extremely large a waves (cannon waves) denote atrial contraction against a closed tricuspid valve. They may occur regularly, as in junctional rhythm, or irregularly as in AV dissociation.

Palpating the skin   In your examination of the patient, palpate the skin for temperature, tenderness, and edema. When checking for temperature changes, use the backs of your fingers, which are more temperature-sensitive than the palmar aspects. Coldness is a reliable sign of pathological vasoconstriction only if you examine the patient in a warm environment and he does not suffer normally from cold extremities. Increased warmth is of less significance than coldness in evaluating the vascular system, although it often accompanies thrombophlebitis. Tenderness or frank pain occurs with thrombosis of superficial or deep veins and with arterial occlusion.

Vascular assessment of bedridden patients should include a check for Homan's sign. To elicit this sign, extend or slightly flex the patient's knee and then dorsiflex the foot. Pain felt in the upper posterior calf (positive Homan's sign) may indicate deep venous thrombosis, although it is a somewhat unreliable sign since it is not experienced by all patients with that affliction and may occur in other conditions.

Edema   Edema is the accumulation of excessive fluid in the interstitial spaces of tissues. Normally, extracellular fluid and other substances move between the capillaries and interstitial spaces because of pressure gradients and capillary permeability. Movement is thought to occur primarily by diffusion, either through pores or the capillary membrane itself. Diffusion is the term that applies to the movement in one direction, filtration the term that describes the balance of outward and inward diffusion, that is, the net fluid movement.

Many years ago, Starling hypothesized that the direction and speed of fluid exchange across the capillary membrane depends upon the interaction of pressures in the capillary fluid and interstitial fluid. The following descriptions of the mechanics of fluid exchange and edema formation are based upon Guyton (1976).

There are four pressures which affect filtration: two pressures exerted by fluid *(hydrostatic pressures)* and two by proteins *(colloid osmotic pressures)*. Hydrostatic pressure tends to "push" fluid out of a compartment and colloid pressure tends to "pull" fluid into a compartment. The effective filtration pressure equals the sum of the forces tending to move fluid in one direction minus the sum of the forces tending to move fluid in the opposite direction. The colloid osmotic pressures and the interstitial hydrostatic pressure are relatively constant. Plasma colloid osmotic pressure approximates 28 mm Hg, interstitial colloid osmotic pressure 5 mm Hg, and interstitial hydrostatic pressure −6.3 mm Hg. In contrast, the capillary hydrostatic pressure varies from 25 mm Hg at the arterial to 10 mm Hg at the venous end.

Figure 5-7 provides a schematic representation of the effects of these pressures. Note that at the arteriolar end of the capillary, the net force causes fluid movement out of the capillary into the interstitial space. At the venular end, the net force causes diffusion of fluid back into the capillary. About 90% of the fluid which leaves the arteriolar end of the capillary is reabsorbed at the venular end. The remainder is reabsorbed by the lymphatic system, which also reabsorbs the small amounts of protein which leak continuously from the capillary. *Starling's law of the capillaries* states that the mean filtration forces at the capillary membrane exist in equilibrium, so that the amount of fluid which leaves the capillaries equals that returned to the capillaries and lymphatics.

The factors affecting capillary dynamics suggest the various causes of edema. Increased capillary hydrostatic pressure occurs with arteriolar dilatation (as in allergic reactions), venous obstruction (as with clots or congestive heart failure), or fluid retention (as in renal failure). Decreased plasma proteins can result from

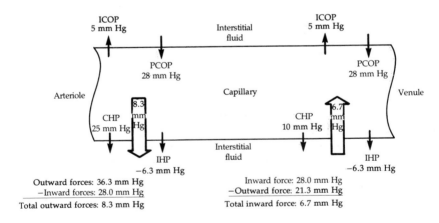

Figure 5-7.   Capillary fluid dynamics. **ICOP,** interstitial colloid osmotic pressure; **PCOP,** plasma colloid osmotic pressure; **CHP,** capillary hydrostatic pressure; **IHP,** interstitial hydrostatic pressure. Values from Guyton (1976).

inadequate nutrition or accelerated protein loss, as in nephrosis. Increased capillary permeability occurs in capillary damage, for example, with burns or endotoxins. Finally, decreased lymphatic drainage can produce edema, for instance following surgical removal of diseased lymphatic glands.

There is a safety zone in which some of these causes can exist without producing clinically obvious edema (Guyton 1976). Interstitial hydrostatic pressure normally is negative. As it becomes more positive, it tends to produce increased lymphatic flow, which not only carries away some of the excess fluid but also some of the tissue proteins, thereby reducing their osmotic pull on capillary fluid. The mean capillary hydrostatic pressure normally is about 17 mm Hg. It must increase 17 mm Hg or the plasma colloid oncotic pressure must decrease 17 mm Hg before edema develops. Edema usually is not detectable until the interstitial fluid volume is 30% above normal; it can reach several hundred percent above normal in severe cases.

Edema may be pitting or nonpitting. A depression (pit) that slowly disappears following fingertip pressure indicates that edema fluid is soft enough to be displaced by outside pressure. Edema that does not pit (brawny edema) indicates that increased capillary permeability has allowed fibrinogen to leak into the interstitial space, where it has coagulated.

Frequently, you can deduce the cause of edema from its characteristics. Edema that occurs bilaterally in dependent body parts (such as the sacrum in the bedridden patient or feet in the ambulatory patient), pits on pressure, and decreases with position changes is dependent (*orthostatic*) edema, caused by increased capillary hydrostatic pressure secondary to gravity. Unilateral or bilateral pitting or *brawny* edema, often associated with skin ulceration, is characteristic of increased hydrostatic pressure caused by venous obstruction or valvular insufficiency. Localized nonpitting swelling of the eyes, lips, tongue, hands, or genitals, or internal swelling (especially of the larynx), often associated with itching or burning sensations, typifies allergic (*angioneurotic*) edema. This type of edema results from increased hydrostatic pressure due to arteriolar dilatation following histamine release from damaged tissues.

Additional signs and symptoms   When examining the patient be alert for additional signs and symptoms which may point to vascular malfunction. Among them are central cyanosis (described in Chapter 9), a diminishing level of consciousness, arrhythmias or angina, and a falling or absent urinary output, all of which may be signs of failing central (core) perfusion. The signs and symptoms of shock are discussed later in this chapter.

Laboratory tests

Laboratory measures of hematopoiesis and coagulation can provide helpful assessment clues when used as adjuncts to the patient's history and physical examination.

CBC and reticulocyte count   A fairly comprehensive evaluation of the blood's formed elements can be obtained by studying the complete blood count (CBC). This common group of laboratory tests measures the blood's formed elements: red blood cells (*erythrocytes*), white blood cells (*leukocytes*), and platelets (Figure 5-8). The following information on CBC interpretation is derived from Guyton (1976), Byrne (1976), and Strand (1976). Red blood cells (RBCs) have three major functions: oxygen transport, carbon dioxide transport, and acid-base buffering. In the normal adult, RBC production occurs in the marrow of flat and short bones, for example, the vertebrae, sternum, ribs, and bones of the hands and feet. Production is stimulated by *erythropoietin,* a glycoprotein formed primarily in the kidneys in response to hypoxia. Normal red blood cell formation requires the presence of amino acids, iron, Vitamin B_{12}, folic acid, and other nutrients.

Red blood cell measures contained in the CBC are the red cell count, hemoglobin level, and hematocrit. The normal *red cell count* varies with sex, age, altitude, and exercise. It usually falls within 4.5–6.0 million per cubic millimeter for males and 4.0–5.5 million per cubic millimeter for females. *Hemoglobin* is an iron-protein complex, formed and carried inside RBCs, which functions both in O_2 transport and in acid-base buffering. Males usually have a hemoglobin level between 14 and 17 gm per 100 ml and females between 12 and 16 gm. The *hematocrit* expresses the volume percentage of red blood cells in whole blood, and normally ranges between 40% and 54% for males and 38–45% for females. The red cell count, hemoglobin level, and hematocrit usually follow the same trend. Elevated values, for instance, occur with dehydration and polycythemia. Decreased values are seen in fluid retention, hemorrhage, and anemia.

Additional information on red cell production can be obtained from a separately ordered reticulocyte count. *Reticulocytes* are immature RBCs, which usually represent 0.5–1.5 percent of the RBC count. An increased reticulocyte count indicates an accelerated rate of RBC production, such as in sickle cell anemia or hemorrhage. A decreased count means depressed bone marrow production of red cells, as in aplastic anemia.

White blood cells (WBCs) or leukocytes are mobile cells which function to protect the tissues from inflammatory agents, remove cellular debris, and also participate in the immune response. The CBC contains both a white cell count and a differential white cell count.

The white cell count normally ranges between 5,000 and 10,000 per cubic millimeter of blood. An increased count is a common, nonspecific finding seen in various types of inflammation and in leukemia. A decreased count, signifying bone marrow depression, occurs in viral infections, hepatitis, radiation therapy, and toxic reactions.

On the basis of their cytoplasmic, nuclear, and staining characteristics, WBCs are subdivided into five major classes, which are reported in the WBC *differential count.* Both the total WBC count and the differential count are important in diagnosis.

Those WBCs formed in the bone marrow are termed *granulocytes* (because their cytoplasm contains numerous granules) or *polymorphonuclear leukocytes* (due

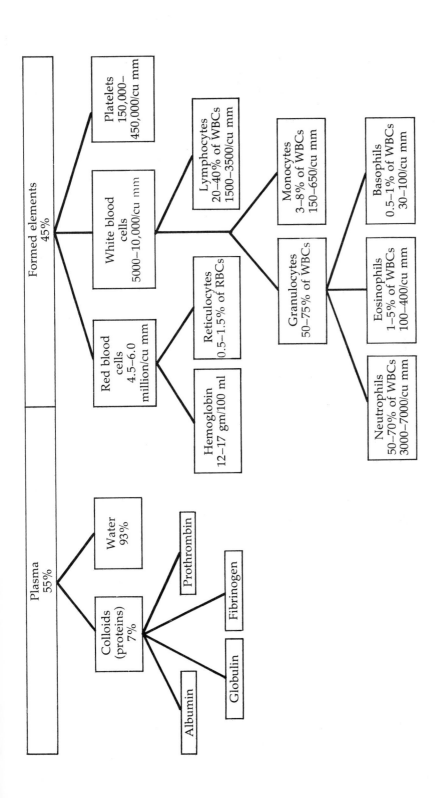

Figure 5-8. Blood constituents.

to the irregular shapes of their nuclei). They represent about 50–75% of the WBCs, and are divided further on the basis of their staining characteristics into neutrophils, eosinophils, and basophils. *Neutrophils* normally represent about 50–70% of WBCs (3,000–7,000/cu mm). Almost any process causing tissue damage, whether or not accompanied by inflammation, attracts neutrophils which phagocytize and digest foreign particles and damaged tissue. Among the conditions in which the neutrophil percentage rises are infection, surgical procedures, and myocardial infarction. A decreased neutrophil count occurs with hepatitis, aplastic anemia, some viral infections, and some medications such as sulfonamides and antihistamines.

Eosinophils represent about 1–5% of WBCs (100–400/cu mm). Although their function is unclear, Guyton suggests they may detoxify foreign proteins in the lungs and intestinal tract and/or enter blood clots and release profibrinolysin to initiate clot dissolution. The eosinophil count rises in administration of foreign proteins, allergic reactions, and parasitic infections. It decreases with high levels of epinephrine and adrenocorticotropic hormone, as in severe stress reactions.

Basophils, normally 0.5–1.0% of the WBCs (30–100/cu mm) also have an unclear role. Since they are very similar to mast cells which release heparin, Guyton speculates they may be precursors of these cells. The percentage increases with splenectomy, radiation therapy, and hemolytic anemia.

In addition to the WBCs formed in bone marrow, some are formed in the lymphoid tissues, which include the lymph glands, thymus, and spleen. These cells, which do not have granular cytoplasm but do have nuclei, are termed *lymphocytes* and *monocytes.* Along with tissue *histiocytes* (which provide the first line of defense against tissue damage), lymphocytes and monocytes are capable of transforming into *macrophages,* the highly powerful cells which ingest and digest foreign substances and cellular debris. Lymphocytes have an additional capability of becoming sensitized against specific antigens and functioning like antibodies. Lymphocytes normally range between 1500 and 3500/cu mm (20–40%), monocytes between 150 and 650/cu mm (3–8%). The lymphocyte count rises in inflammation, viral infections, hepatitis, and lymphocytic leukemia. It drops in radiation therapy and stress reactions. The monocyte count increases in inflammation and monocytic leukemia; decreases are rarely seen.

Platelets (thrombocytes) are formed in the bone marrow by fragmentation of *megakaryocytes,* another type of WBC. The normal platelet count is 150,000–450,000/cu mm. Platelets initiate blood clotting, as explained in detail in the section on blood coagulation. The platelet count is decreased in most leukemias and idiopathic thrombocytopenic purpura and elevated in some anemias, severe hemorrhage, and thrombocytosis.

Blood coagulation values   *Blood coagulation* is an intricate sequence of chemical reactions which remains only partly understood despite years of investigation. The following simplified explanation is based upon Guyton (1976), Anthony and Kolthoff (1975), and Byrne (1977).

When a blood vessel is ruptured, hemostasis occurs in several steps. First, vessel spasm limits the amount of blood loss. Second, a platelet plug forms because platelets adhere to the roughened endothelial surface and cause additional platelets to adhere to them. Third, a blood clot forms. Fourth, fibroblasts invade the clot and organize it into fibrous tissue within 8–10 days, or, less commonly, the clot dissolves.

Instrumental in clotting are prothrombin and fibrinogen, two plasma proteins formed by the liver. Coagulation occurs in three basic steps: the formation of prothrombin activator, the conversion of prothrombin to thrombin, and the conversion of fibrinogen to fibrin (Figure 5-9).

Prothrombin can be activated by either of two systems, the details of which are poorly understood. Damage to the blood itself initiates an intrinsic activator system, while damage to tissue initiates an extrinsic system. Although separated for purposes of analysis, these systems probably interact in the patient.

The factor which initiates the intrinsic pathway is uncertain; at present, it appears to be damage to the blood itself or blood contact with subendothelial collagen. The initiating event causes platelets to release platelet phospholipids. It also activates Factor XII, which in turn activates Factor XI, which subsequently activates Factor IX. Activated Factor IX, in conjunction with Factor VIII, platelet phospholipids, and calcium, activates Factor X.

In the extrinsic system, damaged tissue releases thromboplastin and tissue phospholipids. Thromboplastin interacts with Factor VII to activate Factor X.

From the activation of Factor X, clotting proceeds almost identically for both pathways. Activated Factor X interacts with Factor V, calcium, and platelet or tissue phospholipids to convert prothrombin to thrombin. Thrombin is a proteolytic enzyme which in turn converts fibrinogen to fibrin.

Loose fibrin threads adhere to the vessel wall, forming a network and trapping platelets, RBCs, and plasma. The loose threads are formed into an insoluble clot by Factor XIII. The clot then retracts, squeezing out the plasma and further binding the margins of the vessel rupture. Large numbers of platelets, which apparently bond the fibrin threads together, are needed for retraction.

After tissue growth is underway, fibrinolysis destroys the fibrin matrix. When a clot is formed, it incorporates a plasma protein called plasminogen (profibrinolysin). Although the mechanisms are unclear, plasminogen can be activated by several substances. Activated plasminogen becomes plasmin (fibrinolysin), a proteolytic enzyme which digests the fibrin threads and destroys the surrounding clotting factors.

Endogenous anticoagulants normally prevent both spontaneous blood clotting and clot extension. Among the most important anticoagulants are the smoothness of vascular endothelium and the rapidity of blood flow, which tends to carry clotting factors away from a developing clot and thereby limit clot size. In addition, the clot's fibrin threads trap most of the thrombin. The remainder is inactivated by another plasma protein, antithrombin, and by fibrin degradation products released during fibrinolysis. These products also inhibit platelet aggre-

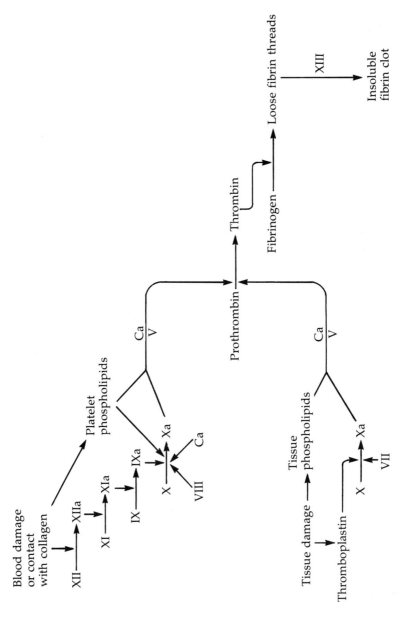

Figure 5-9 Coagulation Process

gation and the formation of the fibrin matrix. Finally, the blood contains heparin. This strong anticoagulant is produced primarily by the mast cells located around the capillaries in the lungs and liver. According to Guyton, heparin prevents the formation of intrinsic prothrombin activator, inhibits thrombin's conversion of fibrinogen to fibrin threads, increases the adsorption of thrombin by the fibrin threads, and accelerates antithrombin's inactivation of thrombin.

This brief explanation of the coagulation process will help you understand the various types of coagulation tests and the kinds of disorders which cause coagulation abnormalities. The following information is derived from Guyton (1976), Strand (1976), and Byrne (1977).

Common coagulation measures are the clotting time, partial thromboplastin time, prothrombin time, and fibrinogen level. (As with other laboratory tests, normal values vary among laboratories.)

The clotting or coagulation time is a general indicator of the blood's ability to clot. It is determined on a venous sample by a number of methods, most commonly the *Lee-White*. Blood is mixed gently at 30 second intervals and the time required for it to clot is noted. Since numerous factors participate in the clotting process, this test is nonspecific for clotting abnormalities. A prolonged clotting time may indicate anticoagulant therapy, liver disease, or a deficiency of Factor I, II, VIII, or IX. Results also are influenced by extraneous factors such as the size of test tubes and room temperature. The normal value range varies greatly with the method used by the laboratory; for the Lee-White method using glass tubes it is 5–15 minutes.

Because standardized results are so difficult to obtain for the clotting time, some physicians prefer the *partial thromboplastin time (PTT)*. It too reflects the general clotting ability of the blood but is faster, more sensitive, and more easily standardized. The range of normal values is 35–45 seconds.

The clotting time and partial thromboplastin time are used primarily to monitor patients on heparin, for which the desired therapeutic values are about twice normal values.

Blood for the *prothrombin time* is a nonfasting, venous sample that is oxalated after drawing to prevent the conversion of prothrombin to thrombin. In the laboratory, calcium is added to neutralize the oxalate, and thromboplastin is added to provoke the conversion of prothrombin to thrombin. The time necessary for fibrin threads to appear then is noted. The test thus measures the activity of prothrombin (Factor I) as well as fibrinogen (Factor II), or Factors V, VII, or X. A control value also is reported, based on the concurrent reactivity of reagents used in the test. The normal prothrombin time is 12–15 seconds. A prolonged prothrombin time may indicate coumarin therapy, liver disease, vitamin K deficiency, or obstructive jaundice (the deficiency of bile salts blocks intestinal absorption of vitamin K). In anticoagulant therapy, the desired level is two times the control.

The *fibrinogen level* is determined on plasma extracted from a venous blood sample. The normal level is 200–500 mg/100 ml. The level is decreased in Factor I deficiency and in disseminated intravascular coagulation. The latter is a coagulopathy with abnormal microcirculatory clotting. It may occur in hemolytic disorders, toxic conditions, surgical trauma, cancers, and other disorders. This clotting consumes platelets and clotting factors and accelerates fibrinolysis. As a result, the patient develops widespread hemorrhage.

Shock

Cardiovascular health is maintained by the interaction of three elements: the heart pump; the blood vessels; and their contents, the blood volume. Shock is an acute process of hemodynamic and metabolic derangements resulting from disruption of one or more factors in this triad. It is an ever-present specter in the care of the critically ill. Because shock can progress so rapidly and has such a high mortality, forestall it whenever you can.

Risk conditions

Conceptualizing three major types of shock, based on the triad components of the cardiovascular system, can assist you in determining which patients are at risk of shock. Major categories of shock (which often overlap) are as follows:

1. *Cardiogenic shock.* Pump failure can produce cardiogenic shock. Patients at risk include those with acute myocardial infarction, severely decreased myocardial contractility, and massive pulmonary embolism.

2. *Vasogenic shock.* Diminished arterial resistance and/or increased venous capacitance may precipitate vasogenic shock. Examples are anaphylactic reactions, intense pain, and sepsis.

3. *Hypovolemic shock.* Depleted blood volume may lead to hypovolemic shock following dehydration, copious diarrhea, excessive diuresis, or profound bleeding.

Take measures to prevent or ameliorate risk conditions. For instance, follow the measures contained in Chapter 10 to prevent pulmonary embolism. Control the patient's pain through the judicious use of narcotics. Monitor the intake, output, serum electrolytes, and osmolality of patients on diuretics. Take particular care to maintain hydration in patients who are unconscious or unable to satisfy their thirst themselves, such as intubated or paralyzed patients. Make sure that all connections in vascular lines are securely fastened and are not left open accidentally after blood samples are drawn.

Early signs of shock

The traditional criteria for shock are a systolic blood pressure below 70 mm Hg; confusion or other signs of diminished cerebral perfusion; pale, cool, clammy skin; a urinary output below 30 ml per hour; and metabolic acidosis. Dependence upon these classic signs, however, will cause you to deprive many of your patients of prompt assistance in the early stages of shock. These signs are late, may not occur in some shock states (especially septic shock); and/or may be inappropriate for a given patient, such as the hypertensive in whom shock can occur within the range of so-called normal systolic pressures.

Because the emphasis increasingly is upon early detection and aggressive management, it is crucial that you be aware that early signs of shock may vary with the underlying disorder. In sepsis, for example, the release of toxins, histamine, and other vasoactive substances initially produces increased cardiac output and decreased peripheral vascular resistance (arteriolar dilatation), especially in the skin and kidneys. Because of this, these patients will have warm, dry skin and an increased urinary output. The increased capillary permeability and filtration pressure which characterize sepsis cause an early fluid shift from the capillaries into the interstitial space, creating an early need for fluid replacement. In contrast, the early stages of some types of cardiogenic shock and of hypovolemic shock are characterized by a compensatory increase in sympathetic stimulation, producing arteriolar and venous vasoconstriction. This sympathetic stimulation is manifested by cool, clammy skin, tachycardia, and a decreased urinary output. It also produces decreased capillary filtration pressure so fluid shifts from the interstitial space to the capillaries, helping to maintain blood volume; this fluid shift is the opposite of that which occurs in early septic shock.

Other relatively early signs of shock include a falling Po_2 and Pco_2, a rising alveolar - arterial oxygen difference ($AaDO_2$), increasing tachypnea, and blood gas changes (Walt and Wilson 1975). The falling Po_2 and increased $AaDO_2$ reflect increased physiologic shunting in the lung. Tachypnea is an appropriate response to the accelerating chemical abnormalities; in fact, its absence may indicate a need for early ventilatory assistance. Early blood gas changes can be confusing. Respiratory alkalosis, reflected by a falling Pco_2, develops early in some patients because of tachypnea. Patients with septic shock, however, may have metabolic alkalosis. The cause is unclear but may be related to inhibited anaerobic metabolism causing decreased lactate and lactic acid production.

Later effects of shock

The early capillary-to-interstitial space fluid shift in sepsis eventually depletes blood volume so that hypovolemic shock complicates the picture. As a result, later developments in shock and associated signs and symptoms are similar in almost all types of shock.

Further fluid shifts   Loss of energy to operate the sodium-potassium pump (see Chapter 2) allows sodium to accumulate inside cells. This intracellular sodium load causes fluid to shift from the vascular compartment into the cells. Loss of cellular integrity due to swelling and lysosomal breakdown also allows fluid and colloids to shift from the vascular compartment into the interstitial space.

Cellular hypoxia   Normally cells receive energy from a highly complex series of chemical reactions, briefly summarized here (Fritz 1974, Guyton 1976, Walt and Wilson 1975). These steps are diagrammed in Figure 5-10. During glycolysis, glucose is split to form pyruvic acid. This step does not require oxygen. In addition to the pyruvic acid, it produces a small number of hydrogen atoms and a small amount of energy, which is used in the synthesis of the high energy bonds of *adenosine triphosphate (ATP)*. These phosphate bonds store energy until the cell needs it. The pyruvic acid is converted to acetyl coenzyme A and enters the Krebs (citric acid) cycle, during which the acetyl portion is broken down into carbon dioxide and hydrogen atoms. These hydrogen atoms plus those released during glycolysis undergo oxidative phosphorylation, in which huge amounts of energy are released and again stored as ATP.

Cellular hypoxia has drastic effects upon energy availability. It is unclear at present whether the energy deficit results from decreased energy production or from adequate energy production accompanied by insufficient formation of ATP causing energy to be lost as heat rather than stored as ATP.

Because glycolysis does not require oxygen, it continues to provide a small amount of energy, as well as pyruvic acid and hydrogen atoms. These cannot be metabolized in the Krebs cycle or undergo oxidative phosphorylation in the absence of oxygen. Instead, the excessive amounts of pyruvic acid and hydrogen atoms combine with each other and produce lactic acid. The lactic acid diffuses

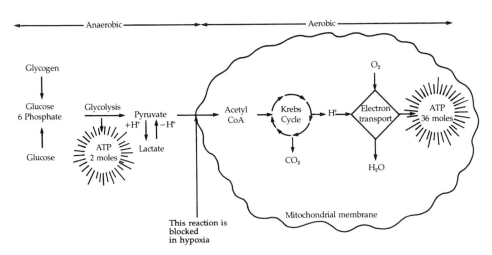

Figure 5-10.   Cellular aerobic and anaerobic energy production. The conversion of pyruvate to acetyl CoA is blocked if not enough oxygen is available to combine with the hydrogen released during the Krebs cycle.

out of the cell into the extracellular fluid, thus allowing glycolysis to continue providing energy for a few minutes. This shift from aerobic to anaerobic metabolism has three important consequences: (a) cellular activities such as protein synthesis are hampered severely due to lack of available energy; (b) the increased demand for glucose causes rapid depletion of glycogen stores; and (c) lactic acidosis deranges the body's acid-base and electrolyte balances.

Metabolic acidosis   By the time metabolic acidosis is detectable in arterial blood gas values, significant physiologic derangement has occurred (Walt and Wilson 1975). Metabolic acidosis thus is a later sign of shock than the respiratory alkalosis or metabolic alkalosis previously mentioned.

If the person resumes adequate oxygenation, the lactic acid can be reconverted to pyruvic acid and utilized in the Krebs cycle. If not, the worsening metabolic acidosis and loss of energy result in cellular destruction.

Cellular destruction   As cells are damaged, disruption of their lysosomes frees proteases and other enzymes, which may hasten cellular destruction. These enzymes also are believed to provoke the release or activation of bradykinin, histamine, and other substances which cause severe vasodilatation and may depress the heart (Walt and Wilson 1975).

Treatment of shock

Emergency measures   Act promptly to identify the type of shock and take appropriate emergency measures:

1. Mentally review the patient's history and quickly do a physical assessment, looking for clues to the cause of shock, such as a site of active bleeding.

2. While summoning medical assistance, take these emergency measures:

A. For hemorrhagic shock, control bleeding if possible. For frank bleeding from hemodynamic lines, reconnect the line or shut it off between the break and the patient. For spontaneous blood vessel ruptures, apply direct pressure and elevate the site.

B. For hypovolemic shock, immediately increase blood volume by speeding up the administration rate of any intravenous solutions that do not contain drugs for which rapid or large dose administration would be harmful. Also place the person in Trendelenburg's position, which increases circulating blood volume 400–800 ml by promoting venous drainage from the legs. Do not use these measures for patients with cardiogenic shock, increased intracranial pressure, or active bleeding from the head and neck. Increasing the circulating blood volume can actively worsen these conditions. Trendelenburg's position also may compromise respiratory excursion.

To put the patient in Trendelenburg, tilt the bottom of the bed 1–3 feet automatically or with shock blocks so the whole body (rather than just the legs) is inclined. Sun (1971) recommends that you also place pillows under the head and left shoulder. The pillow under the head promotes venous drainage from the head and elevates its arterial resistance, thus reducing the possibility that an abrupt rise in arterial pressure will stimulate baroreceptors in the carotid sinus to cause reflex vasodilatation and cardiac deceleration. The pillow under the left shoulder improves drainage of the azygous and hemiazygous veins into the inferior vena cava.

C. Administer oxygen so that the blood that does reach the tissues is oxygenated optimally.

3. Assist the doctor in inserting an arterial line and a central venous or pulmonary artery (PA) line to monitor hemodynamic pressures. Insert a Foley catheter to monitor urinary output. Monitor these parameters every 15 minutes to 1 hour depending on the severity of shock and rapidity of its progression.

4. Establish baseline values and initial diagnostic data by recording a 12-lead ECG and by obtaining routine laboratory studies, such as a complete blood count; type and crossmatch; serum electrolytes; arterial blood gases; and urinalysis. Additional specimens such as blood cultures should be obtained as indicated. Lactate levels may be useful in assessing the degree and progression of shock, although Walt and Wilson (1975) point out that similar information can be obtained more readily with bicarbonate levels.

5. Administer sodium bicarbonate intravenously if ordered to buffer lactic acidosis. The need for bicarbonate should be determined by arterial blood gases; remember that some shock patients may be alkalotic instead of acidotic. Doses ideally should be titrated according to bicarbonate or lactate levels. Preferably administer the drug as a bolus rather than constant infusion, as the solution frequently precipitates if other drugs are added to it.

6. Administer a fluid challenge if the physician orders one. Evaluation of the preceding data frequently identifies the type(s) of shock present. For instance, a history of angina coupled with ECG signs of a recent infarct strongly suggest cardiogenic shock. In many cases, however, the data is equivocal. For example, a low blood pressure, CVP, and urinary output could be present in any type of shock. In such a case, the physician may want you to administer a fluid challenge to evaluate the hemodynamic response to an increased blood volume. Although the details vary among physicians, one common protocol follows. Measure the CVP and arterial pressure and auscultate the lungs immediately before the challenge. Administer 500 ml of colloid (plasma or salt-poor albumin) over 15 minutes. Monitor the pressures and lung sounds at least every 5 minutes during administration and again after its termination. The normovolemic patient responds by accommodating the fluid in his venous system, that is, his CVP

rises but his arterial pressure and urinary output remain constant. The hypovolemic patient, in whom sympathetic stimulation causes venous constriction, will show signs of an increased circulating volume, that is, his CVP will remain stable and his arterial pressure and urinary output will improve.

7. Assist the physician in treating the underlying cause of shock. Such treatment may include sending the patient to surgery to ligate bleeding vessels *(hemorrhagic shock)* or repair a postmyocardial infarction septal rupture *(cardiogenic shock)*, administering antihistamines *(anaphylactic shock)*, or starting intravenous antibiotics *(septic shock)*.

Stabilizing measures   Often, specific correction of the cause of shock is not the first line of defense but rather must wait until the patient's hemodynamic status is stabilized. The following measures are used to stabilize the shock patient and enhance tissue perfusion:

1. Maintain an appropriate circulating blood volume. Jahre, Grace, Greenbaum, and Sarg (1975) recommend that (in the patient without previously elevated cardiac pressures) the CVP be maintained at 12–14 mm Hg and the pulmonary capillary wedge pressure at 16–20 mm Hg to produce maximal stroke output.

Depending upon the patient's condition and the physician's preference, crystalloids, colloids, and/or blood may be given to restore volume. The relative merits and drawbacks of each remain the subject of considerable debate. The amount varies depending upon the volume lost and upon the degree of vascular capacitance; for example, the patient in septic shock may require more volume than normal. Walt and Wilson (1975) advise against the use of Ringer's lactate in conditions where lactate may not be metabolized properly, specifically severe cirrhosis and severe septic or other shock accompanied by metabolic alkalosis.

Whatever fluids are used, remember to closely monitor intake and output, follow the trend of vascular pressures, and watch for the signs of fluid depletion and overload, discussed in Chapter 6.

2. Administer pharmacologic agents ordered by the physician to improve myocardial contractility. *Digoxin* may be given as a loading dose of 0.5 mg IV followed by additional 0.25 mg doses every hour until an optimum therapeutic effect is achieved. The actions of digitalis and related nursing responsibilities are discussed in Chapter 3. Other agents which may improve contractility are *dopamine* and *isoproterenol*, discussed below and in Chapter 3.

3. Titrate to the desired blood pressure intravenous *vasopressors* and *vasodilators* ordered by the physician. A wide variety of pharmacologic agents can be used to promote cardiac output by altering peripheral vascular resistance. These drugs can be classified according to their effect on sympathetic nervous system receptor sites, called alpha and beta receptors. The heart contains only beta receptors and the blood vessels have both types. *Alpha-adrenergic* drugs constrict

peripheral blood vessels. *Beta-adrenergic* drugs dilate peripheral blood vessels and stimulate heart rate and contractility.

Since vasopressors and vasodilators are so potent, they often are given in extremely small dosages called micrograms (μg). They should be administered with a microdrop intravenous administration set and an infusion pump to be sure accidental under- or overdosage does not occur. Monitor the blood pressure every 2–5 minutes at the start and titrate the administration rate (within the limits set by the physician) to maintain the desired blood pressure.

A. For the patient with only slight tachycardia, no signs of myocardial irritability, and elevated peripheral vascular resistance, the agents most frequently prescribed are beta stimulators, such as isoproterenol (Isuprel) and low doses of dopamine (Intropin). Beta stimulators decrease peripheral vascular resistance and increase myocardial impulse formation and myocardial contractility to raise blood pressure.

Isoproterenol usually is given at a rate of 1–4 micrograms per minute, titrated to the desirable blood pressure. To calculate the number of micrograms per drop, first determine how many milligrams of drug are added to 1000 ml of solution. Divide by a thousand to get the number of micrograms per milliliter. From the brand of microdrop administration set used in your unit, determine the number of microdrops per milliliter. Compare that number with the micrograms per milliliter to obtain the microdrops per minute figure.

For example, suppose the physician ordered an isoproterenol infusion to start at 2μg/min. You have on hand ampules of 1 mg in 5 ml. Adding one ampule to 250 ml of 5% dextrose in water IV solution is the same as adding 4 ampules (4 mg) to 1000 ml of solution. Dividing by 1000 gives you 4 μg/ml. If your infusion set administers 60 microdrops per milliliter, and your solution contains 4 μg/ml, each 60 microdrops would contain 4 micrograms, and 30 microdrops per minute would contain the prescribed 2 micrograms.

Dopamine is being used increasingly as the agent of choice in all types of shock. It is an endogenous precursor to epinephrine. Dopamine is particularly valuable because it selectively dilates blood vessels to the kidneys, heart, brain, and mesentery while constricting other vessels. It is a mixed alpha and beta stimulator. At low doses its beta effects predominate, producing vasodilatation and cardiac stimulation. At high doses, its alpha effects predominate, producing increasing vasoconstriction. According to Jahre, Grace, Greenbaum, and Sarg (1975), 30–40 micrograms per kilogram per minute is the dividing line between low and high doses.

Dopamine is available as a 5 mg ampule containing 200 mg of drug. Adding one ampule to 250 ml of 5% dextrose in water gives a concentration of 800 μg/ml. The usual initial dose is 2–5 micrograms per kilogram per minute (2–5 μg/kg/min), with subsequent doses titrated to the patient's response.

When a patient is receiving a beta stimulator, be sure to observe for excessive beta stimulation, such as, tachyarrhythmias; premature beats; and signs of dangerously increased myocardial workload, such as angina or sudden ST–T changes. Headache may occur but is not an indicator for discontinuing these drugs.

B. If the patient has significant tachycardia, myocardial irritability, or low peripheral resistance (as in septic shock), beta stimulators will only worsen his problems. The most appropriate agent for these patients is one which is primarily an alpha stimulator, such as *norepinephrine* (Levophed) or the higher dosage range of dopamine.

To administer norepinephrine, dilute one ampule (4 mg) in 250 ml 5% dextrose in water to get a concentration of 16 μg/ml. The dose is titrated to the desirable blood pressure, with 2–4 μg/min the usual range. Use a long intravenous catheter whenever possible to minimize the danger of tissue infiltration. If infiltration does occur, notify the physician immediately so that he/she can infiltrate *phentolamine* (Regitine) to minimize tissue necrosis.

C. Cardiac output depends not only upon contractility but also upon preload (the length of myocardial fibers at the end of diastole, which depends upon fluid volume in the ventricles) and afterload (the resistance against which the left ventricle ejects blood). In some cases, peripheral vascular resistance may be so high it diminishes cardiac output. The physician then may prescribe phentolamine, an alpha receptor blocking agent, or sodium nitroprusside to dilate the vessels and thus lower peripheral resistance. The resulting venous dilatation reduces cardiac preload and the arterial dilatation reduces afterload (Moskowitz 1975).

Vasodilators are appropriate only for the shock patient with an expanded blood volume. Their use in hypovolemic or normovolemic patients can worsen shock by increasing the disparity between the capacity of the vascular bed and the fluid available to fill it. Therefore, measure pulmonary capillary wedge pressure before implementing afterload reduction therapy; call low or normal values to the physician's attention. During administration, monitor PCWP and arterial pressure. Because vasodilatation will stimulate renin production (see Chapter 7), you may need to increase the dose to maintain the desired effect. Keep the patient as flat as possible during the infusion and for two hours afterward; raising the head of the bed suddenly can precipitate orthostatic cerebral hypoperfusion.

4. If the above measures are ineffective, the physician may resort to more experimental forms of therapy. Devices to implement mechanical support of the cardiovascular system include a pneumatic suit on the lower extremities, an intra-aortic balloon pump, and prolonged cardiopulmonary bypass. Another controversial area is the use of steroids, particularly in massive doses. Some physicians believe steroids may minimize cell damage by stabilizing lysosomes

and may improve myocardial contractility. Others believe they are useless in shock or may promote gastric bleeding and ulceration. Often, many physicians will try steroids when standard therapy fails to produce improvement, on the theory that the patient's adrenal glands may be unable to secrete adequate levels of steroids due to prolonged or severe stress.

Prevention or relief of complications

Prevent or ameliorate the potential complications of shock: respiratory failure, renal failure, paralytic ileus, acute myocardial infarction, disseminated intravascular coagulation, and cardiopulmonary arrest.

Respiratory failure   Acute respiratory failure can result from microatelectasis, microemboli, increased shunting, increased pulmonary congestion, and worsening acidosis. It is particularly troublesome because it superimposes respiratory acidosis on metabolic acidosis, and the combination often is lethal. See Chapter 10 for information on the prevention, detection, and treatment of respiratory failure and Chapter 11 for acid-base abnormalities.

Renal failure   Acute renal failure is discussed in detail in Chapter 7. Briefly, monitor urinary volume and maintain output above 30 ml/hr. In addition to fluid administration, the physician may prescribe diuretics, usually mannitol, furosemide (Lasix) or ethacrynic acid (Edecrin). Monitor patients carefully during diuresis; fluid overload and congestive heart failure may occur with osmotic diuretics, rapid diuresis may provoke cardiovascular collapse, and a variety of electrolyte imbalances may develop during diuresis.

Paralytic ileus   Paralytic ileus may result from autonomic hyperactivity. Even if it does not, it is unwise to create an increased need for blood flow to the digestive organs at the very time blood is shunted preferentially away from them. For the duration of the shock episode, give the patient nothing by mouth. Before resuming oral feedings, be sure bowel sounds are present.

Acute myocardial infarction   Acute myocardial infarction can occur in shock if myocardial demand exceeds myocardial perfusion. See Chapter 4 for nursing care implications.

Disseminated intravascular coagulation (DIC)   Due to hypotension, lysosomal breakdown, acid-base changes, and other abnormalities, the clotting process often becomes deranged in uncontrolled shock. Disseminated intravascular coagulation may occur, first in the microcirculation and later in larger vessels. Factors which predispose to DIC are those which may activate the intrinsic clotting system (such as sepsis, severe prolonged hypotension, acidosis, or tranfusion reactions) or trigger the extrinsic system (such as massive destruction of tumor cells). Although the precipitating factor may vary, the common pathway is the activation of Factor X, conversion of prothrombin to thrombin, and conversion of fibrinogen to fibrin. Because of rapid, widespread clotting, platelets and clotting factors are consumed faster than they can be synthesized, and secondary fibrinolysis releases many fibrin degradation products into the bloodstream.

Suspect DIC when your patient bruises easily or develops acute frank bleeding, occult bleeding, or oozing from multiple sites. Skin lesions (petechiae, purpura, subcutaneous hematomas, or bleeding from incisions or puncture sites) occur in 84% of DIC episodes, according to Colman, Minna, and Robboy (1974). The urinary tract, bowel, and mucosa are other common bleeding sites. Serial laboratory tests reveal a low platelet level, prolonged prothrombin time, a low fibrinogen level, and increased fibrin degradation products.

DIC is attacked on two fronts: correction of the underlying cause and control of bleeding. Correction of the septicemia, hypotension, acidosis, or other underlying cause is vital. To control bleeding, heparin can be administered intravenously to antagonize thrombin. From 50–80 USP units per kilogram are given every 4 hours to prolong the clotting time to 2–3 times normal (Colman, Minna, and Robboy 1974). Fresh-frozen plasma, platelets, or cryoprecipitate may be necessary for patients bleeding severely. Mortality in DIC patients is distressingly high. While patients with mild or moderate bleeding may recover from the DIC episode, they often die from the underlying disease. Patients who bleed severely rarely survive.

Cardiopulmonary arrest   Cardiopulmonary arrest may result from hypoxia, severe hypovolemia, acid-base derangements, or electrolyte imbalances. See Chapter 3 for detailed directions on cardiopulmonary resuscitation.

Outcome evaluation

Evaluate the patient's progress toward vascular health. Without vasopressor or vasodilator support, the patient ideally should maintain these outcome criteria:

- Arterial blood pressure within ± 20 mm Hg of preshock levels
- Adequate perfusion of vital organs, as manifested by a return to preshock level of consciousness, cardiac status, and renal function
- Adequate peripheral perfusion, as manifested by warm, dry skin, and by peripheral pulse volume within the patient's normal limits
- Arterial blood gases and serum electrolytes within the patient's normal limits
- Prothrombin time, platelets, and fibrinogen level within normal limits.

References

American Heart Association. 1972. *Examination of the heart. Part two: inspection and palpation of venous and arterial pulses.* New York: American Heart Association.
Normal and abnormal pulse contours; examination techniques.

Anthony, C., and Kolthoff, N. 1975. *Textbook of anatomy and physiology.* St. Louis: C. V. Mosby Company.
Basic explanations of vascular anatomy and physiology.

Bates, B. 1974. *A guide to physical examination.* Philadelphia: J. B. Lippincott Company.
Techniques of physical assessment; particularly see Chapters 7 and 13 on vascular assessment.

Byrne, J. 1976. A review of the CBC: the quantitative tests.   *Nursing* 6 (10): 11–12.

―――― 1976. A review of the CBC: the differential white cell count. *Nursing* 6 (11): 15–17.

―――― 1977. Tips for interpreting the sedimentation rate and reticulocyte count. *Nursing* 7 (1): 9–10.

―――― 1977. Coagulation studies. Part II: Tests of plasma-clotting factors. *Nursing* 7 (6): 24–25.
These articles, part of a series in the monthly Lab Report column, briefly discuss normal, elevated, and depressed levels of common blood tests.

Colman, R., Minna, J., and Robboy, S. 1974. Disseminated intravascular coagulation: a problem in critical care medicine. *Heart Lung* 3:789–796.
Pathophysiology, diagnosis, prognosis, and problem-oriented approach to the DIC patient.

Fritz, S. 1974. Energy metabolism in shock. *Heart Lung* 4: 615–618.
Review of Krebs cycle; carbohydrate, lactate, lipid, and protein metabolism in shock.

Fowler, N. 1974. Pericardial disease. In *The heart.* 3rd ed., eds. J. Hurst and R. Logue, pp. 1387–1405. New York: McGraw-Hill Books, Inc.
Diagnosis and treatment of pericardial disorders, including possible mechanisms of paradoxical pulse.

Gifford, R., DeWolfe, V., and Young, J. 1974. Diseases of the peripheral arteries and veins. In *The heart.* 3rd ed., eds. J. Hurst and R. Logue, pp. 1598–1635. New York: McGraw-Hill Books, Inc.
Physical examination and differential diagnosis of peripheral vascular disorders, including acute arterial occlusion, aneurysms, and thrombophlebitis.

Guyton, A. 1976. *Textbook of medical physiology.* 5th ed. Philadelphia: W. B. Saunders Company.
Detailed physiology reference; especially see Chapters 5–7 on blood cells, Chapter 9 on hemostasis, and Chapters 18–22 and 26–28 on circulatory dynamics.

Hurst, J., and Schlant, R. 1974. Examination of the arterial pulse. In *The heart.* 3rd. ed., eds. J. Hurst and R. Logue, 170–179. New York: McGraw-Hill Books, Inc.

_____. Examination of the venous pulse. In *The heart*. 3rd ed., eds. J. Hurst and R. Logue, pp. 179–189. New York: McGraw-Hill Books, Inc.
Normal and pathophysiology of arterial and venous pulses; examination techniques. Particularly recommended for greater detail on pulse abnormalities.

Jahre, J., Grace, W., Greenbaum, D., and Sarg, M. 1975. Medical approach to the hypotensive patient and the patient in shock. *Heart Lung* 4: 577–587.
Highly recommended flow charts to guide diagnosis and therapy; pharmacologic agents, including recommended dosages.

Moskowitz, L. 1975. Vasodilator therapy in acute myocardial infarction. *Heart Lung* 4: 939–945.
Physiology and nursing implications related to use of sodium nitroprusside and phentolamine in cardiogenic shock.

Nutter, D., and Paulk, E. 1974. Measuring and recording systemic blood pressure. In *The heart*. 3rd ed., eds. J. Hurst and R. Logue, pp. 205–215. New York: McGraw-Hill Books, Inc.
Biophysics of blood pressure, measurement methods, diagnostic applications.

Schlant, R. 1974. Normal physiology of the cardiovascular system. In *The heart*. 3rd ed., eds. J. Hurst, and R. Logue, pp. 79–108. New York: McGraw-Hill Books, Inc.
Physiology related to arterial and venous pulses, myocardial function, and blood flow.

Schroeder, J., and Daily, E. 1976. *Techniques in bedside hemodynamic monitoring.* St. Louis: C. V. Mosby Company.
Invasive and noninvasive monitoring of cardiovascular dynamics.

Strand, M., and Elmer, L. 1976. *Clinical laboratory tests: a manual for nurses.* St. Louis: C. V. Mosby Company.
Descriptions of common laboratory tests, normal values, and related nursing implications.

Sun, R. 1971. Trendelenburg's position in hypovolemic shock. *Am. J. Nurs.* 71: 1758–59.
Physiological effects of this common antishock measure.

Walt, A., and Wilson, K. 1975. The treatment of shock. *Advances in Surgery* 9: 1–39.
Pathophysiology of early and late shock, diagnosis, and guidelines for treatment.

Supplemental Reading

DeBakey, M., and Beall, A. 1974. Surgical treatment of diseases of the aorta and major arteries. In *The heart*. 3rd. ed., eds. J. Hurst and R. Logue, pp. 1666–1683. New York: McGraw-Hill Books, Inc.
Locations and varieties of aneurysms; diagrams and aortograms before and after surgical repair.

Geske, C. 1972. Anticoagulant therapy in acute myocardial infarction. *Heart Lung* 1: 639–649.

Mechanisms of coagulation, anticoagulant drugs, and related nursing care. Also contains interesting section evaluating past anticoagulant studies against criteria for clinically valid trial of a therapy.

Taggart, E. 1977. The physical assessment of the patient with arterial disease. *Nurs. Clin. North America* 12: 109–117.

Brief review of assessment of symptoms and arterial pulses.

Chapter 6

Fluid and Electrolyte Imbalances

Fluid and electrolyte imbalances are common in the critically ill. This chapter discusses fluid, sodium, potassium, calcium, and magnesium imbalances and provides measures to assist you in nursing your patients more effectively.

Outline

Assessment Fluid intake and output/Body fluid osmolality/Electrolytes

Imbalances Fluid and sodium imbalances/Potassium imbalances/Calcium derangements/Magnesium imbalances

Objectives

- Monitor at least five items routinely in order to detect fluid and electrolyte imbalances
- Given a patient's sex, weight in kilograms, and general body size, state the approximate number of liters present as: a) intracellular fluid, b) plasma, and c) interstitial fluid
- Given a patient's weight loss in kilograms, state the number of liters of fluid he/she has lost
- List average fluid intake from: a) liquids, b) food, and c) oxidation of food and body tissues
- List average fluid output in: a) urine, b) insensible water loss, and c) feces
- Define obligatory fluid loss and give its average daily value

- Describe briefly how antidiuretic hormone, aldosterone, left atrial barorecep-tors, and arterial baroreceptors function to maintain extracellular volume and/or concentration
- Define osmolality and state the normal value for serum osmolality
- Define isotonic, hypotonic, and hypertonic solutions compared to plasma
- Name the primary electrolytes in: a) intracellular fluid, b) extracellular fluid, c) urine, and d) gastric juice
- Name the normal serum potassium, calcium, and magnesium concentrations
- Assess the patient for risk conditions, signs and symptoms of each imbalance
- Plan and implement appropriate nursing care for each imbalance
- Evaluate the patient according to outcome criteria

Assessment

As a critical care nurse, you should develop skill at effective intervention to protect the critically ill from the ravages of fluid and electrolyte imbalances. Such intervention requires you to maintain a high index of suspicion in conditions which increase the patient's vulnerability to such imbalances. You should antici-pate and forestall the development of these disorders whenever possible. If they do occur, you should recognize their signs and symptoms, alert the physician, and help him or her institute treatment early.

Table 6-1 presents a useful format for assessing the patient's fluid and elec-trolyte status. Assessment includes evaluation of serial body weights, fluid in-take and output, serum and urine osmolalites, serum and urine electrolytes, and signs and symptoms.

Serial body weights

Monitor serial body weights (daily in patients susceptible to fluid imbalances).

The proportion of body weight which is body fluid varies with the patient's sex and fat content; the following figures are from Weisberg (1962). In males, 50–70% of body weight is water. The percentage for an obese man is 50%, for an average man 60%, and for a lean man 70%. Women have more fat and less water than men. In females, body water averages 42% of body weight for an obese woman, 50% for an average sized woman, and 60% for a lean woman.

Body fluid is divided into two main compartments: intracellular and extracel-lular. Forty percent of body weight represents intracellular water, while 20% of body weight represents extracellular water. (Estimates of the volumes of fluid compartments vary considerably with the test substance used. The percentages given here are approximate and represent averages of those reported by various

Table 6-1   Fluid and electrolyte assessment format

1. History _____

2. Physical

    Weight _____

    Signs and symptoms _____

    _____

3. Diagnostic procedures and laboratory tests

    Intake and output (24 hr) _____

    Osmolality: serum _____ urine _____

    Electrolytes: serum Na^+ _____ K^+ _____ Cl^- _____

                Ca^{++} _____ Mg^{++} _____

         urine Na^+ _____ K^+ _____ Cl^- _____

    Other _____

4. Other relevant data _____

authors.) The extracellular compartment is subdivided into fluid outside the cells in the vascular system (plasma) and that outside the cells in body tissues and cavities (interstitial fluid). Plasma equals about 5% of body weight and interstitial fluid about 15%. Dynamic fluid exchange occurs continuously among the intracellular, plasma, and interstitial compartments. Of these three, only the plasma can be influenced directly by the intake of fluid from outside the body or by the elimination of fluid from the body. For instance, when you drink water, the first fluid compartment that is affected is the plasma. The intracellular and interstitial compartments then respond to changes in the volume or concentration of the plasma.

A rapid weight change (over 0.5 kg/day) suggests a fluid imbalance and often appears before other, more subtle signs and symptoms. Since a kilogram equals 2.2 lb and a liter of body fluid equals 2.2 lb, a general guideline is that each liter of fluid retained is reflected by a rapid weight gain of 1 kg, and each liter lost by a loss of 1 kg. A patient's weight therefore can serve as a valuable guide to estimating fluid deficit or excess. For example, suppose an average-sized male patient weighed 70 kg prior to surgery. Since 60% of his weight represents body water, his total fluid volume was 42 L. Forty percent (28 L) of his weight was intracellular water, 5% (3.5 L) plasma, and 15% (10.5 L) interstitial fluid. Now suppose his post-op weight is 66.5 kg, a loss of 3.5 kg. This is equivalent to a loss of 5% of his body weight, or 3.5 L from his total body fluid of 42 L.

The appearance of specific signs and symptoms can provide a rough guide to the degree of fluid loss (Weisberg 1962). Thirst, the earliest sign, appears when the fluid depletion is mild (about 2% of body weight). Extreme thirst, dry mouth and tongue, oliguria, and minor personality changes may indicate a moderately severe fluid loss (about 6% of body weight). Intensification of these signs with greatly diminished mental and physical capabilities point to very severe fluid depletion, 7–14% of body weight.

On the basis of the weight change, you could estimate that your patient has suffered a moderate fluid deficit and would require fluid replacement of 3.5 L.

Fluid intake and output

For the internal environment to remain in a steady state from day to day, the intake and output of fluids must be equal. In the healthy adult, intake or output varies between 1500 and 3000 ml daily. The major routes of water intake are ingestion of liquids (500–1700 ml), the ingestion of water in foods (800–1000 ml) and the oxidation of food and body tissues (200–300 ml). The primary normal routes of water output are urine (600–1600 ml), water vapor excreted through the lungs and skin (850–1200 ml), and feces (50–200 ml). There is an obligatory water loss of approximately 1500 ml daily: about 500 ml necessary to excrete metabolic wastes via the kidneys, plus about 1000 ml of water vapor from the lungs and skin (insensible water loss). Vaporization from the lungs and skin occurs even when water intake is zero. Urine is excreted only after the water needs for insensible water loss have been met.

The regulation of water intake and output is a fascinating subject which can be dealt with only briefly in this book. Oral intake is regulated by the thirst center, believed to be located in the anterolateral hypothalamus. When plasma osmolality increases or blood volume decreases, the person becomes thirsty and increases water intake.

Water output is under multiple controls, the most significant of which are antidiuretic hormone (ADH), aldosterone, and baroreceptors. ADH is a hormone made in the supraoptic nuclei and stored in the posterior pituitary gland. On the surface of the anterior hypothalamus are cells called *osmoreceptors* which sense changes in the concentration of the extracellular fluid which bathes them. When osmotic pressure increases, the supraoptic neurons discharge impulses to the posterior pituitary at a faster rate, so there is an increased release of ADH. Conversely, when osmotic pressure decreases, ADH release also falls. ADH travels in the bloodstream to the kidneys. There it alters tubular permeability to water, creating increased reabsorption of water (and therefore decreased urinary output). The retained water dilutes the extracellular fluid, reducing its concentration toward normal. The restoration of normal osmotic pressure then feeds back to the osmoreceptors to inhibit their discharge. The thirst center and supraoptic nuclei are close together, appear to respond to the same stimuli, and seem to be equally important in regulating water balance.

Aldosterone is a hormone secreted by the adrenal cortex in response to many stimuli. The most potent stimuli are a decreased serum sodium concentration or an increased level of angiotensin resulting from increased renin secretion by the juxtaglomerular apparatus in the kidneys. (See Chapter 7 for an explanation of the renin-angiotensin system). Aldosterone also travels in the bloodstream to the kidneys, where it is believed to cause the formation of carrier proteins or enzymes necessary for active sodium transport through the tubular epithelium of the distal tubule and collecting duct (Guyton 1976). An increased level of aldosterone therefore causes increased sodium retention and an obligatory increase in water retention, thus reducing the urinary output. The retained sodium and water serve to increase the volume of extracellular fluid and feed back to inhibit aldosterone secretion. In contrast to ADH, which is the major controller of extracellular fluid concentration, aldosterone is one of the major controllers of extracellular volume.

The other major controllers of extracellular volume are cells which sense pressure or stretch, called baroreceptors or stretch receptors. The following descriptions of baroreceptor function are based primarily upon Koushanpour (1976). Baroreceptors which sense low (venous) pressure changes are located in the left atrium. When left atrial pressure increases (as in fluid overload), these receptors send an increased frequency of impulses via the vagus nerve to the vasomotor center in the medulla, which connects with the supraoptic nuclei. Increased left atrial pressure thus results in decreased synthesis and release of ADH, permitting an increased urinary output to return the blood volume toward normal. Factors which stimulate the left atrial receptors are an absolute increase in blood volume, cold, and a recumbent posture. Cold and recumbency each causes a redistribution of blood volume so that the peripheral blood volume decreases and the central blood volume increases. Both cold and recumbency, therefore, tend to cause diuresis. Koushanpour states that left atrial receptors serve as a first line of defense for up to a 10% loss of total blood volume.

Baroreceptors that sense high (arterial) pressure changes are located in the arch of the aorta and in each carotid sinus, located just above the bifurcation of the internal and external carotid arteries. When arterial pressure drops, these receptors transmit more impulses from the carotid sinuses (via the Hering and glossopharyngeal nerves) and from the aortic arch (via the vagus nerves) to the vasomotor center. They stimulate the sympathetic (cardioaccelerator and vasoconstrictor) center and inhibit the parasympathetic (cardioinhibitor) center. As a result, heart rate accelerates and the peripheral vasculature constricts, increasing the central blood volume. At the same time, sympathetic stimulation constricts the renal afferent and efferent arterioles. This constriction reduces glomerular filtration pressure, so less water is excreted.

Body fluid osmolality

When you consider the concentration of body fluids, it is important to realize that concentration may be expressed in several different ways. The term *concen-*

tration in itself expresses the ratio between dissolved substances (solutes) and dissolving fluid (solvent).

You probably already are familiar with the use of weight and equivalent values to express concentration. Concentration expressed as weight is equal to the grams of solute per 100 ml of fluid; an example is a serum albumin value of 5 gm/100 ml, also reported sometimes as 5 gm/dl or 5 gm%. An *equivalent weight* equals the molecular weight of a substance divided by its valence. In clinical situations, the value is given as milliequivalents per liter of fluid (mEq/L). You are familiar with this method of reporting serum electrolyte values, for example, a serum sodium level of 140 mEq/L.

Concentration values which may be less familiar to you are osmolarity and osmolality. A *mol* is the gram molecular weight of a substance. An *osmol* is the gram molecular weight of a substance multiplied by the number of dissociating ions. For instance, urea does not dissociate in a solvent, so one mol of urea equals one osmol. Sodium chloride consists of two ions (Na^+ and Cl^-) which dissociate incompletely in a solvent, so one mol of sodium chloride equals 1.86 osmols per kilogram of solvent. Because of the small concentrations with which we work in clinical situations, values are expressed in thousandths of an osmol, that is, milliosmols (mOsm). Using this method, concentration can be described in terms of osmolarity or osmolality. The *osmolarity* of a solution is the solute concentration per volume of solution, or mOsm/L. The *osmolality* is the solute concentration per weight of solvent, or mOsm/kg of solvent. Both osmolarity and osmolality are measures of the ability of solutes to cause *osmosis*. Osmosis is the movement of water from a solution with fewer solute particles across a semipermeable membrane into a solution with more solute particles.

In clinical practice, osmolarity or osmolality often are preferred to other measures of concentration, such as specific gravity, milliequivalency, or weight, because they express the number of osmotically active particles without regard to their size, electrical charge, or molecular weight.

Because liquids expand and contract with changes in temperature, osmolarity (mOsm/L) may vary with temperature, but osmolality (mOsm/kg) does not. Normally in the body, solute concentrations are low and temperature is fairly constant. In these circumstances, the difference between osmolarity and osmolality is slight. For instance, the theoretical plasma osmolarity is about 310 mOsm/L, while its osmolality is about 310 mOsm/kg of plasma water. Actual measured osmolality is lower, about 285 mOsm/kg, due to the interaction of other constituents of plasma (Weisberg 1962).

Solute concentration can vary with the volume of a solution or with the amount of solute present in the solution. In the clinical setting, osmolality is the preferred measure of concentration when the state of hydration is undergoing rapid change, such as during the operative period, vomiting, diuresis, or burns.

Normally, the osmotic pressure exerted by nonelectrolytes in plasma can be ignored (Weisberg 1962). Osmolarity becomes important when the volume is relatively constant but there are abnormal amounts of nonelectrolytes in the solution, such as in diabetes mellitus, uremia, or proteinuria.

Urine osmolality is discussed in detail in Chapter 7.

Electrolytes

An *electrolyte* is a substance which will carry an electrical current when it is dissolved. The electrically charged particles into which it dissolves are called *ions*. Negatively charged ions are *anions,* and positively charged ones are *cations.* An ion may have one or more ionic bonds (places where it can bond with another ion). The number of ionic bonds per liter is expressed as milliequivalents per liter of fluid (mEq/L). For example, sodium chloride is an electrolyte. It dissolves into a cation, sodium (Na^+), and an anion, chloride (Cl^-). Each ion has one ionic bond. The normal serum concentration for sodium is 135–144 mEq/L and for chloride 96–106 mEq/L. (The reason sodium concentration is higher than chloride concentration is that additional sodium exists in the serum in forms other than Na Cl, for instance as sodium bicarbonate.)

Often you will hear an electrolyte solution described in terms of its *tonicity,* that is, its osmotic pressure as compared to that of another solution, such as plasma. The tonicity of plasma is about 310 mEq/L. Tonicity is determined by adding the mEq of particles which cannot be ionized (such as urea), the mEq of those which can be but are not (such as undissolved sodium bicarbonate), and the mEq of ionized particles (anions plus cations). If the sum is within the range of 250–375 mEq/L, the solution is said to be isotonic with plasma. If it is less than 250 mEq/L, the solution is called hypotonic, and if it is over 375 mEq/L, it is called hypertonic. The method of calculating tonicity explains why normal saline is isotonic with plasma in spite of the fact that normal saline contains more sodium and more chloride than plasma. (Isotonic saline contains 154 mEq/L each of sodium and chloride. Plasma has about 142 mEq/L of sodium and 102 mEq/L of chloride.) Although plasma contains less sodium and chloride, it includes protein, urea, and other substances which add to its tonicity.

Electrolytes are taken into the body in food and fluids. They are lost normally through sweat, which is hypotonic, and urine, which is hypertonic. They also may be lost through hemorrhage, vomiting, and diarrhea.

The distribution of electrolytes varies considerably within fluid compartments and body fluids. Figure 6-1 depicts these distributions graphically.

The signs and symptoms of fluid and electrolyte imbalances vary considerably. They are discussed under individual disorders below.

Imbalances

This chapter presents fluid, sodium, potassium, calcium, and magnesium imbalances. As you know, fluid balance and sodium balance are related intimately.

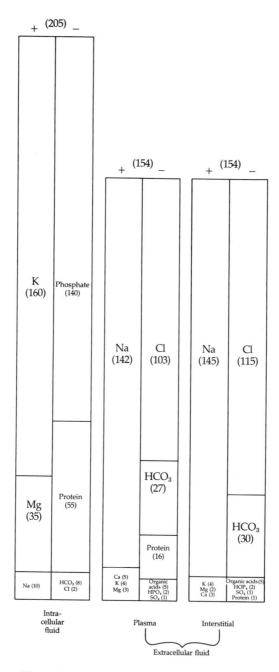

Figure 6-1.   Electrolyte composition of various body fluids. Concentrations given in approximate mEq/L. (Adapted from Fluid and Electrolytes © 1970 Abbott Laboratories.)

Since fluid and sodium imbalances have many common signs and symptoms, they are discussed together. Potassium, calcium, and magnesium imbalances are discussed separately. (For information on phosphate and chloride imbalances, see the supplemental reading section at the end of this chapter. For phosphate depletion, also see Chapter 12.)

Many sources present information on imbalances in a format that first names the condition and then describes its signs and symptoms. This approach is useful from the perspective of cognitive organization. It is difficult to transfer to the clinical setting, however, because it is the reverse of what happens with a patient, where you see the signs and symptoms first and then identify the condition causing them. Accordingly, this section will present the information in an innovative format that will increase its clinical relevance.

Fluid and sodium imbalances

In attempting to understand fluid and sodium imbalances, it is important for you to remember the relationship between the intracellular and extracellular compartments. As mentioned earlier, the normal ratio is for one third of total body water to be in the extracellular space and two thirds in the intracellular space.

The initial change in a fluid or sodium imbalance occurs in the extracellular space, and signs and symptoms of extracellular imbalances are more obvious than those of intracellular imbalances. For these reasons, this chapter categorizes fluid and sodium excesses and deficits first in terms of their extracellular effects. Although fluid intakes or losses initially affect the extracellular space, fluid readily moves across the cell membrane. Thus, you can anticipate that two thirds of a gain or loss of total body water will occur from inside the cells. You also can anticipate that changes in the extracellular sodium concentration will cause changes in intracellular volume. Signs of an intracellular fluid excess are confusion, headache, twitching, convulsions, and coma; signs of an intracellular fluid deficit are restlessness, delirium, weakness, and hyperpnea (Stroot, Lee, and Schaper 1974). With each extracellular imbalance, either an intracellular excess or deficit may coexist.

Extracellular volume deficits   Information on the types of extracellular deficits is summarized in Table 6-2.

1. A weight loss; decreased pulse volume, pulse pressure, and blood pressure; decreased urinary output; tachycardia; and dry skin and mucous membranes indicate the patient has an extracellular fluid deficit. Infants and the elderly are particularly susceptible to this condition, so be especially alert for these signs in them. There are three fluid and electrolyte imbalances which can cause these signs. The first is a decreased volume of isotonic fluid (hypovolemia). The second is true sodium depletion (depletional hyponatremia), and the third is

Table 6-2 Extracellular volume deficits

Predisposing conditions	Signs and symptoms	Disorder	Treatment
Anorexia Lethargy Unconsciousness Blood loss Loss of electrolyte-rich gastrointestinal secretions: vomiting, diarrhea, fistulas, suction Diaphoresis	Weight loss Decreased pulse volume Decreased blood pressure Decreased urinary output Dry skin and mucous membranes *Plus* Restlessness, weakness, delirium, hyperpnea *Plus* Normal serum sodium concentration	Extracellular deficit *Plus* Intracellular deficit *Owing to* Isotonic fluid loss (Hypovolemia)	Addition of fluid and electrolytes: Isotonic fluid replacement (example of isotonic fluid: normal saline)
Adrenal insufficiency Low sodium diet Renal disease	Weight loss Decreased pulse volume Decreased blood pressure Decreased urinary output Dry skin and mucous membranes *Plus* Confusion, headache, convulsions, coma *Plus* Decreased serum sodium concentration	Extracellular deficit *Plus* Intracellular excess *Owing to* Depletional hyponatremia	Addition of sodium: Isotonic or hypertonic fluid replacement (example of hypertonic fluid: 5% NaCl)
Decreased water intake Watery diarrhea Persistent osmotic diuresis Diabetes insipidus	Weight loss Decreased pulse volume Decreased blood pressure Decreased urinary output Dry skin and mucous membranes *Plus* Restlessness, weakness, delirium, hyperpnea *Plus* Increased serum sodium concentration	Extracellular deficit *Plus* Intracellular deficit *Owing to* Hypernatremia from loss of more water than sodium	Addition of fluid: Isotonic or hypotonic fluid replacement (example of hypotonic fluid: 0.45% NaCl)

hypernatremia due to an excessive water loss. These possible causes have radically different etiologies. Differential diagnosis depends upon the patient's history and upon the serum sodium concentration. The serum sodium concentration expresses the relationship between the amount of sodium in the serum and the volume of plasma. When plasma volume decreases without a proportional sodium loss, the sodium concentration rises. The key word here is "proportional": if both plasma and sodium are lost, but the plasma loss is greater than the sodium loss, the sodium *concentration* increases. (Sodium concentration also increases when a person gains more sodium than water. This condition, however, produces an extracellular volume excess and is discussed later in the chapter.) If more sodium is lost than water, the serum sodium concentration decreases. (Serum sodium concentration also decreases when a person gains more water than sodium, but that state also produces an extracellular volume excess and is discussed later.) In all three types of extracellular volume deficit, the urinary sodium concentration is low because the volume loss stimulates avid sodium retention by the kidneys.

2. Additional signs and symptoms will vary with the accompanying intracellular imbalance and with the cause.

A. Restlessness, weakness, delirium, or hyperpnea in addition to the extracellular signs indicate that the patient has an intracellular deficit along with the extracellular one. A normal serum sodium concentration (135–144 mEq/L), indicates that isotonic fluid must have been lost from the extracellular space (hypovolemia). This loss causes fluid and electrolytes to move out of the cell, so that both the extracellular and the intracellular compartments end up with volume deficits. Conditions which predispose to hypovolemia include anorexia, lethargy, unconsciousness, blood loss, and the loss of electrolyte-rich secretions through vomiting, diarrhea, fistulas, and nasogastric suction. As with any fluid or electrolyte disorder, such clues from the patient's history can be invaluable in identifying the imbalance present.

The treatment for hypovolemia requires replacement of both fluid and electrolytes with an isotonic solution. (Of course, one must treat the cause, too. This is such an obvious point that it will not be belabored in the remaining discussions.)

B. Confusion, convulsions, headache, or coma in addition to the manifestations of the extracellular deficit point to an accompanying intracellular excess. A low serum sodium concentration identifies hyponatremia as the cause. A history of diuretic use, adrenal (aldosterone) insufficiency, low sodium diet, or renal disease suggests that the patient has lost more sodium than water from the extracellular space and therefore has a true hyponatremia. Because of the decreased serum sodium concentration which results, only fluid moves from the serum into the cells. True hyponatremia thus produces an extracellular deficit and an intracellular excess. It is treated with isotonic solutions or, if the sodium depletion is severe, with hypertonic solutions.

C. The combination of signs of an extracellular deficit, intracellular excess (confusion, etc.), and elevated serum sodium concentration describes the disorder of hypernatremia secondary to a loss of more water than sodium. Because of the loss of fluid, serum sodium concentration rises. As a result, only fluid moves from the cell into the serum. This type of hypernatremia is characterized by both extracellular and intracellular volume deficits. Causes include decreased water intake, watery diarrhea, persistent osmotic diuresis, and diabetes insipidus. Hypernatremia resulting from a proportionally greater deficit of water than sodium is relieved by administering isotonic or hypotonic solutions.

As you can see, the possible causes of an extracellular volume deficit can be quite different. A constellation of the patient's history, indicators of an accompanying intracellular disorder, and serum sodium level point to a specific etiology and thus determine therapeutic intervention. For outcome criteria by which you can judge the patient's progress, see the end of the next section on extracellular volume excesses.

Extracellular volume excesses   Information on these disorders is given in Table 6-3.

1. Increased weight; increased pulse volume, pulse pressure, and blood pressure; increased urinary output; and edema suggest that the patient has an extracellular fluid excess. Three fluid and electrolyte imbalances can produce these signs and symptoms. The first is an increased volume of isotonic fluid. The second condition is dilutional hyponatremia, and the third is hypernatremia caused by an excessive intake of sodium.

2. Additional signs and symptoms will vary with the accompanying intracellular imbalance and the cause of the disorder.

A. Confusion, headache, twitching, convulsions, or coma indicate that the person has developed an intracellular excess in addition to the extracellular excess. The combination of intracellular and extracellular excesses can occur either as a result of the intake of isotonic fluid into the extracellular space or from dilutional hyponatremia.

Normal serum and urinary sodium concentrations confirm an isotonic imbalance. In this state, an increased volume of isotonic fluid in the extracellular space causes both fluid and electrolytes to move into the cell. The result is both an extracellular and an intracellular volume excess. Pathological conditions which can produce this imbalance include steroid therapy, chronic renal disease, severe congestive heart failure, and hyperaldosteronism. The treatment for isotonic excess is to remove both fluid and electrolytes by

Table 6-3 Extracellular volume excesses

Predisposing conditions	Signs and symptoms	Disorder	Treatment
Steroid therapy Chronic renal failure Severe congestive heart failure Hyperaldosteronism	Increased weight Increased blood pressure Increased pulse volume Increased urinary output Edema *Plus* Confusion, headache, convulsions, coma *Plus* Normal serum and urinary sodium concentrations	Extracellular excess *Plus* Intracellular excess *Owing to* Isotonic fluid overload	Removal of fluid and electrolytes: Limited intake Diuretics Salt-poor albumin Dialysis
Excessive water intake without accompanying salt Inappropriate increase in ADH secretion (certain cerebral and pulmonary disorders) Excessive tap water enemas Irrigation of gastric tubes with water instead of normal saline	Increased weight Increased blood pressure Increased pulse volume Increased urinary output Edema *Plus* Confusion, headache, convulsions, coma *Plus* Decreased serum and urinary sodium concentrations	Extracellular excess *Plus* Intracellular excess *Owing to* Dilutional hyponatremia	Removal of fluid: Restricted intake Diuretics
Excessive sodium intake without accompanying water Salt craving Excessive sodium bicarbonate administration	Increased weight Increased blood pressure Increased pulse volume Increased urinary output Edema *Plus* Restlessness, delirium, weakness, hyperpnea *Plus* Increased serum and urinary sodium values	Extracellular excess *Plus* Intracellular deficit *Owing to* Hypernatremia	Removal of sodium: Decreased intake Diuretics Hypotonic intravenous solutions

limiting their intake and utilizing diuretics, salt-poor albumin, or dialysis. Intravenous fluids usually are not indicated when isotonic excess is present.

B. Signs of an intracellular fluid excess plus low serum and urinary sodium levels implicate dilutional hyponatremia. Dilutional hyponatremia differs from the true hyponatremia discussed in the section on fluid deficits. In true hyponatremia, the patient has lost more sodium than water. In dilutional hyponatremia, in contrast, the patient has not lost sodium, but instead has diluted what he has by increasing the proportion of water to the sodium in his serum. The increased water decreases the serum sodium concentration, which in turn causes only water to move into the cell due to osmotic pull. This process produces both an extracellular and intracellular volume excess. Situations which may produce this state are excessive water intake without accompanying salt replacement (such as after sweating during strenuous exercise), excessive tap water enemas, and inappropriately increased ADH secretion (sometimes seen in lung tumors, pneumonia, cerebral tumors, and cerebral trauma). Dilutional hyponatremia usually responds to limited water intake and diuretic administration.

C. In addition to the signs of an extracellular excess listed above, the patient may have restlessness, delirium, weakness or hyperpnea and an elevated serum and urinary sodium concentration. This constellation of signs indicates that the extracellular excess is accompanied by an intracellular deficit, and points to an excessive sodium intake as the cause. The hypernatremia discussed under fluid deficits differs from the hypernatremia which causes fluid excess. The first type of hypernatremia was caused by the loss of proportionally more water than sodium. This second type results from an intake of more sodium than water, either through meals or hypertonic intravenous solutions. The serum sodium concentration rises, since the amount of sodium is increased in relation to the amount of water in the serum. The increased concentration of sodium outside the cell causes water to osmose to dilute the sodium. The result is an extracellular volume excess and an intracellular volume deficit. Hypernatremia due to excessive sodium intake is treated by restricting sodium intake, and administering diuretics or hypotonic intravenous solutions.

Outcome criteria   Evaluate the patient's progress toward healthy water and sodium balances according to these outcome criteria:

- Weight within normal limits (WNL) for patient
- Blood pressure and pulse volume normal for patient
- Level of consciousness and respiratory rate normal for patient
- Skin warm, dry, and with normal turgor
- Moist mucous membranes

- Urinary volume WNL for patient, ideally 600–1600 ml/24 hr
- Serum sodium normal for patient, ideally 135–144 mEq/L
- Urinary sodium WNL for patient, ideally 50–130 mEq/L
- Serum osmolality WNL for patient, ideally 285–295 mOsm/kg
- Urinary osmolality WNL for patient, ideally 500–800 mOsm/kg

Potassium imbalances

Roles of potassium   Potassium is a cation that functions in neuromuscular activity and in acid-base balance. Nearly 98% of total body potassium is found inside cells, approximately 160 mEq/L. High potassium concentrations also are found in gastric juice (9 mEq/L), bile, and pancreatic secretions. The serum and interstitial compartments contain 3.5–5.3 mEq/L. Although large fluctuations in intracellular potassium are tolerated by the body, even small fluctuations in serum potassium can be toxic.

Potassium is freely filtered at the glomerulus and most of it is reabsorbed in the proximal renal tubule. Potassium excretion varies with sodium retention. Under the influence of aldosterone, the tubule will increase reabsorption of sodium and secretion of potassium. Normal urinary loss averages 40 mEq/L and must be replaced by daily potassium intake. The kidney does not conserve potassium effectively and urinary losses will continue even in the face of a potassium deficit.

Hypokalemia and hyperkalemia   Information on these conditions is summarized in Table 6-4.

Be alert for patients prone to develop potassium imbalances. Conditions which increase susceptibility to hypokalemia are numerous. Broad causes are inadequate dietary intake, loss of gastrointestinal secretions, increased urinary loss, aldosterone excess, and acid-base imbalances. Conditions predisposing to hyperkalemia are excessive potassium intake, cellular breakdown, decreased urinary output, aldosterone deficiency, and acid-base imbalances.

The mechanisms by which acid-base imbalances can cause potassium imbalances require elaboration. Body cells contain buffer systems which can either accept or donate H^+ ions. Hydrogen ions and potassium ions freely exchange across the cell membrane. Since the amount of extracellular potassium is quite small compared to the intracellular amount, even small shifts of K^+ across the cell membrane cause significant changes in the serum level. In acidosis, excess H^+ ions in the serum migrate into the cells, where their buffering displaces K^+ ions. To maintain intracellular electrical balance, the K^+ ions diffuse out into the serum. As a result, acidosis can cause hyperkalemia. In alkalosis, the reverse is true. The intracellular buffers dissociate to release H^+ ions. As they move out of the cells, K^+ ions move in. Thus, alkalosis can cause hypokalemia. These rela-

Table 6-4 Potassium Imbalances

Predisposing conditions	Signs and symptoms	Disorder	Treatment
Lethargy, anorexia, coma, postoperative fasting: inadequate dietary intake Persistent vomiting, diarrhea, gastrointestinal drainage, fistulas: loss of gastrointestinal secretions Diuretics, diabetic acidosis, diuretic phase of renal failure: increased urine output Severe prolonged stress, corticosteroid therapy, adrenal tumor, Cushing's disease: aldosterone excess Alkalosis	Flattened T waves Prominent U waves Peaked P waves Prolonged PR interval Ventricular asystole or fibrillation Digitalis toxicity Hypoactive reflexes Paresthesias Weakness, fatigue Cramps Respiratory arrest Abdominal distention, ileus, anorexia, nausea, vomiting	Hypokalemia	Correction of alkalosis Increased potassium intake: foods, oral supplements, intravenous solutions Treatment of cause
Rapid IV potassium administration: excessive intake Crush injury, burns, stored bank blood transfusions: cellular breakdown Oliguric phase of renal failure: decreased urine output Addison's disease: aldosterone deficiency Acidosis	Tall, peaked T waves Prolonged PR interval Prolonged QRS duration with decreased height of R wave Hyperactive reflexes Weakness Cramps Twitching Abdominal cramps, diarrhea *Later:* Absent P waves Bradycardia, escape rhythms Ventricular asystole or fibrillation Paresthesias, paralysis Intestinal ileus	Hyperkalemia	Correction of acidosis Limited potassium intake Ion exchange resins Dialysis Insulin and dextrose infusion Treatment of cause

tionships are true in the initial stages of the imbalance, *if* the patient's serum potassium level was normal at the start. If not, the acid-base imbalance can mask a potassium imbalance. For example, an initially hypokalemic patient could show a normal serum potassium level during acidosis.

The kidney's sodium/potassium/hydrogen ion exchange mechanism also influences the interrelationship of acid-base and potassium balance. In acidosis, the kidney preferentially retains sodium ions in exchange for hydrogen ions. The excess hydrogen ions block the secretion of potassium ions, causing a potassium excess. In alkalosis, the kidney keeps hydrogen ions and sodium in exchange for potassium. The excretion of potassium ions leads to hypokalemia.

The mechanisms by which potassium imbalances cause acid-base imbalances are discussed in Chapter 11.

Preventive measures   Whenever possible, use the following measures to prevent the development of potassium imbalances. Consult the physician about adding potassium to the intravenous fluids of patients fasting postoperatively, particularly if they have gastrointestinal suction or diarrhea. Monitor serum potassium levels of patients on potassium-wasting diuretics, especially furosemide and ethacrynic acid. Be particularly alert with patients receiving both diuretics and digitalis, since hypokalemia potentiates digitalis toxicity (see Chapter 3 for further details). If it is necessary to transfuse patients in renal failure, use fresh blood; as stored blood ages, its cells break down and release potassium.

Signs and symptoms of hypokalemia   Monitor the patient for the signs and symptoms of potassium imbalances. These are easier to understand and remember if you can recall the effect of K^+ on the resting membrane potential and its role in the sodium-potassium pump. (See Chapter 2 for a review if necessary.)

During hypokalemia, the serum deficit allows K^+ to move out of the cell more easily than normal. The result is an increased negativity inside the cell, which reduces membrane excitability, making depolarization more difficult and altering repolarization. The decreased responsiveness to stimuli may be manifested on the ECG as flattened T waves, prominent U waves, peaked P waves, and prolonged PR intervals (Figure 6-2). Since hypokalemia potentiates the actions of digitalis, you may see rhythms common in digitalis toxicity, such as paroxysmal atrial tachycardia. Ventricular asystole or fibrillation also may occur. Skeletal muscle depression appears as hypoactive deep tendon reflexes, paresthesias, weakness, cramps, and fatigue. Smooth muscle hypoactivity causes the gastrointestinal symptoms of distention, ileus, anorexia, nausea, and vomiting.

Signs and symptoms of hyperkalemia   In hyperkalemia, the excess serum K^+ opposes the normal K^+ leak from the cell in its resting state. As a result, the inside of the cell becomes less negative (more positive) than usual. A fewer

Hyperkalemia

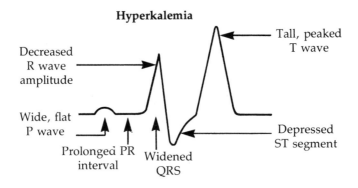

Decreased
R wave
amplitude

Tall, peaked
T wave

Wide, flat
P wave

Prolonged PR
interval

Widened
QRS

Depressed
ST segment

Normokalemia

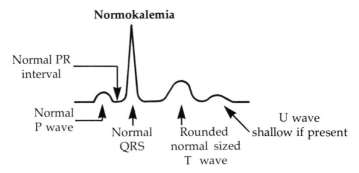

Normal PR
interval

Normal
P wave

Normal
QRS

Rounded
normal sized
T wave

U wave
shallow if present

Hypokalemia

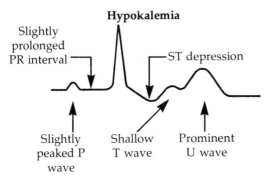

Slightly
prolonged
PR interval

ST depression

Slightly
peaked P
wave

Shallow
T wave

Prominent
U wave

Figure 6-2.   Effects of potassium levels on ECG.

number of positive ions must flow in to initiate depolarization, so the cell fires more easily. Depolarization is prolonged, and repolarization is shortened. As hyperkalemia worsens, however, the cell eventually has too many positive charges inside it to respond to a stimulus. Impulse formation and transmission slow and eventually cease.

Progression of hyperkalemia often is associated with specific ECG signs, according to Wenger and Herndon (1974). The earliest sign, which appears at a serum potassium level of about 5.5 mEq/L, is shortened repolarization, seen as tall, symmetrical, peaked T waves. At 6.5 mEq/L, the decreased rate of ventricular depolarization is manifested by prolonged QRS durations with diminished R wave amplitude (Figure 6-2). Above 7 mEq/L, atrial conduction slows, producing flattened P waves and prolonged PR intervals. Above 8–9 mEq/L, atrial excitability ceases and P waves disappear, although QRS complexes continue. The QRS complexes eventually widen so much they merge with T waves to form sine wave configurations. This abnormality occurs because some areas of the myocardium still are undergoing depolarization while others are being repolarized. Among the arrhythmias which may appear with hyperkalemia are tachycardias, premature beats, atrial fibrillation, bradycardia, escape rhythms, and sinus arrest. Above 10 mEq/L, complete atrioventricular dissociation, ventricular fibrillation, or ventricular asystole occur.

In the earlier stages of hyperkalemia, skeletal muscle excitability is manifested by hyperactive deep tendon reflexes, weakness, cramps, and twitching. Smooth muscle hyperactivity appears as abdominal cramps and diarrhea. During the later stages of hyperkalemia, when cellular excitability diminishes, skeletal muscle depression produces paresthesias and paralysis, and smooth muscle hypotonicity causes intestinal ileus.

Alert the physician promptly if you suspect a potassium imbalance. Obtain serial serum potassium levels to monitor the patient's progress. Remember, however, that the serum potassium is not an accurate indicator of the state of intracellular potassium imbalance.

Treatment   Minimize the effects of the imbalance while you assist the physician to treat the disorder.

For hypokalemia, implement the following measures:

1. Conserve the patient's energy to lessen weakness and fatigue.

2. Relieve gastrointestinal discomfort symptomatically.

3. Be prepared for emergency defibrillation, cardiac massage, and artificial respiration if the person arrests.

4. Assist the physician to treat the underlying cause and to correct alkalosis if present (see Chapter 11 for details).

5. Increase the oral intake of potassium by giving K$^+$ rich foods, such as oranges, bananas, dried figs, and peaches, or oral potassium supplements if ordered. Oral potassium can produce small bowel lesions, so alert the physician if the patient develops abdominal distention, pain, or gastrointestinal bleeding.

6. Administer intravenous potassium as ordered by the physician. Be sure that the patient has an adequate urinary output before giving increased oral or intravenous potassium; decreased renal excretion can quickly convert therapy for hypokalemia into precipitation of hyperkalemia. Dilute intravenous potassium and administer it slowly. Rapid intravenous administration of potassium can exceed the kidney's ability to excrete a surplus, and create hyperkalemia. For

this reason, do not exceed a rate of 20 mEq/hr unless the patient is on a cardiac monitor and the physician specifically orders a faster rate.

7. Teach patients, especially those to be discharged on digitalis or diuretics, the importance of eating potassium-rich foods at home, the signs and symptoms of hypokalemia, and the necessity of prompt medical attention if they appear.

The treatment of hyperkalemia varies with its severity. The following recommendations are based upon Levinsky and Alexander (1976).

Minimal hyperkalemia is characterized by a serum potassium level of 5.5–6.5 mEq/L and a normal ECG. Administer cation exchange resins as ordered by the physician. The one most commonly used is sodium polystyrene sulfonate (Kayexalate), given orally or by retention enema.

Moderate hyperkalemia is present when the serum potassium level is 6.5–7.5 mEq/L and/or the ECG shows peaked T waves. Immediate intravenous therapy is recommended to shift the excess potassium from the serum into the intracellular fluid. A hypertonic glucose and insulin infusion is usually effective within half an hour. The potassium apparently is carried in along with the dextrose, while the insulin facilitates the entrance of dextrose into the cell. If the patient is acidotic but not fluid overloaded, sodium bicarbonate may be added to the infusion; correcting the acidosis will drive some potassium back into the cells.

Severe hyperkalemia is present when the serum potassium level exceeds 7.5 mEq/L, or the ECG shows absent P waves, widened QRS complexes, or ventricular arrhythmias. To relieve cardiac toxicity, potassium can be antagonized by the intravenous administration of calcium gluconate. This treatment does not lower the serum potassium level. Its effects are rapid but transient, so it must be followed by intravenous glucose and bicarbonate therapy.

Levinsky and Alexander point out that dialysis requires several hours to lower serum potassium. It therefore is more useful in the prevention of hyperkalemia than in immediate therapy of moderate or severe hyperkalemia.

Outcome criteria   Use the following outcome criteria to gauge the patient's progress toward a healthy potassium balance:

- Serum potassium WNL for patient, ideally 3.5–5.3 mEq/L
- Arterial blood gases WNL for patient, ideally pH 7.35–7.45, PO_2 70–100 mmHg, PCO_2 35–45 mmHg, and HCO_3 23–28 mEq/L
- ECG normal for patient, ideally with normal sinus rhythm, rounded P waves, PR interval 0.12–0.20 seconds, QRS duration 0.06–0.12 seconds, rounded T waves
- Deep tendon reflexes, neuromuscular irritability, and muscular strength normal for patient
- Gastrointestinal function WNL for patient

Calcium derangements

Roles of calcium   Calcium (Ca^{++}) is important in neuromuscular excitability, muscular contractility, bone and tooth formation, and blood clotting. The following explanations of its roles in neuromuscular excitability and contraction are based upon Guyton (1976). Calcium is believed to bind with cellular membranes, near the openings of sodium channels. Its positive charges theoretically block the entrance of sodium. It thus helps to establish the normal resting membrane potential, in which the cell is more negative on the inside than the outside of the membrane. When a sufficient stimulus occurs, the calcium supposedly is displaced from the pores and sodium enters the cell, initiating depolarization.

Calcium also plays an important role in muscular contractility. Skeletal, cardiac, and smooth muscle all contain myofibrils of protein called actin and myosin. One current theory of contractility postulates that the actin and the myosin are inhibited from interacting in the resting state. When a stimulus causes depolarization, calcium ions are released from their storage sites. In skeletal and cardiac muscle cells, the sites are believed to be in sacs abutting the longitudinal and transverse tubules. In smooth muscle, there may be a storage site in the cell or calcium may diffuse in from the interstitial fluid. The calcium allows actin and myosin to link up in cross-bridges. The subsequent breaking and reforming of the cross-bridges pulls the actin and myosin filaments closer together, producing the muscle contraction.

In blood coagulation, calcium is thought to be essential in the formation of prothrombin activator by the intrinsic and extrinsic pathways, the conversion of prothrombin to thrombin, and possibly the conversion of fibrinogen to fibrin threads.

Most of the calcium in the body is contained in the bones. (Because of this large reservoir, it is unnecessary to add calcium to routine intravenous solutions.) Calcium exists in three forms in the serum: one ionized form and two nonionized forms. The ionized calcium, about 45% of the total plasma calcium, is the form that is important physiologically. The nonionized calcium is bound to plasma proteins or complexes such as citrate. The serum calcium level may be reported in two ways: as ionized calcium or as total calcium. The routine serum calcium level measures total calcium. Its normal value is 8.5 –10.8 mg%. The total plasma calcium report does not indicate the portion which is ionized.

The ionized portion varies with the pH of the blood and with the level of plasma proteins. As the pH becomes more acidic, ionization increases. As it becomes more basic, ionization decreases. The ionized portion also varies inversely with the nonionized, protein bound portion. A deficit of ionized calcium is called hypocalcemia. An excess of ionized calcium is known as hypercalcemia.

Calcium is absorbed from foods in the presence of normal gastric acidity and Vitamin D. About 87% of calcium is excreted in the feces and the remainder is in the urine. The serum calcium is controlled by two feedback loops, one involving parathyroid hormone and the other involving calcitonin. (The parathyroid glands also control the serum phosphorus level inversely with calcium.) When ionized serum calcium drops, the glands secrete increased parathyroid hormone. This hormone causes increased calcium absorption from the gastrointestinal tract and increased calcium reabsorption from the renal tubule and bone. The resulting rise in calcium ion concentration feeds back to lower parathyroid hormone secretion. This control mechanism is slow, taking hours to days to function. When ionized calcium rises excessively, the thyroid gland secretes calcitonin. This substance acts quickly and briefly to inhibit calcium reabsorption from bone. Acute changes in serum calcium also are buffered by the easily exchangeable calcium in the bones and some mitochondria.

Hypocalcemia and hypercalcemia   Information on these conditions is summarized in Table 6-5.

Be alert for conditions which can lead to calcium imbalances. Hypocalcemia occurs in conditions characterized by decreased calcium absorption, decreased calcium ionization, or increased calcium losses. Increased calcium intake, acidotic conditions, increased bone reabsorption, and malignant tumors predispose to hypercalcemia.

Preventive measures   Try to prevent calcium imbalances through such measures as active or passive range of motion exercises for patients confined to bed and prompt correction of prolonged vomiting or other conditions leading to alkalosis.

Signs and symptoms of hypocalcemia   Watch for the signs and symptoms of hypocalcemia and hypercalcemia. As with potassium imbalances, these are easier to remember if you understand the roles calcium plays in the body.

A calcium deficit (hypocalcemia) increases neuronal membrane permeability and allows sodium to enter the cell more easily than usual, facilitating spontaneous depolarization. Although this effect occurs in both the central and peripheral nervous systems, most manifestations appear peripherally. Central nervous system manifestations include irritability and convulsions. Early peripheral nervous system signs are hyperactive reflexes, twitching, and muscular cramps. Smooth muscle hyperactivity may cause diarrhea, nausea, and vomiting. Spasmodic muscular contractions (tetany) may occur. At first, tetany may not be apparent unless you add another stimulus to depolarization, such as tapping the nerve or causing ischemia, or unless hyperventilation worsens the hypocalcemia by reducing calcium ionization. If you tap the facial nerve just below the temporal bone anterior to the ear, the facial muscles on that side of the head may twitch. This result is called a positive Chvostek's sign. Similarly, you can apply a blood pressure cuff to the arm and raise its pressure slightly above the patient's systolic level. If the hand folds in, carpal spasm (tetany of the hand) is present. This spasm following pressure on the nerves and vessels of the upper arm is known

Table 6-5 Calcium imbalances

Predisposing conditions	Signs and symptoms	Disorder	Treatment
Vitamin D deficit, hypoparathyroidism: decreased calcium absorption Alkalosis: decreased ionization of calcium Massive subcutaneous infection, generalized peritonitis: Immobilization of calcium in inflamed tissues Diarrhea, acute pancreatitis: increased gastrointestinal loss Diuretic phase of renal failure: increased urinary loss Massive transfusions of citrated blood: increased calcium binding	Irritability Convulsions Hyperactive deep tendon reflexes Twitching Muscular cramps Diarrhea, nausea, vomiting Positive Chvostek's sign Positive Trousseau's sign Carpopedal spasms Generalized tetany Prolonged QT interval	Hypocalcemia	Seizure precautions Possible emergency tracheotomy Calcium administration Treatment of cause
Vitamin D excess, hyperparathyroidism: increased calcium intake Oliguric phase of renal failure: decreased urinary loss Acidosis: increased ionization Prolonged immobilization: increased reabsorption from bone Malignant tumors (with or without metastasis to bone)	Lethargy Coma Constipation, nausea, vomiting Hypoactive deep tendon reflexes Weakness Shortened QT interval Bradycardia, heart blocks Digitalis toxicity Polyuria, thirst, dehydration Renal calculi, flank pain Deep bone pain, pathological fractures	Hypercalcemia	Gentle handling Ambulation, exercises Intake/output recording Adequate hydration Straining of urine Observation for digitalis toxicity Reduced digitalis doses Phosphate administration Acidification of urine Treatment of cause

as a positive Trousseau's sign and is indicative of latent tetany. As hypocalcemia progresses to approximately 6 mg%, tetany will appear even without added stimuli (Guyton 1976). Generalized tetany eventually leads to death from laryngospasm.

Prolonged ventricular systole, seen on the ECG as a prolonged QT interval, occurs at approximately 5 mg% (Guyton 1971). Hypocalcemia theoretically causes arrhythmias, diminished cardiac contractility, and bleeding due to inadequate clotting. In reality, however, death from tetany usually occurs first at about 4 mg% (Guyton 1976).

Signs and symptoms of hypercalcemia   A calcium excess diminishes neuromuscular excitability theoretically because the extra calcium in the cellular pores repels sodium. Decreased excitability of the central nervous system is seen as lethargy or coma. Gastrointestinal signs include constipation, nausea, and vomiting. The skeletal muscles display hypoactive deep tendon reflexes and weakness. The ECG shows a shortened QT interval, indicative of a shortened ventricular systole. Decreased impulse formation and conduction may appear as bradycardia or heart blocks. Since hypercalcemia potentiates the effects of digitalis, rhythms of digitalis toxcity may occur. Because hypercalcemia impairs glomerular filtration and the kidneys' ability to concentrate urine, polyuria occurs and leads to thirst and dehydration. Renal calculi and flank pain also may appear. In hyperparathyroidism, increased parathyroid hormone causes excessive calcium reabsorption from the bones, and deep bone pain and pathological fractures may bedevil the patient. The effects of hypercalcemia begin at approximately 12 mg% and worsen as the level rises. Near 17 mg%, calcium precipitates in the body tissues themselves (Guyton 1976).

It sometimes is difficult to understand why a decrease in calcium ions causes tetany, yet an increase in calcium ions stimulates the heart during a cardiac arrest. To sort out the confusion, it helps to remember that in general too little calcium is followed by the sequence of increased membrane permeability, increased membrane excitability, weaker membrane action potentials, and weaker contractions. The association of hypocalcemia, tetany, and weak contractions follows logically from this sequence. An increased calcium level causes diminished membrane permeability, decreased membrane excitability, stronger membrane action potentials, and stronger contractions. These effects are put to therapeutic use in the treatment of cardiac arrest, when an intracardiac injection of calcium is administered to reestablish normal cardiac excitability, increase the strength of myocardial contraction, or make ventricular fibrillatory movements coarser so that defibrillation attempts are more likely to be successful.

Serum report   Alert the physician if you suspect a calcium imbalance. An ionized serum calcium reading will confirm the imbalance. A total serum calcium report may not reveal the imbalance, since it does not indicate the proportion that is ionized. There are three situations in which the total plasma calcium report may be misleading:

1. Total serum calcium is low because of a deficit of plasma proteins. As the plasma protein level decreases, the proportion of nonionized calcium also decreases, and the proportion of ionized calcium rises. This patient will not show signs of hypocalcemia, because that condition is a deficit of ionized calcium.

2. Total serum calcium is low, and the patient has acidosis. Since acidosis increases ionized calcium, the patient will not have signs of hypocalcemia until the acidosis is corrected.

3. Total serum calcium is normal, and the patient has alkalosis. Since alkalosis decreases ionized calcium, this patient will show signs of hypocalcemia until the alkalosis is corrected.

Treatment   Prevent complications of the imbalance while you assist the physician in treating it. Implement these measures for hypocalcemia:

1. Minimize the likelihood and effects of seizures by reducing environmental stimuli and placing the patient on seizure precautions.
2. Be prepared to assist with an emergency tracheotomy if laryngospasm occurs.
3. Administer calcium chloride, gluconate, or gluceptate as ordered by the physician. Do not add calcium to intravenous solutions containing bicarbonate or phosphate; it will precipitate.
4. Implement medical orders aimed at removing the cause of the calcium deficit.

For hypercalcemia, your nursing care should include these interventions:

1. Maintain ambulation or active or passive exercises to minimize bone cavitation. Avoid rough handling or trauma, which increase bone pain and can induce pathologic fractures.
2. Record intake and output. Because hypercalcemia impairs the kidney's ability to concentrate urine, urinary output will be high. Be sure intake is at least 1000 ml over output to prevent dehydration.
3. Encourage a fluid intake of at least 4000 ml daily to minimize possible precipitation of calcium as renal calculi. Maintain an acid urine by encouraging the intake of foods which acidify urine (such as cranberry juice) and by preventing urinary infections, which alkalinize the urine.
4. Strain all urine for renal calculi.
5. For patients on digitalis preparations, observe closely for signs of digitalis intoxication. Ask the physician about reducing digitalis doses.
6. Administer intravenous or oral phosphate if ordered by the physician to increase calcium excretion.
7. Aid the physician in treating the cause.

Outcome criteria   Evaluate the patient's progress toward restoration of normal calcium balance according to the following outcome criteria.

- Serum calcium level 8.5–10.8 mg%
- Normal deep tendon reflexes, muscular strength, and irritability (for example, negative Chvostek's sign and Trousseau's sign; no carpopedal spasms or other signs of tetany)
- Gastrointestinal function and urinary output normal for patient
- Signs or symptoms of deep bone pain, renal calculi, or pathologic fractures absent or controlled by therapy

Magnesium imbalances

Roles of magnesium   Magnesium is an essential catalyst for many important enzyme systems, especially those involved with carbohydrate metabolism and protein synthesis. It also is instrumental in the maintenance of normal ionic balance, osmotic pressure, neuromuscular transmission, and bone metabolism.

Magnesium is primarily an intracellular cation; a small amount (1.5–2 mEq/L) is found extracellularly. About half of the body's total is found in bones, with the remainder in muscles, soft tissues, and body fluids. Magnesium must be ingested daily. The body's requirement usually is met through eating chlorophyll-containing vegetables, meat, milk, and fruits. Extracellular magnesium concentration is regulated by the kidneys, though the mechanism is unclear.

Hypomagnesemia and hypermagnesemia   Information on these conditions is summarized in Table 6-6.

Be on the lookout for conditions which increase the patient's susceptibility to these disorders. Conditions disposing to magnesium depletion are those characterized by decreased intake or absorption and those resulting from increased urinary excretion. States predisposing to magnesium intoxication are less frequent: excessive parenteral administration and oliguric renal failure.

Prevention   Take measures to prevent magnesium imbalances. To avoid hypomagnesemia, encourage patients on oral intake to eat magnesium-containing foods. Ask the physician about magnesium supplements for alcoholic or malnourished patients, those suffering from excessive diarrhea or diuresis, and those receiving total parenteral nutrition.

To forestall hypermagnesemia, do not give drugs containing magnesium (such as antacids containing magnesium hydroxide) to patients in oliguric renal failure. When administering magnesium sulfate intravenously, do not exceed the rate recommended by the physician and watch for the signs of magnesium intoxication.

Signs and symptoms   Recognize the signs of magnesium disorders. Magnesium depletion causes increased neuronal excitability and neuromuscular

Table 6-6 Magnesium imbalances

Predisposing conditions	Signs and symptoms	Disorder	Treatment
Malnutrition, severe diarrhea: decreased intake or absorption	Twitches Muscle cramps Convulsions Tetany	Hypomagnesemia	Increased intake of magnesium-rich foods (chlorophyll-containing vegetables, meat, milk, fruits)
Alcoholism: cause unclear			Magnesium supplementation (oral or intravenous)
Diuretic phase of renal failure, diuretics: increased urinary loss			Treatment of cause
Hyperaldosteronism			
Hyperparathyroidism			
Oliguric phase of renal failure: decreased urinary excretion	Flushing Tachycardia leading to bradycardia Prolonged PR interval Prolonged QRS	Hypermagnesemia	Decreased intake of magnesium-rich foods
Excessive parenteral administration	Increased T wave amplitude Loss of deep tendon reflexes Respiratory arrest		Use of non-magnesium antacids
			Slowing or discontinuation of parenteral magnesium
			Dialysis

conduction. At a serum concentration of 1 mEq/L or less, you may see twitches, muscle cramps, convulsions, or tetany. There are no diagnostic ECG signs.

Magnesium intoxication depresses neuronal excitability and neuromuscular transmission. (These depressive effects sometimes are used therapeutically in the treatment of refractory supra-ventricular and ventricular extrasystoles and tachycardias, though magnesium's clinical use is limited by its unwelcome side effects.) During hypermagnesemia, peripheral vasodilatation produces flushing. Tachycardia appears initially and later progresses to bradycardia. Although ECG signs are not diagnostic of this disorder, you may observe certain changes (Wenger and Herndon 1974). At a serum concentration of 5–10 mEq, you may note prolonged PR intervals, longer QRS durations, and increased T wave amplitude. Above 10–15 mEq/L, deep tendon reflexes are lost and respiratory arrest ensues.

Treatment   If signs of magnesium imbalances appear, notify the physician. Magnesium depletion is treated by correcting the underlying disorder and/or administering magnesium supplements. Magnesium intoxication is treated by slowing or discontinuing the administration of magnesium-containing drugs and by dialysis. When appropriate to the patient's condition, teach him/her ways to prevent the reoccurrence of magnesium depletion or intoxication. For instance, provide the renal failure patient with the names of antacids that do not contain magnesium.

Outcome criteria   Use these desirable outcome criteria to evaluate the patient's progress.

- Serum magnesium level 1.5–2 mEq/L
- Normal neuromuscular excitability and deep tendon reflexes
- Spontaneous respirations, at rate normal for patient
- ECG within patient's normal limits
- Magnesium-depleted patient verbalizes knowledge of foods containing magnesium, awareness of importance of eating such, and ability to purchase them at home
- Magnesium-intoxicated (oliguric renal failure) patient states intention to avoid magnesium hydroxide and names acceptable alternative antacids

References

Guyton, A. 1971, 1976. *Textbook of medical physiology.* 4th ed., 5th ed. Philadelphia: W. B. Saunders Company.
Detailed reference on physiology of membrane potentials, muscle contraction, and calcium balance.

Koushanpour, E. 1976. *Renal physiology: principles and functions.* Philadelphia: W. B. Saunders Company.
Outstanding presentation of latest concepts and research findings on advanced topics such as possible hepatic osmoreceptors. Particularly good explanations of fluid and electrolyte regulation in the chapters on body fluids (2 and 3) and renal regulation of extracellular fluid volume and osmolality (12).

Levinsky, N., and Alexander, E. 1976. Acute renal failure. In *The kidney,* eds. B. Brenner and F. Rector, pp. 806–837. Philadelphia: W. B. Saunders Company.
Pathophysiology and therapy of acute renal failure, including hyperkalemia.

Stroot, V., Lee, C. and Schaper, C. 1974. *Fluids and electrolytes: a practical approach.* Philadelphia: F. A. Davis.
Simplified review of fluid, electrolyte, and acid-base imbalances.

Wenger, N., and Herndon, E. 1974. Endocrine and metabolic disorders. In *The heart.* 3rd ed. eds. J. Hurst and R. Logue. New York: McGraw-Hill Books, Inc.

Weisberg, H. 1962. *Water, electrolyte, and acid-base balance.* 2nd ed. Baltimore: Williams and Wilkins Company.
Detailed information of normal and pathologic physiology of water, electrolytes, and acid-base.

Supplemental Reading

Metheny, N., and Snively, W. 1974. *Nurses handbook of fluid balance.* 2nd ed. Philadelphia: J. B. Lippincott Company.
Basic concepts of fluid and electrolyte balance, including functions of individual electrolytes, compositions of body fluid compartments, and considerations in various diseases.

Tripp, A. 1976. Hyper- and Hypocalcemia. *A.J.N. 76:1142–1145.*
Overview of normal calcium function and causes, symptoms, and treatment of imbalances.

Zeluff, G., Suki, W. and Jackson, D. 1977. Depletion of body phosphate—ubiquitous, subtle, dangerous. *Heart Lung 6:519–525.*
Review of causes, manifestations, prevention, and treatment of hypophosphatemia.

Chapter 7

Renal Assessment and Acute Renal Failure

Renal failure can be insidious and life-threatening. The chronic form is well known to most nurses and may be reviewed in any standard nursing text. This chapter will focus on the acute form, which is of particular concern to the critical care nurse because it is both rapid and reversible.

Outline

Renal assessment   History and physical examination / Laboratory tests

Acute renal failure   Risk conditions / Signs and symptoms / Care planning and implementation

Dialysis   Hemodialysis / Peritoneal dialysis

Outcome evaluation

Objectives

- Name the functions of the kidney
- List in order nephron structures for (a) blood flow and (b) urine flow
- Describe the significance of the juxtaglomerular apparatus
- Explain how the renin-angiotensin system functions to maintain blood pressure
- Compare and contrast filtration, reabsorption, and secretion in urine formation
- Define the significance of the countercurrent mechanisms in the loop of Henle and the vasa recta

- Describe the role of antidiuretic hormone in the excretion of concentrated urine
- Explain the significance and normal value range of these tests of renal function: urine osmolality; specific gravity; urine color, clarity, pH, and sediment; BUN; serum creatinine; creatinine clearance
- Define and give examples of prerenal, renal, and postrenal causes of acute renal failure
- Take measures to prevent acute renal failure
- Recognize signs and symptoms of acute renal failure
- Recognize and relieve complications of acute renal failure
- Explain why an AV shunt is preferred for hemodialysis in the previously healthy patient who develops acute failure
- Prevent or relieve common problems with AV shunts
- Describe the principles and technique of (a) hemodialysis and (b) peritoneal dialysis
- Provide nursing care during hemodialysis
- Provide nursing care during peritoneal dialysis
- Evaluate the patient's progress according to outcome criteria

Renal assessment

The kidneys, which measure about 6 by 12 cm, lie retroperitoneally on either side of the vertebral column. The left kidney is slightly higher than the right. The upper border of the left kidney is protected by the eleventh and twelfth ribs and that of the right kidney by the twelfth rib. Their lower borders are at the level of the third lumbar vertebra.

The kidney's gross structures consist of the cortex, medulla, pyramids, papillae, calyxes, and pelvis (Figure 7-1). The cortex, the outermost layer, contains glomeruli arranged like bunches of grapes, proximal and distal tubules and the first parts of the loops of Henle and collecting ducts. The medulla, the middle layer, contains 10–15 wedge-shaped pyramids formed by the loops of Henle and collecting ducts. The apices (papillae) of these pyramids empty into cup-shaped structures called calyxes, which in turn empty into the hollow inner section of the kidney, the pelvis. From the pelvis, urine travels down the ureter into the bladder and is excreted.

The kidneys have excretory, regulatory, and secretory (endocrine) functions. In addition to their well known role in excretion of metabolic wastes, the kidneys function in regulation of extracellular fluid volume and osmolality, electrolyte balance, and partial control of acid-base balance. Endocrine functions are the secretion of renin, which affects blood pressure, and erythropoeitin, which influences production of red blood cells.

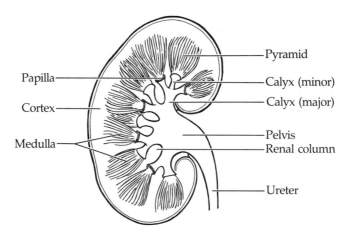

Papilla

Cortex

Medulla

Pyramid

Calyx (minor)

Calyx (major)

Pelvis
Renal column

Ureter

Figure 7-1.   Gross renal anatomy.

Because of the diversity of renal functions, you must evaluate several parameters in order to judge the health of the kidneys. A convenient assessment format is shown in Table 7-1.

History and physical examination

When assessing the patient for renal problems, the history and physical examination often are less informative than laboratory tests, discussed in detail below. Nevertheless, do ask the patient about a history of renal disease, concomitant diseases such as diabetes mellitus, and the presence of such symptoms as dysuria and changes in volume or frequency of urination. Physical signs and symptoms of renal disease often are nonspecific. Often, they are those of fluid and electrolyte imbalances (reviewed in Chapter 6) and those of acid-base imbalances (presented in Chapter 11).

If pain is present, evaluate its characteristics. The renal cortex is surrounded by a capsule which contains pain receptors. Since the capsule is tough and does not expand easily, any process which increases pressure against it may produce pain. Pain associated with kidney inflammation, such as with glomerulonephritis, may be constant, dull, and located over the flanks. The pain of pyelonephritis is sharp and severe. That associated with renal calculi may radiate toward the bladder or scrotum. If the stone becomes lodged in the ureter, severe spasmodic pain (ureteral colic) may occur.

If the patient is unable or unwilling to verbalize his pain, you may be able to detect it by noting his attempts to guard the area when he moves or by other signs of pain such as a drawn facial expression. Sometimes, too, blunt percussion over the lower back will elicit pain. Remember, however, that many renal disorders are not characterized by pain, so its absence is not necessarily indicative of a healthy kidney.

Table 7-1   Renal assessment format

1. History _____

2. Physical _____

3. Diagnostic procedures and laboratory tests

   Urine: volume _____

        sp.g. _____ osmolality _____

        color _____ clarity _____

        pH _____ sediment _____

    BUN _____ Creatinine _____ Creatinine clearance _____

    Other _____

4. Other relevant data _____

Laboratory tests

The most commonly monitored parameters of renal function are the urinary output, urine solute concentration, and ability to excrete nitrogenous waste products. This section describes common tests of renal function and their significance. In order to comprehend the interpretation of these tests, you must have a clear understanding of urine formation. The following paragraphs review the anatomy and physiology of urine formation.

    Urine is an ultrafiltrate of blood, formed by the kidney's microscopic structures. Urinary output depends upon a multiplicity of factors which include integrity of the structures in the nephron, renal blood flow, adequacy of the countercurrent mechanisms, and hormonal influences.

The nephron   The functional unit for urine formation is called the *nephron;* there are about a million in each kidney. Each nephron contains basically two sets of microscopic structures, one for blood flow and one for urine flow (Figure 7-2).

    The renal artery carries blood to the kidney. Blood then flows through increasingly smaller arteries, the interlobar, arcuate, and interlobular arteries. After passing through the renal capillaries, blood returns via the corresponding veins to the renal vein.

    The nephron's structures for blood flow arise from the interlobular artery. Blood travels through the *afferent arteriole* to a tuft of capillaries called the

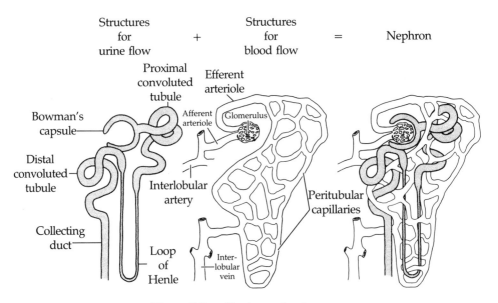

Figure 7-2.   Nephron structures.

glomerulus. The glomerular capillaries recombine to create the *efferent arteriole,* which carries away from the glomerulus arterial blood that was not filtered. Since the glomerular capillary bed is surrounded on both ends by arterioles, it is a high pressure system. (The clinical significance of this fact will be elaborated on later.) From the efferent arteriole, blood enters a second capillary bed, the peritubular system, and then empties into venules. As its name implies, the peritubular system surrounds the renal tubules. Because it lies between an arteriole and a venule, the peritubular system is a lower-pressure capillary bed.

Vasa recta are straight capillary loops which arise from the peritubular capillary network. They descend around the lower parts of the loops of Henle, loop into the medulla, and then return to the cortex. Their role in forming concentrated urine is discussed later.

Urine is filtered from the glomerulus into a surrounding structure called *Bowman's capsule.* From there it travels through the *renal tubule.* The tubule consists of a proximal convoluted section, a U-shaped turn called Henle's loop, and a distal convoluted portion. From the tubule, urine passes through a collecting duct (or collecting tubule); then this duct joins other collecting ducts to empty into the calyx. Several calyces empty into the renal pelvis, from which urine flows down the ureter into the bladder.

There are two types of nephrons, superficial cortical and juxtamedullary. Both have glomeruli and proximal and distal tubules in the cortex, with part of the collecting ducts and loops of Henle in the medulla. The superficial cortical nephrons (about seven-eights of the total) lie in the outer cortex, so their loops of Henle extend only a short distance into the medulla. The juxtamedullary nephrons lie in the inner cortex, near the medulla, so their loops of Henle extend much deeper into the medulla.

Glomerular filtration   Tracing the formation of urine will help you to better understand the interrelationships of these structures. The first step in urine formation is filtration from the glomerulus to Bowman's capsule.

About 20% of the cardiac output, or 1200 ml/min, flows through both kidneys. Of this renal blood flow, 650 ml is the normal renal plasma flow. From the plasma, the kidneys form about 125 ml/min of glomerular filtrate. The portion of the plasma that becomes filtrate is called the filtration fraction; it also averages 20%.

Renal blood flow (RBF) and *glomerular filtration rate (GFR)* remain relatively constant despite mean arterial pressure fluctuations between 80 and 180 mm Hg. This regulation of renal blood flow appears to be relatively independent of outside nervous control and blood-borne hormones as well as arterial pressure. Because control appears to reside within the kidney itself, this phenomenon is called *autoregulation.* Several theories have been advanced to explain autoregulation. Recent studies strongly support the presence of a feedback mechanism involving the juxtaglomerular apparatus (Figure 7-3).

Following is a current explanation for the role of the juxtaglomerular apparatus (Guyton 1976, Koushanpour 1976, Thurau and Boylan 1976). The distal tubule on its way to the collecting duct doubles back past the afferent arteriole leading to the glomerulus. A portion of the early distal tubule is in anatomic contact with the afferent arteriole. The cells in this portion of the distal tubule are called macula densa cells. Those cells in the corresponding portion of the afferent arteriole are called juxtaglomerular cells. The macula densa and juxtaglomerular cells comprise the juxtaglomerular apparatus, so called because it is near the glomerulus.

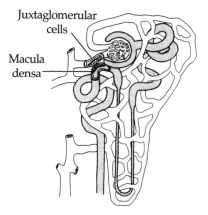

Figure 7-3.   Juxtaglomerular apparatus.

Most current evidence supports the theory that juxtaglomerular cells in the afferent arteriole act as baroreceptors, that is, sense changes in intraluminal pressure or vascular volume. When mean pressure in the afferent arteriole drops sufficiently, the juxtaglomerular cells become stimulated and secrete an enzyme called renin (Figure 7-4). This enzyme acts on a substance called angiotensinogen, which is formed by the liver and circulates in the bloodstream. Renin converts angiotensinogen, an inert substance, into angiotensin I, also inert. Angiotensin I then is converted by converting enzyme to angiotensin II. The origin of converting enzyme is unclear. Although conversion of angiotensin I to II is believed to occur primarily in lung capillaries, recent works suggest that the kidney itself may be able to form angiotensin II.

Angiotensin II has multiple roles in elevating arterial perfusion pressure. It intensely stimulates the adrenal glands to release aldosterone, promoting sodium reabsorption and thus water reabsorption. It is a powerful vasoconstrictor, acting directly on arteriolar smooth muscle to cause contraction. In the kidney, the vasoconstriction of the efferent arterioles reduces sharply the excretion of both salt and water. Angiotensin II also is believed to act on the brain to stimulate thirst. The resulting rise in blood volume and pressure returns afferent arteriolar pressure toward normal.

The role of the macula densa cells is controversial. They currently are believed partially to control renin secretion by the juxtaglomerular cells. They probably respond primarily to sodium chloride entering the distal tubule, although the exact mechanism is unclear.

Also unclear is the role that renin production plays in maintaining blood pressure. At present, it is believed that it plays a minor role, if any, at normal renal perfusion pressures. It probably plays a major role when severe renal hypotension occurs, and also may contribute to some cases of hypertension. Investigation continues into the highly controversial role of excessive renin production in human hypertension.

The kidneys (especially the afferent arteriole) are supplied with autonomic nerve fibers. Sympathetic stimulation constricts the afferent and efferent arterioles. Because it causes a relatively greater reduction in renal plasma flow (RPF) than in glomerular filtration rate (GFR), it usually increases the filtration fraction (GFR/RPF). Sympathetic stimulation also may lead indirectly to renin secretion, by constricting the afferent arteriole, thus reducing glomerular filtration rate and altering the sodium load in the distal tubule. Strong sympathetic stimulation causes such great arteriolar constriction that glomerular blood flow drops severely. The autonomic nerve fibers appear to play little role in the autoregulation of the kidney, since a transplanted kidney is able to function without a nerve supply.

Filtration occurs both because the glomerulus is a high pressure capillary bed and because its membrane is very permeable. As with other capillaries, glomerular filtration depends on the balance between hydrostatic and osmotic pressures on each side of the membrane. All substances except protein and blood cells are filtered, so the filtrate is similar to plasma.

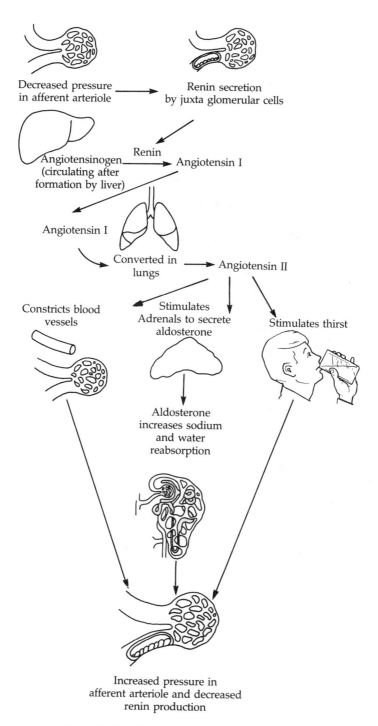

Figure 7-4.   Renin-angiotensin system.

Tubular reabsorption and secretion   From Bowman's capsule, the filtrate enters the tubules, where the processes of reabsorption and secretion separate substances to be conserved from those to be excreted. *Reabsorption* is the movement of solutes and water from the tubule into the peritubular network, that is, from the filtrate back into the bloodstream. *Secretion* is the movement of substances in the opposite direction—from the peritubular network into the tubule.

Reabsorption can occur passively or actively. Passive movement, *diffusion,* results from concentration or electrical gradients. Among substances reabsorbed this way are water, urea, and negative ions such as chloride. Active movement occurs against gradients and requires both chemical carriers and energy. Numerous substances are reabsorbed this way, including sodium, potassium, calcium, and glucose.

There is a maximum rate of reabsorption for each solute, called the *transport maximum.* When it is exceeded by the amount filtered, the remaining solute is excreted in the urine.

Secretion of substances also can be active or passive and is determined by hormones and the concentration of the substance in the extracellular fluid. Substances that may be secreted include hydrogen ion, potassium, penicillin, and x-ray contrast media.

Countercurrent mechanisms   The osmolality of the kidney's interstitial fluid varies from about 300 mOsm/L in the cortex to about 1200 mOsm/L deep in the medulla. As the glomerular filtrate passes through the proximal convoluted tubule, loop of Henle, and distal convoluted tubule, its osmolality also varies. In the proximal tubule, about 65% of the filtered sodium is reabsorbed actively. Water is reabsorbed because of the osmotic gradient established by the reabsorption of sodium. Other substances reabsorbed in the proximal tubule include all of the glucose, nearly all the amino acids, potassium, bicarbonate, and urea. When the fluid leaves the proximal tubule, it is isotonic with the glomerular filtrate.

As the tubular fluid passes through Henle's loop, it is exposed to increasingly hypertonic interstitial fluid in the medulla. The medullary hypertonicity plays an important role in the kidney's ability to concentrate urine, as explained later. The medullary interstitium is hypertonic primarily because of complex countercurrent mechanisms in the loops of Henle and vasa recta (Figure 7-5). The explanation given here is based on Guyton (1976), Pitts (1974), Vander (1975), and Koushanpour (1976).

Guyton explains that a *countercurrent mechanism* is one in which fluid going in and down one arm of a long loop interacts with fluid going up and out the opposite arm to create a high solute concentration at the tip of the loop.

The ascending limb of the loop of Henle actively transports sodium and chloride ions from the tubular fluid into the medullary interstitial fluid. Water is unable to follow the sodium chloride into the interstitial fluid because the ascending limb is highly impermeable to water. Since water does not follow the

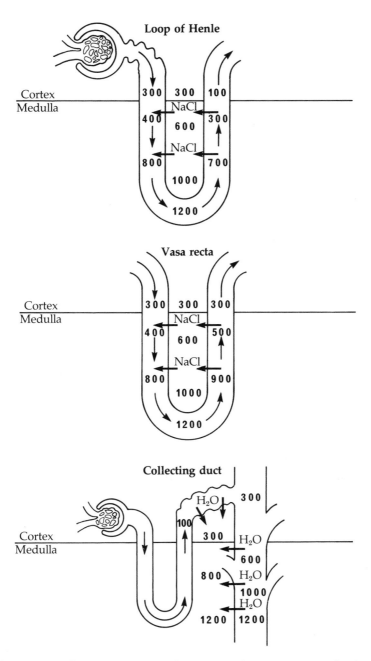

Figure 7-5. Countercurrent mechanisms and concentration of urine. (Adapted from Guyton, 1976. *Textbook of Medical Physiology.* 5th ed. Copyright © 1976 by W. B. Saunders Company, Philadelphia. Used with permission of author and publisher.)

sodium chloride, the medullary interstitial fluid becomes hypertonic. The descending limb of the loop is highly permeable to sodium chloride. As a result, sodium moves from the ascending limb into the interstitial fluid and then into the descending limb. This sodium raises the tonicity of fluid in the descending limb as it flows downward. The sodium flows back around the loop and then again is transported outward of the ascending limb to repeat the countercurrent cycle. In addition, more sodium is added to the cycle as new glomerular filtrate enters the descending limb. As a result of this process, the sodium chloride concentration in the medulla becomes extremely high.

Although the fluid leaving the proximal convoluted tubule is isotonic with the glomerular filtrate, its concentration rises rapidly as it flows down the descending limb of the loop of Henle. This rise occurs both because of the inflow of sodium chloride described above and because water diffuses out into the interstitial fluid to establish an osmotic equilibrium between the fluid in the descending limb and that in the interstitium.

At the bottom of the loop, the tubular fluid is isotonic with the medullary interstitial fluid (but hypertonic compared to the fluid entering the descending limb).

Because sodium chloride is removed from the ascending limb while water remains, the tubular fluid becomes hypotonic as it passes through the ascending limb on its way to the distal tubule and collecting duct. Final adjustment of the concentration of tubular fluid in the distal tubule and collecting duct depends on the presence or absence of antidiuretic hormone (ADH), as explained later.

Most recently, it has been proposed that urea also moves into and out of the medullary interstitium, also increasing the osmolality of the medullary interstitial fluid.

The medullary hypertonicity also is maintained by a countercurrent mechanism in the vascular system, specifically the vasa recta which run parallel to the loops of Henle. Blood flow in the vasa recta is quite sluggish. As blood flows down the descending limbs of the vasa recta loops, sodium chloride diffuses in from the medullary interstitial fluid and water osmoses out. These movements progressively raise the tonicity of the blood until blood at the bottom of the loop is isotonic with the interstitial fluid (but hypertonic compared to the blood entering the vasa recta). As blood flows back up the loop, sodium chloride diffuses back out into the interstitial fluid and water re-enters the bloodstream from the interstitial fluid. The blood leaving the medulla thus is only slightly more concentrated than that entering it and carries very little sodium away from the medulla. The net result of these countercurrent mechanisms in the loop of Henle and vasa recta is to produce and protect the hypertonicity of the medullary interstitial fluid.

Excretion of dilute or concentrated urine   As mentioned earlier, fluid is hypotonic when it enters the distal tubule and collecting duct, where final adjustment of urine concentration takes place. If the body does not need to retain water, no adjustment is necessary. In the absence of antidiuretic hormone, the distal tubule and collecting duct are impermeable to water. As fluid passes through them, sodium and other substances are actively transported out but water is not reabsorbed. The already hypotonic urine becomes even more hypotonic, and a dilute urine is excreted.

Sometimes, however, the body needs to retain water to offset an increased osmolality of the extracellular fluid, such as occurs in dehydration. When this happens, the hypertonicity of the medullary interstitial fluid enables the kidney to concentrate urine as it passes through the distal tubule and collecting duct. The increased extracellular fluid osmolality is sensed by osmoreceptors in the anterior hypothalamus. These stimulate the release of antidiuretic hormone from the posterior hypothalamus. ADH travels to the kidneys, where it increases the permeability of the distal tubule and the collecting duct to water. Because the surrounding interstitial fluid is so hypertonic due to the countercurrent mechanisms, a *concentration gradient* is created. This gradient makes water osmose from the tubule into the interstitial fluid. This mechanism can make the urine in the cortical portion of the collecting duct isotonic with the cortex (300 mOsm/L) and if necessary can make the urine in the medullary portion of the collecting duct isotonic with the medullary interstitial fluid (up to 1200 mOsm/L). As a result, highly concentrated urine can be excreted. The water reabsorbed from the collecting duct re-enters the bloodstream to return serum osmolality to normal. This delicate mechanism fails early in kidney disease and its loss is the reason renal patients often have dilute urine with a fixed osmolality or specific gravity.

In addition to urine concentration being adjusted in the distal tubule and collecting duct, reabsorption and secretion of solutes may occur. Selective reabsorption of sodium will occur in the presence of aldosterone, a hormone secreted by the adrenal cortex in response to decreased serum sodium concentration, increased renin secretion, and other stimuli. Bicarbonate may be reabsorbed and hydrogen, ammonia, and potassium secreted by the distal tubule and collecting duct.

Urine volume   As mentioned earlier, blood flow to the kidneys approximates 1200 ml/min. About 125 ml/min becomes glomerular filtrate. During its journey through the nephron, nearly all of this volume is reabsorbed, producing a urine output of 1 ml/min in the healthy adult.

Simply measuring the volume of urine can indicate the presence of a problem with urine formation but gives very limited information about its cause or about the adequacy of other kidney functions. For these items, you must depend upon the results of more definitive tests of renal function.

Urine osmolality and specific gravity   Evaluate the kidney's ability to concentrate or dilute urine by interpreting the serum and urine osmolalities or the specific gravity of urine. As explained in Chapter 6, osmolality is a measure of the number of osmotically active particles in solution. It is a laboratory determination reported as milliosmols (mOsm) of solute per kilogram of solvent. Normal serum osmolality is about 285–295 mOsm/kg. Normal urine osmolality is 500–800 mOsm/kg (Table 7-2). Although the absolute values for each are important, the relationship between them is more significant. Maximal dilution can make urine osmolality as low as one-sixth of serum osmolality (down to 50 mOsm/kg) and maximal concentration can raise urine osmolality to four times serum values (up to 1200 mOsm/kg). Urine osmolality should vary in the same direction as the serum value. When serum osmolality is increased, indicating an elevated concentration, urine osmolality also should increase because the kidneys should conserve water to return the serum value to normal.

A cruder bedside measurement of the ability to alter urine concentration is the *specific gravity* of urine, which compares the concentration of urine to that of water. To measure it, you place urine in a small cylinder and float a hydrometer in it. The specific gravity is read in thousandths according to the level of the bottom of the fluid meniscus (Figure 7-6). Normal specific gravity of urine is 1.010–1.025.

Urine osmolality is a more accurate measurement than specific gravity. Specific gravity readings reflect not only the concentration of particles but also their size and molecular weight. Falsely high readings occur when protein,

Table 7-2   Composition of the urine of a normal adult human whose diet includes protein.

pH	5.0 to 7.0
Osmolality	500 to 800 mOsm/kg H_2O
Na^+	50 to 130 mEq/L
K^+	20 to 70 mEq/L
NH_4^+	30 to 50 mEq/L
Ca^{++}	5 to 12 mEq/L
Mg^{++}	2 to 18 mEq/L
Cl^-	50 to 130 mEq/L
$H_2PO_4^-$	20 to 40 mEq/L [a]
$SO_4^=$	30 to 45 mEq/L
Organic acids	10 to 25 mM/L [a]
Urea	200 to 400 mM/L
Creatinine	6 to 20 mM/L

[a]At an acid urinary pH of 6.0 or lower, nearly all of the urinary inorganic phosphate exists in the monovalent form. Urinary organic acids (for example, lactic, uric, citric, pyruvic acids) have different valences; the molar concentration listed assumes an average valence of minus two.
From Valtin, H. *Renal function: mechanisms preserving fluid and solute balance in health.* Boston: Little, Brown and Company. © 1973. Used with permission of the author and publisher.

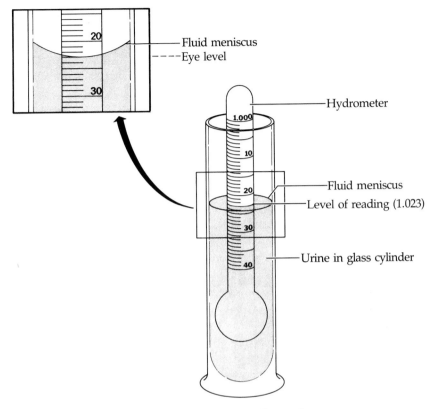

Figure 7-6. Reading specific gravity.

glucose, radiographic contrast media, and other high molecular weight substances are in the urine. In contrast, urine osmolality reflects the concentration of particles without being affected by their size and weight. With both measures, serial determinations are more significant than single ones.

The healthy kidney is able to vary urine osmolality and specific gravity according to the concentration of serum. It does this through the countercurrent mechanism and under the influence of ADH. When kidneys are damaged, the ability to concentrate urine is one of the first functions lost. Urine osmolality becomes fixed within 50 mOsm of the serum value. Specific gravity readings also become fixed, near 1.010.

Routine urinalysis   Routine urinalysis evaluates urine color, clarity, pH, and sediment. The following descriptions are based on Brunner et al (1975) and Papper (1971). Urine usually is yellow or amber, due to the presence of urobilin. When red blood cells are destroyed or die, their hemoglobin is split and the heme portion is converted by reticuloendothelial cells into bilirubin. The bilirubin circulates to the liver, where it is conjugated and excreted into bile. It empties into the intestine, where it is modified into urobilinogen. Some of the urobilinogen is reabsorbed into the blood and is excreted into the urine where it becomes oxidized into urobilin, producing the characteristic color of urine. Abnormal urine colors may be due to the presence of blood, diagnostic media, or therapeutic drugs, or to disease.

Normal urine is clear. Cloudy urine may indicate the precipitation of urates or phosphates on standing or the presence of blood, bacteria, or pus. The pH of urine ranges from 4.5–8.0. Although usually acid, it rapidly becomes alkaline on standing due to bacteria decomposing its urea into ammonia. More acid urine is seen commonly in acidosis and sodium depletion, alkaline urine in alkalosis and infections.

The mechanisms by which the kidneys alter urinary pH include hydrogen ion secretion/bicarbonate retention, secretion of ammonia, and acidification of phosphate salts. They are explained and diagrammed in the chapter on acid-base balance (Chapter 11).

Routine urinalysis includes a microscopic examination for blood cells, crystals, casts, and bacteria. Red blood cells are a sign of pathology or menstruation, while a few scattered white cells are common. A variety of crystals may be included, especially when the urine is concentrated; most are of no significance. Casts are abnormal. They are formed when the lumen of the tubules becomes filled with a material which then hardens, forming a *cast* of the lumen. Bacteria are not significant except in "clean catch" or catheterized urine samples. If present in those samples, they must be identified further through cultures. The urine normally contains no detectable protein, glucose, or ketones. Proteinuria is common in renal disease, glycosuria in diabetes mellitus, and ketonuria in diabetic ketoacidosis and starvation.

BUN   Urea is an end product of protein metabolism, both endogenous protein (muscle) and exogenous protein (meals). According to Guyton (1976), urea is formed primarily in the liver by the process of *deamination*. Amino groups are split off from amino acids, forming molecules of ammonia and molecules of keto acid. The keto acids are metabolized in the citric acid (Krebs) cycle which occurs in all cells, or in some cases are converted to glucose or fat. The ammonia molecules usually are converted to urea and excreted in the urine. The normal *blood urea nitrogen (BUN)* value is 8–20 mg%. Because the level of urea nitrogen in the blood varies with urine output, the BUN level can be a useful indicator of renal function. Its value is limited, however, because factors other than renal function also may affect it: intake of urea precursors, the body's metabolic state, and blood volume. The level decreases in malnutrition or severe liver failure. It increases in conditions with increased urea formation (such as ingestion of protein-rich meals, infection, or administration of glucocorticoids), decreased urea excretion (such as renal disease), or altered relative concentration in the blood (such as dehydration).

Creatinine   Creatinine is an end product of muscle metabolism. Since its production is endogenous, the serum creatinine level is relatively independent of protein intake and metabolic state and therefore is a somewhat better guide to renal function than the BUN. Because serum creatinine concentration depends on lean body mass, the value varies from person to person; the normal range is 0.5–1.2 mg%. Within one person, the value normally is constant, so serial determinations are a useful way to follow the patient's progress.

Normal urine creatinine production is 1–1.8 gm/24 hr. The relationship between plasma and urine creatinine concentrations can be helpful in differentiating two common causes of acute oliguria, as explained later.

Creatinine clearance   One of the kidney's functions is to clear the extracellular fluid of waste products.

Clearance may be defined as the volume of plasma per minute that the kidneys completely clear of a substance. The clearance of a given substance can be a clinically useful indicator of glomerular filtration rate, if the substance is freely filtered at the glomerulus but neither reabsorbed nor secreted. Inulin is such a substance, but inulin clearance tests are expensive, time-consuming, and require careful analysis. The most commonly used substitute for inulin is creatinine. Creatinine is secreted as well as filtered, but because of certain characteristics of the method used to determine creatinine clearance, creatinine clearance actually closely approximates inulin clearance (Brenner, Deen, and Robertson 1976).

Clearance is determined by measuring the plasma concentration of a substance, the urine concentration of the same substance, and the urine flow rate. Logically, the plasma concentration times the glomerular filtration rate equals the urine concentration times the urine flow rate. This relationship can be expressed mathematically as follows, where P_x = plasma concentration, U_x = urine concentration, GFR = glomerular filtration rate, and V = urine flow rate:

$$P_x \times GFR = U_x \times V$$

Rearranging the terms of the equation results in this formula:

$$GFR = \frac{U_x V}{P_x}$$

When creatinine is used to measure glomerular filtration rate, the following formula is derived from the general formula given before:

$$\text{Creatinine clearance} = \frac{\text{Urine creatinine concentration times urine flow rate}}{\text{Plasma creatinine concentration}}$$

To determine creatinine clearance, a 24-hour urine specimen must be collected carefully. Have the person empty the bladder; record the time as the onset of the collection period. Collect *all* urine voided during the next 24 hours. At the end of the collection period, obtain another urine specimen. Add it to the volume and record the exact time. Obtain a blood sample for serum creatinine. The laboratory will measure the serum and urine creatinine concentrations and calculate urine flow by dividing the total volume by the duration of the collection. By entering these figures in the clearance equation, the laboratory will determine the value for creatinine clearance.

Brundage (1976) reports normal creatinine clearance for men as 140 ± 27.2 ml/min and for women 112 ± 20.2 ml/min.

Hemoglobin and hematocrit   When oxygen tension decreases, the healthy kidney secretes erythropoietin, which stimulates the bone marrow to produce red blood cells (Guyton 1976). Patients with kidney disease may not secrete erythropoietin adequately and therefore rapidly become anemic.

Most of the above measures of renal function are done routinely on admission to the hospital as a screening device. Some, such as creatinine clearance, the physician will order only if he or she suspects renal damage.

Acute renal failure

Although a variety of renal disorders may afflict the critically ill, the one seen most frequently and the one you can play the greatest role in preventing is acute renal failure.

Nursing care in acute renal failure begins with assessment of the patient for risk conditions and signs and symptoms.

Risk conditions

Conditions predisposing to acute renal failure can be divided into three categories, prerenal, renal, and postrenal causes.

Prerenal causes are those that diminish renal perfusion without causing tubular damage (Papper 1971). Examples of prerenal causes are as follows:

- Diminished cardiac output owing to arrhythmias, ventricular failure, shock, or cardiac tamponade
- Decreased peripheral vascular resistance owing to vasogenic shock, acidosis, or gram-negative sepsis
- Hypovolemia owing to hemorrhage or severe dehydration
- Obstructed or compromised renal perfusion owing to emboli, renal arterial thrombosis or stenosis, or abdominal aneurysms

Renal causes may manifest interstitial, glomerular, and/or tubular damage. Examples are:

- Glomerulonephritis
- Pyelonephritis

- Nephropathy due to hypertension or diabetes
- Transfusion reactions
- Nephrotoxic drugs such as insecticides, heavy metals, sulfonamides, some antibiotics (gentamycin, streptomycin, kanamycin, neomycin, cephaloride, tetracycline, penicillin)
- Acute tubular insufficiency

Postrenal causes are urinary tract obstructions. Examples are: ureteral stones, benign prostatic hypertrophy, or carcinoma of the bladder.

Prevention   To prevent failure eliminate as many causes as possible. For instance, check for a history of allergic reactions before administering drugs. Follow the measures outlined in other chapters to prevent or treat arrhythmias, ventricular failure, tamponade, shock, acidosis, and extracellular fluid deficit. Maintain strict aseptic technique during urethral catheterization. Do not give Atropine to a patient with benign prostatic hypertrophy. If a patient develops hypotension, maintain renal perfusion with fluids, vasopressors, and diuretics. Promptly restore blood volume. Administer vasopressors, such as dopamine, which promote rather than deprive renal blood flow. Force diuresis by administering mannitol, furosemide, or ethacrynic acid, as ordered by the physician.

Signs and symptoms

The signs and symptoms of acute renal failure vary somewhat in intensity from those of chronic renal failure. For example, hyperkalemia is a major problem in acute failure, but relatively less severe in chronic failure. Signs and symptoms also vary depending upon the cause. In the clinical setting, the most common causes of acute failure are decreased perfusion and acute tubular insufficiency (with or without necrosis). The latter usually is caused by severe ischemia or nephrotoxic agents. Be alert for the following signs of failure.

Urine volume   Urinary output may vary with both the cause and duration of failure. Anuria indicates complete obstruction or total renal shutdown. Oliguria (less than 400 ml/24 hr) is most common in the early stage of failure, the first two weeks. It occurs both in reduced perfusion and in acute tubular insufficiency, though it may be transient in the latter. Polyuria may characterize the later diuretic phase of failure, though it is seen less frequently now because of the trend toward early dialysis.

Urine osmolality and specific gravity   If the cause of failure is diminished perfusion, the urine osmolality will be greater than plasma osmolality and the specific gravity will be elevated because of the kidney's attempts to conserve volume. If the cause is tubular damage, urine osmolality will be within 50 mOsm/kg of serum osmolality and the specific gravity of urine will be low. The reason for this is that when nephrons are damaged, the ability to concentrate urine is one of the first functions lost.

Urinary sodium levels   Urinary sodium levels usually are decreased in pre-renal causes of failure because the healthy tubules respond normally to stimuli for avid sodium retention. In acute tubular insufficiency, urinary sodium usually is increased because the damaged tubules fail to reabsorb sodium.

BUN and creatinine   The trend of BUN and creatinine values varies with the stage of failure. Serum creatinine and BUN rise during the oliguric phase of failure due to diminished glomerular filtration. During the early diuretic phase, although urinary output increases due to the gradual return of renal function, the creatinine and BUN continue to rise because of diminished glomerular function. During the late diuretic phase, the BUN and creatinine fall and stabilize.

U/P creatinine ratio   In prerenal failure, the ratio between urinary and plasma creatinine is high, almost always over 10:1 and usually over 40:1; in acute tubular insufficiency, it almost always is below 10:1 (Levinsky and Alexander 1976).

Potassium imbalances   Evaluation of the ECG and the patient's muscles and reflexes may point to potassium imbalances. Peaked T waves, prolonged PR intervals or QRS durations, twitching, cramps, or hyperactive reflexes suggest hyperkalemia. This condition is a common, major problem in acute failure.

In addition to impaired potassium excretion, hyperkalemia may result from acidosis, increased cellular breakdown, or excessive potassium intake in diet, medications, or intravenous solutions. Flattened T waves, muscle weakness, nausea or vomiting, and hypoactive reflexes implicate hypokalemia. Although this condition is less common than hyperkalemia during renal failure, it can result from vomiting, diarrhea, some diuretics, decreased intake, or increased renal exchange of potassium for sodium.

Other signs and symptoms   Drowsiness, weakness, twitching, convulsions, itchy skin, confusion, mental irritability, slowed thinking, and altered thought processes may result from uremia.

Anorexia, nausea, vomiting, and diarrhea or constipation may indicate metabolic acidosis. This acid-base imbalance may result from decreased reabsorption of bicarbonate and diminished excretion of ammonia and phosphates.

Hypertension, rales, and signs of congestive heart failure or pulmonary edema may result from fluid overload.

Bruising, oozing of blood or frank bleeding, and decreased hemoglobin and hematocrit values may indicate anemia, increased capillary fragility, and/or decreased platelet adhesiveness. Anemia may appear within a few days of renal shutdown due to the diminished synthesis of erythropoietin.

Care planning and implementation

Patient assessment serves as the basis for planning and implementing care to relieve the effects of acute renal failure and to prevent its complications. In addition to taking the following measures, it is of course essential to assist the physician in identifying and treating the cause of the failure. Nursing care during dialysis is discussed later in the chapter.

Diminished drug excretion   Avoid or give reduced dosages of nephrotoxic drugs or those which depend on the kidneys for excretion. For example, if digitalis is prescribed in reduced dosages, monitor closely for signs of digitalis toxicity. Avoid antacids containing calcium or magnesium (such as Maalox). Instead, use antacids containing phosphate binders, such as Amphogel. In addition to being excreted more easily, they help to prevent bone disease, as explained later.

Anemia   Because of the anemia which afflicts renal patients, it is essential to minimize blood loss. Draw minimal amounts of blood for laboratory specimens. Handle the patient gently to avoid bruising due to the increased capillary fragility. Minimize irritation from nasogastric tubes to prevent nosebleeds. Avoid hypodermic injections. Prevent or promptly treat stress ulcers. Use stool softeners to avoid constipation and prevent bleeding from hemorrhoids. Watch carefully for signs of bleeding and alert the physician to them. Administer packed cells when ordered by the physician.

Fluid, potassium, and acid-base imbalances   Follow the plans of care in Chapter 6 for extracellular volume deficit or overload and hypo/hyperkalemia; see Chapter 11 for care in metabolic acidosis.

Infection   Give meticulous attention to asepsis for wounds and invasive catheters. Maintain a vigorous regimen of pulmonary hygiene to prevent pooling of secretions and bacterial growth. Avoid skin breakdown through well-aligned body positioning and frequent turning.

Maintain adequate nutrition with enough calories, carbohydrates, and protein to prevent negative nitrogen balance. Carbohydrates also forestall the production of ketones from fat metabolism and prevent gluconeogenesis from body protein.

Malnutrition   Nutrition is a real challenge in the face of the gastrointestinal symptoms and decreased mental alertness. Maintaining mouth care, giving small portions, and providing social interaction during meals may encourage the oral intake of a high-calorie diet. If oral intake is insufficient to prevent protein catabolism (worsening the uremia) or fat metabolism (worsening the acidosis), the physician may prescribe hyperalimentation. See Chapter 12 for the care related to this type of nutrition.

Uremic pericarditis, cardiac failure, and cardiac tamponade   Uremic pericarditis (see Chapter 4 for details) is a common complication of acute and chronic renal failure. Avoid predisposing factors. The most common ones are bacterial infection (shunt, respiratory, wound, or other) and poor dietary control. Watch for fever, chills, chest pain, a pericardial friction rub, and gallop rhythm. The pericarditis frequently is fibrinous. The most serious acute complications of pericarditis are cardiac failure from myocarditis, and cardiac tamponade. (See Chapter 4 for discussions of prevention, recognition, and treatment of failure and tamponade.) Treatment of uremic pericarditis includes treatment of infection, good dietary control, and increased frequency of dialysis (with regional heparinization). If pericarditis is severe or persistent, pericardiocentesis, creation of a pericardial "window" or pericardiectomy may be necessary.

Bone disease   A troublesome complication of prolonged renal failure is defective bone metabolism. In renal failure, bone disease may occur because of calcium depletion. Since kidney failure impairs tubular excretion of phosphate, the serum phosphorus level rises. Owing to its inverse relationship to the phosphorus level, the serum calcium level decreases. The serum calcium level also decreases because calcium normally is absorbed poorly from the gut and because the kidney is unable to convert Vitamin D to its active form. The low serum calcium stimulates parathyroid hormone secretion. An excess of this hormone leaches calcium from the bones into the serum, and in time the patient may end up with osteodystrophy. Phosphate binders can help to prevent this cycle and thus protect bone integrity.

Pulmonary edema   For nursing care in pulmonary edema, see Chapter 10.

Dialysis

Dialysis is the process by which dissolved particles diffuse from a fluid compartment across a semipermeable membrane into another fluid compartment. In the past, dialysis was prescribed only when more conservative management failed to control uremia, hyperkalemia, acidosis, or other effects of failure. Increasingly, physicians are prescribing it early in the course of failure, as part of an aggressive attempt to forestall the more severe manifestations and complications of failure.

There are two types of dialysis in use: peritoneal dialysis and hemodialysis. In *peritoneal dialysis*, the semipermeable membrane is the peritoneum. The first compartment is the body fluids on the visceral side of the peritoneum, and the dialysate infused into the peritoneal cavity is the second compartment. In *hemodialysis,* the blood is one fluid compartment, the membrane is an artificial one in the dialysis machine, and the dialysate is the second fluid compartment.

Each type of dialysis has advantages and disadvantages. They are summarized in Table 7-3.

Hemodialysis

Nursing care for the hemodialysis patient includes maintaining circulatory access, initiating dialysis, attending to patient status and technical aspects of dialysis, discontinuing dialysis, promoting patient health between dialyses, and coordinating other aspects of care as well as providing standard nursing care.

Dialyzers and dialysate solutions   There are numerous models of dialyzers on the market, generally grouped into coil, parallel plate, and hollow fiber types. There also are several types of dialysate delivery systems. The dialysate consists

Table 7-3   Comparison of hemodialysis and peritoneal dialysis

	Hemodialysis	*Peritoneal dialysis*
Speed	Rapid—up to 8 hours per treatment	Slow—up to 72 hours initially, up to 12 hours per treatment thereafter. Can be advantage in patients who cannot tolerate rapid fluid and electrolyte changes.
Cost	Expensive	Manual—relatively inexpensive; automated—expensive
Equipment	Complex	Manual—simply and readily available; automated—complex
Vascular access	Required	Not necessary, so suitable for patients with vascular problems
Heparinization	Required; systemic or regional	Little or no heparin necessary, so suitable for patients with bleeding problems
Technical nursing skill necessary	High degree	Manual—moderate degree; automated—high degree
Complications (other than fluid and electrolyte imbalances common to both)	Dialysis disequilibrium syndrome (preventable) Mechanical dysfunctions of dialyzer	Peritonitis Protein loss (0.5 gm/liter of dialysate) Bowel or bladder perforation

of specially treated water, electrolytes, sodium acetate, and other substances, depending upon the patient's needs. The solution usually is not sterile, because bacteria and viruses are too large to pass across the dialysis membrane. The concentration of waste products such as urea is zero; they diffuse out because of the concentration gradient between the blood and dialysate. Glucose may be added to the dialysate to create an osmotic gradient enhancing water removal. The concentration of electrolytes depends on the individual patient's needs. To prevent diffusion of substances for which the patient has desirable serum concentrations, an equivalent concentration is added to the dialysate. For example, a higher than usual potassium concentration will be used in the dialysate of a patient on digitalis, to prevent hypokalemia and precipitation of digitalis toxicity. In some cases, it may be advisable to add substances to the dialysate that will diffuse into the bloodstream. Sodium acetate, for example, will be metabolized by the body to bicarbonate ions, which then can buffer the metabolic acids the kidneys are unable to excrete.

Hemodialysis is a highly complex technical procedure. In order to implement it and respond rapidly and effectively to complications, the nurse needs specialized training and practice under the guidance of an experienced practitioner. Even if you yourself do not perform the dialysis, being knowledgeable about the process will help you support the patient and family and enhance your awareness of potential problems.

Circulatory access   Maintain access to the circulation. There are many routes of circulatory access for hemodialysis. In the patient with acute failure, the most common ones are the arteriovenous (AV) cannulae, or shunt, and the femoral catheters.

Femoral catheterization can be accomplished quickly but is suitable for only short-term use (24–48 hours). One catheter may be inserted low in the femoral vein for blood removal and a second one higher in the vein for blood return. Alternatively, a special catheter with a double lumen (Mackintosh catheter) may be used. Infection, clotting, and hemorrhage are potential complications of femoral catheterization.

The AV *cannulae* or *shunt* (Figure 7-7) is more permanent. Average life expectancy is 8–10 months although some last for longer periods of time. It is inserted under local anesthetic in the operating room or occasionally at the bedside. Common sites of insertion are the radial artery and cephalic vein in the forearm and the posterior tibial artery and saphenous vein in the leg. Hard Teflon vessel tips are placed in an artery and vein. Soft cannulae made of Silastic are attached to these tips and tunneled subcutaneously to skin exit sites 2–4 cm from the vessel tips. Between dialyses, the cannulae are connected with a Teflon connector and blood flow is maintained directly from the artery to the vein.

Common problems with an AV shunt include thrombosis, hemorrhage, ischemia of the extremity, and infection. Forestall them with the measures described in the following sections.

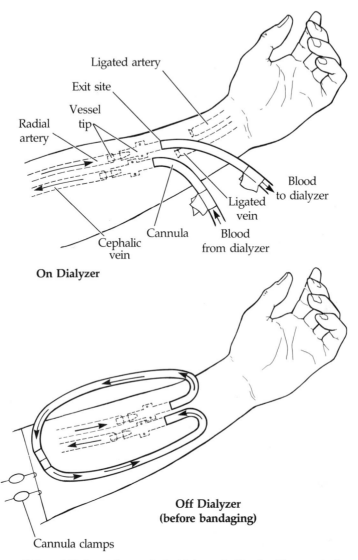

Figure 7-7.   AV shunt (cannulae). (Adapted. Used with permission of Ann Holmes, RN, Herrick Memorial Hospital, Berkeley, Ca.)

Thrombosis   Thrombosis (clotting) is a serious complication that frequently can be prevented by meticulous nursing care. The following measures will assist in prevention of clots:

1. Inspect, palpate, and auscultate the shunt at least every two hours, more often if the shunt is new or there are problems with flow. Blood in the shunt

should be uniformly red, warm, and pulsatile to the touch. Distal to the shunt (on the venous side), you should hear a bruit (murmur) and feel a thrill, caused by the turbulence resulting from the transmission of arterial pressure to the vein.

2. Prevent thrombosis by maintaining arterial blood pressure and avoiding trauma and infection at the shunt site. Elevate the extremity for the first 2–3 days and handle it and the tubing gently. Limit activity on the extremity. Avoid taking blood pressures on or drawing blood samples from that limb. Warn the patient not to fall asleep with the limb bent. Do not apply constrictive dressings. Be careful to maintain cannulae alignment when you manipulate the cannulae or change the dressing. Misalignment can cause kinks or epithelial damage which enhance clotting.

3. The decrease of a bruit, thrill, or pulse in the shunt may portend its clotting; notify the physician. Very dark blood or blood that has separated into serum and red blood cells indicates thrombosis of the shunt. Notify the physician or hemodialysis nurse promptly, as the success of declotting attempts depends on how rapidly they are instituted. The physician or nurse will try to aspirate the clot, irrigate both cannulae tips with a heparinized solution, or strip the vessel with a Fogarty catheter. Even if declotting is successful, thrombosis may recur unless the precipitating factor is corrected.

4. Minimize trauma to other vessels, which may be needed later for placement of another shunt, a graft or arteriovenous fistula. For example, whenever possible, draw blood samples from the shunt rather than piercing another potential access site.

Hemorrhage   Hemorrhage can be lethal within a matter of minutes. Make sure cannulae connections are secure. Keep bulldog clamps instantly available. If the cannulae separate, immediately clamp them to prevent massive blood loss and then reconnect them. If a cannula or the whole shunt falls out, you may need to control bleeding with a tourniquet. Emergency surgery will be necessary to ligate the vessels.

Ischemia   ischemia to the extremity may occur if collateral supply is inadequate. Periodically, palpate the limb's pulses and observe skin color and temperature. (In the artery containing the cannula, the pulse distal to the cannula will be absent.) Alert the physician if ischemia develops; it may be necessary to reposition the shunt.

Infection   Prevent infection by scrupulous attention to sterile technique. Shunt care should be given only by nurses specially trained in the cleaning, positioning, and dressing of shunts, to prevent accidental damage. The following measures are especially important in shunt care:

1. Keep the dressing dry and check periodically for drainage. Inspect the exit sites for erythema, edema, or tenderness whenever the dressing is changed or dialysis is performed.

2. When cleaning the sites, use separate sterile supplies for each site. Start the cleaning at the exit site and move outward to avoid contaminating the site with organisms from the distal epithelium. Apply an antibiotic ointment if the physician or unit procedure calls for it.

3. If you observe signs of infection, culture each site and notify the physician or hemodialysis nurse. An infected site is a serious problem, because it predisposes toward thrombosis, embolism, systemic spread of the infection during hemodialysis, bacterial endocarditis, and septic shock. The infection is treated with appropriate antibiotics. Sometimes the shunt is removed, although maintenance of dialysis usually is more important than infection at the access site.

Fistulas and grafts   If chronic hemodialysis is necessary, the surgeon may create an arteriovenous fistula or implant a graft. A *fistula* (Figure 7-8) is formed by a subcutaneous anastamosis of an artery and vein, which may be connected end to end, side to side, or end to side. The pressure from the artery causes the vein to dilate. After several weeks, the vein can be used for dialysis. A *graft* is a

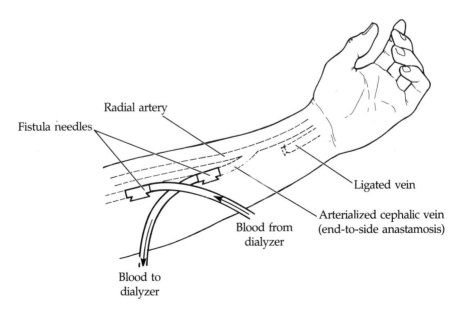

Figure 7-8.   AV fistula. (Adapted. Used with permission of Ann Holmes, RN, Herrick Memorial Hospital, Berkeley, Ca.)

vessel implant anastamosed between an artery and vein. A fistula or graft can be used for hemodialysis by inserting large gauge needles for blood flow into and out of the patient. Potential problems include thrombosis, hemorrhage, infection, ischemia of the extremity, and aneurysm formation.

Preparation for hemodialysis   Specific procedures for initiating dialysis vary but include the steps discussed below:

1. Reinforce the physician's explanation of the procedure. Explain the upcoming sequence of events to the patient and family, and answer their questions about it.

2. Assess the patient physically and review the clinical record and laboratory reports. Particularly assess the fluid and electrolyte imbalances present. Record baseline values for the patient's weight, blood pressure, pulse, respirations, temperature, emotional state, and any other indicated parameters.

3. Draw blood samples for serum electrolytes, BUN, hematocrit, and clotting time.

4. Begin heparinization. Heparin is used to prevent clotting in the extracorporeal circuit. There are two techniques of heparinization: systemic and regional. In *systemic heparinization,* the clotting times of both the dialyzer and the patient are increased to the values appropriate for the dialyzer model in use. The heparin may be administered intermittently or continuously in the arterial line. *Regional heparinization* is preferred if the patient is bleeding already (such as in gastrointestinal bleeding) or is at high risk for bleeding (such as with recent surgery, pericarditis, intracranial hematoma). In this method, the clotting time of the dialyzer, but not that of the patient, is increased by adding heparin to the dialyzer but neutralizing it with protamine sulfate before blood returns to the patient.

Heparin doses are individualized by body weight. Clotting times are monitored if the patient is acutely ill or has a potential bleeding problem. If an infusion is used, check its rate frequently.

Observe the patient closely for gastric bleeding, cardiac tamponade, and other signs of bleeding. These observations are particularly important if the patient has been on heparin before dialysis, for example, for a myocardial infarct. If bleeding occurs, protamine sulfate usually is administered to return the clotting time to the desired range. Dialysis may be discontinued if bleeding is severe.

5. Connect the patient to the dialyzer. For an AV shunt, clamp the arterial and venous cannulae and disconnect them. Connect the arterial line to the dialyzer, discard the saline in the dialyzer as it fills with blood, and then connect the venous line.

For an AV fistula or internal graft, you may want to infiltrate the puncture sites with xylocaine to reduce patient discomfort. For the arterial line, insert a large-gauge needle or catheter directed toward the fistula or graft. The tip should be at least 2 cm away from the fistula or graft (Figure 7-8). For the venous line, direct a second needle away from the fistula or graft in the direction of venous flow. Although past technique called for a tourniquet between the needles to prevent dialyzed blood from re-entering the arterial line, current practice utilizes a blood pump to achieve this end and obviates the need for a tourniquet.

Anchor the lines so there is no tension on them or kinking.

6. Begin blood flow to the dialyzer slowly to avoid precipitating hypotension. Monitor the blood pressure every two to five minutes while the dialyzer fills and the flow rate is increased.

7. Set alarm limits for blood flow rate, and dialysate concentration, flow rate, and temperature. Also activate the monitors for air bubble and blood leak detection.

Monitoring hemodialysis   Monitor the patient closely during the dialysis and respond promptly to problems. The major potential problems during dialysis are volume depletion, fluid overload, electrolyte imbalances, dialysis disequilibrium syndrome, mechanical dysfunction, and immobility. These problems are described in the following sections.

Volume depletion   Hypotension, tachycardia, falling CVP, and/or thirst indicate volume depletion. The most common causes are antihypertensive or diuretic drugs, excessive volume removal for dialysis, and excessive ultrafiltration (water removal). (Accidental disconnection of the lines will not cause these signs; the alarms go off early enough to prevent the amount of blood loss which would produce them.) Before the dialysis, check with the physician about omitting any diuretic agents and antihypertensives (unless the patient is in hypertensive crisis). If sudden hypotension occurs anyway, immediately give normal saline intravenously through the extracorporeal circuit. Excessive volume removal for dialysis is a problem particularly with smaller patients and those who are hypovolemic before dialyses. To forestall this problem, a small-volume dialyzer may be employed, little pressure may be used to enhance fluid removal, and normal saline may be given intermittently or continually via the venous line to replace excess fluid loss. *Ultrafiltration* is the process of removing water from the circulation by manipulating pressure in the blood compartment and/or the dialysate compartment to increase the blood-to-dialysate pressure gradient. Ultrafiltration pressure is individualized according to the weight loss desired during dialysis. If the patient on ultrafiltration becomes hypotensive secondary to hypovolemia, the pressure gradient can be reduced. Fluid removal during dialysis can be monitored easily if bed scales are used.

Fluid overload and electrolyte imbalances   Hypertension; weight increase; headache; ankle, sacral, and/or periorbital edema; wet rales in lungs; or symptoms of pulmonary edema suggest fluid overload. They can be corrected by increasing the pressure gradient and thus increasing ultrafiltration.

Arrhythmias, muscle weakness or cramps, hypoactive or hyperactive reflexes, or other signs of electrolyte imbalances call for a prompt check of serum electrolytes and consultation with the physician for possible orders regarding changes in the dialysate solution.

Dialysis disequilibrium syndrome   Headache, nausea, vomiting, hypertension, confusion and/or seizures may indicate the dialysis disequilibrium syndrome. This syndrome, seen primarily at the completion of dialysis or shortly thereafter, may be due to too-rapid removal of urea from the bloodstream. One explanation of the syndrome holds that because of the blood-brain barrier, rapid removal of urea from the bloodstream is not accompanied by equivalent removal from brain tissue. The hypertonic cerebrospinal fluid may cause water to shift from the plasma into brain tissue until equilibration occurs, and this cerebral edema may produce the signs of the syndrome. The syndrome may be prevented by early dialysis (before the BUN becomes excessively high), by dialyzing the acutely uremic patient gradually over two to three days, or by using the less efficient peritoneal dialysis. If the symptoms appear during hemodialysis, the blood flow rate may be reduced, medications may be administered to control seizures, or dialysis may be discontinued.

Mechanical problems   Mechanical problems include changes in dialysate concentration, flow, or temperature; blood flow or pressure; and many others. Although these items usually are monitored mechanically, the availability of such aids should not replace astute nursing observation and intervention. Follow these measures:

1. Before each dialysis, use a chloride meter or chloride test to measure the number of chloride ions present in the solution. Since most positive ions are combined with chloride when added to the mixture, this check is an indicator of the correct dialysate mixture. This is the only specific dialysate electrolyte test that can be performed at the bedside.

2. Maintain dialysate flow within the optimal range by checking the flowmeter and making necessary adjustments hourly.

3. Maintain the dialysate temperature near body temperature. Too high a temperature causes hemolysis, fever, and pain; too low, chills, and vessel spasm.

4. Quickly investigate when alarms are triggered. Pressure alarms on the extracorporeal circuit's arterial and venous blood lines monitor changes in blood flow into and out of the dialyzer. They may indicate obstructions, separations, clots, vessel spasm, hematomas, or many other problems with blood flow.

5. If a blood leak alarm occurs, look at the dialysate and check it with a blood indicator dipstick since air bubbles can cause false alarms. A small blood leak may seal over and allow continuation of dialysis. A large blood leak usually calls for immediate cessation of dialysis.

Immobility   The reduced mobility necessitated by dialysis contributes to discomfort, boredom, thrombosis, and atelectasis. Change the patient's position and give back rubs and range of motion exercises. Establish with the patient a schedule of deep breathing and coughing exercises. Provide diversion with books, television, crafts, or visits from family or friends. Remember to continue other regular treatments such as intermittent positive pressure breathing.

Discontinuing dialysis   When dialysis is completed, discontinue it in the following manner.

Discontinue heparinization (if not already done). When needles are used with internal access routes, heparin may be discontinued 1–2 hours before the dialysis is stopped so that puncture sites can clot more readily.

Clamp the arterial line but leave the venous line open for blood return to the patient. Rinse the venous line with saline and discontinue it.

For an AV shunt, reconnect the cannulae and dress the sites as described earlier. For an AV fistula, use a gloved finger to apply direct pressure as the needles are removed and maintain it until bleeding stops. Use just enough pressure to prevent bleeding but not enough to occlude flow.

Problems between dialyses   Be alert for problems between dialyses. Post-dialysis, anticipate that the patient's weight, blood pressure, and urinary output (if any) will be decreased. Since serum potassium will have been returned to normal, be alert for conditions which could provoke hypokalemia, such as diarrhea, persistent vomiting, or nasogastric drainage. Also observe for the dialysis disequilibrium syndrome, as outlined above.

Peritoneal dialysis

Peritoneal dialysis uses the peritoneum as the dialyzing membrane. One surface of the peritoneum lines the abdominal cavity; the other covers the abdominal viscera. The space between is the peritoneal cavity into which the dialyzing fluid is instilled. On the other side of the membrane is extracellular fluid. From it, the dialysate removes fluid through osmosis and metabolic wastes through diffusion and filtration. Peritoneal dialysis is contraindicated in adhesions of the peritoneal cavity. Unless it is being used to treat peritonitis, it is contraindicated in that condition also.

Preparation for peritoneal dialysis   To prepare the patient for peritoneal dialysis, follow these steps.

1. Assist the physician in explaining the necessity of dialysis and the technique involved. Inform the patient of common sensations associated with dialysis, such as pressure during catheter insertion and fluid instillation.

2. Record baseline vital signs and weight.

3. Assist the physician to insert the peritoneal catheter. Bring to the bedside skin prep supplies, dressing supplies, the size and type of catheter the physician prefers, its trocar, and the dialysis delivery system. Peritoneal dialysis may be done either with bottles of solution run in via gravity or by a machine which mixes the dialysate and delivers it via a pump. The dialysate should be at body temperature to minimize discomfort and optimize clearance of waste products. Add to the solution any prescribed medications such as potassium or heparin.

Immediately prior to catheter insertion, have the patient empty his bladder to minimize the risk of bladder perforation. Clean and shave the abdomen. Drape it with sterile towels. The physician will anesthetize the area just below the umbilicus and make a small incision. Through this, he or she will insert the trocar into the peritoneal cavity. After the catheter is passed through the trocar, the trocar is removed and the catheter is sutured in place. Urine, feces, or blood dripping out the catheter indicate perforation of the bladder, intestine, or abdominal blood vessels. If no such catastrophe occurs, connect the administration set to the catheter.

4. Begin dialysis. The physician will specify the type and amount of fluid to be instilled and the length of the infusion, equilibrium, and drainage periods. One common order is 2 liters of fluid per cycle with an inflow time of 10 minutes, equilibrium time of 30 minutes, and outflow period of 20 minutes. If you are using an automated delivery unit, it will cycle by itself. If you are not, clamp the outflow tubing and infuse the dialysate over a 10 minute period. When it has run in, clamp the tubing before air can enter the peritoneal cavity. The equilibration period (dwell time) may last 15–45 minutes. At the end of the period, unclamp the outflow tubing to permit the dialysate to drain by gravity into the closed drainage system. During this time, turning the patient from side to side may help to facilitate drainage. Fluid drained from the first cycle after catheter insertion may be slightly bloody.

Monitoring peritoneal dialysis   During and after the dialysis respond promptly to problems. The potential complications of peritoneal dialysis are fluid retention, pain, peritonitis, dyspnea and/or atelectasis, hyperglycemia, bladder or bowel perforation, and protein loss. These complications are described in the following sections.

Fluid retention   Inadequate fluid drainage, hypertension, and signs and symptoms of fluid overload or congestive heart failure indicate fluid retention. Be sure that the bottles of dialysate contain exactly the amount ordered for infusion; some manufacturers add an extra small amount, which you should pour off.

Keep a running record of inflow, dwell, and outflow times; volume instilled; volume drained; and the cumulative fluid balance. The amount drained should equal or exceed the amount instilled. Frequently, the patient may retain some of the dialysate, running a positive fluid balance. The amount of positive fluid balance allowable varies with the patient and should be specified in the doctor's orders for the procedure. In some cases, as in the patient with congestive heart failure, it may be as low as a few hundred milliliters. Incomplete drainage can result from pooling of fluid due to body position, obstruction to the catheter if it is buried in the omentum or clogged with fibrin clots, or escape of the fluid via a bowel or bladder perforation. When drainage is less than expected, try these measures. Turn the patient from side to side, elevate the head of the bed, and/or massage the abdomen gently. Should the problem continue and the patient continually retain fluid on each exchange, consult with the physician before initiating another cycle. He may attempt to clear the catheter by rotating it or probing it to dislodge any fibrin clots.

Pain   Prevent the common effect of pain by making sure the dialysate is at body temperature and by promoting effective drainage of fluid. If pain persists, notify the physician since it may indicate peritonitis. Once peritonitis has been ruled out, the doctor may prescribe the instillation of a local anesthetic at the start of each cycle, decrease the volume instilled, or have you administer analgesics. Serving meals in small portions and providing diversion through family visits, television, and radio may also help reduce the discomfort.

Peritonitis   Abdominal pain, fever, rebound tenderness, and/or cloudy return fluid suggest peritoneal infection. Prevent peritonitis by scrupulous attention to sterile technique. Observe the outflow fluid; it should be pale yellow and clear. Routinely culture fluid drained from the first cycle and one cycle daily thereafter. If you note signs of infection alert the physician. Antibiotics will be given in the dialysate and/or systemically in the hope of maintaining use of the catheter.

Dyspnea or atelectasis   Dyspnea or atelectasis may result from restricted diaphragmatic descent due to the pressure of the fluid. Elevate the head of the bed. Prevent atelectasis by promoting deep breathing and coughing. If the patient develops acute dyspnea, drain the dialysate immediately and summon medical assistance.

Hyperglycemia   Confusion and lethargy may result from fluid overload or hyperglycemia. Measures to prevent fluid overload are discussed above. When the dialysate fluid has a high glucose concentration, hyperglycemia may occur if glucose crosses the peritoneal membrane. To forestall hyperglycemia, make sure that the dialysate fluid has the ordered dextrose concentration (1.5%, 3%, or 4.25%) and drain dialysate promptly at the end of the specified equilibration period. Place diabetics on routine urine and/or blood tests for sugar and acetone.

Bowel or bladder perforation   Diarrhea and diminished or fecal colored peritoneal drainage imply bowel perforation. Notify the physician because laparoscopy may be necessary to repair the perforation and minimize peritonitis. Bladder fullness, increased urinary output, and decreased peritoneal drainage suggest bladder perforation. Confirm your suspicion by testing both the drainage fluid and the urine for sugar; in perforation, they will have the same concentration (Richard 1975). Alert the physician, who will repair the bladder surgically.

Protein loss   Protein loss has been estimated at 0.2–0.5 gm/L of drained fluid. Since dialysis often includes 24–48 cycles initially, this loss can be significant. High-protein meals and intravenous protein infusions may be contraindicated because of the diminished urea excretion. Because patients with low protein intake will develop edema, poor resistance to infection, and wasting after several months of peritoneal dialysis, some physicians prefer a high-protein diet to minimize catabolism.

With proper management, patients may be sustained on intermittent home peritoneal dialysis for up to five years.

Outcome evaluation

To evaluate the patient's progress, use these outcome criteria:

- Urine output within normal limits (WNL) for patient, ideally 600–1600 ml/24 hr
- Urine osmolality WNL for patient, ideally 500–800 mOsm/kg
- Serum osmolality WNL for patient, ideally 295–395 mOsm/kg
- Plasma and urine electrolytes WNL for patient
- BUN WNL for patient, ideally 8–20 mg%
- Creatinine concentrations WNL for patient, ideally 0.5–1.2 mg% for plasma and 1–1.8 gm/24 hr urine
- Level of consciousness unchanged or improved from that before onset of acute renal failure
- Nutrition and elimination WNL for patient
- Vital signs, ECG, and arterial blood gases WNL for patient
- No signs or symptoms of fluid overload/deficit, anemia, infection, malnutrition, or uremic pericarditis

References

Brenner, B., Deen, W., and Robertson, C. 1976. Glomerular filtration. In *The kidney*, eds. B. Brenner and F. Rector, pp. 251–271. Philadelphia: W. B. Saunders Company.
Detailed explanations of glomerular filtration and of clearance. This and other chapters represent the most current, comprehensive source of highly detailed information on normal renal function; body fluid disturbances; pathogenesis, pathophysiology, and management of renal disease. Extensive bibliographies. Highly recommended.

Brundage, D. 1976. *Nursing management of renal problems*. St. Louis: C. V. Mosby Company.
Renal function, renal failure, dialysis procedures, home dialysis and renal transplantation.

Brunner, L., Emerson, C., Ferguson, L., and Suddarth, D. 1975. *Textbook of medical-surgical nursing*. 3rd ed. pp. 619–668. Philadelphia: J. B. Lippincott Company.
Basic descriptions of renal physiology, patient assessment, renal disorders, and nursing care.

Guyton, A. 1976. *Textbook of medical physiology*. 5th ed. Philadelphia: W. B. Saunders Company.
Guyton, Pitts, and Vander are moderately detailed references on renal physiology.

Koushanpour. E. 1976. *Renal physiology: principles and functions*. Philadelphia: W. B. Saunders Company.
Comprehensive, current information on renal clearance, tubular functions, and other aspects of renal physiology. Detailed presentation of theories of renin release in Chapter 12.

Levinsky, N., and Alexander, E. 1976. Acute renal failure. In *The kidney*, eds. B. Brenner and F. Rector, pp. 806–828. Philadelphia: W. B. Saunders Company.
Etiology, pathophysiology, clinical course, and treatment of acute renal failure.

Papper, S. 1971. *Clinical nephrology*. Boston: Little, Brown, and Company.
Concise, clinically-oriented reference.

Pitts, R. 1973. *Physiology of kidney and body fluids*. 3rd ed. Chicago: Year Book Medical Publishing Company.

Richard, C. 1975. Nursing implications in prevention of complications in peritoneal dialysis. *Heart Lung* 4:890–893.
Brief review of complications and related nursing care.

Thurau, K., and Boylan, J. 1976. Acute renal success. *Am. J. Med.* 61:308–315.
Role of the juxtaglomerular apparatus in sensing tubular reabsorption and adjusting glomerular filtration rate to protect body's fluid volume.

Vander, A. 1975. *Renal physiology*. New York: McGraw-Hill Books, Inc.

Valtin, H. 1973. *Renal function: mechanisms preserving fluid and solute balance in health*. Boston: Little, Brown, and Company.
Basic, concise explanations of renal, fluid, and electrolyte physiology; oriented toward medical students.

Supplemental Reading

American Association of Nephrology Nurses and Technicians. 1977. *Standards of clinical practice for the nephrology patient. Section IV: acute renal failure.* Park Ridge, Illinois.
Objectives, standards and assessment factors stated clearly and specifically.

Dhar, S., and Smith, E. 1975. Renal transplantation. *Heart Lung* 4:894–899.
Donor and recipient selection, pre- and postoperative care, diagnosis, and management of rejection episodes.

Dolan, P. 1975. Renal failure and peritoneal dialysis. *Nursing 75* (July):40–49.
Case study approach including brief review of anatomy and physiology and pictures of peritoneal catheter insertion.

Visel, J. 1975. Clinical aspects of renal biopsy. *Heart Lung* 4:900–902.
Indications, technique, and nursing implications.

Chapter 8

Thermal Regulation: Therapeutic Hypothermia

Therapeutic hypothermia, the deliberate lowering of body temperature, can be achieved in two ways: by cooling the blood with a pump oxygenator or by cooling the body surface. Extracorporeal cooling is often used during major cardiac surgery and neurosurgery. In the critical care unit, surface cooling may be achieved with ice or a hypothermia blanket. Since ice is messy, impractical, and a potential electrical hazard, most units rely on a hypothermia blanket when a critically ill patient must be cooled.

Outline

Uses of Hypothermia

Inducing hypothermia   Nursing measures / Prevention of complications

Rewarming   Possible complications

Objectives

- Recognize patients who may benefit from hypothermia
- Initiate hypothermia with a cooling blanket
- Anticipate the effects of hypothermia on patient comfort, vital signs, absorption and detoxification of medications, sensorium, aeration, and acid-base balance
- Implement measures to prevent each of these complications of hypothermia: skin breakdown and frostbite; drift, after-fall and shivering; arrhythmias; and thromboemboli
- Anticipate patient problems which may appear during rewarming

Uses of hypothermia

Patients who may benefit from hypothermia fall into two main categories. The first includes those who have a temperature above normal due to heat stroke, thyroid crisis, or infection, and who remain febrile in spite of antipyretics and conservative measures such as tepid baths, cooling fans, and ice packs. These patients are candidates for hypothermia because each degree centigrade of temperature elevation above normal raises metabolism approximately 7%; this increases physiologic stress in a patient whose resources may be nearing depletion due to the critical nature of his illness. The second group of patients includes those who are normothermic and who suffer an insult whose effects can be minimized by reducing the normal metabolic demand. Examples are patients with craniotomies, acute cerebral ischemia or edema, severe gastrointestinal bleeding, or persistent coma following cardiac arrest. Both groups may be helped by moderate hypothermia, which can reduce the total metabolic demand by 50%. The effect on the function of individual organs varies, with some, such as the brain, being affected profoundly and others, such as the kidney, being affected minimally.

Inducing hypothermia

When you recognize a situation in which hypothermia may be beneficial, suggest its use to the patient's physician. If the physician orders hypothermia, assist him/her in explaining its benefits and risks, as well as the sensations the patient will experience, to the patient and the family.

To initiate hypothermia, bring the following items to the bedside: a hypothermia blanket, a plastic blanket containing coils through which a cooling solution can flow; a hypothermia machine; a rectal thermometer probe; a glass rectal thermometer; a bath blanket; and two bed pads.

Connect the machine to the blanket and turn it on to inspect for leaks. Check the thermometer probe by simultaneously measuring the temperature of a glass of water with the probe and the glass thermometer.

Place the blanket on the bed. Place one bed pad at the top of the blanket where the head will rest and the other at the bottom where the feet will be. Cover the bedpads and hypothermia blanket with a single layer of a bath blanket, which will absorb skin perspiration and provide a softer surface on which the patient can lie.

Place the patient on the blanket. Prepare the skin and extremities as explained later. Insert the rectal probe at least two inches, making sure it is not embedded in feces. Tape the probe in position; if it falls out, it will register the cold blanket temperature and cause the machine to heat the patient. Set the blanket temperature several degrees centigrade lower than the body temperature. Adjust the machine to automatically shut off when the desired hypothermic level is detected by the probe. Since many probes and machines are inaccurate, it is a wise precaution to periodically check the patient's temperature with a rectal thermometer during hypothermia induction and maintenance.

Nursing measures

Monitoring   Monitor the patient for the expected effects of hypothermia. The range of temperature associated with the greatest physiologic benefit and least hazard is the moderate range of hypothermia, 28–32° C. Since this is the range used most commonly at the bedside, this chapter will focus on effects of moderate hypothermia and not those of deep hypothermia (below 28° C). Expected effects at 28–32° C include discomfort, vital sign changes, altered response to drugs, decreased sensorium, and a tendency toward respiratory and/or metabolic acidosis.

Alleviating discomfort   Hypothermia is an unpleasant experience for the patient, both physically and emotionally. When the patient complains of being cold, let him express his discomfort and reinforce the value of the cooling. Help him focus on the fact it is temporary. Be patient if he becomes irritable from his continuing discomfort. Follow the measures listed in later sections to prevent shivering, which worsens the discomfort.

Anticipating vital sign changes   The following descriptions of vital sign changes in response to cold are based on Hendee and Hudak (1973). During the first 20 minutes of hypothermia, the pulse rate rises, blood pressure increases, and respiratory rate accelerates. The body initially responds to the cold stimulus by conserving body heat and increasing heat production. Peripheral vasoconstriction minimizes surface heat loss, and skin pallor occurs. The increased venous return due to the vasoconstriction causes the blood pressure to rise. Increased heat production is achieved by the intense muscular activity known as shivering, estimated to occur in more than 95% of people exposed to intense cold (Abbey et al 1973). Pulse rate, respiratory rate, and temperature all rise initially due to this increased metabolic activity.

After about 20 minutes, vasoconstriction ceases and superficial blood flow reoccurs. Reactive hyperemia causes reddened skin. As body heat continues to be lost, all vital signs decrease. They stabilize at lower levels when the desired degree of hypothermia is maintained. At moderate hypothermia, the cardiac refractory period and ventricular relaxation are prolonged. The heart rate slows, coronary arterial filling is proportionally enhanced, and ventricular contractility improves.

Urinary output does not change significantly. Although a moderate decrease in glomerular filtration occurs, secretion of antidiuretic hormone is inhibited. Thus, the output will increase and the urine osmolality and specific gravity may decrease; however, electrolyte excretion by the kidney is unchanged.

It is crucial that you interpret the patient's vital signs and urinary output in light of the expected changes. For example, a pulse rate of 90 at 30° C is an abnormal finding that requires prompt investigation. Similarly, a progressive drop in urinary output may signal the onset of hypovolemia or renal failure.

Considering altered drug absorption   Because of the altered absorption of drugs produced by decreased perfusion, avoid subcutaneous and intramuscular injections; give medications intravenously instead. If a medication must be given intramuscularly, use a deep injection technique.

Although few liver functions are decreased by moderate hypothermia, the ability to detoxify morphine and some barbiturates is reduced. The physician may prescribe reduced doses or substitutes for these drugs.

Remembering decreased sensorium   Cerebral metabolism drops more than the rest of the body, approximately 6.7% per degree centigrade. Cerebrospinal fluid pressure drops 5.5% per degree centigrade with moderate hypothermia. Cerebral blood flow decreases about a third while cerebral metabolic demand diminishes about 54% (Zinn 1973). Since the decrease in cerebral metabolism is greater than the decrease in cerebral blood flow, cerebral perfusion is relatively improved.

At normal temperatures, the brain is slightly colder than the rest of the body. With surface cooling, it becomes 1–2 degrees centigrade warmer than the body core. Highly integrated centers are depressed first by hypothermia, providing a valuable cerebral protective mechanism even at moderately hypothermic levels. The sensorium, including hearing, fades at a body temperature of 33–34° C.

Nursing implications related to the decreased sensorium include applying artificial tears and taping the eyelids shut if blinking becomes infrequent. To evaluate changes in the level of consciousness, avoid assessing higher integrative responses (such as response to a simple command); instead, check the more primitive responses, such as those elicited by painful stimuli.

Minimizing the development of acidosis   The respiratory system undergoes several significant changes during hypothermia. Carbon dioxide production decreases, but ventilation decreases more rapidly (Zinn 1973). This imbalance between carbon dioxide production and excretion can lead to respiratory acidosis. Oxygen uptake increases, but cold shifts the oxyhemoglobin dissociation curve to the left, reducing the dissociation of O_2 from the red blood cells. This effect contributes to tissue hypoxia, which can precipitate ventricular irritability. If the hypoxic patient shivers, the cells must rely more heavily on anaerobic metabolism for energy production, which produces lactic acid and ketone bodies as by-products. Since circulation is reduced, these by-products accumulate and metabolic acidosis can occur.

Minimize the risk of acidosis by monitoring the blood gases closely. Prevent shivering, and promote ventilation through elevating the head of the bed, turning the patient frequently and implementing a program of chest physiotherapy to enhance CO_2 elimination and removal of secretions. The physician may prescribe the addition of 2–5% CO_2 to the patient's ventilation. This treatment induces respiratory acidosis, which shifts the oxyhemoglobin dissociation curve back toward normal (the Bohr effect), thus promoting the release of oxygen to the tissues. It also dilates the cerebral vasculature.

Prevention of complications

The possible complications of hypothermia are skin breakdown and frostbite; drift, after-fall and shivering; arrhythmias; and thromboemboli.

Skin breakdown and frostbite   Skin breakdown and frostbite can result from both diminished perfusion to the skin and the patient's decreased awareness of skin damage. Take the following steps to avoid these problems.

Keep the face, hands, and feet off the blanket. Place lamb's wool between the fingers and toes. Cover the hands and feet loosely with cotton and wrap them with stretch gauze. When bathing the patient, use tepid water and massage the skin gently to avoid producing heat. Turn the patient at least every two hours to relieve pressure points. To maintain the hypothermia, turn the blanket with the patient.

Drift   Minimize the interrelated problems of drift, after-fall and shivering. Cold receptors in the skin appear to be affected markedly by the rate of temperature change (Hensel 1970) and the core temperature seems to follow the sensors (Hardy 1970): the faster the change in skin temperature, the faster the change in core temperature. Drift is defined as a sudden change in body temperature greater than one degree centigrade in 15 minutes. Many nurses have observed that drift precedes frank shivering, shock, and arrhythmias.

After-fall   After-fall is the phenomenon of continuing drop in core temperature after the hypothermia machine is turned off. (Some people call this phenomenon drift, also.) It occurs because even though the machine is turned off, the chilled coolant in the blanket remains in contact with the patient's body. In addition, during hypothermia the periphery cools more than the core, so that even after hypothermia is discontinued, the warmer core continues to lose heat to the superficial tissues. At present, most nurses turn off the machine when the rectal temperature is 0.5 degrees centigrade above the desired temperature. The patient usually shows an after-fall of 1–5 degrees centigrade. The more rapid the drift, the greater the after-fall. Drift and after-fall are intensified when the patient is obese. Muscle tone, thermoregulatory and vascular responses, and ambient temperature and humidity also affect drift and after-fall (Abbey et al 1973) so that you cannot predict the extent to which these phenomena will develop in a given patient.

Shivering   Shivering is a normal physiologic response to cold. Shivering is produced by stimulation of the shivering center in the posterior hypothalmus. This center appears to respond to changes in skin temperature receptors and the temperature of the anterior hypothalamus (Ogata and Murakami 1972).

It is important to prevent or minimize shivering in the hypothermic patient for several reasons. Shivering increases the patient's and family's discomfort. It also accelerates the metabolic rate, pulse, arterial pressure, venous pressure, cerebrospinal fluid pressure, oxygen consumption, carbon dioxide production, and production and accumulation of lactic acid. These effects occur at a time when perfusion to the core organs already is reduced. Since blood flow to the muscles is increased during shivering, the temperature gradient between the core and periphery steepens, and core heat loss worsens. Shivering therefore is only a short-term mechanism for coping with hypothermia, with numerous undesirable effects.

Measures to minimize complications   To minimize drift, after-fall, and shivering (without resorting to drugs), take the following steps:

1. Prevent rapid cooling of the distal limbs. Since the hands and feet are most distal from the body, they lose heat very rapidly. Slowing their rate of heat loss appears to slow the change in core temperature. Wrap the upper extremities from fingertips to elbows and the lower extremities from toes to knees, until the patient has stabilized at the desired temperature. A pilot study by Abbey et al (1973) on the efficacy of this measure found that by itself it decreased the incidence of frank shivering from the usual 95% to 24%. The investigators used three thicknesses of new terry cloth toweling in order to maintain a constant insulation factor during the study. The thicknesses were not overlapped; instead, wooden clothespins held the edges together. These clothespins provided for easy access to the extremity and rapid resumption of the wrapping afterwards. The wraps were changed when damp. Although the sample size for the pilot study was small (17 patients), results from a larger group of patients will be published in the future.

2. During induction of hypothermia, initially set the blanket temperature to provide a steep gradient between it and the patient (15° C is a common initial setting). Monitor the rectal temperature. If it drops more than one degree centigrade per 15 minutes, reduce the gradient between the patient and blanket by increasing the setting for the blanket temperature.

3. Observe the patient for shivering. Premonitory signs of frank shivering are tensing or clenching of the masseter muscles, which close the jaw (Figure 8-1). Actual shivering begins in the masseters as a twitch and moves to the neck or pectoral areas. Frank shivering in the extremities and chattering teeth are later signs which usually necessitate pharmacologic intervention.

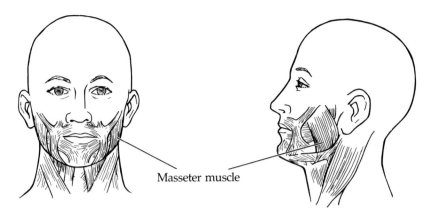

Masseter muscle

Figure 8-1.   Location of masseter muscle.

4. If shivering occurs, try reducing the rate of temperature decline by in-creasing the blanket temperature. If this action is contraindicated by the gravity of the patient's condition, the physician may prescribe chlorpromazine (Thorazine) in 10–25 mg doses. The effect of chlorpromazine on shivering is unpredictable. In addition, it causes vasodilatation, which produces hypoten-sion, tachycardia, and increased core heat loss.

5. To minimize after-fall, control drift as described above. Also consult the physician about using a range of desired temperature rather than an absolute value. Turn the machine off at 0.5 degrees centigrade above the upper limit of the range.

Arrhythmias   Be alert for arrhythmias. Arrhythmias (other than sinus bradycardia, which is an expected response) are unlikely to occur with moderate hypothermia if precautions are taken to ensure slow cooling and to avoid unin-tended deep hypothermia. During hypothermia, the total cardiac refractory period lengthens. The proportion of relative refractory period to absolute refrac-tory period also increases, so the vulnerable period is prolonged (Zinn 1973). The length of the vulnerable period is of concern, since an ectopic ventricular beat falling during the vulnerable period of the ventricles may initiate ventricular tachycardia or fibrillation. The likelihood of ectopic beats producing ventricular tachycardia or fibrillation does not increase dangerously during hypothermia until the temperature drops below 28° C. To minimize ventricular irritability, limit the temperature drop to one degree centigrade per 15 minutes and prefera-bly do not allow the core temperature to go below 28°C.

Hypothermia prolongs all intervals on the ECG. In addition, it often causes a slowly inscribed terminal portion of the QRS, called a J wave or Osborn wave (Clements and Hurst 1972). This wave, illustrated in Figure 8-2, does not signify any danger; it is an incidental finding. It is most pronounced in leads V_3–V_6.

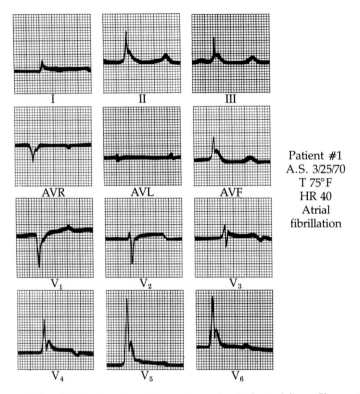

Patient #1
A.S. 3/25/70
T 75°F
HR 40
Atrial
fibrillation

Figure 8-2. ECG of accidental hypothermia. (Adapted from Clements, S., and Hurst, J. Diagnostic value of electrocardiographic abnormalities observed in subjects accidentally exposed to cold. *American Journal of Cardiology* 29:729, 1972. Used with permission of the author and publisher.)

Other electrocardiographic findings may include a fine muscle tremor and, at lower hypothermic levels, atrial fibrillation with a slow ventricular response (Gilbert 1974).

Thrombosis and embolization   During hypothermia, fluid shifts from the intravascular space into the intracellular and interstitial spaces. This shift leaves the blood more concentrated, and thrombosis and embolization may occur. In addition to frequent turning and range of motion exercises, see Chapters 5 and 10 for suggestions on avoiding this complication.

Rewarming

When hypothermia is no longer needed, rewarm the patient gradually. Although surface rewarming can be used, it carries the danger of warming the periphery before the core. The still cold heart then may be unable to produce a cardiac output adequate for the metabolic demands of the warmer areas. Dilatation of the surface vessels causes blood pooling, a diminished venous return, and a further decrease in cardiac output. These conditions may lead to shock.

For these reasons, natural rewarming is preferred. Simply turn the machine off, remove the cooling blanket, and place a bed blanket over the patient. (To avoid damaging the hypothermia blanket or losing cooling fluid, disconnect the hoses from the machine and attach them to each other. Roll rather than fold the blanket to store it.)

Possible complications

Shock and acidosis   During the rewarming period, which may take up to 8 hours, observe for shock and acidosis. Shock may result from too rapid warming, as explained above; this can occur even if the rewarming is achieved naturally. Acidosis may result from inadequate perfusion of the warmer areas or a release of the lactic acid which accumulated during shivering. During rewarming, the level of consciousness, pulse, blood pressure, and respiratory rate should increase proportionally to the core temperature. When any decrease or disporportionate increase occurs, alert the physician, who may want to investigate other possible causes (such as a bleeding ulcer), prescribe vasopressors, or initiate recooling.

Cumulative drug effects   During the rewarming phase, remember to observe for the cumulative effects of previously administered drugs, particularly those given intramuscularly. Also, remember that hearing will return at about 34° C; you can use this knowledge to gradually reorient the patient to his surroundings.

Ulcers   Another problem that may appear during rewarming is gastritis or peptic ulceration. During hypothermia, pepsin production continues, although the secretion of gastric juice diminishes. When rewarming occurs and gastric juice flow increases, it contains an increased concentration of pepsin. Notify the physician if signs of gastritis or ulceration appear.

Overhydration   Rewarming causes fluid to shift from the intracellular and interstitial spaces back into the intravascular compartment. If fluids were not given cautiously during hypothermia, signs of overhydration may appear during rewarming. Fluid overload is discussed in detail in Chapter 6.

References

Abbey, J., Andrews, C., Avigliano, K., Blossom, R., Bunke, B., Clarke, E., Engberg, N., Healy, P., Halliburton, P., Peterson, J., Shirley, C., and Waers, C. 1973. A pilot study:

the control of shivering during hypothermia by a clinical nursing measure. *J. of Neurosurg. Nurs.* 5(2) 78–88.
Report of pilot study on efficacy of wrapping extremities to prevent shivering. Highly recommended reading.

Clements, S., and Hurst, J. 1972. Diagnostic value of electrocardiographic abnormalities observed in subjects accidentally exposed to cold. *A. J. of Cardiol.* 29:729–734.
Report and illustrations of ECG findings, including J (Osborn) wave.

Gilbert, C. 1974. Temperature and humidity, radiation, underwater environment, hyperbaric oxygen, and the cardiovascular system. In *The heart.* 3rd ed. eds. J. Hurst and R. Logue. pp. 1572–1579. New York: McGraw-Hill Books, Inc.
Effects of these diverse factors on cardiovascular function. ECG changes with hypothermia.

Hardy, J. 1970. Thermal comfort: Skin temperature and physiological regulation. In *Physiological and behavioral temperature regulation.* eds. J. Hardy, A. Gagge, and J. Stolwijk. pp. 856–893. Springfield, Ill.: Charles C. Thomas.

Hendee, R., and Hudak, C. 1973. Pathophysiology of the central nervous system and management modalities. In *Critical care nursing.* ed. C. Hudak, B. Gallo, and T. Lohr. pp. 268–282. Philadelphia: J. B. Lippincott Company.
Brief review of increased intracranial pressure, cerebral concussion/contusion, cerebral edema, and other cerebral disorders. Phases of hypothermia and related nursing care.

Hensel, H. 1970. Temperature receptors in the skin. In *Physiological and behavioral temperature regulation.* eds. J. Hardy, A. Gagge, and J. Stolwijk. pp. 442–453. Springfield, Ill.: Charles C. Thomas.

Ogata, K., and Murakami, N. 1972. Neural factors affecting the regulatory responses of body temperature. In *Advances in climatic physiology.* pp. 50–67. New York: Springer-Verlag.

Zinn, W. 1973. Hypothermia in the critical care unit. *Heart Lung* 2(1) 58–61.
Organ responses to hypothermia, method of induction, and clinical application.

Chapter 9

Aeration Assessment

Aeration is a process which includes three major phases. The first phase is the movement of air into and out of the alveoli, called *ventilation*. The second phase is the exchange of gases between the alveoli and pulmonary capillaries, called *alveolar-capillary diffusion*. The third phase is the *transport of gases* in the blood, to and from the cells.

Your ability to assess the adequacy of your patient's aeration is vital in assisting him to maintain adequate oxygenation and ventilation. Table 9-1 presents a suggested format for nursing assessment of aeration.

Outline

History and Physical Examination   The lungs and thorax/Description of examination findings/Inspection/Palpation, percussion, and auscultation/Extra-thoracic signs of respiratory distress

Bedside pulmonary function tests   Inspiratory force/Airway resistance/Compliance/Lung volumes and capacities/Deadspace/V_D/V_T ratio

Blood gas values   Obtaining the blood gas sample/Interpreting blood gas values

Chest x-ray   Normal characteristics/Abnormal signs/Easily identifiable abnormalities

Objectives

- Describe the boundaries of the lungs in relation to external chest markings
- Inspect the thorax for shape, respiratory rate, respiratory rhythm, and chest expansion

Table 9-1   Aeration assessment format

1. History _____

   _____

2. Physical

   A. Inspection

      Thoracic shape _____

      Respirations: rate _____ rhythm _____

      Chest expansion _____

   B. Palpation

      Trachea _____

      Tactile fremitus _____

   C. Percussion _____

   D. Auscultation

      Breath sounds _____

      _____

      Adventitious sounds _____

      _____

      Voice and whispered sounds _____

- Describe respiratory stimuli and controls
- Describe the mechanics of chest movement
- Palpate for tracheal position, chest expansion, and tactile fremitus
- Percuss the chest, identifying normal percussion notes for specific areas of the chest
- Describe the characteristics and normal locations of bronchial, bronchovesicular, and vesicular breath sounds
- On chest auscultation, differentiate normal from adventitious sounds
- Describe the normal characteristics of voice and whispered sounds and indicate the significance of changes
- Describe the significance of common extrathoracic signs of respiratory distress

Table 9–1 *(continued)*

E. Extra-thoracic signs

Cyanosis _____ Clubbing _____

Use of accessory muscles _____

Other _____

3. Diagnostic procedures and laboratory tests

Pulmonary function tests _____

Inspiratory force _____ Compliance _____

FEV_1 _____ TV _____ RV_____

FRC _____ TLC _____ VC _____

V_D/V_T ratio _____

Other _____

Arterial blood gases _____

FIO_2 _____ PO_2 _____ PCO_2 _____

A-a gradient _____ Shunt _____

Chest x-ray _____

Other _____

- Interpret common bedside pulmonary function tests
- Define anatomic, alveolar, and physiologic deadspace
- Obtain an arterial blood sample that will facilitate accurate analysis
- Describe factors affecting diffusion across the alveolar-capillary membrane, specifying normal values for alveolar and capillary PO_2 and PCO_2
- Describe the differences between atmospheric and alveolar air
- Define four possible ventilation/perfusion relationships
- Define anatomic, capillary, and physiologic shunts; define venous admixture
- Differentiate these terms: O_2 carrying capacity, O_2 content, PO_2, and O_2 saturation
- Describe the significance of the oxyhemoglobin dissociation curve

- State the range of normal PO_2 and O_2 saturation for a patient with normal temperature and acid-base balance
- Explain the measurement of the A-a gradient, give its normal value, and describe its usefulness in pulmonary assessment
- Explain the use of iso-shunt lines for estimating virtual shunt and determining desirable FIO_2
- Give the range of normal values for P_aCO_2 and identify the meaning of abnormal values
- Interpret chest x-ray reports related to acute aeration disorders

History and physical examination

The scope and depth of your history-taking in the critical care setting depend upon the urgency of the situation and whether the physician has already examined the patient. Pertinent factors to note include smoking history, exposure to inhaled toxins, chest trauma, past respiratory illnesses, thoracic surgery, and development of symptoms such as easy fatigability, dyspnea, and hemoptysis.

The physical examination provides information about the patient's current aeration status. The following sections describe in detail aeration physical assessment skills useful for the critical care nurse.

The lungs and thorax

The physical examination must be based on a clear understanding of the relationships between external chest landmarks and the underlying respiratory structures (Figure 9-1). The following information on these relationships is derived from Bates (1974). The apices of the lungs extend about 2-4 cm above the inner portion of each clavicle. Anteriorly, the bases of the lungs extend down to the diaphragm, which is located at about the sixth rib on the left and about the fifth or sixth rib on the right. Posteriorly, the bases extend to about the level of the tenth thoracic spinous process and descend to the level of the twelfth spinous process on deep inspiration.

The right lung has three lobes, the left lung two. Each lung is divided by the major, oblique fissure. This fissure goes from the third thoracic spinous process in the back, to the fifth rib in the midaxillary line, to the sixth rib at the midclavicular line. In the left lung, this fissure separates the left upper and lower lobes. In the right lung, it separates the upper and lower lobes posteriorly, but the *middle* and lower lobes anteriorly. For this reason, one examines much more of the upper lobe in the anterior chest than in the posterior chest, while the lower lobe is primarily a posterior organ. In the right lung, the upper and middle lobes are separated by the minor, horizontal fissure which runs from the fifth rib

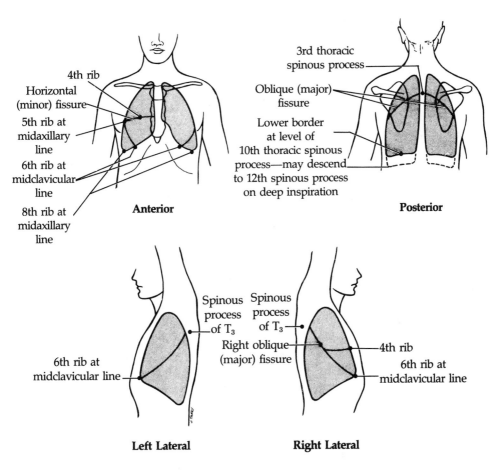

4th rib

Horizontal
(minor) fissure

5th rib at
midaxillary
line

6th rib at
midclavicular
line

8th rib at
midaxillary
line

Anterior

3rd thoracic
spinous process

Oblique (major)
fissure

Lower border
at level of
10th thoracic spinous
process—may descend
to 12th spinous process
on deep inspiration

Posterior

6th rib at
midclavicular line

Spinous
process
of T_3

Spinous
process
of T_3

Right oblique
(major) fissure

4th rib

6th rib at
midclavicular line

Left Lateral   **Right Lateral**

Figure 9-1.   Lung boundaries. (Adapted from Bates, B., 1974. *A Guide to Physical Examination.* Philadelphia: J. B. Lippincott Co.)

in the midaxillary line across to the fourth rib at the sternum. The lobes are further subdivided into ten segments in the right lung and eight in the left.

The right and left mainstem bronchi subdivide into the five lobar bronchi, then into eighteen segmental bronchi, and then into numerous nonrespiratory (terminal) bronchioles. All these structures conduct air but do not participate in gas exchange. Terminal bronchioles (which do not have alveoli) give rise to respiratory bronchioles, which do have alveoli opening onto them. Respiratory bronchioles subdivide into alveolar ducts, each of which leads to several alveolar sacs. Some alveoli line the walls of the respiratory bronchioles, more lie along the alveolar ducts, and the greatest number cluster around the alveolar sacs.

All the air passages beyond a terminal bronchiole are referred to collectively as an acinus. An acinus thus includes several branchings of respiratory bronchioles; alveolar ducts; alveolar sacs; and alveoli. Each acinus contains about five primary lobules. A primary lobule consists of a single respiratory bronchiole; its alveolar ducts, sacs, and alveoli; and its vascular supply structures.

Accompanying the respiratory bronchiole into the lobule are a branch of the bronchial artery carrying oxygenated blood to the tissues and a branch of the pulmonary artery carrying unoxygenated blood which participates in gas exchange. After it is oxygenated, the blood enters a branch of the pulmonary veins, which ultimately empty into the left atrium.

Description of examination findings   Describe the location of your findings in reference to the closest intercostal space or rib and the imaginary chest reference lines. Anteriorly, it is fairly easy to number ribs and spaces by using the angle of Louis as the reference point. (See Chapter 2 if you wish to review the technique.) Remember that only the costal cartilages of ribs 1–7 attach to the sternum. Those of ribs 8–10 attach to the cartilage immediately above each of them, and ribs 11 and 12 have free anterior tips. The reference lines on the anterior chest are the midsternal and midclavicular; on the lateral chest, the anterior, mid, and posterior axillary lines.

Posteriorly, numbering ribs is difficult, since the spinous processes of T_4-T_{11} overlie the vertebral body of the next lower rib (for example, the T_7 spinous process is near the attachment of the eighth rib). It is possible to number the ribs by having the patient flex his neck; the prominent bump at the base of the neck usually is the seventh cervical spinous process. From there down you can palpate and count the thoracic processes. The imaginary reference lines on the posterior chest are the vertebral and midscapular.

When you examine the thorax and lungs, use your senses of sight, touch and hearing to examine the anterior, posterior and lateral chest.

Inspection

Evaluate thoracic shape   The normal thoracic shape is symmetrical, with the anteroposterior (AP) diameter less than the lateral diameter. When the AP diameter is equal or greater than the lateral, the patient is said to have a barrel chest, which frequently is seen in chronic pulmonary disease. Other important observations include curvature of the spine and asymmetry of the chest wall.

Note respiratory rate and rhythm   The rate and rhythm of respiration are controlled by the respiratory center. According to Guyton (1976), the respiratory center is a group of neurons dispersed in the medulla and pons. It is subdivided into the medullary rhythmicity center, the apneustic center, and the pneumotaxic center. The rhythmicity center receives input from the spinal cord, cerebral cortex, pons, and vagus and glossopharyngeal nerves. The rhythmicity center in the medulla sets the basic rhythm, which is smoothed and strengthened by the apneustic and pneumotaxic centers in the pons. The Hering-Breuer reflex also plays a role in controlling respirations. It is thought that the lung tissue itself contains receptors which respond to inflation. When stretched, they send inhibitory impulses via the vagus nerve to the respiratory center. This reflex causes inspiration to stop and allows expiration to begin.

The most potent stimulus to respiration is the partial pressure of CO_2 in arterial blood (P_aCO_2) as explained later in the chapter. The partial pressure of oxygen in arterial blood probably is not a strong stimulus to respiration within the normal P_aO_2 range (70 mm Hg or above). As P_aO_2 drops, the chemoreceptors in the aortic and carotid bodies become excited and stimulate the respiratory center by reflex action. Below a P_aO_2 of about 50 mm Hg, the respiratory centers become hypoxic and depressed.

To a limited extent, respirations can be controlled voluntarily by the cerebral cortex; an example is singing. Other lesser stimuli to respiration include pain, cold, exercise, fear, and some drugs such as acetylsalicylic acid (aspirin).

The respiratory rate normally is 14–18 breaths a minute. The rhythm should be regular with inspiration shorter than expiration, that is, an I:E ratio of 1:1.5 or 1:2. Abnormal rhythms and their physiologic causes are discussed in detail in Chapter 15 on assessment of stimulation.

Chest expansion   Next, inspect chest expansion to evaluate the muscular work of breathing. Muscular movement depends on both the adequacy of neural impulses from the respiratory center to the muscles and on the integrity of the muscles and bones of the thorax. The chief nerves involved in inspiration are those innervating the external intercostal muscles, and the phrenic nerve which innervates the diaphragm. Motor stimuli from the respiratory center cause these muscles to contract. Contraction of the diaphragm causes it to flatten, thus expanding the thorax downward. Contraction of the external intercostals elevates the ribs, expanding the chest laterally.

The lungs expand because their coverings (the visceral pleura) closely approximate the lining of the chest (the parietal pleura). The space between the visceral and parietal pleurae is a potential space, with a thin layer of pleural fluid to allow gliding movement between the pleural layers. It is important to remember that each lung has a separate pouch of pleura (and pleural space) which surrounds it except at its attachment to the mainstem bronchi and pulmonary vessels (its hilum). Expiration usually occurs passively due to elastic recoil of the lungs, chest wall, and abdominal musculature.

While inspecting the chest, note whether breathing is thoracic, abdominal, or both. Normally, inspiration causes both expansion of the thorax and outward movement of the abdomen. Predominantly thoracic breathing may be either normal (as in late pregnancy) or abnormal (as in abdominal pain or distention). Predominantly abdominal breathing also may be either normal (as in healthy males) or abnormal. Chronic obstructive lung disease patients often use a mixture of thoracic and abdominal breathing, with upper thoracic effort prominent on inspiration. They may use forceful abdominal contraction on exhalation, because the diaphragm is depressed and relatively immobile, and in some cases (emphysema) the lung has lost its elastic recoil.

Observe, too, for signs of increased work of breathing, such as the use of accessory muscles in the neck or upper chest, retraction or bulging of the intercostal muscles, and active contraction of the abdominal muscles.

Also note whether the ribs and sternum move symmetrically. One abnormal sign occurs when one part of the chest wall moves paradoxically, that is, moves in on inspiration and out on expiration. Such movement can be a sign of underlying pleural disease. Flail chest, the term for the entire sternum moving paradoxically, results from rib fractures and causes severe respiratory distress.

The depth of chest expansion can be classed only crudely by inspection as normal, increased, or decreased. Accurate evaluation of the depth of expansion must be made with a spirometer.

Palpation, percussion, auscultation

The remaining steps of palpation, percussion, and auscultation enable you to assess the vibrations transmitted by the thoracic contents. You will recall that air enters the lungs through the nose and mouth, which filter, humidify, and warm it. It then passes through the glottis to the trachea, which is highly vascular and supported by C-shaped cartilagenous rings. The trachea bifurcates into the mainstem bronchi at the carina, which is heavily innervated. The carina is located anteriorly at the level of the angle of Louis and posteriorly at the level of T_4. The right mainstem bronchus is shorter, wider, and at a greater angle to the trachea than the left mainstem bronchus. The bronchi subdivide into the lobar branches, then into the segmental bronchi, terminal bronchioles, respiratory bronchioles, and finally into the alveolar ducts. In palpation, you will use your hands to feel the vibrations created by the movement of air through these structures when the patient speaks. In percussion, you will feel the vibrations created when you tap on the chest. In auscultation, you will use a stethoscope to exclude extraneous noise while you listen to the vibrations created by the patient breathing or speaking.

Sound transmission   While performing these steps, it is useful to remember some principles of sound transmission. Solid structures conduct sound better than air, unless they are too big or too compressed to respond to sound. Air in the pleural space will conduct sound very poorly.

Sounds are described according to their intensity, pitch, quality, and duration. Intensity refers to loudness and pitch to the frequency of vibrations. Quality refers to the unique characteristics of a sound that enable you to identify it again once you have heard it, such as the quality of a fingernail scraping a blackboard.

To date, different authorities have used a bewildering array of terms to describe findings on palpation, percussion, and auscultation. Recently a Joint Committee on Pulmonary Nomenclature, consisting of members of the American College of Chest Physicians and the American Thoracic Society (1975), has recommended a simplification of pulmonary labels. This chapter presents both the terms currently used by most practitioners and the latest recommendations from the Joint Committee.

Palpation   To continue the examination, palpate the chest to assess the position of the trachea, chest expansion, and tactile fremitus. The trachea should be midline; tracheal deviation can result from such conditions as pneumothorax and atelectasis. To evaluate chest expansion further, stand in back of the patient and place your hands on the lower rib cage so that you grasp the lateral ribs. Instruct the patient to exhale completely and then inhale deeply (using his abdominal muscles) to try to move your hands. As the patient breathes in, note whether your thumbs move apart equally. *Tactile fremitus* is the name given to palpable vibrations caused by speaking; the Joint Committee recommends the term "transmitted sounds." To palpate for fremitus, use the most sensitive part of your hands; this part may be either the pads of your fingertips or the part of your palm that overlies the heads of the metacarpal bones. Ask the patient to say "ninety nine" several times while you palpate the chest wall bilaterally. Normally, you will be able to feel vibrations like the purring of a cat over the trachea and bronchi. These vibrations should be equal bilaterally, except over the heart. Since solids conduct vibrations better than air, any condition that consolidates the lung close to the chest wall will increase fremitus. Decreased or absent fremitus occurs when a condition blocks the passage of air (such as an obstructed bronchus) or moves the lung tissue away from the chest wall (such as a pneumothorax).

Percussion   Next, percuss the chest, to evaluate the density of structures just below the chest wall. To do this, press the terminal phalanx of your middle finger on the chest wall and strike it on the knuckle with the tip of your other middle finger. Be sure to press only the terminal phalanx on the chest wall; if you allow contact between the rest of your hand and the chest, it will damp the vibrations. Strike the phalanx quickly at almost a 90° angle by cocking your wrist.

There are five sounds you may hear; you can learn four of them by percussing your own body. The sound normally heard over the lungs is medium loud, low-pitched, and relatively long; it is called *resonant*. Increased density of the lungs (as in pulmonary edema or pleural effusion) produces dull or flat sounds. A *dull* sound results from a moderate increase in density. It is soft, short, and high-pitched and is the sound heard when you percuss the liver. A *flat* sound is due to a severe increase in density. It is soft, high-pitched, and very short; you can reproduce it by percussing your thigh. Decreased density (such as in pneumothorax or emphysema) causes either *hyperresonant* or *tympanitic* sounds. A moderate decrease in density produces a loud sound which is lower-pitched and longer than resonance, called hyperresonant; you can not reproduce this sound in yourself, although you can mimic it somewhat by percussing your chest while you hold a deep breath. A large decrease in density produces a loud, long, high-pitched, drum-like sound described as tympanitic; you can reproduce it by percussing over your stomach. This term usually is not used in describing findings on lung percussion since it is heard commonly over air in an enclosed space. The Joint Committee recommends that instead of these five notes, percussion notes be described simply as normal, dull, or tympanitic.

Begin at the apices and percuss side to side down the chest until you reach the diaphragm. Listen for the sounds and feel for the vibrations produced.

Normally on percussing the chest you will hear resonance except in a few locations. On the posterior chest, you will hear dullness over the vertebrae, scapulae, and below the diaphragm. On the anterior chest, you will hear dullness over the sternum and heart; dullness starting at about the fifth or sixth intercostal space on the right (the upper border of the liver): and tympany at about the sixth rib on the left, where the stomach begins.

If you hear an abnormal percussion note, localize the finding by percussing from an area of resonance to the abnormal area.

Auscultation   Finally, use the diaphragm of a stethoscope to auscultate the chest from side to side. Ask the person to breathe through his mouth a little more deeply than normal.

Listen first for breath sounds. The following descriptions are from Bates (1974). The sounds normally heard over the trachea are called bronchial or tubular. They are loud and have a short inspiration, pause, and a longer, louder expiration. The sounds heard over the bronchi (that is, over the apices, below the clavicles anteriorly, and between the scapulae posteriorly) are called bronchovesicular. They are medium sounds with inspiration followed by a short pause, and an equally loud, equally long expiration. The sounds heard over the rest of the lungs are called vesicular. They are soft, with a long inspiration, no pause, and a shorter, softer expiration.

Decreased or absent sounds are caused by any condition that reduces air flow (such as an obstructed bronchus) or moves the lungs away from the chest wall (such as a pneumothorax). Increased breath sounds occur when an abnormal process fills air spaces with fluid (for example, pneumonia) or compresses lung tissue (for example, atelectasis), while the bronchus remains open. Increased breath sounds will be heard as bronchovesicular sounds where vesicular ones should be present, or bronchial sounds where you should hear vesicular or bronchovesicular ones.

The Joint Committee suggests that breath sounds be described only as normal, decreased, absent, or bronchial.

Next, listen for abnormal (*adventitious*) sounds, which are superimposed on breath sounds. To identify them, decide whether they are discrete or continuous and more prominent on inspiration or expiration. Since abnormal sounds may vary greatly in pitch and intensity, those characteristics are not particularly helpful in identifying them. In the past, an adventitious sound has been labelled as a fine, medium or coarse rale, a rhonchus, or a wheeze. Confusion has arisen since various authorities give conflicting definitions of these terms.

The Joint Committee recommends the use of only two terms, and their definitions are the ones included here. Discontinuous crackling sounds are called rales, and continuous musical sounds are called rhonchi; wheezes are included with rhonchi. (Although not included in the Joint Committee definitions, the following characteristics of rales and rhonchi are useful to know. Rales are more prominent on inspiration and rhonchi on expiration. Rales usually result from air passing through partially closed, compressed or fluid-filled alveoli, while rhonchi result from airway narrowing due to bronchospasm, secretions, and so on.) At present, to avoid misinterpretation by others, report your findings by describing their characteristics rather than just by labeling them. You also may detect a pleural friction rub; it is a grating, continuous sound that is associated with breathing.

Abnormal voice and whispered sounds rarely are checked by the critical care nurse. They are included here primarily so you will understand their significance when noted in a physician's work-up. Voice sounds are the auscultatory equivalent of the vibrations palpated during tactile fremitus. The patient is asked to say "ninety-nine" repeatedly. Normally, the sounds are heard indistinctly over the large airways and are equal bilaterally. Absent voice sounds occur when air flow is blocked (as in an obstructed bronchus) or the lung and chest wall are separated (as in a pneumothorax). Increased voice sounds are due to consolidation (solidification) of the lung. Increased sounds are detected when the syllables are heard more clearly than normal although still muffled; this finding is called bronchophony. A related finding, also due to consolidation, occurs when the patient's spoken E is heard as A; this phenomenon is called egophony. Whispered sounds normally are heard only faintly over the mainstem bronchi. In consolidation they are heard clearly; this occurrence is called whispered pectoriloquy. Again, the Joint Committee recommends a much simpler classification. It suggests that findings be reported as voice or whispered sounds that are normal; decreased or absent; or increased in intensity or clarity.

Significance of your findings   To interpret the significance of your findings from inspection, palpation, percussion, and auscultation, consider them in association with each other; some of the common groupings are included here, based on Bates (1974). A barrel chest, bilaterally decreased tactile fremitus, hyperresonance, decreased breath sounds, and rales or rhonchi suggest chronic obstructive lung disease. Asymmetrical chest expansion, unilaterally decreased fremitus, hyperresonance, decreased or absent breath sounds, and no adventitious sounds indicate a pneumothorax. Increased fremitus, dullness, and increased breath and voice sounds indicate consolidation. Decreased fremitus, dullness, and decreased breath and voice sounds are seen in atelectasis.

When you assume responsibility for a patient, it is useful to at least inspect and auscultate the chest so you have a basis for comparison as you later evaluate the effects of your nursing care. For instance, you might note when you come on duty that your patient is restless and slightly tachycardic. Auscultation might reveal diffuse rales and rhonchi. After chest physiotherapy and suctioning, you would again auscultate the chest; the absence of the adventitious sounds would indicate the effectiveness of your intervention to improve oxygenation. Your skill at chest diagnosis can be a valuable tool in assessing, planning, implementing, and evaluating the care you give patients.

Extra-thoracic signs of respiratory distress

Cyanosis   One of the extra-thoracic signs of respiratory distress is cyanosis. Cyanosis results from the presence of at least 5 gm of desaturated hemoglobin per 100 ml of blood. In the normal person, this amount is equivalent to about one-third of the hemoglobin; however, the presence of cyanosis is due not to the proportion but to the absolute amount of unsaturated Hgb. For this reason, the anemic patient may not show cyanosis because he or she does not have enough hemoglobin to accumulate five desaturated grams; the polycythemic patient may display cyanosis even though he or she has an adequate O_2 content. Thus, cyanosis is an unreliable indicator of the degree of oxygen deficit.

There are two basic causes of desaturation of hemoglobin. In the first, hemoglobin is saturated normally in the lungs but slowed passage through the tissues allows it to unload more O_2 than normal. This type is called peripheral cyanosis and may be seen in the extremities, particularly in the nailbeds. Its presence may be due to such factors as cold, nervous excitement, or cardiac failure. In the second type of cyanosis, the hemoglobin never becomes adequately saturated because it is not exposed to enough O_2, that is, the arterial O_2 saturation is below normal. This type is called central cyanosis because it is seen centrally as well as peripherally, for instance on the lips, under the tongue, and in the buccal mucosa. It is more serious than peripheral cyanosis as it usually is not seen until the O_2 saturation has decreased to about 75–80%.

Clubbing   Clubbing may be seen in the terminal phalanges of the fingers and toes. To recognize it, examine the angle between the base of the nail and the skin. The normal angle is about 160°; the increase of this angle to 180° or more is called clubbing.

Pulse   Note the patient's pulse rate for abnormal rate or rhythm. Tachycardia is an early compensatory response to hypoxia, and various arrhythmias may result from an oxygen deficit.

Other extra-thoracic signs   Other signs of respiratory distress include the use of accessory neck muscles or abdominal muscles to facilitate breathing; nasal flaring; pursed lips; and coughing. Confusion and disorientation may be seen in hypoxia or CO_2 retention; drowsiness may indicate CO_2 retention. Peripheral edema, jugular venous distention, and liver tenderness may be seen in cor pulmonale.

Bedside pulmonary function tests

Bedside pulmonary function tests are gaining increasing importance in assessment of the critically ill patient. Although they usually are performed by a respiratory therapist, understanding their results can help you plan, implement, and evaluate your nursing care. The following information on bedside pulmonary function tests is based on Comroe et al (1962). Brunner et al (1975), and Shapiro, Harrison, and Trout (1976).

Inspiratory force

Air enters the lungs because muscular expansion of the chest creates subatmospheric intra-alveolar pressures. The inspiratory force is measured by having the patient breathe in against a negative pressure manometer while his airway is occluded. The normal inspiratory force is about −60 to −100 cm H_2O pressure. If the inspiratory force is less than −25 cm H_2O, the person cannot maintain a normal sigh volume or cough effectively.

Airway resistance

In order for air to move in and out of the lungs, a variety of non-elastic and elastic resistances must be overcome. The non-elastic resistances consist of non-elastic tissue resistance and airway resistance. Guyton (1976) defines non-elastic tissue resistance as the resistance of the tissues of the lungs and thoracic cage to the molecular rearrangements necessary for lung expansion and contraction. Non-elastic tissue resistance normally comprises only a small portion of non-elastic resistance; airway resistance is much more important.

Airway resistance to gas flow depends on the lumen size, velocity of air flow, and gas characteristics. In normal quiet breathing, airway resistance is slight. Airway resistance can be evaluated by measuring the relationship between pressure and air flow. It is not feasible to measure airway resistance directly in the critically ill, but indirect measurements can be obtained by measuring expiratory flow rates. The patient is asked to breathe in as much air as possible and then to expel it as hard and fast as possible. This forced expiratory volume is recorded on a graph containing a time scale. The volume expired in one second is called the FEV_1. The ratio between it and the vital capacity is an indicator of resistance in the larger airways. The normal person is able to expel about 83% of his vital capacity in the first second and 97% in three seconds.

Compliance

The tissues of the lung and thorax also have elastic resistances, which must be overcome during inspiration. The lung tissues resist inspiration because they contain elastic fibers and because of the surface tension of fluids lining the alveoli, as explained below. These factors make the lungs tend to recoil (deflate). The thoracic muscles, tendons, and connective tissue also have elastic properties which make them resist expansion.

The distensibility of the lungs and chest wall is called total pulmonary compliance. It can be evaluated by measuring the relationship between pressure and volume, and can be expressed as the change in volume (V) per unit of change in pressure (P)

$$C = \frac{\Delta V}{\Delta P}$$

In the critically ill person, effective (dynamic) compliance is calculated by dividing the peak airway pressure into the tidal volume; the normal value is about 35–45 ml per cm pressure. Total pulmonary compliance decreases in conditions that (a) increase the resistance of the chest wall, such as scoliosis, tight dressings, or musculoskeletal diseases such as polio, or that (b) reduce the distensibility of the lung, such as pulmonary congestion, atelectasis, restrictive diseases, or disorders characterized by decreased surfactant.

The surface between the alveolar gas and alveolar wall has the property of surface tension. This property tends to make the alveoli collapse, therefore making expansion very difficult. Surfactant, a phospholipid made by the large alveolar cell, counters this tendency. It progressively increases surface tension on inspiration and decreases it on expiration, thus helping to control alveolar volume and prevent alveolar collapse. When surfactant decreases (as in shock lung), alveolar surface tension increases. Because of the resulting decrease in lung distensibility and increase in elastic recoil, compliance decreases.

Lung volumes and capacities

The air in the lungs can be subdivided into several volumes and capacities. A lung volume cannot be subdivided further. Two or more volumes combine to make a capacity.

Figure 9–2 presents the volumes and capacities graphically and gives examples of normal values. It must be stressed that these normal values are variable and are predicted on the basis of sex, age, height, weight, activity, and barometric pressure. The "normal" values given here apply only to a healthy young male with a surface area of 1.7 m², lying at rest and breathing air at sea level. They are taken from Comroe et al (1962).

Tidal volume   *Tidal volume* (V_T) is the amount of gas inspired or expired with a normal breath. It is measured with a spirometer. Its normal value is 500 ml.

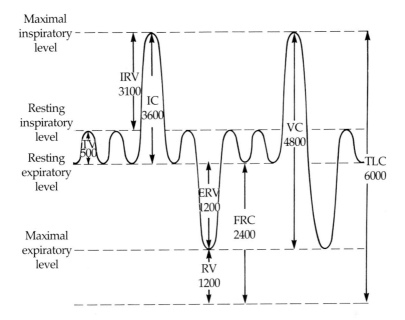

Figure 9-2.   Lung volumes and capacities. *ERV,* expiratory reserve volume; *FRC,* functional residual capacity; *IC,* inspiratory capacity; *IRV,* inspiratory reserve volume; *RV,* residual volume; *TLC,* total lung capacity; *TV,* tidal volume; *VC,* vital capacity. (Based on data from Comroe, J. H., Jr., et al. *The Lung: Clinical Physiology and Pulmonary Function Tests.* 2nd ed. Copyright © 1962 by Year Book Medical Publishers, Inc., Chicago. Used by permission.)

The inspiratory reserve volume is the volume that can be inspired above tidal volume; the normal value is 3100 ml. The expiratory reserve volume is the amount that can be expired below tidal volume; the normal value is 1200 ml. These two volumes do not give a great deal of information about pulmonary function.

Residual volume, functional residual capacity, and total lung capacity   The *residual volume* is the amount of gas that always remains in the lungs, that is, that cannot be expelled even with a maximal expiration. It cannot be measured directly. Instead, the patient breathes in a known percentage of an insoluble gas. His expired gas is collected for several minutes and analyzed for the amount of expired air and concentration of the gas. The residual volume can then be calculated; a normal value is 1200 ml. This test measures only the air in parts of the lung that communicate well with the airways. It is not accurate for completely trapped gas, as in emphysema. For such patients, a body plethysmograph ("body box") must be used to measure residual volume in the laboratory.

As mentioned above, two or more volumes combine to make a lung capacity. The residual volume plus the expiratory reserve volume represent the volume of air in the lungs at the end of a normal expiration. This amount is called the *functional residual capacity (FRC)*. A usual value is 2400 ml. It is measured by the gas washout method used to measure residual volume. The FRC functions to maintain a constant alveolar PCO_2. It increases in hyperinflation, such as in emphysema or asthma. An increased FRC increases the muscular effort of breathing, because it increases thoracic size. It also impairs the ability to increase ventilation and to alter quickly the composition of alveolar gas.

The total amount of air in the lungs is called the *total lung capacity* and measures about 6000 ml. It consists of the FRC and the inspiratory capacity. The *inspiratory capacity* is the maximal volume that can be inspired starting from a resting expiratory level; in other words, the tidal volume plus the inspiratory reserve volume. The inspiratory capacity measures about 3600 ml and usually represents 75% of the vital capacity.

Vital capacity   The *vital capacity (VC)* is very important clinically. It equals the total lung capacity minus the residual volume and is a measure of the person's ability to take a deep breath. To measure it, the patient is told to take a deep inspiration and then expel as much air as possible. The exhaled volume is measured with a spirometer. Normal vital capacity is about 4800 ml. Since there is a wide variety of normal values, Comroe et al recommend that a reading not be considered abnormal unless it is more than 20% below the predicted value. A decreased vital capacity is a helpful but nonspecific sign, since it may be caused by depression of the respiratory center, obstructive diseases, or restrictive conditions. It is important to recognize that a normal vital capacity does not rule out the presence of pulmonary disease, such as pulmonary embolism.

Significance   To interpret the patient's pulmonary volumes and capacities, group the data into the broad categories of obstructive or restrictive pulmonary diseases. Obstructive diseases are those associated with obstructions to airflow, such as asthma and emphysema. Restrictive diseases are those which limit lung expansion. Examples are neuromuscular diseases, chest deformities, pain, restricted diaphragmatic descent, and space-occupying lesions of the thorax. Increased total lung capacity, increased functional residual capacity, and decreased expiratory flow rates characterize obstructive pulmonary diseases. Decreased total lung capacity and vital capacity typify restrictive pulmonary diseases. Shapiro, Harrison, and Trout (1975) point out that acute restrictive pulmonary disease is the most common respiratory problem in the critically ill, as this category includes atelectasis, the acute respiratory distress syndrome, and the postoperative patient.

When interpreting lung measurements, remember that the trend of values is more important than one particular reading. Also remember that changes in lung volumes are not as significant as changes in alveolar ventilation, capillary perfusion, and alveolar-capillary diffusion.

Deadspace

The total volume of air that ventilates the lungs per minute is called the *minute ventilation*. It is the product of the tidal volume (V_T) times the respiratory rate (f), and is symbolized as V. (V alone stands for flow. With a dot over it, it means flow per unit time, assumed to be one minute unless stated otherwise.) Part of the minute ventilation merely fills the tracheobronchial tree and does not participate in gas exchange; it is called deadspace (V_D). The volume of gas per minute that actually reaches the alveoli and participates in gas exchange is called alveolar ventilation (V_A).

There are two types of deadspace: anatomic deadspace and alveolar deadspace. Anatomic deadspace is the air in the tracheobronchial tree up to the terminal bronchioles. Alveolar deadspace is that air in the alveoli which does not participate in gas exchange (because the alveoli containing it are without capillary blood flow). The sum of anatomic deadspace and alveolar deadspace is called physiologic deadspace.

Alveolar ventilation equals the tidal volume minus deadspace, times respiratory rate; that is $V_A = (V_T - V_D)$ f. A normal value is about 5200 ml assuming V_T = 500, V_D = 150, and f = 15. Alveolar ventilation can be estimated or measured. To estimate it, you must know the tidal volume, respiratory rate, and weight of your patient. Then assume that the anatomic deadspace equals 2 ml/kg (1 ml/lb) of body weight, subtract that value from the tidal volume, and multiply by the rate. Note that this formula does not take into account alveolar deadspace, and will not be accurate for patients with increased alveolar deadspace (as in pulmonary embolism), nor altered anatomic deadspace (as in a tracheostomy). Alveolar ventilation can be calculated more accurately by measuring physiologic deadspace. The patient's expired air is collected for several minutes and analyzed for expired PCO_2 (P_ECO_2). The arterial PCO_2 (P_aCO_2*) is measured from an arterial blood sample. A modified Bohr equation is used:

$$\frac{P_aCO_2 - P_{\bar{E}}CO_2}{P_aCO_2} \times V_T = V_D$$

The value obtained for deadspace then can be subtracted from tidal volume. The resulting number is multiplied by rate to calculate alveolar ventilation.

In the normal lung, deadspace is minimized by a protective reflex. When alveolar deadspace increases, the lack of matching perfusion causes local bronchoconstriction, which redirects ventilation to better perfused areas.

V_D/V_T ratio   More commonly in the clinical setting, we are less interested in the amount of alveolar ventilation per se than in the ratio between deadspace

---

*Note that P stands for partial pressure. A subscript written with a capital letter means the gas is in the gas phase; one written with a lower case letter signifies the gas in a liquid phase. Thus, P_ACO_2 means alveolar PCO_2, while P_aCO_2 means arterial PCO_2. A dash above a symbol signifies a mean value.

and tidal volume. This V_D/V_T ratio indicates what proportion of the tidal volume is being wasted as deadspace. As explained later, the PCO_2 of arterial blood is a useful indicator of tidal volume. Comparing the PCO_2 of arterial blood and the PCO_2 of expired gas indicates the amount of wasted ventilation. Rearranging the terms of the modified Bohr equation gives the equation for the ratio:

$$\frac{V_D}{V_T} = \frac{P_aCO_2 - P_{\bar{E}}CO_2}{P_aCO_2}$$

The usual V_D/V_T ratio is approximately 0.3; above 0.6, it is unlikely that the person can maintain spontaneous ventilation.

Blood gas values

The adequacy of gas exchange in the lungs can be evaluated by arterial blood gas analysis. The blood sample is obtained by withdrawing it from an existing arterial line or by percutaneous puncture of an artery. The following steps describe how to obtain an arterial blood sample. For either procedure, you will need the following equipment:

1. A heparinized syringe and 21–24 gauge steel needle. Use a syringe large enough to hold the amount of blood your laboratory requires. Draw up 1.5 cc of heparin 1:1000. After you remove the needle from the vial, pull back on the plunger to "rinse" the inside of the syringe. Then hold it with the needle upright and expel the air and heparin.

2. A bucket of ice large enough to hold the syringe after the sample is obtained.

3. A label for the syringe and a laboratory request slip with pertinent information such as the patient's name, date, time, concentration of inspired oxygen, and clinical status.

Obtaining the blood gas sample

To withdraw blood from an arterial line in order to analyze blood gases, follow this procedure. Use a second unheparinized syringe to withdraw the arterial line's flush solution until the line is filled with blood. This step will remove the flush solution in the line which otherwise would dilute the sample. Discard this syringe and solution. Use the heparinized syringe to withdraw the blood from the line. Then close the stopcock port. Remove the syringe. Immediately expel any air which may be in the syringe, cap the syringe, immerse it in ice, and have it taken promptly to the blood gas laboratory. Flush the stopcock port from which you obtained the sample so that a clot will not form. Also flush the arterial line.

An alternate method of obtaining an arterial blood sample is to perform a direct arterial puncture. Explain the procedure to the patient. Warn him he will feel a brief sharp pain when the artery is pierced. Choose an easily palpable artery. The brachial, radial, and femoral are the common sites; the radial is preferred because of fewer documented complications. Before puncturing the radial artery, be sure to perform an Allen's test. Occlude both the radial and ulnar arteries with your thumbs and ask the patient to open and close his hand several times. When the hand is white, release the ulnar artery but continue occluding the radial artery. Prompt pinkening of the hand demonstrates ulnar artery patency, indicating that the hand will be perfused even if the radial artery becomes occluded as a result of the procedure.

Hyperextend the site by placing a rolled-up towel under it. Prepare the skin according to your unit's procedure. If the patient is very tense, you may want to infiltrate only the skin with 1% xylocaine. (This will reduce skin pain but not eliminate the pain of the arterial puncture.) If infiltrated deeply, a vessel spasm could be provoked causing loss of the pulse and a very difficult procedure. Disinfect the first two fingers of your left hand. Use them to palpate and stabilize the artery. Hold the needle at a 45° or 90° angle. Pierce the skin and artery just until blood spurts into the syringe. After the sample is obtained, quickly withdraw the needle. Have someone apply firm pressure on the site for at least 5 minutes, while you expel any air; cap the sample, place it on ice, and send off the specimen. After the pressure is released, check the site in five minutes to make sure that a hematoma is not forming.

Interpreting blood gas values

The laboratory report of arterial blood gases will state the PO_2, PCO_2, and a measure of bases in the body (either bicarbonate or base excess). A convenient progression in analyzing these values is first to analyze the partial pressures reported and then to analyze the acid-base values. The chapter on acid-base balance will present the interpretation of acid-base values. This chapter will review the interpretation of partial pressures, which are reported in mm Hg or torr (1 torr = 1 mm Hg at 0°C).

Diffusing capacity   Before discussing factors related to interpretation of only PO_2 or only PCO_2, it is helpful to review those factors affecting exchange of both gases. The ability of the alveolar-capillary membrane to exchange a gas is called its diffusing capacity. Guyton (1976) defines diffusing capacity as "the volume of a gas that diffuses through the membrane each minute for a pressure difference of 1 mm Hg." The diffusing capacity for a given gas is affected by the pressure gradient across the membrane, the area of the membrane, the thickness of the membrane, and the diffusion coefficient of the gas.

Pressure gradients   The pressure gradients for O_2 and CO_2 are major determinants of gas exchange. In a mixture of gases, such as atmospheric or alveolar air, the pressure exerted by each gas is independent of the other gases and proportional to its percentage of the total gas (Dalton's law). The pressure exerted by each gas is called its *partial pressure*. The total pressure of the air inspired is the *barometric (atmospheric) pressure*. This pressure varies in relation to distance above or below sea level; at sea level, it is 760 mm Hg. The partial pressure of a gas is calculated by multiplying the total pressure by the percentage of the gas. Table 9–2 presents the approximate percentages and partial pressures for inspired air, which consists primarily of nitrogen, oxygen, carbon dioxide, and water vapor. Note that to obtain the partial pressures of inspired gases, the pressure exerted by water vapor must be subtracted first. The reason for this subtraction is that gases in the airways are completely humidified; this means that at 37°C the other gases can exert a maximum partial pressure of 713 mm Hg. Water vapor pressure varies with body temperature.

Alveolar air differs somewhat from atmospheric air. Nitrogen, which accounts for the greatest percentage, readily establishes equilibrium across the alveolar-capillary membrane and therefore can be disregarded. The remaining gas consists of about 14% oxygen, 5% CO_2, and 6% water vapor. Thus, alveolar air contains less oxygen and more carbon dioxide and water than atmospheric air.

The partial pressure of O_2 in atmospheric air is 150 mm Hg; in alveolar air, it is about 100 mm Hg. The partial pressure of CO_2 is 0.2 mm Hg in atmospheric air and 40 mm Hg in alveolar air. Blood in the pulmonary capillaries has a PO_2 of 40 mm Hg and PCO_2 of 45 mm Hg. The resulting pressure gradients cause oxygen to diffuse from the alveoli into the capillaries, and carbon dioxide to diffuse from the capillaries into the alveoli. Although the pressure gradient for CO_2 is small, it diffuses faster than oxygen because its solubility is much greater.

Surface area and thickness of membrane   In addition to the pressure gradients, factors affecting gas exchange in the alveoli are the alveolar surface area and the thickness of the alveolar-capillary membrane. The alveolar surface area

Table 9-2   Composition of inspired gas at sea level

Total barometric pressure		760	mm Hg
− Water vapor at 37° C		47	
Corrected barometric pressure		713	

Gas	Percentage		Partial Pressure
Nitrogen	79.03% × 713	=	563.5 mm Hg
Oxygen	20.94% × 713	=	149.3
Carbon dioxide	0.03% × 713	=	0.2
Total	100%		713.0

varies with age, body size, lung volume, presence of surfactant, and other factors. It decreases with emphysema and pneumonectomy.

The thickness of the alveolar-capillary membrane occasionally becomes clinically important, because increased thickness reduces the diffusing capacity. The membrane's thickness increases with pulmonary edema and pulmonary fibrosis.

Diffusion coefficient   The diffusion coefficient expresses the rate of gas transfer across the membrane. According to Guyton, the coefficient depends both upon the gas' solubility and its molecular weight. The diffusion coefficient of carbon dioxide is approximately twenty times that of oxygen.

Ventilation/perfusion relationships   Of the four factors affecting diffusing capacity, changes in pressure gradients are most important clinically. Pressure gradients depend on the relationship between ventilation and blood flow in alveolar-capillary units.

The relationship between ventilation (V) and perfusion (Q) has a critical influence on gas exchange. The lungs are perfused by two circulations: the bronchial and the pulmonary. The bronchial circulation provides oxygenated blood to supply the lung structures down to and including the terminal bronchioles (but not the alveoli). The pulmonary circulation provides deoxygenated blood to participate in gas exchange and incidentally nourishes the alveoli. After the pulmonary blood is oxygenated, it travels through pulmonary veins, which ultimately empty into the left atrium.

It is clinically significant that there are four possible relationships between ventilation and perfusion for a given alveolar-capillary unit (Thomas 1972). The normal unit is both ventilated and perfused. A so-called silent unit is neither ventilated nor perfused. A deadspace unit is ventilated but not perfused; this concept has already been discussed. The fourth type, a shunt unit, is perfused but not ventilated. The significance of shunt will be discussed later in the chapter.

It is important to realize that even in the normal lung there is an uneven distribution of ventilation in relation to perfusion. The normal overall ventilation/perfusion (V/Q) ratio is about 0.8 (4 L of alveolar ventilation to 5 L of cardiac output), but in any given part of the lung, the ventilation and perfusion may not match. Some areas of the lung have too much ventilation in relation to perfusion, others too little. These regional V/Q mismatches are unimportant in the healthy person.

The previous sections discussed factors common to exchange of both oxygen and carbon dioxide and therefore common to interpretation of P_aO_2 and P_aCO_2. The following sections will discuss individual factors related to interpretation of P_aO_2 as an indicator of oxygenation and P_aCO_2 as an indicator of alveolar ventilation.

PO₂ and other indices of oxygenation   In order to interpret PO$_2$ as an indicator of oxygenation, you need a clear understanding of the relationship between PO$_2$ and other indices of oxygenation. Since the distinctions among these measurements can be confusing, they are defined in the following sections.

Oxygen is carried in the blood in two ways: most is bound to hemoglobin; a small amount is dissolved in the blood. The total amount that can be dissolved in the blood is about 0.3 ml/100 ml blood. The amount that can be carried on the hemoglobin is 1.34 ml O$_2$/gm hemoglobin. If you assume a normal hemoglobin level of 15 gm/100 ml, the hemoglobin could carry 15 × 1.34 ml, or 20.1 ml of O$_2$ in each 100 ml of blood. The total amount Hgb could carry (20.1 ml) plus the dissolved amount (0.3 ml) is called the O$_2$ carrying capacity. The actual amount of oxygen the blood is carrying (the O$_2$ content) would be valuable to know but is difficult to measure.

Instead, a widely used index of oxygenation is the *partial pressure of oxygen (the PO₂)*. It expresses not the amount of oxygen carried in the blood but rather the pressure of the O$_2$ dissolved in the blood. The reason that PO$_2$ is so widely used is that the PO$_2$ is the major determinant of O$_2$ saturation, which in turn provides a close estimate of the actual amount of O$_2$ carried in the blood (the O$_2$ content). O$_2$ saturation is a percentage expressing the relationship between the amount of O$_2$ the hemoglobin is carrying and the amount it could carry, that is, between the O$_2$ content and the O$_2$ carrying capacity.

Oxyhemoglobin dissociation curve   The relationship of PO$_2$ to O$_2$ saturation is expressed in the *oxyhemoglobin dissociation curve* (Figure 9-3). This relationship is not linear; a given amount of change in PO$_2$ may be associated with varying amounts of change in O$_2$ saturation.

When you know your patient's PO$_2$, you can consult the oxyhemoglobin dissociation curve to learn his O$_2$ saturation. First, however, you must ask yourself, "Are any conditions present which alter the hemoglobin dissociation curve for the patient?" Examples are fever or acidosis, which shift the curve to the right, indicating that hemoglobin has less affinity for O$_2$. A subnormal temperature or alkalosis will move the curve to the left, causing a higher than usual O$_2$ saturation, which indicates that hemoglobin has more affinity for O$_2$. Thus, if you want to know the O$_2$ saturation, you must consult the curve appropriate to your patient's condition. In most cases, you do not need to know the precise O$_2$ saturation for nursing purposes. It is helpful, however, to realize the implications of the oxyhemoglobin dissociation curve. A few examples will show its great clinical importance. At high PO$_2$s (such as that in lung capillaries), hemoglobin becomes almost completely saturated with O$_2$, producing a normal O$_2$ saturation of 95–100% for arterial blood. This fact enables it to carry O$_2$ to areas of low PO$_2$ such as the tissue capillaries. There, PO$_2$ is about 40 mm Hg; as a result, hemoglobin becomes less saturated, giving up its O$_2$ to the tissues which need it for cellular metabolism. The normal saturation for venous blood is about 70–75%.

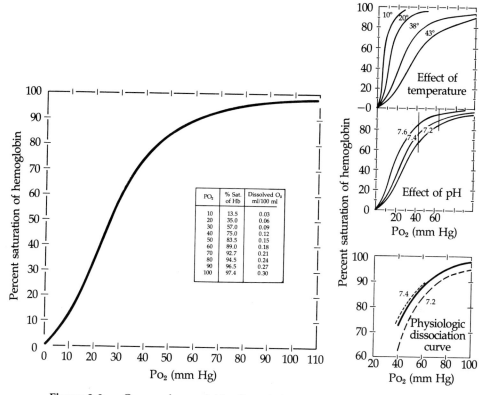

Figure 9-3.   Oxygen hemoglobin dissociation curve. Based on data of Dill. The large curve applies when the blood's pH is 7.4 and temperature is 37°C. The curve shifts with temperature (upper small box) or pH changes (middle small box). The physiologic dissociation curve (lower small box) expresses the change from pH 7.37 to pH 7.40 which normally occurs when the PCO₂ of mixed venous blood decreases as it passes through the pulmonary capillaries. (From Comroe, J. H., Jr. et al.: *The Lung: Clinical Physiology and Pulmonary Function Tests.* 2nd ed. Copyright © 1962 by Year Book Medical Publishers, Inc., Chicago. Used by permission.)

You will notice that the upper portion of the curve is relatively flat while the middle and lower part are steep. At the upper end of the curve, a large change in PO_2 is associated with only a small change in O_2 saturation. This fact is the reason we are not very alarmed when a patient's arterial PO_2 drops from 90 to 70; his hemoglobin still will be well saturated and therefore able to carry O_2 to his tissues. On the steep portion of the curve, however, a change in PO_2 is associated wih a much greater effect on O_2 saturation. A drop in arterial PO_2 from 60 to 40, for instance, indicates a significant reduction in the amount of O_2 carried by hemoglobin to the tissues.

Another important implication of the curve is that an arterial PO_2 over 100 mm Hg does not really benefit a patient, since hemoglobin saturation cannot exceed 100%.

A knowledge of what PO_2 and other indices of oxygenation represent will help you avoid erroneous conclusions based on them. For instance, you will recognize that PO_2 or O_2 saturation alone does not tell you how much oxygen actually is being carried to the blood. In order to calculate the amount of O_2 a given patient's blood is carrying, you must know both the O_2 saturation and the hemoglobin level; 95% saturation of 15 gm is considerably different from the same saturation of 10 gm. Similarly, even an adequate O_2 content in the blood does not mean the tissues are well oxygenated; the patient could be in shock and have a cardiac output too low to carry the O_2 to the peripheral areas of the body. In other words, adequate tissue oxygenation depends upon an adequate PO_2 for optimal hemoglobin saturation, a normal level of hemoglobin to carry the oxygen, and satisfactory circulation to carry the oxygen to the tissues.

The previous sections discussed the significance of the P_aO_2 as the most clinically useful laboratory index of oxygenation. The following paragraphs will describe the technique of interpreting the P_aO_2 and related measures.

P_aO_2 interpretation   When evaluating P_aO_2 data from the laboratory, make the following observations:

Note the measured P_aO_2 and the percentage of inspired oxygen at the time the sample was obtained. This percentage usually is expressed as the fractional inspired oxygen concentration, or FIO_2; the value is given as a decimal. An FIO_2 of 0.4, for instance, means 40% O_2 concentration. The FIO_2 of room air is 0.21.

Compare the actual P_aO_2 and FIO_2 to the desired P_aO_2 and FIO_2 for that patient. Ideal values are P_aO_2 of 80–100 mm Hg on an FIO_2 of 0.21 (room air).

Mixed venous blood values   So far, we have been discussing analysis of arterial blood samples. Since arterial blood has not yet reached the systemic tissues, it does not give a full picture of what is happening on the cellular level. In some situations, it is helpful to analyze samples of mixed venous blood. Mixed venous blood cannot be obtained from peripheral veins. The PO_2 of peripheral venous blood represents the arterial-venous O_2 difference of only that area of tissue, and varies depending on the area sampled, its metabolic activity, and distance from the heart. By the time blood reaches the pulmonary artery, venous drainage from various peripheral areas, the coronary sinus, and Thebesian veins have become blended. Mixed venous blood thus is obtained from a catheter in the pulmonary artery.

Normal values for mixed venous PO_2, O_2 saturation, and O_2 content all are lower than for arterial blood:

	Arterial	*Mixed Venous*
PO_2	80–100 mm Hg	35–40 mm Hg
O_2 saturation	95% or above	70–75%
O_2 content	19.8 ml O_2/100 ml blood	15.5 ml O_2/100 ml blood

If venous values are normal, it is possible to conclude that tissue oxygenation is adequate. Increases in these values imply that less O_2 than normal is being used by the tissues or that there is an abnormal source adding O_2 to venous blood (such as a left to right cardiac shunt). Decreases imply that more O_2 is being unloaded in the tissues, such as in slowed circulation due to decreased cardiac output, which allows more time for O_2 extraction by the tissues.

Alveolar-arterial O_2 difference   Because the diffusing capacity of carbon dioxide is believed to be about twenty times that of oxygen, damage to the alveolar-capillary membrane affects oxygen diffusion long before it affects carbon dioxide diffusion.

In the clinical setting, oxygen diffusing capacity can not be measured directly. Instead, the adequacy of diffusing capacity can be inferred from the alveolar-arterial oxygen difference ($AaDO_2$), sometimes called the alveolar-arterial (A-a) gradient.

Often, a critically ill person will have a low P_aO_2. Identification of the cause is essential for optimal therapy.

A decreased P_aO_2 can occur in two general ways: First, the alveolar PO_2 may be low, as in hypoventilation or, rarely, decreased FIO_2 in high altitudes. Second, alveolar PO_2 may be normal but diffusion into the capillaries may be impaired, as in ventilation/perfusion mismatch, increased shunting, or rarely, a diffusion block at the alveolar-capillary membrane. To differentiate shunting (the most common cause of hypoxemia) from hypoventilation, V/Q mismatch, and diffusion block, the patient can be given 100% O_2 and the $AaDO_2$ can be calculated. The procedure is as follows:

1. Place the patient on 100% O_2 for 15 minutes to wash nitrogen out of the alveoli.
2. Draw an arterial blood sample and have it analyzed.
3. Measure the patient's temperature and look up the water vapor pressure for that temperature.
4. Subtract the water vapor pressure from the barometric pressure to get the total pressure of the carbon dioxide and oxygen in the alveoli.
5. Assume that the measured arterial PCO_2 equals alveolar PCO_2, since the values for CO_2 usually are about equal.
6. From the total pressure of alveolar O_2 and CO_2 obtained in step 4, subtract the assumed alveolar PCO_2 to get the estimated alveolar PO_2.
7. From the alveolar PO_2, subtract the arterial PO_2 to get the A-a gradient ($AaDO_2$).

The normal $AaDO_2$ on 100% O_2 is less than 50 mm Hg (Bushnell 1973); in other words, the alveolar and arterial PO_2 are similar.

If the hypoxemic patient has a normal A-a gradient, the cause of the hypoxemia probably is an inadequate alveolar PO_2, that is, hypoventilation. If the patient has an increased A-a gradient, his hypoxemia probably results from a problem at the alveolar-capillary level. Although theoretically such a problem could be due to uneven ventilation, alveolar-capillary block, or shunt, using 100% O_2 almost completely eliminates the first two causes. Therefore, an increased A-a gradient on 100% O_2 most likely is due to an increased shunt. Because the A-a gradient does not take into account changes in FIO_2, cardiac output, or metabolic rate, Shapiro, Harrison, and Trout (1975) state that they do not like to use it with critically ill patients.

Shunt and increased $AaDO_2$ Earlier, the concept of deadspace was introduced (ventilation without perfusion). Shunt refers to the opposite situation— perfusion without ventilation. Physiologic shunt is the percentage of cardiac output which is wasted perfusion because it does not exchange with gas in the alveoli. It accounts for the fact that arterial PO_2 normally is slightly lower (95 mm Hg) than alveolar PO_2 (100 mm Hg).

Physiologic shunt is subdivided into anatomic shunt and capillary shunt. Anatomic shunt is that portion which anatomically bypasses the pulmonary capillaries and returns unoxygenated to the left atrium. Normally, it results from venous drainage from the bronchial, pleural, and Thebesian veins and represents 2–4% of cardiac output (Thomas 1972). (Abnormal venoarterial communications such as right to left cardiac shunts increase anatomic shunt). Capillary shunt is that portion that goes through pulmonary capillaries but does not exchange with alveolar gas and so also returns unoxygenated to the left atrium. According to Shapiro, Harrison, and Trout (1975), capillary shunt consists of true capillary shunt, due to nonventilated alveoli (such as in atelectasis) and venous admixture, due to underventilated alveoli (such as in pulmonary edema and chronic obstructive lung disease). Because these latter alveoli have more perfusion than ventilation, they represent a type of failure of gas exchange. Increased capillary shunt is a common, serious problem in critically ill patients.

Shunting is minimized in the normal lung by a protective reflex. When shunting increases, diminished or absent local ventilation causes a low P_AO_2. The local blood vessels constrict, redirecting flow to better ventilated areas. Shunt, the most common cause of hypoxemia, may be due to failure of this protective reflex, decreased cardiac output, or diffuse disease of the lung or vasculature which prevents adequate matching or compensation.

Isoshunt lines for determining degree of shunt   It is helpful to estimate the degree of shunt both to follow changes in the patient's condition and to plan oxygen therapy. One promising approach is the use of isoshunt lines presented by Benatar, Hewlett, and Nunn (1973). They derived curves showing the relationship between FIO_2 and P_aO_2 for various degrees of shunt, and validated the curves with 44 clinical observations.

These lines are presented in Figure 9-4. They enable you to estimate the degree of shunt from initial simultaneous measurements of FIO_2 and P_aO_2. They

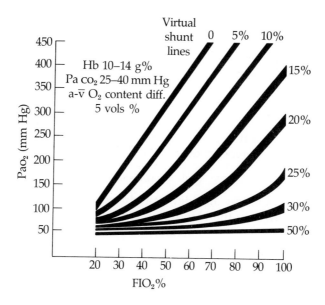

Figure 9-4. Shunt lines. (From Benatar, S., Hewlett, A., and Nunn, J.: 1973. The use of isoshunt lines for control of oxygen therapy. *British Journal of Anesthesia* 45:711–718. Used with permission of John Sherratt and Son, Ltd.)

also enable you to predict the P_aO_2 which would result from a lower FIO_2. The relationship between FIO_2 and P_aO_2 is very complex. According to the authors, it depends upon the hemoglobin level, displacement of the oxyhemoglobin dissociation curve, P_aCO_2, arterial/mixed venous oxygen content difference, and shunt. The authors state that the first three variables are of relatively minor importance and that changes in the arterial/mixed venous O_2 content difference do not alter the pattern of the relationship between FIO_2 and P_aO_2. To present the simplified relationship between FIO_2 and P_aO_2, they assume the arterial/mixed venous O_2 content difference to be 5 ml/100 ml and define the shunt at this value as *virtual shunt*.

The authors caution that these curves apply only to patients whose hypoxemia results from venous admixture, whose PCO_2 ranges between 25 and 40 mm Hg, whose hemoglobin level is between 10 and 14 gm/100 ml, and who are in a relatively steady state.

To use the graph, place the patient on a known FIO_2 between 0.6 and 1.0 (60–100%) and measure P_aO_2. Next determine the curve on which the patient's FIO_2 and P_aO_2 values fall and identify the percent of shunt. By making serial determinations you can observe whether the degree of shunt is lessening or worsening over time.

Isoshunt lines for guiding FIO$_2$ selection   An increased P$_a$O$_2$ frequently is seen in patients receiving supplemental O$_2$. It usually is an indication to reduce the FIO$_2$ since high oxygen tensions contribute to oxygen toxicity and should not be used longer than absolutely necessary. The FIO$_2$ can be reduced by 0.05, blood gases rechecked after 15–30 minutes, and the process repeated until an FIO$_2$ yielding a normal P$_a$O$_2$ is reached.

An easier method is to identify the shunt line appropriate for the patient, follow it down to the point opposite the desired P$_a$O$_2$, and read the FIO$_2$ below that point. This value represents the FIO$_2$ which should yield the P$_a$O$_2$ desired for that patient.

Evaluating P$_a$CO$_2$ Carbon dioxide is produced by cellular metabolism and eliminated by the lungs. In the blood, it is carried in three forms (Keyes 1974). About 60% is converted to bicarbonate in this reaction:

$$CO_2 + H_2O \rightleftarrows H_2CO_3 \rightleftarrows H^+ \text{ and } HCO_3^-$$

In other words, carbon dioxide combines with water to form carbonic acid, which then dissociates to a hydrogen ion and a bicarbonate ion. An enzyme called carbonic anhydrase facilitates the formation of carbonic acid. Since much more carbonic anhydrase is contained in red blood cells than in plasma, most of the body's bicarbonate is formed in the red blood cells. It then diffuses out of the cells into the plasma, where it is carried. About 30% of the CO$_2$ is carried on hemoglobin. The last 10% is physically dissolved in the blood. It is the pressure of this dissolved CO$_2$ that is measured in the P$_a$CO$_2$.

The normal P$_a$CO$_2$ is 35–45 mm Hg. The P$_a$CO$_2$ varies with both the production of carbon dioxide and its elimination by the lungs. Altered P$_a$CO$_2$ levels most frequently reflect changes in alveolar ventilation. A decreased P$_a$CO$_2$ usually indicates hyperventilation, as in hypoxia or compensation for metabolic acidosis. An increased P$_a$CO$_2$ (hypercapnia or hypercarbia) indicates hypoventilation, as in respiratory center depression, increased V$_D$/V$_T$ ratio, or compensation for metabolic alkalosis. The P$_a$CO$_2$ is a better indicator of alveolar ventilation than is the patient's P$_a$O$_2$. The reason for this is that hypoventilation is but one cause of hypoxia, while it is the only cause of hypercarbia.

As mentioned earlier in the chapter, the P$_a$CO$_2$ is the body's most potent stimulus to respiration. This stimulus is mediated primarily by central chemoreceptors in the medulla and secondarily by peripheral chemoreceptors in the aorta and carotid bodies.

CO$_2$ affects the central chemoreceptors through its influence on the acidity of cerebrospinal fluid, which bathes the medulla. CO$_2$ diffuses freely across the blood brain barrier. It then combines with water to form carbonic acid, which dissociates into a hydrogen ion (H$^+$) and a bicarbonate ion. The increased H$^+$ concentration lowers the pH of cerebrospinal fluid. The resulting stimulation of the respiratory center causes an increase in the rate and depth of ventilation (hyperventilation). Similarly, a decrease in PCO$_2$ causes a decrease in ventilation (hypoventilation). Peripheral chemoreceptors are sensitive to PCO_2 and pH of arterial blood, as well as its PO_2.

Chest x-ray

Reading the chest x-ray report is the final step in assessing a patient's aeration status. A basic understanding of chest x-ray interpretation is useful in reading x-ray reports and understanding medical discussions of your patient's condition. Occasionally, too, you may be the first person to see an abnormal film; your ability to spot abnormalities needing urgent attention may enable you to obtain medical therapy immediately for your patient. The following information on chest x-ray interpretation is based on Felsen (1973) and Tinker (1976).

Different substances allow varying amounts of x-ray energy to pass through them and strike the film, producing four x-ray densities. Because metal density absorbs most of the energy and allows very little to strike the film, it produces a white color. Water density is darker, fat density still darker, and air density the darkest (in other words, black) because it allows most of the energy to pass through. Lungs appear as air density; soft tissue and blood as water density; and bone as metal density. When the x-ray beam traverses several structures of different densities, it will produce an image combining their densities.

In examining a film, follow a logical sequence such as the one indicated here. The most significant principle to remember is that you can see a structure only if its edge is of a density that contrasts with the surrounding density.

Normal characteristics

The normal chest film has the following pulmonary characteristics (Figure 9-5). Cardiac abnormalities visible on the chest x-ray were presented in Chapter 2.

The ribs are intact and can be traced starting from their more superior attachment to the spine. The spine is straight. The clavicles, visible in the upper thorax, are intact and equidistant, indicating the person was centered properly.

The hemidiaphragms appear rounded. The upper edge of each hemidiaphragm is visible (because of the contrast between air and water densities). The right hemidiaphragm usually is slightly higher than the left (because of the liver). On the left hemidiaphragm, the lower edge may be visible because the stomach often contains air. The lower edge of the right hemidiaphragm should not be visible. If it is, it signifies free air in the abdomen, such as from a perforated ulcer. The angles between the diaphragm and ribs (the costophrenic angles) should be clear.

The pleura is not visible.

The trachea is midline. The aortic knob, which is formed by the arch of the aorta, is seen as a knob-like water density.

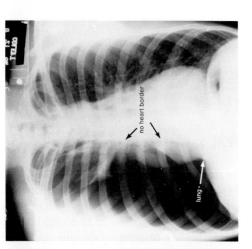

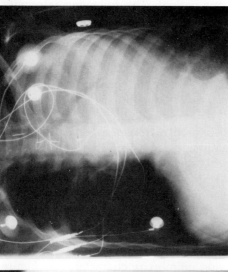

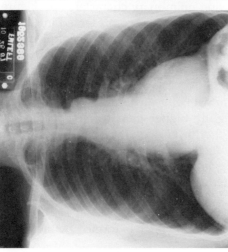

Figure 9-5. Chest x-rays. **A,** Normal posteroanterior (PA) chest film taken from 6 feet away, with the patient standing, and with as much of the anterior chest touching the plate as possible. Note that the normal heart is really quite small. **B,** A problem in the left lung is obvious in this x-ray; note the air bronchogram sign on the left indicating atelectasis. The air bronchogram clearly delineates the bronchus as it passes into the lower lobes of the left lung; left upper lobe bronchus is not visible indicating the probable presence of a mucus plug in that area. Vigorous endotracheal suctioning with ventilatory therapy produced significant clearing in 24 hours in this four-year-old girl. X-ray was taken two days post open heart surgery. Note endotracheal tube and wires used to close the sternum. **C,** The pneumothorax here is very extensive. Note that pressure in the right hemithorax must be greater than in the left, because the heart and other mediastinal structures are shifted away from the free air. This is a tension pneumothorax. Air entering the right pleural space is unable to escape because of a ball-valve effect, and each inspiration increases the intrapleural pressure. Prompt diagnosis and treatment, perhaps even with a large bore needle at first, are essential, often lifesaving. (From John H. Tinker, "Understanding Chest X-Rays," *American Journal of Nursing* 76(1):54–58, 1976. Courtesy, John H. Tinker, MD, and American Journal of Nursing.)

The heart appears solid, since the blood in it and its walls are the same density. The edges of the heart are clear because of the contrast with the surrounding air density of the lung.

Just above the heart, small bilateral water densities are visible. These densities mark the hila, where the pulmonary vessels and bronchi join the lungs. The left hilum usually is slightly higher than the right because the left main pulmonary artery is higher and more posterior than the right. The hilum consists primarily of the major pulmonary vessels. Lesser vascular markings (also called lung markings) are seen out to the edge of the lung fields; they are more prominent in the lower lungs when the person is upright. Because the vascular markings are water density, they cause the lung fields to look like a fuzzy air density. Beyond a small amount of mainstem bronchus visible to about one inch out from the hila, the bronchi usually can not be seen. They have thin walls and since they are filled with air, they do not contrast with the air density of the surrounding lung.

Individual lobes of the lung can be identified because the lobes are separated by fissures (also called septa). These interlobar septa are visible in different projections. Septa between lobules (interlobular septa) normally can not be seen.

Abnormal signs

Three important signs you may see or hear discussed are the silhouette sign, the air bronchogram, and Kerley's B lines.

Silhouette sign   You will recall that in order for a structure to be visible, the density of its edge must contrast with the surrounding density. This contrast produces the silhouette. The loss of the contrast is called the silhouette sign; it indicates that the densities of the two structures have become the same. This sign is useful in localizing processes that increase the water content of the lung, such as pneumonia and infiltrates. For instance, since the heart is an anterior organ, the complete loss of the right cardiac silhouette implies that the pathology lies in the anterior lobes (the upper or middle lobes) in an area in anatomic contact with the heart. A shadow overlapping a border without obliterating a silhouette implies that the process is located in the lower (posterior) lobes, the posterior mediastinum, or the posterior pleural cavity.

Air bronchogram sign   Another sign of a process that is making part of the lung water density is the air bronchogram sign. You will remember that the bronchi normally cannot be seen because they and the surrounding lung are both air density. When a process (such as pneumonia or pulmonary edema) makes the lung tissue water density, the contrast makes the bronchi visible, unless the bronchi themselves are filled with secretions or destroyed. The appearance of the air bronchogram identifies the disorder as intrapulmonary. Areas that do not have bronchi (such as the pleural space) cannot show an air bronchogram sign.

Kerley's B lines   Kerley's B lines are short linear shadows perpendicular to the pleural surface. They are thought to represent fluid in or thickening of the interlobular septae. They are seen frequently in pulmonary edema and mitral valve disease; pulmonary fibrosis or inflammatory exudate also may cause them.

Easily identified abnormalities

Differential diagnosis of chest x-ray finding is a complex science beyond the scope of this book. However, there are some abnormalities you will encounter so frequently they are worth reviewing here.

Collapse   Collapse of a part of the lung has many causes. It may be due to bronchial obstruction followed by absorption of the air remaining in the lung (atelectasis). Another cause may be compression, such as by air in the pleural space. A third cause is contraction, such as in pulmonary fibrosis.

Collapse is diagnosed by displacement of the septa, crowding of the vascular markings or air bronchograms, and increased radiopacity of the lung tissue. Other signs sometimes seen are shift of the trachea (if upper lobes are involved), displacement of the hilum, increased closeness of the ribs, elevation of the diaphragm on the affected side, and compensatory overexpansion of the adjacent parts of the lung causing increased radiolucency in those areas.

Pneumothorax   If you see an area of clear blackness (that is, no lung markings), it probably results from a pneumothorax. Since air rises, look at the apices for this sign on an upright or semirecumbent film. Other signs you may see are increased radiopaqueness of the collapsed lung tissue, depression of the diaphragm, and tracheal and mediastinal shift away from the pneumothorax. The findings may be more apparent on an expiratory film, because the smaller size of the thorax makes the pneumothorax proportionately larger. Also, the normal clouding of the lung fields on expiration (due to less air in the chest) will not be as evident in pneumothorax.

Consolidation   Areas of increased density (whiteness) are referred to as areas of consolidation. They can result from numerous causes. Broadly, causes of consolidation can be grouped into those that collapse the lung tissue, thereby making it more dense, and those that increase the fluid content of the lung. Increases in density due to fluid accumulation may be diffuse or localized. Diffuse increases are seen in pulmonary edema and pneumonia, as well as other disorders. They can be differentiated on the basis of associated signs, such as air bronchograms, Kerley's lines, and the pattern of fluid distribution.

Localized increases due to fluid are usually pleural (such as effusions or hemothorax). Fluid that causes partial or complete obliteration of the costophrenic angle on an upright film probably is free pleural fluid. When a film is taken with the patient on his side or back, this fluid will appear in the dependent part of the chest cavity. Fluid that does not shift with position is called encapsulated or loculated.

The above descriptions, although brief, will enable you to better interpret chest x-ray film reports and spot common abnormalities on chest films.

References

American College of Chest Physicians and American Thoracic Society Joint Committee on Pulmonary Nomenclature. 1975. Pulmonary terms and symbols. *Chest* 67:583–593.

Bates, B. 1974. *A guide to physical examination.* Philadelphia: J. B. Lippincott Company.
Step by step graphic guide to respiratory assessment in Chapter 25.

Benatar, S., Hewlett, A., and Nunn, J. 1973. The use of isoshunt lines for control of oxygen therapy. *Brit. J. Anaesth.* 45: 711–718.
Derivation, discussion, and clinical use of isoshunt lines.

Brunner, L., and Suddarth, D. 1975. *Textbook of medical-surgical nursing.* 3rd ed. Philadelphia: J. B. Lippincott Company.
Chapter 3: Physical assessment; Chapter 16: Measurements of pulmonary function.

Bushnell, L. 1973. Physiology of the respiratory system. In *Respiratory intensive care nursing.* ed. S. Bushnell. pp. 15–32. Boston: Little, Brown, and Company.
Compliance, resistance, volumes, deadspace, indices of oxygenation.

Comroe, J., et al 1962. *The lung.* 2nd ed. Chicago: Year Book Medical Publishers, Inc.
Concise discussion of pulmonary function tests.

Felsen, B. 1973. *Chest roentgenology.* Philadelphia: W. B. Saunders Company.
Comprehensive, logical resource with numerous illustrations of abnormal x-rays.

Keyes, J. 1974. Blood gases and blood-gas transport. *Heart Lung* 3: 945–954.
Review of pertinent gas laws and mechanisms of oxygen and carbon dioxide transport.

Thomas, A. 1972. Respiratory care. *The cardiac patient: a comprehensive approach.* ed. R. Sanderson. Philadelphia: W. B. Saunders Company.
Simplified review of pulmonary physiology.

Tinker, J. 1976. Understanding chest x-rays. *A.J.N.* 76: 54–58.
Brief review of the essentials, with illustrations of common acute disorders.

Chapter 10

Acute Aeration Disorders

This chapter will help you anticipate, prevent, recognize, and alleviate the effects of five acute aeration disorders: acute respiratory failure, atelectasis, acute pulmonary edema, pulmonary embolus, and pneumothorax. It also will include nursing care related to six therapeutic modalities: oxygen therapy, chest physiotherapy, artificial airways, tracheal suction, mechanical ventilation, and chest tubes.

Outline

Artificial airways   Types of artificial airways / Prevention of complications / Treatment of complications / Removal of artificial airways / Outcome evaluation

Tracheal suctioning   Prevention of complications / Treatment of complications / Outcome evaluation

Mechanical ventilation   Procedure for mechanical ventilation / Prevention of complications / Treatment of complications / Discontinuation of mechanical ventilation / Outcome evaluation

Chest drainage   Techniques of chest drainage / Maintenance of chest drainage / Prevention of complications / Removal of chest tubes / Outcome evaluation

Objectives

- Recognize the patients at risk of developing each disorder
- Take measures to prevent each disorder when possible
- Recognize the signs and symptoms of each disorder
- Implement nursing measures to relieve the effects of each disorder
- Use specified outcome criteria to evaluate the patient's progress
- Identify patients who might benefit from each therapeutic modality discussed in the chapter
- Correctly perform or assist with implementation of each modality
- Prevent complications of each intervention when possible
- Respond appropriately if complications do occur

Acute respiratory failure

Acute respiratory failure may be defined as the sudden onset of an abnormally low arterial PO_2 (usually less than 60 mm Hg) and/or abnormally high PCO_2 (usually above 60 mm Hg, except in chronic obstructive pulmonary disease [COPD] or compensated metabolic alkalosis).

Risk conditions

Recognize the conditions that increase the patient's risk of developing acute respiratory failure. The major causes of acute failure are alveolar hypoventilation, increased shunt, increased alveolar deadspace, and impaired alveolar-capillary diffusion.

Alveolar hypoventilation may result from respiratory center depression, impaired neuromuscular transmission, increased airway resistance, or decreased compliance. Following are examples of conditions which increase the risk of developing alveolar hypoventilation:

1. Respiratory center depression may result from increased intracranial pressure; narcotic, sedative, or anesthetic overdose; or severe central nervous system hypoxia.
2. Impaired transmission of neuromuscular impulses is seen in Guillain-Barré disease; myasthenia gravis; or fractures of cervical vertebrae.
3. Increased airway resistance may result from neck flexion in a patient with decreased mental alertness; laryngospasm; or asthma.
4. Decreased compliance of lungs or chest wall occurs with pneumothorax; hemothorax; interstitial pulmonary edema; atelectasis; pneumonia; abdominal distention; or thoracic or abdominal pain.

   Increased physiologic shunt usually results from atelectasis; pneumonia; or pulmonary edema.
   Increased alveolar deadspace severe enough to cause respiratory failure may result from a massive pulmonary embolism.
   Impaired alveolar-capillary diffusion may be seen in severe pulmonary edema; pulmonary fibrosis; or emphysema.

Implement ways to prevent the preceding conditions when possible. For example, maintain a patent airway if the patient is unable to do so independently; hyperextend the head and neck, insert an oral airway, and/or position the patient with his head turned to the side to decrease the possibility of aspiration of vomitus. Minimize respiratory infections by such measures as washing your hands before suctioning, using sterile technique for endotracheal suctioning, and so on. Clear airway secretions through turning; deep breathing and coughing exercises; stimulation of the cough reflex with a nasal catheter; postural drainage; and/or chest physiotherapy.

Signs and symptoms

Early detection of acute respiratory failure can be accomplished by observing the patient for signs and symptoms of failure.

Signs of hypoxia   Observe the patient for signs of hypoxia. Hypoxia may result from alveolar hypoventilation, ventilation/perfusion (V/Q) abnormalities, increased shunting, or impaired alveolar-capillary diffusion. Watch for the pulmonary signs of hypoxia: tachypnea, shortness of breath, and sometimes central or peripheral cyanosis. Also, monitor for compensatory cardiovascular signs due to sympathetic stimulation: tachycardia, mild hypertension, and peripheral vasoconstriction. It is important to be aware that the patient may show no sympathetic response in which case you may observe bradycardia and hypotension instead.

Signs of hypercarbia   Also monitor the patient for signs of hypercarbia (hypercapnia, CO_2 narcosis) due to alveolar hypoventilation. Observe for central nervous system signs: headache because of cerebral vasodilatation, and depressed mentation, ranging from drowsiness to coma. Be alert for additional signs of vasodilatation: reddened skin, sclera, and conjunctiva due to increased blood flow, and sweating. Watch also for signs of a sympathetic response to the increased PCO_2, particularly hypertension and tachycardia. Monitor the patient for signs of acidosis due to CO_2 retention, such as increased serum K+, pH below 7.35, or ECG signs of hyperkalemia.

Be particularly alert with the patient recovering from acute hypoxia. During the acute phase of respiratory failure, the patient hyperventilates to maintain an adequate PO_2. This hyperventilation eliminates any excess CO_2 which otherwise might accumulate, such as from an increased shunt. As the hypoxia is corrected and the ventilatory rate slows, signs of hypercarbia may appear.

Nursing interventions

If you observe signs of hypoxia or hypercarbia, notify the physician and act promptly to restore adequate oxygenation and ventilation. Depending upon the patient's arterial blood gases, A-a gradient, inspiratory force, tidal volume, vital capacity, and other clinical factors, the physician may prescribe oxygen therapy, aggressive chest physiotherapy, or intubation and mechanical ventilation to support the patient's aeration while the causes of failure are being identified and treated. Nursing care related to these therapeutic interventions is discussed in detail later in this chapter. If the patient is apneic, institute emergency life support measures while summoning the physician. Establish a patent airway as explained later in this chapter and in Chapter 3. Ventilate the person mouth-to-mouth or with a hand ventilating bag and mask, as explained in Chapter 3 in the section on cardiopulmonary resuscitation.

Outcome evaluation

Judge the patient's progress according to these outcome criteria:

- Spontaneous respirations 12–18 times a minute
- Blood pressure and pulse WNL for patient
- Skin warm and dry (and pink if the patient is Caucasian)
- Arterial blood gases WNL for patient
- Arterial blood gases WNL for patient

Atelectasis

Atelectasis means collapsed alveoli in part or all of the lung. Although the term may be used to refer to collapse due to compression (as with a tumor), it commonly refers to collapse caused by airway obstruction followed by absorption of gas in the alveoli.

Risk conditions

Recognize the conditions increasing the risk of developing atelectasis. These conditions are shallow breathing (as with pain), dehydration, aspiration of foreign objects, retained secretions (mucous plugs), bronchospasm, ciliary depression, or decreased surfactant (usually due to decreased alveolar expansion).

Preventive measures   Take measures to prevent atelectasis:

1. Auscultate the lungs to determine the need for, frequency of, and effectiveness of the interventions that follow.

2. Preoperatively, establish rapport with the patient and teach her about deep breathing, coughing, turning, suctioning, chest physiotherapy, and intermittent positive pressure breathing. Emphasize the importance of these techniques in maintaining pulmonary function. Encourage the patient to practice breathing and coughing exercises several times a day preoperatively. Observe that she performs them correctly. Praise her for her participation in her own care, and tell her that during her stay in the critical care unit you will remind and assist her with these measures. Postoperatively, give adequate analgesics and wait enough time for them to take effect. Then capitalize on the preoperative relationship to motivate the patient to perform breathing exercises in spite of any remaining discomfort.

3. Position the patient to facilitate lung expansion. Avoid pronounced compression of the diaphragm.

4. Turn her every 1–2 hours to lessen pooling of secretions and prevent regional atelectasis.

5. Help her to deep breathe every 1–2 hours to reexpand closed alveoli. If she is unable to deep breathe, sigh the lungs with a hand ventilating bag about 10 times. Deliver a volume 2–3 times her tidal volume. (Patients on continuous ventilation with high tidal volumes do not need to be sighed.)

6. Encourage oral fluids (if permitted) to reduce viscosity of secretions. If only intravenous fluids are allowed, maintain adequate hydration.

7. Mobilize secretions by performing chest physical therapy periodically.

8. Help her to cough effectively by splinting abdominal or thoracic incisions with a sheet. If necessary, stimulate the cough reflex by passing a nasal catheter down the trachea or by pressing over the trachea. If the patient has increased secretions and is unable to raise them, suction the trachea and bronchi.

9. Assist with intermittent positive pressure breathing if ordered by the physician.

Signs and symptoms

Recognize the signs of developing atelectasis. If the airways to major atelectatic areas are open, bronchial breathing and increased tactile fremitus, voice sounds and whispered sounds may be present. If the airways are plugged, these signs will be absent. The chest x-ray may show patches or larger areas of consolidation, an elevated diaphragm, and a mediastinal shift, depending upon the site and extent of the collapse. Most postoperative atelectasis, however, is microatelectasis (random alveolar collapse not detectable on chest x-ray). Signs and symptoms usually are subtle, and may include restlessness; tachypnea; tachycardia; decreasing P_aO_2 or increasing $AaDO_2$; or dullness on percussion over areas that should be resonant.

Nursing interventions

Atelectasis results in increased physiologic shunting (explained in Chapter 9) and often in pulmonary infection as the retained secretions are an excellent medium for bacterial growth.

Relief of hypoxia Relieve the hypoxia which results from increased physiologic shunting by taking these measures.

1. Implement steps 3–10 listed under the goal of prevention.
2. Provide supplemental O_2 as ordered by the physician.
3. If the obstruction is massive, it may be necessary for the physician to bronchoscope the patient.
4. Monitor the $AaDO_2$ to gauge the effectiveness of therapy.

Relief of bacterial growth Prevent or treat bacterial growth in the retained secretions and collapsed alveoli.

1. Monitor the patient's temperature every four hours.
2. Observe the quality of secretions. Send a daily specimen to the laboratory for examination.
3. Use scrupulous sterile technique with suctioning, fluid lines, and incisions to avoid introducing bacteria into the patient's body.

4. Administer prophylactic or therapeutic antibiotics as ordered by the physician.

Outcome evaluation

Use these outcome criteria to judge the patient's progress:

- Respiratory rate 12–18 times a minute
- Pulse rate 60–100 times a minute
- P_aO_2 80–100 mm Hg on room air
- $AaDO_2$ less than 50 mm Hg on 100% O_2
- Lung physical examination normal (no bronchial breathing over lung fields; normal voice sounds and whispered sounds; resonance on percussion; normal tactile fremitus)
- Chest x-ray normal (no consolidation, diaphragmatic elevation, or mediastinal shift)

Pulmonary edema

Pulmonary edema results from altered pulmonary capillary dynamics due to elevated capillary pressure, decreased plasma proteins, altered membrane permeability, and/or impaired lymphatic drainage.

Risk conditions

Recognize the patients at risk for acute pulmonary edema; prevent it when possible.

The conditions that increase the patient's risk are grouped here under the four broad causes of pulmonary edema just mentioned.

1. Increased pulmonary capillary pressure results from fluid overload, acute myocardial infarct, severe mitral stenosis, advanced aortic stenosis or insufficiency, severe hypertension, massive pulmonary embolism, and severe tachycardia.
2. Decreased plasma proteins usually result from malnutrition or liver disease.
3. Increased capillary membrane permeability occurs in severe shock, microemboli, disseminated intravascular coagulation, inhalation of a toxic gas, and acute heroin overdose.
4. Decreased lymphatic drainage characterizes pneumonia, pulmonary contusion, microemboli, and increased central venous pressure (because lymphatics empty into systemic veins).

Prevention of risk   Consider ways to prevent the above conditions. Some examples follow. Closely monitor intake and output to avoid circulatory overload. Minimize physical and emotional stress to decrease left ventricular workload and tachyarrhythmias. Teach the stable patient with chronic heart disease the importance of continuing his medications at home, the symptoms of congestive heart failure, and the need for prompt medical attention if symptoms occur. Prevent acute myocardial infarction and shock as outlined in earlier chapters.

Signs and symptoms

The signs and symptoms of pulmonary edema are those of dyspnea, hypoxia, and fluid-filled alveoli.

Observe for signs of dyspnea due to decreased lung compliance, for example, use of accessory muscles, intercostal and supraclavicular retractions, expiratory wheeze, and increased anxiety. Check for signs of hypoxia, such as tachypnea, tachycardia, hypertension, severe apprehension, diaphoresis, and peripheral vasoconstriction. Note signs of transudation of fluid into alveoli—profuse, frothy, pink sputum; cough; and rales.

Nursing interventions

Take measures described in the following paragraphs to relieve symptoms as promptly as possible.

Decreasing venous return   Decrease venous return promptly by taking action as follows:

1. While summoning the physician, elevate the head of bed 45°–90°, and lower the legs to pool blood in the periphery.
2. Give IV morphine sulfate as ordered by the physician to decrease respiratory rate, apprehension, and sympathetic stimulation (thereby decreasing peripheral arterial resistance and increasing venous capacitance). Morphine will decrease the circulating blood volume, so be alert for early signs of shock. It also decreases respiratory center sensitivity to PCO_2, so watch for respiratory depression and possible respiratory arrest.
3. Administer rapid-acting diuretics as ordered by the physician.
4. The physician may order rotating tourniquets to temporarily decrease the circulating volume while slower therapeutic measures take effect. Apply them as follows.

    A. Explain the procedure to the patient, and let him know his limbs will be swollen and discolored during the treatment.

B. Take the blood pressure and pulse before applying the tourniquets and at least every 15–30 minutes during the treatment.

C. Check the peripheral pulses, color, and temperature of each limb. Do not apply a cuff on a limb that already is ischemic or infected or if peripheral vascular disease, peripheral blood clots, or an intravenous line is present. Mark the peripheral pulses with a pen to facilitate checking during use of the rotating tourniquets.

D. Preferably use an automatic rotating tourniquet machine, since it provides better control of pressures and timing cycles. If an automatic machine is unavailable, use portable blood pressure cuffs. In either case, wrap the cuffs high on each extremity.

E. If all limbs are healthy, apply pressure to three cuffs at a time. Most authorities recommend setting the pressure slightly above the diastolic blood pressure. Such a pressure will retard venous return but not occlude arterial blood flow. If you have selected an appropriate pressure, the peripheral pulses distal to the cuffs will be palpable at all times; the limb will be cool and mottled when the cuff is inflated but promptly will become warmer and pinker when the cuff is deflated.

F. Rotate the cuff inflation systematically. With portable cuffs, develop a definite sequential cycle of rotation on paper and follow it to ensure that pressure is released on the proper limb at the correct time. Usually, each limb is compressed for no more than 45 minutes at a time and is free of compression for about 15 minutes at a time. A rotating tourniquet machine will cycle automatically, usually at shorter intervals. Be sure to check that the cuffs are inflating and deflating properly.

G. During the treatment, observe for shock and for signs of pulmonary or arterial emboli. If shock occurs, notify the physician and remove the cuffs as described below. If a limb loses its pulse or becomes hot, cold, tender, or painful, alert the physician and rotate the tourniquets only among the unaffected limbs.

H. When the treatment is discontinued, do *not* remove all the tourniquets at once since the abrupt increase in venous return could again precipitate pulmonary edema. Instead, release the pressure on one limb at a time and remove the cuff. Wait 15 minutes between each release. With an automatic machine, clamp each cuff as it deflates and remove it.

I. During tourniquet removal, observe for signs of recurring pulmonary edema as described earlier. If they occur, consult the physician about continuing the rotating tourniquets.

5. Assist with a phlebotomy if the physician elects to perform such a procedure.

Improving oxygenation and ventilation   To improve oxygenation and ventilation, take these steps. Administer supplemental O_2 as described later in the chapter. The patient will need particular emotional support to accept an oxygen mask, since it often reinforces the sensation of smothering. Also, administer intermittent positive pressure ventilation, as ordered by the physician. This treatment increases intrathoracic pressure, thereby decreasing venous return and helping to shift fluid out of the alveoli.

Relief of anxiety   Take action to relieve the patient's anxiety. Stay with patient and try to provide a calm environment and brief, clear explanations. Also, administer morphine to relieve anxiety.

Additional measures   Work with the physician to alleviate the cause of the attack. For example, administer digitalis if the problem is poor myocardial contractility; assist with cardioversion if tachycardia precipitated the attack.

Outcome evaluation

Evaluate the patient's progress according to these outcome criteria:

- Unlabored respirations 12–18 times a minute
- BP and pulse WNL for patient
- Lungs clear on auscultation
- Skin warm and dry (and pink if the patient is Caucasian)
- No cough or sputum
- Ability to tolerate level of anxiety or apprehension as indicated verbally or nonverbally (by facial expression and body posture)
- Arterial blood gases WNL for patient

Pulmonary embolus

An embolus is an undissolved mass that travels in the blood stream and occludes a blood vessel. Emboli to the lungs include venous thromboemboli, air emboli, fat emboli, and catheter emboli.

Risk conditions

Anticipate and prevent emboli whenever possible. Conditions increasing the likelihood of different types of emboli are stated on the following page to enhance your ability to identify patients at risk.

1. Thromboemboli may result from blood stasis, venous wall abnormalities, clotting abnormalities, or irrigation of clotted catheter tips. In 1846, Virchow identified blood stasis, venous wall abnormalities, and clotting abnormalities as factors promoting venous thrombosis. Remembering this triad can help you to recognize risk conditions for thromboemboli. For example, blood stasis may be caused by obesity, congestive heart failure, immobilization (bedrest), atrial fibrillation or standstill, or severely decreased myocardial contractility. Venous wall abnormalities can result from venous punctures or incisions, trauma, or atherosclerosis. Disorders causing abnormal blood clotting include thrombocytosis and dehydration.

The critical care nurse also must be aware that forceful irrigation of clotted catheter tips can dislodge the clots, creating emboli.

2. Air emboli may result from surgery on the peritoneal cavity, air in intravenous lines, or breakage of a pulmonary artery catheter balloon.

3. Fat emboli can result from long bone fractures (especially the femur and tibia), sternal splitting incisions, use of a pump oxygenator during cardiopulmonary bypass, or trauma to subcutaneous fat. The exact mechanism of fat embolization is unclear; fat release from bones and tissues, alteration of circulating fats, and other causes have been implicated.

4. Catheter emboli may also occur. Many polyethylene intravenous catheters have a surrounding short steel needle to facilitate venipuncture. After venipuncture, the catheter is advanced through the needle, which is withdrawn and covered by a protective shield. If the catheter is advanced and then manipulated while the needle is unshielded, a portion of the catheter can be sliced off and embolize to the lung.

Preventive measures   Take measures to reduce the likelihood of embolization.

Virchow's triad of factors contributing to thromboemboli has numerous implications for nursing prevention. Follow these measures to reduce risk of thromboemboli.

1. Decrease venous stasis as follows:

A. Consult with the physician about the use of antiembolic stockings to maintain venous flow.

B. Ensure that active or passive exercises are performed, since muscular activity promotes venous flow by alternately compressing and releasing the veins. See Chapter 14 for recommended exercises.

C. Some physicians recommend elevating the legs about 15° in the supine patient to aid venous flow without causing inguinal pooling. Avoid constant Fowler's position whenever not required by other conditions (such as acute pulmonary edema).

2. Reduce venous wall trauma as follows:

   A. Avoid venous punctures on the legs whenever possible.

   B. Observe vascular catheter insertion sites for inflammation and phlebitis. If they occur, discontinue the line (unless no other sites are available) and restart elsewhere.

3. If you suspect a line has clotted, first try to aspirate blood; reposition the tip; and then irrigate gently. Do *not* irrigate forcefully.

4. Prevent dehydration to help maintain normal coagulability.

Take preventive action against air emboli. According to Schlant (1974), the lethal dose of air is believed to be 5–15 ml/kg. Although this is a sizeable amount (350–1050 ml for a 70 kg person), lesser amounts can occlude small vessels. Always remove air from vascular lines when assembling them. If you note a bubble once the line is in use, you can remove it with a needle and syringe without breaking continuity of the line. To prevent air embolization from breakage of a pulmonary artery catheter balloon, see the chapter on cardiac assessment and hemodynamic monitoring lines.

Reduce the risk of catheter emboli by implementing the following measures. If it is necessary to reposition a catheter during insertion, withdraw the catheter and unshielded needle simultaneously. Once a catheter is positioned properly, withdraw the needle and cover it with the protective shield.

If a venous catheter is sliced off accidentally, it is imperative that you try to prevent it from reaching the heart. Immediately clamp your hands around the limb between the insertion site and the heart, and obtain immediate medical assistance to remove the catheter.

Signs and symptoms

Detect the occurrence of pulmonary embolism promptly. Signs and symptoms vary depending on the type, size, and hemodynamic consequences of the embolus. Frequently, signs of hypoxia, acute right ventricular failure, and/or decreased cardiac output will be present.

Signs of hypoxia   Watch for signs of hypoxia resulting from the increased alveolar deadspace. The signs include dyspnea, tachypnea, restlessness, and irritability. This wasted ventilation is reduced somewhat by the constriction of distal airways due to alveolar hypocapnia, causing a redirection of ventilation to better perfused areas.

Signs of acute right ventricular failure   Monitor for signs of possible acute right ventricular failure (cor pulmonale). This condition may result from increased pulmonary vascular resistance following a large embolus and produce an accentuated P_2, atrial arrhythmias, increased CVP readings, distended neck veins, or liver engorgement.

Signs of decreased cardiac output   Observe for indications of potential decreased cardiac output. Signs resulting from decreased left ventricular filling are tachycardia, hypotension, dizziness or confusion, shock, or angina. The angina is a result of decreased coronary artery perfusion coupled with an increased right ventricular workload.

Signs of air embolism   A churning noise upon auscultation of the right ventricle is a sign of air embolism to the ventricle. It is accompanied by sudden dyspnea, shock, and cyanosis.

Signs of fat embolism   Suspect fat embolism if you see petechiae along with the signs and symptoms of increased deadspace, right ventricular failure, or decreased cardiac output. Petechiae are most common on the anterior chest, neck, and axillary folds.

Signs of pulmonary infarction   Be alert for symptoms of a possible pulmonary infarction. The signs are those indicated above plus fever over 39°C; transient or persistent pleuritic pain and/or pleural friction rub; cough; and hemoptysis. A chest x-ray 12–24 hours postembolization frequently will show a localized density in the periphery with a rounded edge facing the hilum.

Infarction occurs in only about 10% of the known episodes of embolization. The probable reason for this fact is the dual blood supply to the lungs. There are numerous anastamoses between the bronchial and pulmonary capillaries and veins producing a network facilitating collateral flow in the event of an embolus. Authorities hypothesize that infarcts occur only when middle-sized pulmonary arteries are occluded and collateral flow also is decreased by such conditions as pulmonary venous hypertension or systemic hypotension (Dexter and Dalen 1974).

Other diagnostic aids   Keep abreast of the results of other diagnostic maneuvers. Additional tests may or may not be helpful in detecting an embolus. The ECG occasionally shows signs of right axis deviation and right ventricular strain. The routine chest x-ray may show nothing or may show an elevated diaphragm due to pneumoconstriction, decreased or absent vascular markings, or dilatation of the main pulmonary artery and right ventricle. Pulmonary angiography may show a filling defect due to an embolus or a cutoff due to a complete occlusion. Ventilation/perfusion scans usually show an area of normal ventilation with decreased or absent perfusion. However, emboli smaller than those lodging in the segmental arteries cannot be detected during angiography or scans (Moser 1975). Blood gases may be normal or show an increased $AaDO_2$.

Nursing interventions

Relieve symptoms of pulmonary embolism promptly. The following paragraphs describe nursing interventions to alleviate the symptoms of a pulmonary embolus. If you suspect an air embolus in the right ventricle, immediately place the patient on his left side with the head dependent. This will prevent the air from obstructing the right ventricular outflow tract or migrating to the pulmonary artery. The air will be displaced to the apex, where a physician can aspirate it.

For any type of embolus reaching the pulmonary artery, the goals of care are to relieve the hypoxia resulting from the increased alveolar deadspace, combat any significant decrease in cardiac output, and treat shock vigorously if present.

1. Measures to relieve hypoxia are the following:

   A. Place the person on complete bedrest.

   B. Assist the patient with bathing, eating, and any other activities that worsen the dyspnea.

   C. Administer supplemental O_2 as ordered by the physician.

   D. Raise the head of the bed to the point where dyspnea decreases.

2. Combat the potential decrease in cardiac output as follows:

   A. Decrease additional insults to the left ventricle by reducing its workload: provide physical rest; reduce emotional stress by providing as calm an atmosphere as possible, administering analgesics to control pain, and relieving anxiety as much as possible.

   B. If shock occurs, follow measures outlined in the care plan for shock (Chapter 5).

   C. For persistent shock from a centrally located embolus, embolectomy may be attempted. After the patient is placed on cardiopulmonary bypass, the main pulmonary artery is incised and the embolus removed.

3. Prevent recurrent embolization. Continue prophylactic measures outlined above. Administer fibrinolytic agents if prescribed. (The value of these agents, streptokinase and urokinase, is still under study.) Implement anticoagulant therapy as prescribed by the physician. Protect the patient against excessive anticoagulation by monitoring clotting and/or prothrombin times, observing for signs of internal or external bleeding, minimizing intramuscular injections, testing bowel movements for occult blood, and consulting with the clinical pharmacist on interactions between anticoagulants and the patient's other medications.

   If anticoagulation is contraindicated or emboli persist despite anticoagulation, either the common femoral veins or the vena cava may be ligated; alternatively, an umbrella-shaped device may be inserted in the vena cava to trap further emboli.

When the patient's condition permits, teach him how to prevent, recognize, and respond to symptoms post-discharge. Emphasize the importance of exercise, hydration, measures to promote venous flow, and medical follow-up. Oral anticoagulants may be continued as long as the risk remains, permanently if necessary.

Outcome evaluation

Judge the patient's progress according to these outcome criteria:

- Unlabored respirations 12–18 times a minute
- Pulse, BP, and temperature WNL for patient
- No signs of right ventricular failure (undistended neck veins, normal CVP readings, no liver engorgement)
- Alert and oriented
- No churning noise when right ventricle auscultated
- No cough, hemoptysis, or pleural friction rub

Pneumothorax

A pneumothorax is a collection of free air within the pleural space.

Risk conditions

Anticipate and prevent a pneumothorax whenever possible, by first recognizing the patients at risk for developing a pneumothorax. Predisposing conditions are as follows:

1. Chest trauma, especially penetrating injuries or rib fractures;
2. Pneumonia, because it leads to lung abcesses;
3. Diseases causing degenerative changes in lungs, such as emphysema and bronchitis;
4. Airway obstruction due to bronchospasm, inflammation, or retained secretions;
5. Catheterization of subclavian vein, because it rests on the apical pleura;
6. Thoracentesis;
7. Pericardial tap;
8. Violent vomiting leading to esophageal perforation;

9. Positive pressure ventilation. Risk of a pneumothorax from positive pressure ventilation increases if additional factors are present which increase intra-thoracic pressure. If the patient has chronic obstructive lung disease or is fighting the ventilator, pressure inside the thorax may rise dangerously. The risk of pneumothorax also increases if the tidal volume is over 10 ml/kg, the peak inspiratory pressure is over 35–40 cm H_2O, or positive end expiratory pressure is applied.

10. Pneumothorax also occurs in previously healthy people, for unknown reasons.

11. The likelihood of pneumothorax escalates with increasing numbers of risk conditions. For example, the emphysematous patient on mechanical ventilation who develops retained secretions is more likely to develop a pneumothorax than the previously healthy person on mechanical ventilation whose nurses keep his airway clear.

Preventive measures   Take whatever steps are possible to prevent the predisposing conditions. For example, encourage turning, deep breathing and coughing exercises to clear secretions. If the patient is unable to raise secretions through these methods, stimulate the cough reflex, perform chest physiotherapy, or suction the airway as a last resort.

Administer bronchodilators, steroids, and antibiotics prescribed by the physician to minimize airway obstruction, and antiemetics to control vomiting. Use Trendelenburg's position and have the patient perform a Valsalva maneuver during subclavian catheterization.

Signs and symptoms

Detect the pneumothorax promptly. Signs and symptoms will vary depending on the size and type of pneumothorax. The types are: open, with a continued communication between the pleural space and the outside; closed, with closure of the pleural tear as the lung collapses; or tension, with the opening acting as a one-way valve to let air in but not out. The key signs and symptoms are pain, dyspnea, hypoxia, chest x-ray changes, and sometimes mediastinal shift.

Watch for chest pain which is abrupt, sharp, and constant, and usually appears unilaterally. Signs of dyspnea and hypoxia include tachypnea; nasal flaring; cyanosis; accessory muscle use; retractions; and decreased P_aO_2. On physical examination, the affected side may appear larger with decreased movement, decreased tactile fremitus, hyperresonance or tympany, depressed diaphragm, and decreased breath sounds. Check the chest x-ray for loss of lung markings peripherally, compression collapse centrally, or possible mediastinal shift.

Observe for signs of mediastinal shift away from the pneumothorax (if the pressure is great enough) as follows.

1. Check for tracheal deviation.
2. Auscultate the precordium for deviation in heart sound locations. A crunching sound with the heartbeat (Hamman's sign, resulting from pneumomediastinum) may also be present.
3. Monitor for signs of decreased venous return, such as jugular venous distention, increased CVP readings, liver tenderness, and dependent edema.
4. Observe for signs of decreased cardiac output, such as mental confusion, angina, oliguria, tachycardia, hypotension, and peripheral vasoconstriction.

Nursing interventions

Relieve the pain, dyspnea, hypoxia, and mediastinal shift with the measures described in the following paragraphs.

Stabilization of thoracic cage   Stabilize any associated rib fracture or flail chest. Initially, place the patient on his affected side; obtain medical help for further stabilization, such as positive pressure ventilation following chest tube insertion.

Relief of chest pain   To reduce the chest pain, consult with the physician about type, dosage, and frequency of analgesics. If the pain persists in spite of analgesics, consult with the physician about intercostal nerve blocks. Since the pain usually is abrupt, sharp, constant, and unilateral, call to the attention of the physician any chest pain with different characteristics as a possible indicator of an additional disorder, such as acute myocardial infarction.

Relief of positive intrapleural pressure   Reduce the positive intrapleural pressure which caused the lung collapse and interferes with its reexpansion. Methods of reducing the pressure vary with the type and size of pneumothorax.

1. For a small closed pneumothorax, the physician may prescribe bedrest and supplemental O_2. The air will be reabsorbed slowly, because of the pressure gradient between it and the surrounding blood and tissue.
2. For a tension or larger closed pneumothorax, assist with emergency decompression with a needle, stopcock and syringe, or chest tube. (See later in the chapter for information on the technique and nursing responsibilities related to chest tubes.)
3. Elevate the head of the bed 30° to facilitate expansion of the lung and evacuation of air via the chest tube. Use a footboard to keep the patient from slipping down in bed and restricting diaphragmatic movement.
4. For recurrent pneumothoraces, the physician may elect to create adhesions between the lung and chest wall via injection of an irritating substance into the pleural cavity under local anesthesia or via parietal pleurectomy under general anesthesia.

Compensation for altered lung volumes   Compensate for the effects of the collapse on lung volumes, specifically an increased functional residual capacity and a decreased vital capacity. Follow this procedure:

1. Initially, place the patient on bedrest and assist with eating and bathing.
2. Increase activity when the patient is able to tolerate it without increased pain, respiratory rate, or pulse.
3. Administer supplemental O_2 as prescribed by the physician.

Outcome evaluation

Use these outcome criteria to evaluate the patient's progress:

- No chest pain
- Unlabored spontaneous respirations 12–18 times a minute
- Chest symmetrical in size and expansion
- Normal tactile fremitus and breath sounds
- Involved area of chest resonant on percussion
- Trachea midline
- Heart sounds in normal location; no Hamman's sign
- Venous return normal (neck veins undistended, CVP readings normal, no liver tenderness or dependent edema)
- BP, pulse, and urinary output WNL for patient
- Alert and oriented
- Skin warm and dry (and pink if the patient is Caucasian)
- Chest x-ray—normal peripheral lung markings, no central compression collapse, no mediastinal shift

So far, this chapter has presented the nursing care for the most common acute disorders of aeration. The remaining sections will discuss the therapeutic techniques utilized to combat these disorders.

Oxygen therapy

Recognize the patients who could benefit from supplemental oxygen. Specific signs indicating a possible need for supplemental oxygen are decreased mental status (confusion, impaired thought processes, drowsiness, or lethargy), tachycardia, arrhythmias, hypotension, pale cool extremities, decreased urinary output, dyspnea, fatigue, respiratory depression, cyanosis, or decreased PaO_2. The physician is responsible for prescribing the type of therapy, its frequency and duration, FIO_2 (fractional inspired oxygen), and liter flow. In an emergency (such as shock, severe respiratory depression, impending myocardial infarction, or serious arrhythmias), the nurse should be empowered to start oxygen therapy under standing unit guidelines.

One can estimate the FIO_2 required to achieve a normal PaO_2 in this way (Bushnell 1973):

1. Measure the $AaDO_2$ on 100% O_2, as described in Chapter 9.
2. Add to it 100 mg Hg.
3. Divide the sum by the barometric pressure. For example, if the calculated alveolar PO_2 on 100% O_2 is 673 mm Hg and the measured PO_2 is 373 mm Hg, the $AaDO_2$ is 673 minus 373, or 300 mm Hg. Assuming that in this instance the barometric pressure is 760 mm Hg, the following calculation can be made:

$$\frac{AaDO_2 + 100}{\text{barometric pressure}} = FIO_2$$

$$\frac{300 + 100}{760} = 0.53$$

In this case, an FIO_2 of about 0.53 is required to achieve a normal PaO_2. To avoid such cumbersome calculations, most physicians use nomograms to determine the initial FIO_2 and subsequent adjustments. The use of isoshunt lines for FIO_2 determination is described in Chapter 9.

Methods of oxygen therapy

The following information on methods of oxygen therapy is based primarily on Shapiro, Harrison, and Trout (1975) and secondarily on Bushnell (1973).

The ideal O_2 delivery system would deliver a consistent FIO_2 that could be controlled easily, allow accurate measurement of inspired FIO_2, be comfortable for the patient, convenient for the therapist, and inexpensive. Unfortunately, no current method meets all these criteria. One must choose from a variety of devices the one that will best meet the patient's needs. They may be classified into low-flow and high-flow systems. (Oxygen flow is *not* synonymous with oxygen concentration, because concentration depends on the relationship between O_2 flow *and* total air flow.)

Low-flow systems   If the patient has a normal tidal volume (300–700 ml), a respiratory rate below 25, and a reasonably regular, consistent ventilatory pattern, a low-flow system is suitable. A nasal cannula, nasal catheter, face oxygen mask, and oxygen mask with a reservoir bag are classified as low-flow systems. In a low-flow device the gas flow is not sufficient to meet all requirements for inspiration. Room air must also be inspired. Again, low flow does *not* necessarily mean low concentration; the concentration may vary from 21% to above 90%, depending upon the liter flow, the capacity of the oxygen reservoir, and the rate and depth of ventilation. (A low oxygen concentration is below 35%, a moderate concentration 35–60%, and a high concentration above 60%.) Low-flow systems have an oxygen reservoir which is diluted with room air. The cannula, catheter, face tent, and mask use the nose, nasopharynx, and oropharynx as an anatomical reservoir. The mask with reservoir bag adds an additional O_2 reservoir. Because there is a special valve between this bag and mask, the patient may inspire from the reservoir as necessary (partial rebreathing mask). The types of equipment and their approximate FIO_2s at given liter flows are listed in Table 10-1. These values assume a normal ventilatory pattern. The advantages of low-flow systems are their cost, patient comfort, and familiarity. Their disadvantages are significant. An unstable ventilatory pattern can cause the FIO_2 to fluctuate widely. Variations in respiratory rate or tidal volume will affect the inspired oxygen concentration. The slower the rate or the lower the tidal volume, the higher the FIO_2; the faster the rate or the higher the tidal volume, the lower the FIO_2. This fact has great clinical significance. Consider the patient with chronic lung disease, started on a nasal cannula at 2 L/min. If his tidal volume drops below 300 ml, the FIO_2 may increase to the point where it suppresses his hypoxic ventilatory drive, and you may have an apneic patient on your hands!

For these reasons, monitor the respiratory rate and *measure* the tidal volume every four hours. If the tidal volume decreases below 300 ml, the respiratory rate increases above 25, or the ventilatory pattern becomes irregular or inconsistent, alert the physician, who may want to switch to a high-flow system.

Another disadvantage is that since the patient is breathing air from outside as well as inside the system, the temperature and humidity cannot be controlled.

High-flow systems   In a high-flow system, the patient breathes only the gas it supplies. A high-flow system can deliver an O_2 concentration of 24–100%, that is, a low, moderate, or high concentration. High-flow systems include Venturi masks and nebulizers using the Venturi principle. This principle is based on the Bernoulli principle, which states that as the velocity of gas flow increases, its lateral pressure decreases. In a device using this principle, the oxygen flows through a small orifice at a high velocity. Just after the oxygen leaves the orifice, the low lateral pressure pulls in or "entrains" room air. By varying the size of the orifice and the flow of oxygen, one can provide a precise FIO_2. The high-flow systems have several advantages over low-flow devices. The FIO_2 remains consistent in spite of variations in the patient's ventilatory pattern. Since the patient breathes only the system's air, its temperature and humidity can be controlled. Finally, the FIO_2 can be directly measured with an oxygen analyzer. The disadvantages of these systems are cost and decreased patient comfort.

Complications

Prevent the complications of oxygen therapy: dehydration of mucosa, hypoventilation, absorption atelectasis, and acute oxygen toxicity. Preventive measures are described in the following paragraphs.

Table 10-1 Oxygen Delivery Systems

Equipment	Liter Flow of 100% O_2	Inspired O_2%	Estimating Inspired O_2%	Nursing Precautions
Nasal cannula or catheter	1–6	24–44	For each L above 1, add approximately 4%	Make sure the nares are patent. May use even with a mouth-breather, since oropharyngeal air flow creates Bernoulli effect, pulling in O_2 through nasopharynx. Do not increase L above 6 because it will not increase FIO_2; switch to a mask.
Oxygen mask	5–8	40–60	For each L above 5, add 10%.	Do not run below 5L, as exhaled CO_2 will not be washed out. To increase FIO_2 above 0.60, do not increase liter flow; switch to a bag with reservoir.
Mask with reservoir bag	6–10	60–99+	For each L above 6, add 10%.	Maintain flow rate sufficient to keep bag from completely collapsing on inspiration.
Venturi mask	4–8 (set according to flow rate specified on mask)	24–40%	Look on mask (24%, 28%, 35%, or 40% mask)	To increase FIO_2, switch to a higher-concentration mask.

Data from: Shapiro, B., Harrison, R., and Trout, C., 1975. *Clinical Application of Respiratory Care*. Chicago: Yearbook Medical Publishers; and Bushnell, S., 1973. *Respiratory Intensive Care Nursing*. Boston: Little, Brown and Company.

Dehydration of mucosa   Always humidify oxygen because it is a dry gas which can quickly dehydrate the mucosa. Humidification can be achieved with humidifiers or nebulizers. Heated humidifiers deliver fully saturated water vapor, while nebulizers deliver aerosols (tiny water particles).

Hypoventilation   Avoid provoking hypoventilation in chronic lung disease patients. These patients depend upon the hypoxic stimulus to ventilation rather than the normal hypercapnic stimulus. When you relieve the hypoxia, you may cause apnea. To prevent this problem, use only very low O_2 flows (1–2 L/min.) if the patient is not mechanically ventilated. Monitor the ventilatory pattern closely. Be especially alert if the patient is breathing slowly or shallowly, since as mentioned earlier these will increase the FIO_2 in a low-flow system.

Absorption atelectasis   Prevent absorption atelectasis. This complication can occur because oxygen washes out the nitrogen in the alveolus. Nitrogen normally maintains the residual volume that keeps the alveolus open because it is poorly absorbed, in equilibrium, and, at ambient pressures, metabolically inert. When it is replaced by oxygen, which is readily absorbed, the residual volume decreases and the alveolus collapses. This process occurs when the patient has a low tidal volume, a normal tidal volume without sighing, or early airway closure which traps alveolar gas, as in emphysema. Therefore, prevent this problem by limiting the duration of 100% inspired O_2 to 30 minutes and, even at lower concentrations, maintaining a patent airway, mobilizing secretions, sighing the patient, or providing constant high tidal volumes.

Acute oxygen toxicity   Prevent acute oxygen toxicity. The toxicity depends both on the alveolar oxygen pressure (not alveolar O_2 concentration or arterial PO_2) and duration of exposure. Its manifestations occur in two phases (Bushnell 1973). The exudative phase is characterized by alveolar edema, intra-alveolar hemorrhage, pulmonary congestion, and the formation of hyaline membranes. The slightly later proliferative phase consists of worsened alveolar edema, inter-alveolar septal edema, hyperplasia of alveolar cells, and fibrosis.

Shapiro, Harrison, and Trout (1975) recommend these guidelines:

1. Maintain FIO_2 below 50% if possible. Even prolonged use at these lower concentrations rarely causes acute O_2 toxicity.
2. Limit the duration of 100% inspired O_2 to 24 hours. (Remember that within 30 minutes, absorption atelectasis may begin.)
3. Limit the use of inspired concentrations above 60% to 3 days.

In addition, it may be helpful to increase the FIO_2 gradually and provide intermittent air exposure, if possible.

These guidelines of course must be considered in light of the patient's need for relief of hypoxia. With many critically ill patients, the dangers of this therapy are outweighed by the need for high inspired oxygen concentrations over prolonged periods to maintain adequate tissue oxygenation.

Outcome evaluation

Evaluate the effectiveness of O_2 therapy by using these outcome criteria:

- Improved level of consciousness, ideally alert and oriented
- BP, pulse rate, and cardiac rhythm WNL for patient
- Spontaneous, unlabored respirations 12–18 times a minute
- Urinary output WNL for patient
- Extremities warm and dry (and pink if the patient is Caucasian)
- P_aO_2 WNL for patient, ideally 80–100 mm Hg

Chest physiotherapy

Be alert for patients who can benefit from chest physiotherapy. Used prophylactically, chest physiotherapy can benefit patients who have had a history of thoracic or abdominal surgery, smoking, coma, endotracheal or tracheostomy tube, or chest wall deformity. Therapeutic use of chest physiotherapy can benefit patients with respiratory depression, thoracic or abdominal incisions, atelectasis, copious or viscous secretions, pneumonia, bronchitis, or emphysema. Chest physiotherapy will provide no benefit for patients with pneumothorax, hemothorax, or pleural effusion (because the pleural space does not connect with bronchi); pulmonary edema; or congestive heart failure.

To assess the need for chest physiotherapy (chest PT), examine a variety of indicators. Physical examination may reveal increased respiratory rate or effort, decreased chest excursion, decreased or bronchial breath sounds, rales or rhonchi. Arterial blood gases may show decreased PO_2 and/or increased PCO_2. Pulmonary function tests may reveal a decreased tidal volume or vital capacity. The chest x-ray may show consolidation, atelectasis, or infiltration.

Prevent patient apprehension and pain. Explain to the patient the benefits and techniques of chest PT. (Demonstrate them on yourself or gently on him or her.) Administer analgesics before starting, unless contraindicated by his or her pulmonary or systemic status.

Techniques of chest PT

A repertoire of chest PT techniques includes: postural drainage, percussion, vibration, huffing, diaphragmatic breathing, localized expansion, and belted breathing.

Postural drainage   Use the diagrams in Table 10-2 to position the patient to drain the desired segments. Note that 12 positions drain all 18 pulmonary segments. Leave the patient in the position for at least 20 minutes to obtain effective drainage.

Table 10-2   Postural drainage positions

Upper lobes		
*Segment to be drained**	*Patient position*	*Area for chest physiotherapy*
Apical segment (right apical, or left apical/posterior segment)		
Anterior portion	Sitting upright and slightly backward	Just below clavicle with fingers curving slightly over clavicle
Posterior portion	Sitting upright and slightly forward	Behind clavicle with fingers curving slightly over shoulders

Anterior portion   Posterior portion

Right lung   Left lung

Anterior segment (right or left)	Supine with pillow under knees	Just below clavicle

Left lung

Right lung

Posterior segment Right	On left side; place pillow in front of shoulder and roll patient forward until 45° from prone	Over right scapula

*Schematic lungs (not in anatomic perspective) show bronchus drained.

(continued)

Table 10-2 *(continued)*

Upper lobes		
Segment to be drained*	*Patient position*	*Area for chest physiotherapy*
Left apical/posterior	On right side, 45° from prone; raise head of bed 12 inches (or use 3 pillows to raise shoulder)	Over left scapula

Right lung

Left lung

Right posterior segment

Left apical/posterior segment

Middle lobe and lingula		
Segment to be drained	*Patient position*	*Area for chest physiotherapy*
Right (lateral or medial segment)	On left side; place pillow behind back from right shoulder to hip; roll backward until 45° from supine; raise whole bed (not just feet) so feet 12 inches higher than head	Over right nipple area

Right middle lobe

Right lung

Left lung

(continued)

Table 10-2 (*continued*)

Upper lobes		
Segment to be drained*	*Patient position*	*Area for chest physiotherapy*
Lingula (superior or inferior segment; lingula is that part of the left upper lobe that is analagous to the right middle lobe)	On right side; place pillow behind back from left shoulder to hip; roll backward until 45° from supine; elevate bed so feet 12 inches higher than head	Over left nipple area

Left lung

Right lung

Lower lobes		
Segment to be drained	*Patient position*	*Area for chest physiotherapy*
Superior segment (right or left)	Prone with pillow under abdomen	Below scapula

Left lung

Right lung

(*continued*)

Table 10-2 *(continued)*

Upper lobes		
*Segment to be drained**	*Patient position*	*Area for chest physiotherapy*
Lateral basal segment (right or left)	On opposite side; place pillow under hips; raise bed so feet 18 inches higher than head	Over lower lateral ribs
Medial basal segment (right lung only)	On right side; place pillow under hips; raise bed so feet 18 inches above head	Over lower ribs

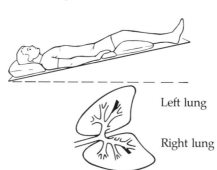

Right lung

Left lung

Right lateral basal segment

Left lung

Right lung

Left lateral basal segment and right medial basal segment

Anterior basal segment (right anterior basal or left anterior medial basal)	Supine; place pillow under knees; raise bed so feet 18 inches higher than head	Over lower anterior ribs

Left lung

Right lung

(continued)

Table 10-2 *(continued)*

Upper lobes		
*Segment to be drained**	*Patient position*	*Area for chest physiotherapy*
Posterior basal segment (right or left)	Prone with pillow under hips; raise bed so feet 18 inches higher than head	Over lower posterior ribs

Left lung

Right lung

Percussion   Use the postural drainage diagrams to position the patient according to the area you want to treat. Cover the skin with a thin towel. Do not percuss over bony prominences or female breasts.

Cup your hands. Relax your shoulders and elbows. Move your hands from the wrists (Figure 10-1) to produce a hollow percussion note rather than a slapping sound. The object is to trap and compress the air between your hand and the chest wall, thus transmitting an energy wave to the lung tissue to loosen mucus.

Work with gravity, that is, percuss from the least dependent to most dependent area. Do not percuss in the opposite direction but instead return your hands to the starting position and repeat the movement.

Begin percussing slowly and gently to accustom the patient to the sensation. Increase the percussion until you are percussing vigorously about 200 times a minute. Percuss for 2–3 minutes in the same area to loosen secretions.

Vibration   Place one hand over the desired area. Place the other hand on top of and parallel to the first. Flex your elbows slightly. Using your shoulder muscles, vibrate your hands on the chest wall throughout exhalation. Repeat for at least five exhalations. Aim at delivering a vibration frequency of about 200 per minute.

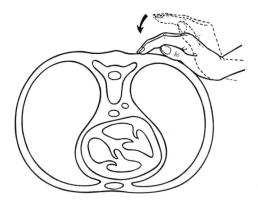

Figure 10-1.   Chest percussion.

Huffing   Place the patient in a comfortable upright position. Tell the patient to take a deep breath, blow part of it out in a short huff by contracting his abdominal muscles, and continue huffing until he must inspire.

Diaphragmatic breathing   Place the patient in Fowler's position with slight knee flexion to facilitate diaphragmatic descent and relax the abdomen. Instruct the patient to use only his abdominal muscles, and reinforce the instruction by having him place his hands on his abdomen to obtain feedback. Have him breathe in by trying to push his hands apart and breathe out by letting them come back together.

Localized expansion   It is possible to improve the expansion of a general area of the lung, such as the apex, base, or lateral lung, with localized expansion techniques. Place one hand anteriorly and the other posteriorly over the area for treatment. Tell the patient to take a deep breath. As the patient inspires, compress the area with the anterior hand. At the height of inspiration, release the pressure suddenly.

Belted breathing   Use a piece of upholstery webbing or fold a drawsheet into a belt. Wrap it around the base of the lungs and cross one end over the other. As the patient exhales, pull on the ends to increase the pressure of the belt against the chest. As he inhales, release it slightly so that the chest is expanding against resistance; release the pressure completely by full inspiration.

Coordinating techniques and treatment goals   From the preceding techniques, select those appropriate to the goal of treatment and your patient's condition.

1. To mobilize secretions, use percussion, vibration, or huffing, in conjunction with postural drainage. To improve tidal volume and exhalation, use diaphragmatic breathing, localized expansion, belted breathing, or huffing.

2. Do not use percussion at all if the patient has acute cardiac disease, thoracic inflammation, hemorrhage, or a very low platelet count. Percuss gently on patients who have or are prone to rib fractures, such as those with osteoporosis, bone cancer, or hypocalcemia. Do not percuss over an incision or area of pain, but percuss normally over the rest of the chest. Brace the incision or painful area with a sheet folded into a belt or with your hand.

3. Modify postural drainage for patients with increased intracranial pressure, orthopnea, or poor cardiovascular reserve.

If the problem is increased intracranial pressure, do not lower the head. Keep it flat (unless contraindicated by the patient's condition or the physician's order). Keep the feet flat and raise the hips on pillows. By doing so, you position the lungs to facilitate drainage but do not increase blood flow to the head because you encourage venous pooling in the legs. If the patient has orthopnea or diminished cardiovascular reserve, lower the head as much as tolerable.

4. Modify PT for the intubated patient. To perform chest PT on an intubated patient, work with another therapist. One person hand ventilates the patient, delivering a slow deep inspiration. Just before the end of inspiration, the second person begins vibration. The ventilator holds inspiration briefly and then releases it quickly while the second person continues vibration throughout exhalation. Repeat several times and suction the patient.

5. Coordinate the duration and frequency of the treatments to achieve the therapeutic goal without exhausting the patient. In general, perform chest PT prophylactically every 2–4 hours, rotating treatment sites. Perform it therapeutically every 1–4 hours, rotating unaffected sites and treating the involved area every other time. Limit treatments to 10–20 minutes. Do not perform them within 30 minutes of oral feedings.

Outcome evaluation

Evaluate the effectiveness of your treatments according to these outcome criteria:

- Lungs clear on auscultation
- Arterial blood gases WNL for patient
- Tidal volume and vital capacity WNL for patient
- Chest x-ray clear

Artificial airways

Patients who can benefit from an artificial airway are those with an upper airway obstruction, profuse secretions, a need for mechanical ventilation, or a likelihood of aspirating gastric secretions.

The most common cause of upper airway obstruction in the nonalert patient is the tongue, which falls back and occludes the hypopharynx. For this reason, whenever possible place the nonalert patient on his side or prone. Do not leave him unattended in the supine position, especially with a pillow under his head.

If the previously alert patient develops apnea or noisy breathing with diminished air movement, immediately open the airway. Following are methods of initial airway establishment.

1. In the patient without a neck injury, hyperextend the head. Place one hand on the forehead, the other under the neck, and tilt the head backward until the chin is in a line with the earlobes. If the head tilt is ineffective, repeat the maneuver as incorrect positioning is the primary reason it sometimes does not open the airway.

2. Should the airway remain obstructed, use a series of chest or abdominal thrusts and back blows to dislodge any foreign objects that may be present. These techniques are explained in the cardiopulmonary resuscitation section of Chapter 3.

3. For persistent obstruction, try the triple airway maneuver (Figure 10-2). Stand slightly behind the head. Place the tips of your fingers behind angles of the mandible, your palms on the patient's temples, and your thumbs just lateral to the corners of the mouth. Tilt the head back with your palms. Displace the jaw upward with your fingers. Retract the lower jaw with your thumbs.

4. The head tilt is dangerous in the patient with a cervical injury. In this case, open the airway with the jaw thrust (Figure 10-3). Use the same technique as the triple airway maneuver but delete the head tilt.

The preceding maneuvers are only temporary measures for maintaining the airway and should be followed by placement of an artificial airway.

Types of artificial airways

For more secure maintenance, insert an artificial airway or assist a physician to do so. The three categories of artificial airways are the pharyngeal airway, the endotracheal tube, and the tracheostomy tube (Figure 10-4).

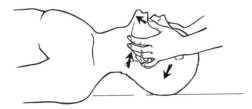

Figure 10-2   Triple airway maneuver. Hyperextend the head by pressing down with your palms on the temples. Lift the mandible with your fingers and open the mouth with your thumbs.

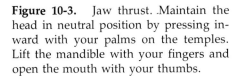

Figure 10-3.   Jaw thrust. Maintain the head in neutral position by pressing inward with your palms on the temples. Lift the mandible with your fingers and open the mouth with your thumbs.

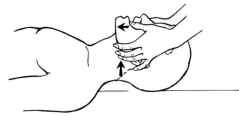

Pharyngeal airways   There are two types of pharyngeal airways: the oropharyngeal and the nasopharyngeal. Often, the nurse may insert these in an emergency at her own discretion. The oropharyngeal or oral airway extends from the lips to the pharynx and therefore displaces the tongue anteriorly. It is made of curved, rigid plastic. To insert one, select a size suitable for the patient. Open the mouth with a tongue depressor or by inserting your crossed thumb and index finger into the corner of the mouth and crossing them further to force the mouth open. Turn the airway sideways and slide it along the buccal mucosa until the flange on the end touches the lips. Then turn it so the curve fits over the tongue. Tape it in position.

A nasopharyngeal airway is a soft rubber tube that extends from the nare to the pharynx. The end of the tube is funnel shaped to prevent it from entering the nostril. Select the largest diameter tube that will fit the nostril. Choose the appropriate length by holding the tube against the patient's cheek, with the funnel-shaped end at the nostril and the other end pointing toward the back of the throat. The end of the tube should be about one inch beyond the earlobe. Lubricate the entire length with water soluble jelly and insert it gently.

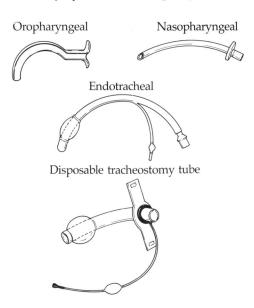

Oropharyngeal   Nasopharyngeal

Endotracheal

Disposable tracheostomy tube

Figure 10-4.   Artificial airways.

Endotracheal tube   An endotracheal tube extends from the nose or mouth into the trachea. The orotracheal route is preferred in emergencies. While the tube can be inserted rapidly by this route, it is more difficult to stabilize the tube and kinking develops more easily than with the nasotracheal route. The nasotracheal route of insertion is more difficult and the diameter of the tube is limited by the size of the nares. An endotracheal tube may be inserted at the bedside by the physician or specially trained nurse or respiratory therapist. To assist with intubation:

1. Bring the following equipment to the bedside: laryngoscope with several sizes of curved and straight blades, extra bulb and battery; assorted sizes of endotracheal tubes; a stylet; topical anesthesia; Yankauer pharyngeal suction tip; suction apparatus; sterile catheters and gloves; syringes; needles; intravenous muscle relaxants (succinylcholine or pancuronium bromide); water soluble lubricant; Magill forceps; benzoin; tape; a bite block or oral airway; and the ordered delivery system for oxygenation and/or ventilation.

2. Snap the size and type of blade preferred by the physician onto the laryngoscope handle. Make sure the light works; if not, replace the bulb or the battery in the laryngoscope handle.

3. Connect the Yankauer suction tip to the suction apparatus. Suction and preoxygenate the patient.

4. Position the head in moderate dorsiflexion. If the patient is conscious, the physician may apply topical anesthesia to the trachea and administer a muscle relaxant.

5. The physician will insert the blade, visualize the vocal cords, and then ask for a specific tube size. Inflate the cuff to test for symmetry of the cuff and any possible leak in the cuff. Then deflate it.

6. Bend the stylet to a curve with a radius of about 30°. Insert it in the tube until it reaches half an inch proximal to the tube's end (if you protrude it past the tip, it may damage the trachea).

7. Lubricate only the tip of the tube; if you lubricate the whole tube, the physician will have difficulty handling it. Hand the tube to the physician.

8. Using her hand or the Magill forceps, the physician will pass the tube between the vocal cords, through the larynx, and into the trachea. When she indicates, quickly inflate the cuff. She will remove the stylet and laryngoscope and hold the tube in place.

9. Connect the tube's opening to the ventilating device and begin ventilation. Insert an oral airway or bite block, paint the skin with benzoin, and tape the tube securely.

Tracheostomy tube   A tracheostomy tube must be inserted by a surgeon. A *tracheostomy* is an artificial opening into the trachea; *tracheotomy* is the operative procedure that creates it. A tracheostomy is indicated when the anticipated time interval for an artificial airway exceeds 48–72 hours, when an upper airway obstruction prevents the use of an endotracheal tube, when radical neck surgery is performed, or as a measure to decrease anatomic dead space.

Ideally, the tracheotomy rarely is performed in an emergency. For emergency airway establishment, the patient should be intubated at the bedside and transferred to the operating room, where the technically more difficult tracheotomy can be performed under calmer, sterile conditions. General anesthesia is administered and the head and neck extended. A horizontal incision is made between the second and third tracheal rings, and a window the size of the tracheostomy tube excised. The largest cannula that will fit the trachea is inserted. A fabric tape is placed around the neck and tied to the flange of the tube. The tube is not sutured to the skin.

If the patient has a severe upper airway obstruction precluding intubation before tracheotomy, an emergency cricothyrotomy may be performed at the bedside. The physician palpates the thyroid cartilage and cricoid ring. He then uses a scalpel or scissors to incise the cricothyroid membrane. A tracheostomy tube is inserted and the patient transported to the operating room for tracheotomy and closure of the cricothyrotomy.

Prevention of complications

The critical care nurse plays a crucial role in forestalling possible problems with an artificial airway. Such complications include: apprehension, malposition or loss of the airway, airway obstruction, infection, and tracheal damage.

Incorporate the following guidelines into your routine care of the person with an artificial airway. Many of them apply to any type of artificial airway. When one applies only to a specific type of airway, it is so stated.

Apprehension   Relieve the patient's apprehension due to his fear of the unknown, discomfort, and inability to talk. Whenever possible before insertion, prepare the patient psychologically. In many cases, you will have to delay this preparation until the airway has been established. Insertion of any of these airways is uncomfortable; the conscious patient will experience an unpleasant sensation of pressure or choking. The endotracheal tube is probably the most uncomfortable. The newly tracheotomized patient may require medication for the pain of the incision. Most patients learn to tolerate an artificial airway. The patient is justifiably anxious when he realizes the airway interferes with speech and he cannot call for help. Explain that he will be able to speak again when the airway is removed. In the meantime, establish a communication system (see Chapter 13) and call it to the attention of all staff caring for him.

Malposition or loss of the airway   Prevent inadequate ventilation due to malposition or loss of the airway. Take these preventive measures:

1. After an endotracheal or tracheostomy tube is inserted, obtain an x-ray to verify placement. Also auscultate both lung fields at least every four hours. Sometimes the tube is placed improperly or migrates so that it enters the right mainstem bronchus rather than remaining above the carina as is necessary for bilateral ventilation. In this case, breath sounds will be present in only one lung.

2. Have readily accessible within the unit a laryngoscope, extra tubes, and tracheotomy tray. At the bedside, keep a hand ventilation bag; in addition, for a tracheostomy tube, keep the obturator (if one was used) and a tracheal dilator.

3. Avoid accidental extubation. For a tracheostomy tube, be sure the tapes holding it in place are tied firmly. For an endotracheal tube, measure from the patient's lip to the tube's junction with the connector (from "lip to tip") every 2–4 hours. Record the distance, and call any displacement promptly to the physician's attention.

Airway obstruction   Forestall obstruction of the airway. Follow these steps to avoid obstruction:

1. Eliminate airway obstruction due to kinking of the endotracheal tube. Position the patient's head normally; avoid flexing it. Support the ventilator tubing with a pillow or suspend it from an intravenous hanger attached to the ceiling over the bed. Some patients will bite an orotracheal tube, thereby occluding it. Prevent this by inserting an oral airway or bite block. If your unit does not stock commercial bite blocks, you can fashion a bite block yourself by wrapping adhesive tape into a rectangle that will fit comfortably between the patient's teeth. Be sure to leave a small tab protruding from the mouth so you can remove it for mouth care.

2. Prevent obstruction due to herniation of the cuff over the tip of the tube. Avoid overdistending the cuff or using a tube whose cuff is not bonded to it.

3. Prevent airway obstruction due to retained secretions. Since these tubes bypass the humidification provided normally by the upper airway, provide artificial humidification. Also maintain adequate systemic hydration. For a tracheostomy, remove the inner cannula (if there is one) at least every eight hours and clean it with half-strength hydrogen peroxide. Since secretions also collect outside the tube, consult with the physician about changing it every 3–7 days.

Institute a vigorous program of coughing, turning, and chest physiotherapy to mobilize secretions. A tube in the trachea, of course, prevents normal coughing, so meticulous attention to removal of secretions is vital. See later sections of this chapter on suctioning and chest physiotherapy for details.

4. Inhibit the formation of tracheal granulation tissue. While this tissue will not cause obstruction during intubation, it may cause obstruction after extubation. To minimize the development of granulation tissue, reduce factors which irritate

the trachea. Remove the secretions that accumulate above the cuff, causing chemical irritation of the trachea. Do not use aerosol sprays where the patient can inhale them. Keep cotton fibers from entering the airway by using non-cotton gauze around a tracheostomy stoma. If your sterile gloves are powdered on the outside, rinse them with sterile solution before suctioning.

Infection   Because the upper airway defense mechanisms are bypassed, pulmonary infection frequently occurs. Follow this procedure to prevent infection:

1. Use meticulous sterile technique during suctioning and tracheostomy care. Keep the skin around a tracheostomy tube free of secretions by cleaning it with hydrogen peroxide and applying a dry sterile dressing around the stoma. Use sterile suctioning technique with a fresh sterile catheter for each episode of suctioning.

2. Give thorough mouth care at least every eight hours to reduce the potential of the oropharynx as a focus of infection.

3. Drain the water that condenses in the ventilator tubing by disconnecting the tubing and letting it empty into a basin. Do *not* drain the condensed water back into the patient's lungs or the reservoir of the humidifier.

4. Follow a prescribed schedule of changing ventilatory equipment. Selecky (1974) suggests that you change the sterile water in the humidifier every eight hours and replace the humidifier or nebulizer and ventilatory tubing every 24 hours.

5. Tie tracheostomy tapes snugly but not tight enough to irritate the skin. Reduce chafing by tying the tape so that there are no knots at the sides of the flange and by changing the tape when it becomes soiled. To eliminate knots at the sides of the flange, loop the tape through one side of the flange, pass both ends behind the patient's neck, and loop the bottom piece of tape through the other side of the flange. Then tie a knot several cm away from the flange so that the knot is on top of the lower piece of tape. This method provides a smooth surface against the skin.

Upper airway damage   Avoid pressure necrosis of the nare by cleaning around a nasotracheal tube and by changing it to the opposite nostril every 8–24 hours. To prevent oral necrosis, reposition an orotracheal tube every eight hours. Have one person hold the tube while you deflate the cuff and remove the tape securing the airway. Move the tube to the opposite side of the mouth, check that the correct distance from lip to tip has been maintained, tape it in position, and reinflate the cuff.

Also forestall tracheal damage from cuffed tubes. Tracheal damage may consist of necrosis, stenosis, tracheoesophageal fistula, distension, or tracheomalacia (loss of cartilage). Numerous factors have been implicated in the genesis of tracheal damage. Among them are infection; the length of intubation; improper size or placement of the tube; cuff size, pliability and shape; and intracuff pressure. After studying autopsy specimens, Cooper and Grillo (1969) reported that tracheal damage is related directly to time, progressing from mild tracheitis at 48 hours to fragmentation of cartilage at 12–16 days. The following paragraphs describe measures which will reduce tracheal damage.

Minimize cuff pressure. Numerous studies have been reported on the relationship between cuff pressure and tracheal damage. Most have utilized animal models and their conclusions are controversial and confusing. After surveying the current literature, Shapiro, Harrison, and Trout (1975) conclude that in the patient with a normal perfusion state and uninfected trachea, cuff pressure over 5 mm Hg obstructs lymphatic flow, producing edema; pressure over 18 mm Hg obstructs venous drainage, producing congestion; and pressure in excess of 30 mm Hg impedes arterial flow, causing ischemia. Cuff pressures over 50 mm Hg create ischemic and necrotic acreas within 48 hours, but these areas are patchy. Permanent damage does not seem to occur unless the sloughing is circumferential, which it usually is not. The potential for damage is increased with a small, rigid, unevenly inflating cuff; such a cuff may necessitate up to 145 mm Hg pressure against the tracheal wall to effect an airtight seal. Mucosal damage does not appear to be countered sufficiently by the ritual of deflating the cuff five minutes each hour.

The current literature has significant clinical implications. To minimize cuff pressure, take these steps:

1. Encourage physicians to use large diameter, high residual volume cuffs. Carroll and Grenvik (1973) recommend that such cuffs measure no more than 20 mm Hg during expiration.

2. Leave the cuff deflated whenever possible. Inflation is necessary for mechanical ventilation, feedings, and swallowing dysfunction.

3. Inflate the cuff with the minimal leak technique. To do this, inflate the cuff while listening over the trachea with a stethoscope. Inflate it until you hear only a slight hiss at the peak of inspiration.

4. Check the cuff pressure initially and every eight hours. To do this, disconnect a blood pressure cuff from a syphgmomanometer. Use a three-way stopcock to connect the manometer and the inflation line for the cuff. Turn the stopcock off to the manometer. Use a syringe to inflate the cuff through the third stopcock port; note the volume of air you insert. Next turn the stopcock to connect the cuff and manometer. As the patient expires passively, read the cuff pressure on the manometer and record it. Disconnect the manometer and allow the cuff to deflate completely. Then reinflate it, following the procedure described in step 3. Call to the physician's attention pressures over 20 mm Hg or progressive increases in the pressure or volume.

5. Tracheal necrosis is more common when both an endotracheal or tracheostomy tube and a large nasogastric tube are in place. If nasogastric drainage is necessary, use as small a size nasogastric tube as is effective.

Watch for other ways to reduce tracheal damage. Observe for bleeding around the tube or pulsations of the tube. Bleeding around the tube usually is minor and due to trauma. Pulsations of the tube when none were present previously may indicate imminent hemorrhage through the tube due to erosion of the tip into the innominate artery. This complication is rare but life threatening. If you spot new pulsations, obtain immediate medical evaluation. It may be necessary to reposition the tube or replace it with a shorter or narrower tube.

Observe for the appearance of oral feedings or tube feedings in the tracheal aspirate. Their presence suggests either a tracheoesophageal fistula or, more commonly, swallowing dysfunction. This dysfunction occurs because the tracheostomy tube prevents the upper esophageal sphincter from relaxing as it normally does during swallowing (Bonnano 1971). You cannot prevent this dysfunction but can minimize it by inflating the cuff and elevating the head of the bed during feedings and for 30 minutes afterward. Both swallowing dysfunction and a tracheoesophageal fistula will cause a positive methylene blue test. When this dye is added to the feeding, its appearance in tracheal secretions confirms the connection between the esophagus and trachea. Differentiating the two causes requires radiology or endoscopy. A fistula usually takes 2–4 weeks to develop, so a positive dye test before then probably indicates swallowing dysfunction. The dysfunction usually will disappear after the airway is removed.

Watch for puffed-up tissues which crackle when palpated, indicating subcutaneous emphysema. Possible causes include air escaping from the stoma into the tissues or a bronchopleural fistula. Call this finding to the physician's attention, as it will necessitate treatment if it continues and compresses the trachea. Once the source is controlled, the air is reabsorbed slowly. If the subcutaneous emphysema is severe, the physician may decompress the tissues by inserting several 18 gauge needles or making small incisions under local anesthesia. Stroking the skin towards the needles or incisions causes the air to escape.

Treatment of complications

The previous section stressed the role you can play in preventing the complications of an artificial airway. If complications do occur, you must recognize them promptly and respond appropriately.

Relief of airway obstruction   Retractions, increased inspiratory pressure on a ventilator, severe apprehension, and decreased or absent air movement signify acute airway obstruction. This life threatening problem can be caused by mucous plugs or herniation of the cuff over the tube's end. Herniation may occur if a cuff is overinflated or if a separately attached cuff slips over the end of the tube.

If you suspect acute airway obstruction, first try to suction the airway. Next, deflate the cuff. If the airway is a tracheostomy with an inner cannula, remove the inner cannula. If the obstruction persists, summon medical help immediately while trying to ventilate through the tube with a bag, tube connector, and 100% O_2. Should you be unable to ventilate through the tube, place a mask on the bag and try to ventilate around the tube; the pressure may force some air around the tube and into the lungs.

Relief of bleeding   Profuse frank bleeding from the endotracheal or tracheostomy tube indicates erosion of the tube into the innominate artery. Summon medical assistance immediately. Hyperinflate the cuff to tamponade the bleeding. If the patient has a tracheostomy tube, the physician may try to insert an endotracheal tube, remove the tracheostomy tube, insert his finger through the tracheostomy, and compress the artery (Utley et al 1972). An immediate operation is necessary to suture the site of the erosion.

Response to accidental extubation   If accidental extubation occurs, *do not panic*. For a tracheostomy, use a tracheal dilator to maintain the stoma and attempt to reinsert the tube (using its obturator if it has one). For other airways, open the airway by hyperextending the head or using the jaw thrust maneuver. Call a physician immediately to reintubate the patient.

Treatment of infection   Purulent or colored secretions or an elevated temperature may indicate a pulmonary infection. Culture the secretions to identify the specific organism, and consult with the physician about drug therapy.

Removal of artificial airways

When the airway is no longer needed, prepare the patient for its removal. Pharyngeal airways are removed in one step. An endotracheal or tracheostomy tube is removed in several steps. First, the patient must maintain spontaneous ventilation for several hours if he has been on a mechanical ventilator; this step is discussed in greater detail under the section on mechanical ventilation. His gag reflex and swallowing ability must be intact. When these criteria are met and it is time to remove the tracheostomy or endotracheal tube, first preoxygenate the patient and suction the lungs. Then suction the oropharynx and deflate the cuff. The physician will remove the tube. Observe the patient closely for signs of recurrent respiratory distress. A sore throat and hoarse voice are common after extubation and require no treatment other than an explanation to the patient and humidification. Inspiratory stridor occurring upon extubation or more commonly about 24 hours later indicates laryngeal edema. Alert the physician, who may reintubate the patient or order further observation, humidification, and local application of a steroid and vaconstrictor (racemic epinephrine) to reduce the edema.

Outcome evaluation

Evaluate the effectiveness of the artificial airway and your care according to these outcome criteria:

- Patient able to communicate needs to staff
- Calm, relaxed appearance
- Unlabored respirations within limit desired for patient
- Arterial blood gases WNL for patient
- Lungs clear to auscultation
- No signs of necrosis or bleeding around the airway
- Tracheal cultures without pathologic flora
- No oral feedings or tube feedings in tracheal aspirate

Tracheal suctioning

Be alert for patients who need tracheal suctioning. Conditions that indicate difficulty with spontaneous clearing of secretions include the following:

1. Increased viscosity of secretions;
2. Weak or paralyzed thoracic or abdominal muscles, for example, owing to thoracic surgery or paraplegia;
3. Depressed ciliary activity such as after general anesthesia;
4. Increased production of secretions;
5. Ineffective cough; a patient is unable to cough effectively if he has an endotracheal or tracheostomy tube, or if his vital capacity is less than 20 ml/kg or three times predicted tidal volume (Shapiro, Harrison, and Trout 1975).

Prevention of complications

Prevent the potential complications of tracheal suctioning: hypoxia, laryngospasm or bronchospasm, arrhythmias, and infection.

Avoidance of routine suctioning   Avoid routine suctioning by capitalizing whenever possible on the patient's ability to remove secretions.

1. Teach the cooperative and able patient how to cough effectively. Tell him to take in a deep breath and close his glottis on a count of "one," contract his thoracic and abdominal muscles on "two," and open his glottis on "three." Demonstrate the sound of an effective cough versus an ineffective one with the glottis open and no abdominal movement. An effective cough can generate an estimated velocity of 600 miles an hour.

2. Maintain adequate systemic hydration (and airway humidification if an artificial airway is in place).

3. Implement a program of chest PT and postural drainage to assist the patient to raise secretions.

4. If necessary, utilize cough stimulation techniques to enhance secretion removal by the patient. Following are some methods of cough stimulation. Press firmly over the lower trachea until the patient coughs. If recommended in your institution, instill at least 5–10 ml of sterile saline down the endotracheal or tracheostomy tube to loosen secretions and initiate a cough. This practice is controversial, because unless you take strict precautions to keep the bottle of fluid sterile, it rapidly becomes contaminated and you will introduce a source of infection. Pass a suction catheter until it reaches the carina. In most patients, this contact will initiate a forceful cough. Consult with the physician about placing a polyethylene catheter through the tracheal wall (cricothyroid cannulation). The instillation of normal saline through such a catheter can liquify secretions and provoke coughing.

Assess the effectiveness of these techniques by auscultating the lung fields every 1–4 hours for rales and rhonchi, examining serial lung x-ray reports (looking for infiltrates or atelectatic areas), and evaluating the blood gases.

Recommended suctioning technique   Suction when secretions are retained in spite of the measures outlined above. Obtain a suctioning order from the physician and prevent or minimize complications by adhering closely to these recommendations:

1. Explain to the patient the purpose, technique, and sensations involved. Warn him that he may feel out of breath or may feel like choking. Suctioning is not a pleasant experience; patients deserve to know this, as well as that the discomfort will be brief. The properly prepared patient is less likely to panic during the procedure. It helps for you to convey a positive rather than punitive attitude. For example, say "I'm going to suction you so you can breathe more easily" rather than "I'm going to suction you because you just won't cough as I showed you before your surgery."

2. Do not suction if you note signs of laryngospasm (crowing respirations), bronchospasm (severe wheezing), or bradycardia.

3. Bring to the bedside single sterile gloves, sterile saline in a small cup, sterile suction catheters, sterile saline in a 10 cc syringe without a needle, sterile water soluble lubricant, a hand ventilating bag connected to 100% oxygen and a mask or endotracheal/tracheostomy tube adaptor, and tissues. Turn the suction apparatus on to 80–120 mm Hg.

4. Wash your hands.

5. Preoxygenate the patient with 100% O_2 for 4–5 deep breaths.

6. Open the catheter package sterilely. Designate one hand as sterile, to handle the catheter only. Place a sterile glove on it. Designate the other hand as unsterile, to connect the suction and occlude the vent. To minimize resistance and trauma while passing the catheter, do not connect it to suction yet and leave the vent open. Apply sterile water-soluble lubricant or sterile saline to the catheter.

7. If the patient has an endotracheal or tracheostomy tube, disconnect the airway from the adaptor on the hand ventilating bag with the unsterile hand. This is tricky; if you cannot do it rapidly, use an assistant to hand ventilate and to disconnect and reconnect the airway.

8. If the patient does not have an endotracheal or tracheostomy tube, facilitate catheter entry into the trachea by placing him in Fowler's position. Put a pillow behind his shoulders and tilt the head backward. Do not turn the head to the right to enter the left bronchus or vice versa; these positions are not as effective as has been thought in the past, since it is very difficult to enter the more sharply angled left bronchus without a specially curved (coudé) catheter. Grasp the tongue with a gauze square and pull it forward gently. To retract the epiglottis, have the patient cough or breathe deeply while you pass the catheter only on inhalation. When the catheter enters the trachea, the patient may become very restless and apprehensive. Talk to him soothingly, reminding him the procedure will be over soon.

9. Advance the catheter gently and rapidly as far as it will go; then withdraw it 1–2 cm to avoid traumatizing the tracheal wall. Since the carina is very sensitive to mechanical stimulation, the patient may cough forcefully at this point.

10. Place your ear over the free end of the catheter and listen for respirations to confirm that the catheter is in the trachea.

11. Connect the catheter to the suction source. Occlude the vent and suction no more than 10 seconds. (Hold your breath while you are suctioning, and you will not forget about the time because of your own urge to breathe!) Rotate the catheter gently as you withdraw it. Watch the cardiac monitor for the development of arrhythmias.

12. Oxygenate the patient again with 100% O_2 for five breaths. If secretions are thick, rinse the catheter with sterile solution.

13. Repeat the suctioning and oxygenating until the secretions are removed.

14. Next, suction the oropharynx using the same catheter. (Note: it is acceptable to use the same catheter to suction first the sterile trachea and then the oropharynx, but *not* the reverse.)

15. Discard the glove, catheter, and cup after *each* suctioning session.

Treatment of complications

Recognize and respond promptly to complications. Restlessness, cyanosis, and sometimes worsened arrhythmias usually indicate hypoxia secondary to depletion of alveolar PO_2. Terminate the suctioning and oxygenate the patient. For future suctioning episodes, increase the duration of preoxygenation and decrease the duration of each suctioning episode.

Worsened arrhythmias may result from hypoxia, catecholamine release during anxiety, or mechanical stimulation of the vagal fibers innervating the trachea. Remove the suction catheter, oxygenate the patient, and calm him if apprehensive. If the arrhythmia persists, notify the physician.

Crowing, wheezing, or resistance to catheter removal indicates laryngospasm or bronchospasm. If the catheter can move freely, remove it and do not attempt to suction again; otherwise, disconnect the suction and leave the catheter in the trachea. Oxygenate the patient and summon a physician immediately.

Purulent or foul-smelling secretions suggest infection. Inform the physician and send a specimen for culture and sensitivity.

Outcome evaluation

Evaluate the effectiveness of suctioning against these outcome criteria:

- Toleration of suctioning without panic
- No restlessness, cyanosis, or worsened arrhythmias during or after suctioning
- No crowing, wheezing, or resistance to catheter removal
- Tracheal cultures without pathologic flora
- Improved breath sounds
- Improved arterial blood gases

Mechanical ventilation

Be alert for patients in need of mechanical ventilation. The physician's decision to institute mechanical ventilation is based not on the disease entity per se but rather on the physiologic stress it imposes on the patient. Shapiro, Harrison, and Trout (1975) have recommended the following indications for mechanical ventilation. Objective signs that a person probably cannot maintain adequate ventilation for a prolonged period of time include a vital capacity of less than 13 ml/kg or twice a predicted tidal volume; a negative inspiratory force of less than -20 cm of water within 20 seconds; arterial PCO_2 below 30 mm Hg or above 50 mm Hg; a shunt of greater than 30%; and/or a deadspace/tidal volume (VD/VT) ratio greater than 80%. The broad indications for mechanical ventilation are apnea, impending or actual acute ventilatory failure, and some cases of hypoxemia. Impending acute ventilatory failure is best documented by progressively increasing P_aCO_2 values and decreasing pH values. Mechanical ventilation may be indicated for hypoxemia due to decreased functional residual capacity, severely increased work of breathing, or an inadequate pattern of breathing.

Procedure for mechanical ventilation

Prepare the patient psychologically. If time and the patient's condition permit, help the physician explain to both the patient and family the purpose of mechanical assistance before it is instituted; otherwise, as soon afterward as feasible. Briefly, explain the equipment involved and the care the patient will receive, for example suctioning and blood gas checks. Emphasize the sensations the patient will experience—those of having something breathe for him or her and those related to the artificial airway. Establish a system by which the patient can summon help immediately. Assure the patient that the ventilator has mechanical alarms; demonstrate the noises the alarms make and explain how the staff will respond. Also assure the patient that a nurse will always be at the bedside or within hearing distance. This psychological preparation will not only reduce the patient's apprehension but also have physiological benefits. The properly prepared patient is less likely to fight the ventilator. Fighting the ventilator is detrimental because it increases catecholamine release, oxygen consumption, and the need for paralyzing drugs.

Bring to the bedside the necessary equipment. From the respiratory therapy department, order the type of ventilator and the settings specified by the physician. Place at the bedside a hand-ventilating bag, mask and oxygen tubing, and sterile suction supplies.

Types of ventilators The ventilators most commonly used are those that produce IPPV (inspiratory [not "intermittent"] positive pressure ventilation). Positive pressure ventilators come in two basic types: pressure limited and volume limited. Pressure limited ventilators include the Bird Mark 7 and Bennett PR II. Since the pressure is predetermined, the dependent variable is the volume of gas delivered. For example, when the airway is clear, the desired volume will be delivered; but if it becomes obstructed, the set pressure will be reached much earlier and only part of the volume will be delivered. Volume preset ventilators include the Bennett MA-1, Ohio 560, Emerson, and Engstrom ventilators; in these, the dependent variable is the pressure.

The type of ventilator chosen depends upon the patient's need and in some cases the availability of the ventilator, since volume ventilators are considerably more expensive than pressure ventilators. The patient with normal compliance is a suitable candidate for the pressure ventilator, since one can be reasonably sure of the delivered volume for a given pressure. The patient with poor or variable compliance needs a volume ventilator, since it is more difficult to predict from a given pressure whether the patient will receive the desired volume.

Inspiratory modes   Either type of ventilator can be used in a variety of inspiratory modes: assist, control, or assist/control. In the assist mode, the patient triggers the machine by starting to inspire; the machine then delivers the set pressure or volume. This mode is suitable for the person with a normal respiratory drive but weak musculature. In the control mode, the machine delivers a set number of ventilations per minute without regard to the patient's efforts. This mode is appropriate for the apneic patient. The patient with an irregular respiratory drive is ventilated best in the assist/control mode: the machine will assist him if he initiates the breath or will provide one if he fails to do so.

Another inspiratory maneuver is intermittent mandatory ventilation (IMV), used with the spontaneously ventilating patient. The patient breathes on his own but intermittently is forced to take a deeper breath by the machine. It is used most commonly during weaning from the ventilator. Since the ventilation is delivered at a predetermined frequency, it may occur out of phase with the patient's own efforts.

Expiratory maneuvers   The physician may order a variety of expiratory maneuvers. Since their distinctions can be confusing, they will be described in relation to their pressure curves (Figure 10-5). The following descriptions are based on Shapiro, Harrison, and Trout (1975).

1. *CPAP*   First note the curve for spontaneous breathing—a negative inspiratory phase followed by a positive expiratory phase and a return to atmospheric pressure. If a positive pressure is added at the end of expiration for someone breathing spontaneously, it raises the baseline pressure but does not disturb the configuration of the curve. In other words, the patient is under continuous positive airway pressure (CPAP).

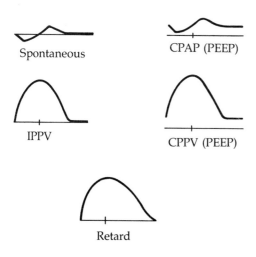

Spontaneous

CPAP (PEEP)

IPPV

CPPV (PEEP)

Retard

Figure 10-5.   Typical airway pressure curves. Typical airway pressure curves during various airway pressure maneuvers (see text). The zero line represents ambient pressure; the small vertical line separates inspiration from expiration. (From Shapiro, B. A., Harrison, R. A., and Trout, C. A. *Clinical Application of Respiratory Care.* Copyright © 1975 by Year Book Medical Publishers, Inc., Chicago. Used by permission.)

2. *CPPV* Now look at the curve created by inspiratory positive pressure ventilation (IPPV). Instead of a negative inspiratory phase, it is positive. The expiratory phase also is positive, and airway pressure returns to atmospheric at the end of expiration. If a positive pressure is added at the end of expiration, it also increases the baseline pressure but does not disturb this curve's configuration. Since the airway pressure is always positive and never returns to atmospheric pressure, this type of ventilation is called continuous positive pressure ventilation (CPPV). This type of ventilation sometimes is called positive end expiratory pressure (PEEP), but restricting the term PEEP to this type (as some therapists have done) is misleading. In reality, the term PEEP could be applied both to CPAP and CPPV, since both are established by adding a positive pressure at the end of expiration. In other words, CPAP and CPPV are subdivisions of PEEP— CPAP in the spontaneously ventilating patient, CPPV in the mechanically ventilated patient.

3. *Retard* The last maneuver that may be used with positive pressure ventilation involves adding a resistance to the expiratory line. It does not disturb the baseline pressure, thus allowing the patient to reach atmospheric pressure at the end of exhalation. All it does is retard the expiratory phase, analogous to the pursed lip breathing used by patients with chronic obstructive lung disease. The maneuver therefore is called retard.

4. *Therapeutic effects of PEEP* PEEP has several significant physiologic effects. Recall that critically ill patients often suffer alveolar collapse, due to the loss of surfactant, absorption atelectasis during the administration of oxygen, or early small airway closure.

When alveoli collapse during expiration, the continuing pulmonary capillary blood flow is not oxygenated; that is, increased shunting occurs. The alveolar collapse also causes a decreased residual volume and therefore a decreased functional residual capacity (FRC). In addition, alveolar collapse causes decreased lung compliance, because it takes a higher than normal airway pressure to reopen the alveoli. Thus, alveolar collapse causes both hypoxia and increased work of breathing. The application of PEEP causes airways to stay open longer, decreasing shunt and increasing FRC. As a result, the patient can oxygenate his blood more readily.

Ventilator settings Initially, ventilator settings are approximate. Inspiratory pressure is set at that necessary to deliver the desired tidal volume; it may range from 15 cm H_2O in the patient with high compliance (such as in emphysema) to 50 cm H_2O or greater in the poorly compliant patient. Ideally, a slow ventilatory rate (8–14 per minute) and high tidal volume are chosen. Shapiro, Harrison, and Trout (1975) recommend multiplying the ideal body weight by 5 ml/lb and adding 100 ml (for ventilator tubing deadspace) to arrive at the initial tidal volume setting. Patient observation and evaluation of blood gases must be used to refine these settings to the patient's need.

Large tidal volumes with slow rates have several physiologic advantages. The effects of deadspace are minimized. Mean airway pressure is lower with slow rates; as a result, venous return is not diminished as much as with faster rates. Ventilation with normal tidal volumes removes the normal sigh mechanism, which prevents collapsed alveoli and promotes surfactant production, so patients on normal tidal volumes need to be given periodic deep inflations. Large tidal volumes obviate the need for sighing and so are more effective in preventing microatelectasis.

Prevention of complications

Prevent the potential complications associated with mechanical ventilation. The primary complications are insufficient or excessive oxygenation and/or ventilation, water imbalances, decreased cardiac output, pneumothorax, infection, atelectasis, and gastrointestinal hemorrhage or dilatation. Prevent them by incorporating the actions described in the following sections into your care of any ventilated patient.

Incorrect ventilation or oxygenation   Monitor the ventilator settings and the delivered values at least hourly. (Ventilator settings often are slightly inaccurate; it is important to note *both* the machine settings and the delivered values.) Make the following checks or, if the respiratory therapist performs them, keep yourself informed of the values.

1. Monitor the exhaled tidal volume. The machine's gauge estimates only the set tidal volume. Delivered tidal volume is measured with a spirometer attached to the exhalation port.

2. Peak inspiratory pressure can be read from a dial on the ventilator. Also note the maximum inspiratory pressure—the setting of the pressure pop-off valve.

3. Count the delivered respiratory rate by observing the patient's chest. Compare it to the set ventilator frequency.

4. Observe the FIO_2 setting and the delivered oxygen concentration. Note the machine setting, especially after the patient has been placed on an FIO_2 of 1.0 prior to suctioning or blood gas sampling. If you fail to reset the FIO_2 after these procedures, the person may develop oxygen toxicity. To determine the delivered oxygen concentration, use an oxygen analyzer and place its tip at the patient's airway.

5. Monitor the ratio between inspiration and expiration (I/E ratio). Inspiration must be shorter than expiration to prevent trapping air in the chest.

6. Keep the alarms *on*. Most ventilators have a delay button you can press to prevent the alarm from sounding when you need to disconnect the patient

temporarily, for example to suction or to drain condensed water from the tubing. Use this delay feature whenever possible. If you do turn the alarm off, be *absolutely* sure to turn it back on when you are finished.

Water imbalances   The patient may develop dehydration or a positive water balance. Dehydration may result from high temperature or low humidity of the inspired gas. To prevent dehydration, be sure there is a thermometer dial in the inspiratory tubing. Visually check it every two hours to maintain the temperature between 32° and 35°C. Also maintain the specified level of fluid in the humidifier. The etiology of positive water balance in mechanically ventilated patients is not clear; factors implicated include humidification of inspired air, reduced lymphatic flow, and inappropriate ADH (antidiuretic hormone). Nebulizers may add up to 500 ml fluid intake per 24 hours; in addition, nebulizers and humidifiers prevent the usual loss of water via the lungs (approximately 300–500 ml/24 hours). Place the patient on intake and output recording. When calculating water balance, consider both the retention of fluid normally lost and the addition of fluid from the equipment. Also monitor the patient's weight, compliance, hematocrit, serum sodium, and chest x-ray for signs of water retention.

Decreased cardiac output   Positive pressure ventilation increases intrathoracic pressure and therefore decreases venous return to the heart. This effect is increased when PEEP is used. Most patients can tolerate this effect, increasing their peripheral venous tone to compensate. Patients with conditions that diminish sympathetic responses (for example, hypovolemia, drugs interfering with sympathetic tone, or old age) cannot compensate for increased intrathoracic pressure. Monitor the heart rate, arterial blood pressure, peripheral perfusion, and venous pressure to detect the patient's response to the increased intrathoracic pressure; notify the physician promptly if you observe signs of falling cardiac output.

Pneumothorax   Pneumothorax may occur due to rupture of a bleb in the lung, disruption of lung sutures, or procedures such as CVP line insertion while the patient is on the ventilator. Its incidence is increased in the patient with PEEP. See the care plan on this condition earlier in this chapter for ways to prevent, recognize, and respond to this complication.

Infection   Minimize the ventilator as a source of infection. Respiratory therapy should follow a regular program of decontaminating equipment. Change ventilator tubing once every 24 hours. When water condenses in the tubing, empty it externally rather than draining it back into the patient's lungs or into the humidifier reservoir.

Atelectasis   Prevent atelectasis by following the measures outlined in the care plan dealing with it. In addition, if normal tidal volumes are being used, periodically sigh the patient to prevent microatelectasis. If the ventilator does not have a sigh button, hand ventilate the patient with a tidal volume larger than the ventilator's. Once the patient has developed microatelectasis, the sigh will not reopen collapsed alveoli. To promote reexpansion, deliver a deep breath and hold the inflation momentarily, that is, "yawn" the patient (Shapiro, Harrison, and Trout 1975). Some ventilators have an "inflation hold" button; if yours does not, hand ventilate the patient and briefly hold inspiration to mimic a normal yawn.

Gastrointestinal complications Prevent gastrointestinal complications. Hemorrhage occurs in about 25% of patients with prolonged mechanical ventilation. Consult with the physician about administering antacids and minimizing the use of steroids. Test fecal matter for occult blood and notify the physician if present. Avoid gastric dilatation (caused by air swallowing) by consulting with the physician about using prophylactic nasogastric decompression.

Treatment of complications

Recognize and respond promptly to the problems of loss of ventilation, cardiovascular deterioration, and/or a struggling patient.

Whenever adequate ventilation fails abruptly, immediately disconnect the ventilator and hand ventilate the patient while you evaluate the problem further. A sudden increase in inspiratory pressure often accompanied by release of the pop-off valve signifies obstruction. Check for kinks in the tubing and suction the airway. A falling pressure in a volume-limited ventilator or a rapidly decreasing tidal volume in a pressure-limited ventilator indicates a leak in the system. Check the tubing connections.

If these simple actions fail to correct the problem, summon the assistance of another nurse, respiratory therapist, or physician.

The cause of cardiovascular deterioration usually is increased intrathoracic pressure. If the decompensation is acute, hand ventilate the patient. Obtain immediate medical reevaluation of the therapy.

A restless or struggling patient may indicate hypoxia or emotional panic. Bag breathe the patient while his blood gases are checked; the ventilator settings may have been inadequate for him. If the gases are abnormal, inform the physician, who may want to alter the settings. If the gases are normal, the problem may be that the patient is terrified of the sensation of being unable to ventilate himself. When this occurs, hand ventilate him, starting at his spontaneous rate and slowly decreasing the frequency until he reaches the desired rate. Then, reconnect him while you coach him to breathe in synchrony with the ventilator. The attitude you convey during this maneuver is very important. If your tone or actions are critical or demeaning, you will only increase his anxiety. If you verbally acknowledge his fright and convey calmness, especially if the patient has developed trust in you before the episode, you will be considerably more effective in helping him adapt to his dependence on the ventilator. If the problem continues, consult with the physician about revising the ventilator settings. If all other measures fail, the physician may order the patient sedated with morphine or paralyzed with small doses of curare or pancuronium bromide.

Discontinuation of mechanical ventilation

Assist with discontinuation of mechanical ventilation as ordered by the physician. First, note how well the patient meets discontinuation criteria. Shapiro, Harrison, and Trout (1975) have identified guidelines for ventilator discontinuance. They point out that the primary criterion for ventilator discontinuance is improvement or reversal of the underlying disease process. Objective signs that the ventilator probably may be discontinued safely include the following: the vital capacity is greater than 13 ml/kg or twice a predicted tidal volume; inspiratory force is better than -20 cm H_2O in 20 seconds; shunt is less than 20%; and VD/VT (deadspace/tidal volume) ratio is less than 60%. If the shunt is 20–30% or the VD/VT ratio is 60–80%, the ventilator may be discontinued providing cardiovascular, hepatorenal, and central nervous system function is satisfactory. Most patients do not need to be weaned from the ventilator gradually.

To discontinue the ventilator, first assist the physician in explaining the impending events to the patient. Let him know he may feel short of breath initially and you will be monitoring him closely. Explain that if he has difficulty, mechanical ventilation will be resumed and discontinuation tried again later.

Connect the airway to a T-piece rather than the ventilator. In addition to the arm that connects to the patient, another arm of the T connects to wide-bore oxygen tubing; the third arm is an exhalation port. Always make sure the patient receives oxygen when the ventilator is discontinued.

Monitor pulse, blood pressure, peripheral perfusion, and ease of breathing for the first 15 minutes. A mild increase in pulse and BP are normal. Suction as necessary.

After 15 minutes, evaluate the blood gases, vital capacity and cardiopulmonary status. If they are satisfactory, continue oxygen, deep breathing and coughing exercises, and chest PT. If the patient remains stable for several hours, the artificial airway then may be discontinued.

When the patient can not maintain spontaneous breathing after the ventilator is discontinued, the cause may be physical or psychological. The possible reasons require careful evaluation by you and the physician. The process of gradual discontinuation (weaning) often is facilitated by IMV and in some cases by CPAP.

Outcome evaluation

Evaluate the effectiveness of mechanical ventilation according to these outcome criteria:

- Calm, relaxed, not struggling against ventilator
- Arterial blood gases within desired limits for patient, usually P_aO_2 60–110 mm Hg and P_aCO_2 35–45 mm Hg
- No signs of dehydration or fluid overload
- BP, pulse rate, venous pressure, and peripheral perfusion WNL for patient
- Tracheal aspirate without pathologic flora
- No hematemesis or blood in fecal matter; hemoglobin and hematocrit levels WNL for patient

Chest drainage

In order for the lungs to expand properly, the pleural space must remain a potential space, with a pressure more negative than the intrathoracic pressure. In addition, there must be no accumulation of fluid or air in the mediastinum which could interfere with lung expansion or produce cardiac tamponade.

When air and/or fluid accumulates in the pleural space or mediastinum, the increased pressure interferes with lung expansion. A chest tube will relieve the pressure, drain the fluid, and thereby facilitate resumption of normal pulmonary dynamics.

Techniques of chest drainage

Recognize patients who could benefit from chest drainage, that is, those with pneumothorax causing respiratory embarrassment; hemothorax; pneumomediastinum; or hemomediastinum. Examples are the patient with a rib fracture and pleural tear and the thoracic surgical patient.

Obtain medical consultation and assist with chest tube insertion. Whenever possible, before starting explain to the patient the purpose and technique of chest drainage.

Gather the necessary equipment. Bring to the bedside a sterile tube thoracotomy tray (containing drapes, scalpel blade and handle, etc.), a sterile chest tube and obturator of the size and type (straight or right-angle) specified by the physician, sterile gloves, local anesthetic, skin cleansing solution, sterile gauze squares, adhesive tape, sterile connecting tubing, sterile solution (water or saline), two rubbershod Kelly clamps, a 50 ml syringe, and the sterile drainage system. The drainage system may be one-, two- or three-bottle drainage (Figure 10-6) or a disposable system such as the Pleurevac (Figure 10-7).

Increasingly, hospitals are using a disposable system because it is simpler to use, less cumbersome, and less prone to breakage than the older bottle system. The principles of chest drainage will be explained using the Pleurevac; correlations with the bottle system will be included.

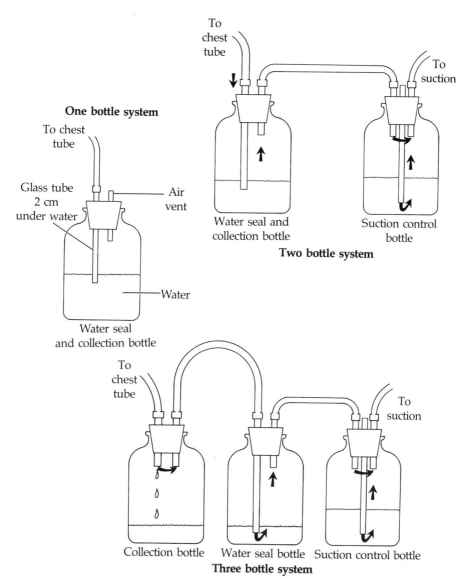

Figure 10-6. Bottle chest drainage systems.

Setting up chest drainage   Before the tube is inserted, unwrap the sterile covering on the drainage system. While maintaining sterility, set up the type of drainage ordered by the physician. The three-bottle system and the Pleurevac have three chambers: a collection chamber, a water seal chamber, and a suction control chamber. Depending on which chambers are used, you have the options

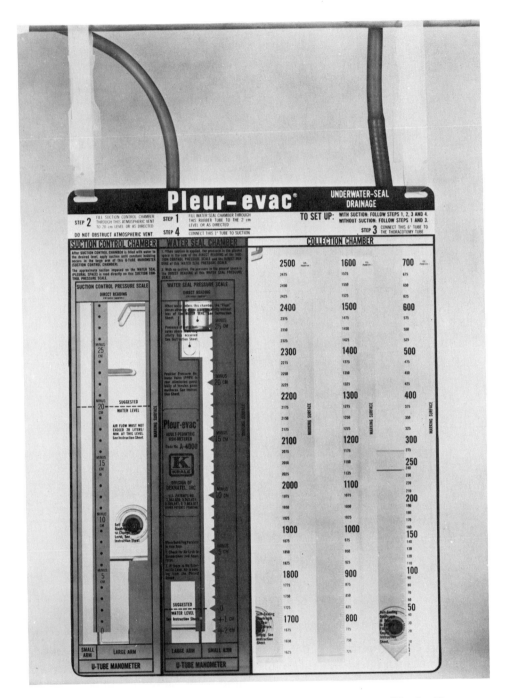

Figure 10-7. Pleurevac disposable chest drainage system. (Used with permission of Deknatel Division of Howmedica, Inc.)

of straight gravity drainage or drainage under low suction (from an external suction source). Fluid drainage accumulates in the *collection chamber.* The *water seal* allows displaced air from the collection chamber to escape but prevents atmospheric air from entering the pleural space. The *suction chamber* controls the amount of suction exerted on the chest. Displaced air leaves the system through a vent.

Directions for setting up the various types of drainage follow. Use a pen to mark all fluid levels with the date and time.

1. For straight drainage without suction—

    A. Pleurevac. Remove the plunger from a 50 ml syringe. Insert the tip of the syringe into the rubber tubing of the water-seal chamber. Pour sterile solution up to the 2 cm mark on the water seal chamber.

    B. One-bottle system. In the one-bottle system, the glass bottle serves as both the collection and water seal chambers. Set up the system by adding sterile water to the bottle until the tip of the long glass tube is 2 cm under water. Add sterile connecting tubing to the free end of this tube, to be attached later to the chest tube. Leave one vent in the bottle cap open to air. Close off any other vents in the cap.

2. To apply low suction—

    A. Pleurevac. First establish the water seal, as above. Then remove the cap from the suction control chamber. Fill the chamber to the level ordered by the physician (usually 10–25 cm), by using the 50 ml syringe without the plunger. Replace the cap, which has a small air vent in it. Attach the external suction source (wall outlet or portable pump) to the tubing connected to the water seal chamber.

    B. Two-bottle system. With the glass bottle system, either a two-bottle or three-bottle system can be used for low suction. In the two-bottle system, the first bottle still serves as the collection and water seal chamber; the second as the suction control chamber. Establish the water seal as with the one-bottle system. Connect the air vent from that bottle to one opening in the cap of the suction bottle. Connect a long glass tube to another opening in that cap; leave the upper end of that tube open to air. Attach the external suction source to the third cap opening. Pour sterile solution into the bottle until the tip of the long tube is under the amount of suction ordered.

    C. Three-bottle system. The three-bottle system has separate bottles for the collection, water seal, and suction chambers. Set up the water seal and suction control chambers as above, but do not connect the water seal chamber to the chest tube. Instead, connect the water seal chamber to an opening in the cap of the collection bottle. Add sterile connecting tubing to another opening in the collection bottle cap (this tubing eventually will connect with the chest tube). Occlude any other vents in the cap. Do not add any fluid to this chamber.

Assisting with chest tube insertion   Assist with bedside chest tube insertion by acting as the unsterile person and by monitoring the patient's condition. The physician will insert one or more tubes depending upon the problem. To evacuate air from the pleural space, he will insert the tube anteriorly at the second intercostal space (Figure 10-8). To remove fluid from the pleural space he will insert it in the eighth or ninth intercostal space in the midaxillary line.

(To evacuate air or fluid from the mediastinum, the tubes usually are inserted in the operating room. One tube is placed anteriorly at the base of the pericardium. The other is placed anteriorly just below the xiphoid process.)

When the tube is inserted and the obturator removed, connect the tube to the drainage system. The doctor will suture the tube to the chest wall and dress the site. If suction has been ordered, turn the suction source on until you see gentle bubbling in the suction chamber. Tape all connections securely. Tape in a circular fashion except at the connection between the chest tube and the connecting tubing. There, tape longitudinally, leaving a narrow space so you can observe the drainage.

Maintenance of chest drainage

Once the system is established, maintain its patency and effectiveness.

Amount, rate, and quality of drainage   Observe the collection chamber for the amount, rate, and quality of drainage. Mark the level of drainage each hour. Call a rate over 100 ml per hour or frank bleeding to the attention of the physician.

Decreased drainage may result from obstructions in the system, pooling of secretions, or reexpansion of the lung. Keep the tubing free of kinks by taping connections to tongue blades to stabilize them. Loosely coil the tubing flat on the

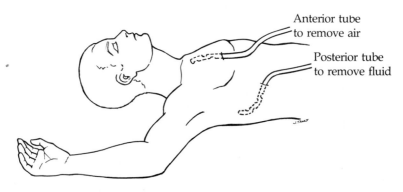

Anterior tube to remove air

Posterior tube to remove fluid

Figure 10-8.   Pleural chest tube locations.

bed; dependent loops cause increased pressure. Unless contraindicated, place the patient in Fowler's position to facilitate both air and fluid removal. Turn him regularly. Most importantly, if fluid is being evacuated, strip and milk the tubes every 15 minutes to one hour. To strip the tube, lubricate about 12 inches at a time with hand cream. Pinch the tube shut proximal to the chest. Maintain the occlusion while you pinch the tube with your other thumb and forefinger and slide them away distally. Then, maintain the distal occlusion while you release the proximal one, creating suction. Finally, remove the distal pinch. Strip the tube down to the collection chamber, to suck fluid and clots into it. Milking is another method to move fluid and clots. To milk the tube, start proximally. Squeeze it with one hand, place your other hand distally and squeeze it, and then release the proximal hand. Continue hand over hand to the collection chamber.

Water seal fluid level   Observe the water seal chamber for the level of fluid once every 8 hours. Too little fluid may allow air to enter the chest; too much means the intrapleural pressure will have to rise excessively before air or fluid can be expelled. Add or remove water as necessary.

Water seal fluctuations   Also observe the water seal chamber for fluctuations. The fluctuations ("tidaling") result from changes in intrapleural pressure with respiration. Normally, the Pleurevac's water seal will show fluid movement upward on inspiration and downward on expiration. (If the patient is on a positive pressure ventilator, the direction will be reversed.) In the bottle system, the fluid in the glass tube will move upward on inspiration and downward on expiration. Excessive fluctuations indicate coughing or respiratory distress. Decreased fluctuations may indicate an obstruction to drainage or reexpansion of the lung. Tidaling is less marked with mediastinal tubes.

Bubbles in water seal   Observe the water seal chamber for bubbles. Bubbles result from air displaced from the collection chamber that passes through the water seal before leaving the system. Thus, they reflect the rate of air and fluid drainage. You should see occasional bubbles in the seal. You should not see continuous bubbles. Persistent continuous bubbling indicates an air leak in either the system or the patient. To identify which, briefly clamp the tube near the patient. If the bubbling stops, you know the leak is at the insertion site or inside the patient. Palpate around the insertion site to see if the leak is there. If it is, notify the physician, who can put in a pursestring skin suture. If the leak is inside the patient, notify the physician and consult with him about switching to a Pleurevac with an air leak meter. On the other hand, if the bubbling does not stop when you clamp the tube, you know the leak is in the system itself. Continue clamping along the system to localize the leak. If it is in the tubing, replace it or tape the connections more firmly. If the leak is in the bottle or Pleurevac, replace it.

Fluid level and bubbling in suction control chamber   Observe the suction control chamber for fluid level and bubbling. Note the level of fluid in the suction control chamber and the rate of bubbling, once every eight hours. The amount of sucion depends on the amount of fluid in the suction control chamber, not the setting on the external suction source or the rate of bubbling. Maintain a gentle constant stream of bubbling; vigorous bubbling simply promotes evaporation of the fluid. Whenever the level of the water decreases, add more to maintain the desired suction. With a Pleurevac, minimize evaporation of fluid from the suction chamber by using the rubber cap with the small air vent to cover the large opening of the suction control chamber.

Placement of system   When using bottles, place them in holders and warn visitors and staff not to kick them accidentally. Pleurevacs may be hung from the bedside or placed in a holder on the floor. Keep the system below the patient's chest, even while transporting him. If necessary when turning the patient, the collection chamber may be lifted over the chest momentarily.

Prevention of complications

Utilize preventive measures described in the following sections to avoid complications.

Pneumothorax   Prevent a tension pneumothorax by keeping the system vented and by clamping only when appropriate.

The drainage system must always be vented to air in order to prevent a dangerous buildup of pressure in the chest. When suction is applied with a Pleurevac, make sure the small hole in the rubber cap of the suction control chamber is not occluded. In the two- or three-bottle system, be sure the upper end of the vent tube in the suction control chamber is not occluded. If it is necessary to interrupt the suction (to transport the patient or if the external source fails), be sure to vent the *water seal* chamber.

Keep two clamps at the bedside, and learn the principles underlying when to clamp and when not to clamp the chest tube. You may clamp the system to locate the source of an air leak. You also may clamp the chest tube near the thoracic wall when changing the collection chamber or when the chamber breaks, *unless* the patient has an air leak.

Ankylosis and discomfort   Prevent shoulder ankylosis and discomfort. Assist the patient with range of motion exercises several times daily. Splint the insertion site while turning or coughing.

Removal of chest tubes

Assist with chest tube removal when the lung has expanded or drainage has become minimal. Signs of lung expansion are cessation of bubbling in water seal fluid, normal physical examination, and a chest x-ray showing fully aerated lungs. Explain the procedure to the patient and premedicate him if possible, since removal is moderately painful. Bring to the bedside a suture removal set, sterile vaseline gauze, dressing supplies, and newspaper. Spread the paper over the bed so the tube can be placed on it after removal. Remove the dressing. The physician will cut the suture and hold the vaseline gauze over the insertion site. He will tell the patient to take a deep breath and bear down, while he quickly pulls out the tube and covers the site firmly with the gauze, to seal it off. Secure the vaseline gauze with gauze squares and tape. (Some physicians prefer to place a suture around the tube on insertion, and have you tighten it as the tube is removed. Also, some believe vaseline gauze is unnecessary and instead use dry gauze squares to cover the site.) A small amount of serosanguinous drainage may occur after removal. If necessary, simply reinforce the dressing for the first 48–72 hours; then it can be changed.

Outcome evaluation

Evaluate the effectiveness of chest drainage according to these outcome criteria:

- Calm, relaxed appearance
- Unlabored respirations WNL for patient
- Performs range of motion and breathing exercises and moves about willingly
- Lungs fully aerated, as manifested by chest x-ray and physical examination

References

Bonnano, P. 1971. Swallowing dysfunction after tracheotomy. *Ann. Surg.* 174:29–33.
Detailed study of 43 patients with tracheostomy tubes: reversible swallowing dysfunction found in three, owing to tube's interference with relaxation of hypopharyngeal sphincter.

Bushnell, S. 1973. *Respiratory intensive care nursing.* Boston: Little, Brown and Company
Useful chapters on respiratory failure, airways, chest PT, oxygen therapy, and mechanical ventilation.

Carroll, R., and Grenvik, A. 1973. Proper use of large diameter, large residual volume cuffs. *Crit. Care Med.* 1:153–154.
Recommended techniques for use of these cuffs.

Cooper, J., and Grillo, H. 1969. The evolution of tracheal injury due to ventilatory assistance through cuffed tubes: a pathologic study. *Ann. Surg.* 169:334–348.
Data and photographs of 30 autopsy specimens of human tracheas demonstrating universal damage at site of tracheostomy tube cuff.

Dexter, L., and Dalen, J. 1974. Pulmonary embolism and acute cor pulmonale. In *The heart*. 3rd ed., eds. J. Hurst and R. Logue, pp. 1264–1274. New York: McGraw-Hill Books, Inc.
Pathophysiology and treatment of various types of emboli.

Moser, K. 1975. Diagnostic measures in pulmonary embolism. *Basics of R.D.* 3:1–4.
Ventilation/perfusion scans.

Schlant, R. 1974. Special types of embolism. In *The heart*. 3rd ed., eds. J. Hurst and R. Logue, 1274–1276. New York: McGraw-Hill Books, Inc.
Air, fat, amniotic fluid, and other rare emboli.

Selecky, P. 1974. Tracheostomy: a review of present day indications, complications, and care. *Heart Lung* 3:272–283.
In-depth discussion of tracheostomy.

Shapiro, B., Harrison, R., and Trout, C. 1975. *Clinical application of respiratory care.* Chicago: Yearbook Medical Publishers, Inc.
Superb, clinically relevant reference. Highly recommended for inclusion in your personal library.

Utley, J., et al. 1972. Definitive management of innominate artery hemorrhage complicating tracheostomy. *J.A.M.A.* 220:577–597.

Virchow, R. 1846. Weitere Untersuchungen uber die Verstopfung der Lungenarterie und Ihre Folgen. *Beit. Exp. Pathol. Physiol.* 2:21.
Cited in Fitzmaurice, J., and Sasahara, A. 1974. Current concepts of pulmonary embolism: implications for nursing practice. Heart Lung 3:209–218.

Supplemental Reading

General

Brunner, L., and Suddarth, D. 1975. *Textbook of medical-surgical nursing.* 3rd ed. Philadelphia: J. B. Lippincott Company.
Chapters 14 and 15—nursing care principles and methods in several respiratory disorders.

Pulmonary embolism

Daly, C., and Kelly, E. 1972. Prevention of pulmonary embolism: intracaval devices. *A.J.N.* 72:2004–2006.
Balloon, spring, and umbrella devices to stop migration of clots to pulmonary artery.

Fitzmaurice, J., and Sasahara, A. 1974. Current concepts of pulmonary embolism: implications for nursing practice. *Heart Lung* 3:209–218.
Review of signs and symptoms, prevention, and treatment.

Grollman, J. 1974. Radiological diagnosis of pulmonary thromboembolism. *Heart Lung* 3:219–226.
Chest x-ray scans, and pulmonary angiography; many reproductions of films.

Wilson, A., Surprenant, E., and Zucker, M. 1974. Radioisotopic diagnosis of pulmonary embolism. *Heart Lung* 3:227–232.
Technique of ventilation and perfusion scans. Table of usual chest x-ray and ventilation/ perfusion findings for several pulmonary diseases.

Acute respiratory failure

Kauffman, L. 1972. Complications of respiratory failure. *Annals of Family Practice* 5:111–118.
Overview of recognition and treatment of complications.

Rogers, R., and Juers, J. 1975. Physiologic considerations in the treatment of acute respiratory failure. *Basics of R.D.* 3(4):1–6.
Definition, signs and symptoms, treatment.

Pulmonary edema

Hurst, J., and Spann, J. 1974. Treatment of heart failure. In *The heart.* 3rd ed., eds. J. Hurst and R. Logue, pp. 465–491. New York: McGraw-Hill Books, Inc.
Therapy in heart failure, including recommendations for treatment of acute pulmonary edema.

Schlant, R. 1974. Altered physiology of the cardiovascular system in heart failure. In *The heart.* 3rd ed., eds. J. Hurst and R. Logue, pp. 416–429. New York: McGraw-Hill Books, Inc.
Pathophysiology and medical therapy of cardiac failure.

Vismara, L., Mason, D., and Amsterdam, E. 1974. Cardiocirculatory effects of morphine sulfate: mechanisms of action and therapeutic application. *Heart Lung* 3:495–499.
Effects of morphine on peripheral vascular resistance, systemic venous bed, cardiac contractility, and respiratory function.

Pneumothorax

Cumming, G., and Semple, S. 1973. *Disorders of the respiratory system.* Oxford: Blackwell Scientific.
Diagnosis and treatment of pneumothorax.

Killen, D., and Gobbel, W. 1968. *Spontaneous pneumothorax.* Boston: Little, Brown and Company.
Signs and symptoms, treatment, complications.

Lake, K., Rumsfeld, J., and Van Dyke, J. 1974. Infraclavicular subclavian catheterization: another caution. *Chest* 65:457–458.
Danger of creating pneumothorax.

Saha, S., Arrants, J., Kosa, A., et al. 1975. Management of spontaneous pneumothorax. *Ann. Thorac. Surg.* 19:561–564.
Results of varying treatments in 136 pneumothoraces.

Steier, M., Ching, N., Roberts, E. et al. 1974. Pneumothorax complicating continuous ventilatory support. *J. Thorac. Cardiovasc. Surg.* 67:17–23.

Walston, A., Brewer, D., Kitchens, C. and Krook, J. 1974. The electrocardiographic manifestations of spontaneous left pneumothorax. *Ann. Intern. Med.* 80:375–379.
Differential electrocardiographic diagnosis of left pneumothorax and acute myocardial infarction.

Chest physiotherapy

Gaskell, D., and Webber, B. 1973. *The Brompton hospital guide to chest physiotherapy.* Oxford: Blackwell Scientific.
Suggestions for maneuvers appropriate in various diseases.

Kurihara, M. 1965. Postural drainage, clapping, and vibrating. *A.J.N.* 65(11):76–79.
Review of diaphragmatic breathing, postural drainage, clapping and vibrating; chart correlating lung segments, postural drainage positions, and areas to be clapped or vibrated.

Artificial airways

Tyler, M. 1973. Artificial airways: suctioning, tubes and cuffs, weaning, and extubation. *Nursing '73* 3(2):21–36.
Phototext of airway care.

Mechanical ventilation

Votteri, B. 1976. Respiratory management. In *Mosby's comprehensive review of critical care,* ed. D. Zschoche. St. Louis: C. V. Mosby Company.
Includes criteria for initiation and optimal level of PEEP.

Chest tubes

Kersten, L. 1974. Chest tube drainage system: indications and principles of operation. *Heart Lung* 3:97– 101.
Conceptual comparison of Pleurevac and bottle systems.

Van Meter, M. 1974. Chest tubes: basic techniques for better care. *Nursing '74* 4:48–55.
Photographic presentation of nursing care.

Chapter 11

Acid-base Balance

Acid-base imbalances are common in the critically ill. In order to participate effectively in caring for the patient with such an imbalance, you must have a sound understanding of acid-base physiology and its application in the clinical setting.

Outline

Assessment   Key physiologic concepts / History / Signs and symptoms / Electrolyte imbalances / Other laboratory data / Arterial blood gases

Treatment planning and implementation   Respiratory acidosis / Metabolic acidosis / Respiratory alkalosis / Metabolic alkalosis / Mixed disorders / General nursing care measures

Outcome evaluation

Objectives

- Define volatile acid, fixed acid, base, and pH
- State the significance of the Henderson-Hasselbach equation
- Name the four major chemical buffers
- Describe the respiratory buffer system
- Describe the renal buffer system
- Explain the difference between respiratory and metabolic acid-base imbalance

- Explain the difference between a single uncompensated imbalance, a compensated imbalance, and a mixed imbalance
- Recognize conditions making a patient prone to respiratory acidosis, metabolic acidosis, respiratory alkalosis, and metabolic alkalosis
- Recognize signs and symptoms suggesting an acid-base imbalance
- Describe the interrelationships between acid-base balance and electrolyte balance
- Define anion gap, explain how to compute it, and state its significance
- Use a systematic method of interpreting acid-base values
- Assist with treatment of acid-base imbalances
- Evaluate the patient's progress according to specified outcome criteria

Assessment

Acid-base imbalances are ubiquitous in the critically ill. Their causes, signs, and symptoms can be subtle and confusing. A hasty or simplistic interpretation of arterial blood gas values can cause you to identify acid-base disorders incorrectly. It is essential that you develop a systematic method to detect these imbalances and that you interpret blood gas values only in the context of the clinical situation.

The approach recommended in this chapter (Table 11-1) is a clinically useful one. It is an expansion of the approach recommended by McCurdy (1972). This approach consists of the following steps:

1. Consider the patient's history, noting conditions which predispose to imbalances.

Table 11-1   Acid-base assessment format

1. History _____

2. Physical _____

3. Diagnostic procedures and laboratory tests

    Serum electrolytes: Na^+ _____ K^+ _____ Cl^- _____ CO_2 _____

    Anion gap _____

    Arterial blood gases: pH _____ PCO_2 _____ HCO_3 _____ BE _____

4. Other _____

2. Next note signs and symptoms suggesting acid-base imbalances.
3. Examine the serum electrolyte values for clues to imbalances.
4. Examine other laboratory data for additional clues.
5. Interpret the blood gases.

In order to utilize this approach, you must have a sound understanding of normal acid-base physiology as well as acid-base pathophysiology. Accordingly, the first portion of this assessment section is devoted to a review of key concepts in acid-base physiology.

Key physiologic concepts

Acids, bases, and pH   An *acid* is a substance that can release a hydrogen ion (H+) when it dissociates; a *base* is a substance that can accept a hydrogen ion. Clinically, the H+ concentration is expressed as pH. Since pH is the negative logarithm of the H+ concentration, pH and H+ concentration are related inversely. In other words, as H+ concentration rises, pH falls; a low pH thus indicates the blood is more acid than normal. Similarly, a high pH indicates the blood is less acid (more alkaline) than normal.

Our metabolic processes produce several acids. The Krebs cycle, our major source of energy, forms carbon dioxide and water as end products. Carbon dioxide and water combine to form carbonic acid (H_2CO_3), which is the most plentiful body acid. Because carbon dioxide can be excreted as a gas, carbonic acid sometimes is referred to as a *volatile* or respiratory acid. Other less plentiful body acids, such as sulfuric acid and phosphoric acid, are breakdown products released by the metabolism of proteins or fats for energy or by other body processes. Since they cannot be excreted as a gas but instead must be excreted in water, they are called nonvolatile, fixed, or metabolic acids. Other metabolic acids are lactic acid, formed by anaerobic metabolism when tissues are hypoxic, and keto acids, commonly the result of metabolic pathways used when insulin is lacking.

The primary base in our bodies is bicarbonate. Lesser bases include forms of hemoglobin, protein, and phosphate.

To maintain the various life processes, our cells can tolerate only minor deviations in the concentration of hydrogen ions. Three primary systems interact to maintain the pH range most suitable for cellular processes. These systems are the chemical buffers in body fluids; the lungs; and the kidneys.

Chemical buffers   A chemical buffer consists of a weak acid and its salt. Chemical buffers are important because they are the body's first line of defense against an acid-base imbalance. When excessive acid or base is present, the chemical buffer system combines with it immediately, thus preventing pronounced changes in H^+ concentration.

There are four major chemical buffers in the body fluids (Reed and Sheppard 1977). The most important extracellular buffers are the bicarbonate/carbonic acid system and the plasma sodium proteinate/protein system. Intracellular buffers include the oxyhemoglobin/reduced oxyhemoglobin system (in red blood cells), the disodium phosphate/monosodium phosphate system, the bicarbonate/carbonic acid system, and intracellular proteins.

A variety of bicarbonate salts participates in the carbonic acid/bicarbonate system. Extracellularly, sodium bicarbonate is most important. Lesser salts in the extracellular fluid and those present in the intracellular fluid are potassium bicarbonate, calcium bicarbonate, and magnesium bicarbonate.

Carbonic acid/bicarbonate buffer system   As mentioned previously, carbonic acid is formed from carbon dioxide and water. It tends to dissociate into its ions: hydrogen and bicarbonate. This system can be expressed as follows:

$$H^+ + HCO_3^- \rightleftarrows H_2CO_3 \rightleftarrows CO_2 + H_2O$$

An important expression of acid-base balance is the Henderson-Hasselbach equation, which applies to the carbonic acid/bicarbonate buffer system. This equation states that the pH equals the sum of a constant value (pK) plus the logarithm of the ratio of bicarbonate to carbonic acid:

$$pH = pK + \log \frac{HCO_3^- \text{ (mEq/L)}}{H_2CO_3 \text{ (mEq/L)}}$$

Carbonic acid is a weak acid and does not dissociate readily. Since carbonic acid exists in the body mostly as CO_2 gas, you can substitute a PCO_2 value in the denominator. Clinically, PCO_2 is measured in mm Hg; to convert that value to mEq/L, multiply by 0.03.

$$pH = pK + \log \frac{HCO_3^- \text{ (mEq/L)}}{PCO_2 \text{ (mmHg)} \times 0.03}$$

The normal ratio between bicarbonate and carbonic acid is 20:1. Since the log of this value is 1.3 and the pK equals 6.1, their sum gives the value of 7.4 as the normal pH. The normal range is considered to be 7.35–7.45. It is essential to remember that the pH is determined by the *ratio* between the two values rather than the absolute amount of HCO_3^- or carbonic acid. This fact has great clinical importance as shown later.

Respiratory buffer system   When the chemical buffers are unable to maintain balance, the respiratory and renal buffer systems come into play to control the concentrations of CO_2 and HCO_3^-, respectively.

The respiratory buffer system responds to an imbalance within minutes to hours. This system controls the level of CO_2 in the blood, and therefore the level of carbonic acid. When carbonic acid increases, the lungs increase their excretion of CO_2 gas by increasing the rate and depth of ventilation. If the body needs more acid, the lungs can decrease ventilation, thereby retaining CO_2 and increasing the amount of carbonic acid.

Renal buffer system   The renal buffer system responds slowly (within hours to days) but powerfully to an acid-base imbalance. It affects pH primarily by controlling the concentration of bicarbonate ion in the extracellular fluid. It also excretes fixed acids (which the lungs cannot eliminate).

Bicarbonate is filtered freely at the glomerulus and "reabsorbed" in the proximal and distal tubules, collecting ducts and thick part of the loops of Henle. (Note that while the term "reabsorbed" is used, the bicarbonate ion which is in the tubular fluid at the start of the process is not the same bicarbonate ion which is in the extracellular fluid at the end of the process.) The following explanation of reabsorption is based on Guyton (1976) and shown in the upper portion of Figure 11-1.

The process of bicarbonate reabsorption begins with carbon dioxide present in the renal tubular cell. In a reaction catalyzed by carbonic anhydrase, carbon dioxide combines with water to form carbonic acid. The carbonic acid immediately dissociates into H^+ and HCO_3^- ions. The H^+ ion is actively transported into the tubular fluid. At the same time, a sodium ion is actively transported from the tubular fluid into the cell. This ion comes from sodium bicarbonate in the tubular fluid, which has dissociated into Na^+ and HCO_3^- ions.

The HCO_3^- ion remaining in the tubular fluid combines with the H^+ secreted by the cell to form carbonic acid, which dissociates into water and carbon dioxide. The water is eliminated by the kidneys, while the carbon dioxide reenters the cell. There it combines with water to form more carbonic acid.

As mentioned above, each time carbonic acid dissociates inside the cell to form H^+ and HCO_3^- ions, the H^+ ion is transported into the tubule. The corresponding HCO_3^- ion combines with the Na^+ ion reabsorbed from the tubule to form sodium bicarbonate. This sodium bicarbonate then diffuses into the extracellular fluid. The kidney thus has "reabsorbed" bicarbonate from the tubular fluid into the extracellular fluid.

Each day, some of the body's bicarbonate is used to buffer non-volatile acids. This bicarbonate must be replaced or the extracellular fluid would soon become so acidic that cells would perish. Fortunately, the kidney has two important systems for creating new bicarbonate and at the same time excreting hydrogen ions: the ammonia buffer system and the phosphate buffer system. The following paragraphs describing these systems also are based on Guyton.

The ammonia buffer system is shown in the middle portion of Figure 11-1. The tubular fluid contains ammonia (NH_3), which is made by the tubular cells primarily from glutamine. In the tubule, the ammonia combines with hydrogen ions to form ammonium ions (NH_4). The hydrogen ions which participate in this reaction come from the dissociation of carbonic acid within the tubular cell, as described above. This dissociation frees a bicarbonate ion which is reabosrbed

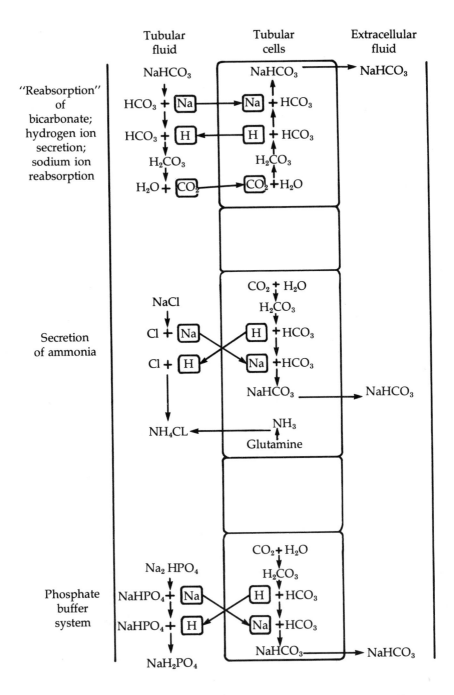

Figure 11-1. Renal mechanisms for reabsorbing and creating bicarbonate.

into the extracellular fluid along with a sodium ion from the tubular fluid. The ammonium ions are excreted with chloride or other anions. The ammonia buffer system thus results in both the secretion of hydrogen ions and the generation of bicarbonate.

The phosphate buffer system is shown in the lower portion of Figure 11-1. Disodium phosphate (Na_2HPO_4) normally is present in the tubular fluid, dissociated into two sodium ions and a phosphate ion. As described earlier, a hydrogen ion enters the tubular fluid from the dissociation of carbonic acid inside the cell. This hydrogen ion combines with the phosphate ion and one sodium ion to form monosodium phosphate (NaH_2PO_4). At the same time, a sodium ion moves into the cell and is reabsorbed into the extracellular fluid along with a bicarbonate ion. The phosphate buffer system thus also results in the excretion of hydogen ions and creation of bicarbonate.

Acidosis and alkalosis   So far this chapter has discussed the body's mechanisms for maintaining acid-base balance. The remainder of the chapter will discuss the various acid-base imbalances you may encounter in caring for your critically ill patients.

The classification of acid-base abnormalities can be confusing, so the basic terms will be reviewed. Two general processes can cause the pH to deviate from normal: an acidosis or alkalosis. An *acidosis* is a process which causes acidemia, a state in which the blood is more acid than normal. An *alkalosis* is a process which causes alkalemia, a state in which the blood is more alkaline (less acidic) than normal. Information about acidoses and alkaloses is shown in Tables 11-2 and 11-3 and discussed in the remainder of the chapter.

History

The patient's history can provide valuable information in identifying acid-base disorders. Tables 11-2, 11-3, and 11-4 give examples of significant conditions to note when reviewing the patient's history. The following paragraphs relate the types of acid-base disorders to predisposing conditions.

Single disorders   An acidosis is present when there is an acid excess or a base deficit in the body, causing the blood's pH to be below 7.35. The acid excess can be a carbonic acid excess (in which case the condition is called respiratory acidosis) or a metabolic acid excess (metabolic acidosis). Mechanical hypoventilation is an example of a condition which causes carbon dioxide retention and respiratory acidosis. An example of a metabolic acidosis is that produced by lactic acid accumulation during cardiac arrest. An acidosis produced by a base deficit can occur only from metabolic causes, such as the loss of alkaline fluids via a fistula of the lower gastrointestinal tract.

An alkalosis is present when there is either an acid deficit or a base excess in the body, causing the pH to be above 7.45. The acid deficit can be a carbonic acid

Table 11-2 Respiratory and metabolic acidosis

Predisposing conditions	Signs and symptoms	Disorder	Treatment
Carbon dioxide retention			
Bronchial obstruction, chronic obstructive pulmonary disease Inadequate mechanical ventilation Central nervous system depression (example: narcotic poisoning) Neuromuscular disorders affecting respiration (example: poliomyelitis)	Hypoventilation (primary) Confusion, coma Acute respiratory failure Hyperkalemia (peaked T waves, twitching, etc.) Hypercalcemia (weakness, lethargy, etc.) pH $\downarrow$, $PCO_2 \uparrow$, HCO_3^- normal or $\uparrow$	Respiratory acidosis	None (if compensated in chronic pulmonary disease) Treatment of cause Mechanical ventilation (cautiously to avoid alkalosis) Bicarbonate replacement Treatment of electrolyte imbalances
Excessive metabolic acids			
Starvation Diabetic ketoacidosis Lactic acidosis Renal failure Hyperkalemia	Hyperventilation (compensatory) Confusion, coma Hyperkalemia Hypercalcemia pH $\downarrow$, PCO_2 normal or $\downarrow$, HCO_3^- $\downarrow$	Metabolic acidosis	Treatment of cause Bicarbonate replacement Treatment of electrolyte imbalances
Loss of alkali			
Diarrhea Fistulas of lower gastrointestinal tract Chloride excess			

Table 11-3 Respiratory and metabolic alkalosis

Predisposing conditions	Signs and symptoms	Disorder	Treatment
Increased CO_2 excretion			
Hypoxia Excessive mechanical ventilation Central nervous system stimulation (examples: pain, anxiety, hysteria)	Hyperventilation (primary) Giddiness, dizziness, convulsions, coma Hypokalemia (weakness, paresthesias, etc.) Hypocalcemia (twitching, paresthesias, carpopedal spasms, tetany, convulsions, etc.) Cardiac arrhythmias pH $\uparrow$, $PCO_2 \downarrow$, HCO_3^- normal or $\downarrow$	Respiratory alkalosis	Treatment of cause Increased CO_2 retention: (by decreased mechanical ventilation or breathing into paper bag) Treatment of electrolyte imbalances
Loss of metabolic acids			
Nasogastric drainage Vomiting Hypokalemia	Hypoventilation (compensatory) Hypokalemia Hypocalcemia Cardiac arrhythmias pH $\uparrow$, PCO_2 normal or $\uparrow$, HCO_3^- $\uparrow$	Metabolic alkalosis	Treatment of cause Chloride administration Treatment of electrolyte imbalances
Excessive intake or retention of alkali			
, Excessive sodium bicarbonate administration Chloride depletion Diuretics Low salt diet without chloride supplementation			

Table 11-4   Mixed disorders

Combination	Examples	Mechanisms
Mixed acidoses	Cardiac arrest Severe hypoventilation	Absent ventilation or hypoventilation→respiratory acidosis Hypoxemia→anaerobic metabolism→metabolic (lactic) acidosis
Mixed alkaloses	Patient with compensated respiratory acidosis rapidly and excessively mechanically ventilated	Elevated bicarbonate level→metabolic alkalosis Hyperventilation→respiratory alkalosis
Respiratory acidosis and metabolic alkalosis	Chronic obstructive pulmonary disease plus diuretics or low salt diet without chloride replacement	COPD→respiratory acidosis Chloride depletion→obligatory bicarbonate retention→metabolic alkalosis
Respiratory alkalosis and metabolic acidosis	Hepatic and renal failure	Liver failure→ toxic metabolites→ hyperventilation→ respiratory alkalosis Kidney failure→ ↓ H^+ excretion and ↓ bicarbonate production→metabolic acidosis

deficit (respiratory alkalosis) or a metabolic acid deficit (metabolic alkalosis). For example, a hyperventilating patient can blow off enough CO_2 to produce a respiratory alkalosis. The loss of metabolic acids, for example via nasogastric suction, produces a metabolic alkalosis. An alkalosis from a base excess can occur only from metabolic causes (such as increased bicarbonate retention because of a chloride deficit) or from an exogenous source, for example, excessive infusion of sodium bicarbonate.

Respiratory acidosis, metabolic acidosis, respiratory alkalosis, and metabolic alkalosis are called the four single acid-base disorders.

Compensation   When a single disorder first occurs, it will cause an abnormal pH and also an abnormal value for the parameter associated with the system causing the imbalance. For instance, a respiratory acidosis causes an abnormal increase in PCO_2 and a resultant decrease in pH. The other value (in this case, HCO_3^-) will be normal initially. At this point, the disorder is called *uncompensated*. As time goes on, the system not causing the problem will try to compensate for it by altering its parameter to return the ratio of bicarbonate/carbonic acid to the normal 20:1. If the alteration is not sufficient to return the pH to normal, compensation is incomplete. At this point, the pH, PCO_2 and HCO_3^- all will be abnormal. If the alteration is sufficient to restore a more normal ratio and hence a normal pH, the condition is called *compensated*. In this stage, the pH will be normal but both the PCO_2 and HCO_3^- values still will be abnormal. Although their ratio will cause the pH to be within the normal range, the pH usually will tend more toward the acidic or alkaline end of the range, depending on the primary process.

In general, the pulmonary and renal system compensate for each other. The renal system also compensates for metabolic acid-base imbalances, providing renal disease itself is not the cause of the imbalance. In respiratory acidosis, the kidneys compensate by increasing bicarbonate retention and accelerating hydrogen secretion. In respiratory alkalosis, the kidneys decrease bicarbonate retention and hydrogen secretion.

The lungs compensate for metabolic acid-base imbalances by varying CO_2 excretion. In metabolic acidosis, stimulation of the respiratory center increases the rate and depth of ventilation, so increased CO_2 is blown off. This compensation is limited, however: a falling PCO_2 eventually causes respiratory depression, returning PCO_2 toward normal. If the kidneys are not the cause of the acidosis, they excrete more hydrogen and retain more bicarbonate. In metabolic alkalosis, the lungs decrease ventilation and therefore retain CO_2. Respiratory compensation for metabolic alkalosis also is limited, however. At a PCO_2 of about 60 mm Hg in most people, the hypoxic stimulus to respiration becomes dominant. This stimulus causes ventilation to increase toward normal. If renal disease is not the cause of the metabolic alkalosis, the kidneys inhibit hydrogen excretion and HCO_3^- retention.

As mentioned earlier, the lungs respond to acid-base imbalances within minutes, while the kidneys take hours. As a result, compensation for metabolic imbalances occurs faster than compensation for respiratory imbalances.

Mixed disorders   If two single disorders occur simultaneously, the patient suffers from a mixed disorder (mixed disturbance). There are four mixed disturbances (Table 11-4). Mixed disturbances result from either two processes with similar effects on the pH (such as respiratory and metabolic acidosis in cardiac arrest) or two processes with opposite effects on the pH (such as respiratory acidosis and metabolic alkalosis in the patient with chronic lung disease who is on diuretics).

Signs and symptoms

Assess the patient for the clinical signs and symptoms of acid-base imbalances as described in the following sections.

Changes in cerebral status   Cerebral status changes result from alterations in cerebrospinal fluid pH. Confusion and coma often are present in acidosis, while dizziness and giddiness are more characteristic of alkalosis. Since CO_2 crosses the blood-brain barrier more quickly than HCO_3^- ions, these symptoms occur sooner in respiratory disorders than metabolic ones.

Assess cerebral status by checking orientation to day, time, and location; ability to follow simple commands; and presence of dizziness or lightheadedness.

Hypoventilation or hyperventilation   Evaluation of ventilatory changes can be confusing, since hypoventilation or hyperventilation may either cause or compensate for acid-base imbalances. Hyperventilation can cause respiratory alkalosis or compensate for metabolic acidosis, in each case by increasing CO_2 elimination. Hypoventilation can cause respiratory acidosis or compensate for metabolic alkalosis, in each case by increasing CO_2 retention. Acid-base imbalances affect the respiratory center by altering the pH of arterial blood and cerebrospinal fluid. Acidosis lowers the pH, stimulates the respiratory center, and produces hyperventilation. Alkalosis raises cerebrospinal fluid pH and produces hypoventilation. To detect hypoventilation or hyperventilation, evaluate the rate and depth of respiration. Because only gross changes in depth of respiration are detectable on physical examination, use a spirometer to check the tidal volume.

Respiratory failure may occur in acute respiratory acidosis when the PCO_2 reaches 60 mm Hg. A patient with chronic hypercapnia, however, may tolerate a PCO_2 above 60 mm Hg without developing acute respiratory failure. Because the slow development of hypercapnia has allowed time for the kidneys to increase the serum bicarbonate level in compensation, the chronic patient can maintain a more normal pH than an acutely afflicted person.

Arrhythmias, angina, or shock   Arrhythmias, angina, or shock may result from hypoxia or from the electrolyte imbalances discussed later. Both acidosis and alkalosis cause shifts of the oxyhemoglobin dissociation curve. This curve is shown in Figure 9-3. In alkalosis, the curve shifts to the left, causing decreased dissociation of oxygen from hemoglobin. This effect contributes to tissue hypoxia. Acidosis causes the curve to shift to the right, so that oxygen is released more readily from hemoglobin. However, acidosis also causes decreased responsiveness to catecholamines, which in turn can cause decreased myocardial contractility and decreased peripheral vasoconstriction. As a result, less efficient circulation of the blood may counterbalance the increased availability of oxygen in the blood.

To detect arrhythmias, angina, or shock, implement the following measures. Auscultate the apical pulse for irregularities and the presence of gallops or murmurs. Monitor the electrocardiogram for signs of new or increasing atrial or ventricular arrhythmias. Also monitor perfusion to the brain, heart, kidneys, and extremities.

Electrolyte imbalances

Accurate diagnosis of acid-base imbalances requires arterial blood gas values, as explained later in the chapter. However, a certain amount of information about acid-base imbalances can be gleaned from signs and symptoms of electrolyte imbalances and from the serum electrolyte panel routinely obtained on patients. This panel typically includes values for serum sodium, potassium, chloride, and CO_2 content. The following sections describe the complex interrelationships between acid-base balance and electrolyte balance.

Sodium (Na^+)   Because there is so much sodium in the extracellular space, shifts in acid-base balance do not affect sodium balance significantly. An increased serum sodium level also does not affect acid-base balance much. A decreased serum sodium level, however, can be associated with great derangements in acid-base balance. The sodium deficit does not cause the derangements directly; the culprit is the accompanying chloride deficit. You may remember that the kidney can reabsorb sodium in three ways: with the negative chloride ion, with the negative bicarbonate ion, or in exchange for the positive potassium or hydrogen ion. In the presence of a depletion of both sodium chloride and water (such as in hypovolemic shock), the kidney will have a potent stimulus for sodium reabsorption. Since relatively little chloride will be available in this situation, the kidney will reabsorb an increased percentage of the sodium with bicarbonate and an increased percentage in exchange for H^+ or K^+. Thus, hyponatremia, through its relationship to hypochloremia, may be associated with alkalosis and hypokalemia.

Potassium (K^+)   Acid-base and potassium balance profoundly affect each other. Acidosis often is accompanied by hyperkalemia and alkalosis by hypokalemia. These associations are due to two mechanisms: exchange of potassium and hydrogen ions across the cell membrane, and altered renal excretion of potassium and hydrogen.

As explained in Chapter 6, the body's cells contain buffer systems which can either accept or donate H^+ ions. Hydrogen ions and potassium ions freely exchange across the cell membrane. Since the amount of extracellular potassium is quite small compared to the intracellular amount, even small shifts of K^+ across the cell membrane cause significant changes in the serum level. In acidosis, excess H^+ ions in the serum migrate into the cell, where their buffering displaces K^+ ions. To maintain intracellular electrical balance, the K^+ ions diffuse out into the serum. As a result, acidosis can cause hyperkalemia. In alkalosis, the reverse is true. The intracellular buffers dissociate to release H^+ ions. As they move out of the cell, K^+ ions move in. Thus, alkalosis can cause hypokalemia. These relationships are true in the initial stages of the imbalance, *if* the patient's serum potassium level was normal at the start. (This point is emphasized because the serum potassium level can be misleading if a hypokalemic patient becomes acidotic. In such a case, the serum potassium level may be normal.)

Conversely, in potassium imbalances ionic shifts across the cell membrane can produce acid-base imbalances. Hyperkalemia causes more potassium ions to move intracellularly, displacing hydrogen ions into the serum and producing acidosis. Hypokalemia favors the shift of potassium ions in the opposite direction—from the cell into the serum. To maintain intracellular electrical balance, more hydrogen ions then move into the cell, leaving the serum alkalotic.

The sodium/potassium/hydrogen exchange mechanism also plays a role in the interrelationships of potassium and acid-base imbalances. In the kidney, sodium ions normally are retained in exchange for potassium or hydrogen ions. In acidosis, because hydrogen ions are more abundant, the kidney tends to exchange hydrogen ions rather than potassium ions for sodium. Since the excess hydrogen ions block the secretion of potassium, hyperkalemia develops. In alkalosis, the kidney exchanges potassium ions rather than hydrogen ions for sodium. This preferential retention of hydrogen ions helps to compensate for the alkalosis, but at the expense of causing hypokalemia.

The $Na^+/K^+/H^+$ exchange mechanism also helps to explain how potassium imbalances cause acid-base imbalances. In hyperkalemia, more potassium ions than hydrogen ions are exchanged for sodium, and acidosis develops. In hypokalemia, fewer potassium ions are available for exchange. More hydrogen ions are excreted, and alkalosis develops.

The signs, symptoms, and treatment of potassium imbalances are discussed in detail in Chapter 6.

Calcium (Ca^{++})   Serum calcium exists in both ionized and non-ionized forms. The ionized form is the physiologically active one. Calcium ionization increases in acidosis and decreases in alkalosis. As a result, an acidotic patient may have signs of hypercalcemia, while an alkalotic person often shows signs of hypocalcemia. Acidosis can mask hypocalcemia because of its ability to increase calcium ionization. When the acidosis is treated and pH returns to normal, twitching, convulsions, paresthesias, carpopedal spasms, tetany, and other signs of hypocalcemia may become evident.

For a complete discussion of signs, symptoms, and treatment of calcium imbalances, refer to Chapter 6.

Chloride (Cl^-)   Chloride is primarily an extracellular anion. Its serum concentration varies inversely with bicarbonate for two reasons: (a) it shifts across the cell membrane during buffering in exchange for bicarbonate (the chloride shift); and (b) renal reabsorption of chloride varies inversely with reabsorption of bicarbonate. For these reasons, hypochloremia can cause metabolic alkalosis, and vice versa; hyperchloremia can cause metabolic acidosis, and vice versa. The interrelationship of hypochloremia and metabolic alkalosis is particularly important clinically. As mentioned in the section on sodium, if insufficient chloride is present in the renal tubules, the kidney will reabsorb an increased proportion of sodium with bicarbonate, causing a metabolic alkalosis.

If the hypochloremic, alkalotic patient also has a stimulus for avid sodium retention, he may well develop a vicious cycle in which the electrolyte and acid-base imbalances feed upon each other. A clinical example is the person with chronic congestive heart failure who is on a low-salt diet without adequate chloride replacement. His abnormal volume regulation causes an intense stimulus for sodium reabsorption. Since he is chloride depleted, an increased percentage of sodium will be reabsorbed with bicarbonate; the stimulus for sodium retention overrides the body's need to reduce alkali, and his alkalemia worsens. Since there also may be an increased renal exchange of potassium for sodium, his hypokalemia may worsen, too.

Serum electrolyte summary   Because the changes in electrolyte balance are hard to remember, they are summarized here.

The normal serum sodium level is 136–144 mEq/L. Hyponatremia, through its relation to hypochloremia, often is associated with alkalosis.

The usual serum potassium concentration is 3.5–5.5 mEq/L. Hyperkalemia often is present in acidosis or recovery from alkalosis. Hypokalemia may be associated with alkalosis or recovery from acidosis. A normal serum potassium may be present in the previously hypokalemic patient who has become acidotic.

The normal serum calcium level is 8.5–10.8 mEq/L. Hypercalcemia may be present in acidosis and hypocalcemia in alkalosis. A normal serum calcium level may be present in the previously hypocalcemic patient who has become acidotic.

The normal serum chloride concentration is 96–106 mEq/L. Hyperchloremia may be present in acidosis; hypochloremia frequently is associated with alkalosis.

CO_2 content   As mentioned earlier, the serum electrolyte panel usually includes a measurement of CO_2 content. CO_2 content consists of about 95% bicarbonate and 5% carbonic acid. It thus can reflect metabolic and/or respiratory activity. The normal CO_2 content is 24–30 mEq/L. CO_2 content is increased in respiratory acidosis and metabolic alkalosis. It is decreased in metabolic acidosis and respiratory alkalosis. Because of its relatively nonspecific nature, the CO_2 content value can indicate only that an acid-base abnormality is present. It cannot indicate whether that abnormality is an acidosis or alkalosis, nor can it pinpoint whether respiratory or metabolic dysfunction is at fault. To identify the type of imbalance, arterial blood gas values should be analyzed.

Anion gap   The serum electrolyte report can provide you with another useful clue to acid-base imbalance, called the *anion gap* or delta.

The anion gap is an expression of the difference between unmeasured cations and unmeasurable anions in the body (Oh and Carroll 1977). To derive the value, add the bicarbonate and the chloride values to get a sum of the measured anions and subtract this sum from the measured cation, Na+. The normal difference is 8–16 mEq/L. For example, if Na is 140, HCO_3^- 20, and chloride 100:

$$20 + 100 = 120$$

$$140 - 120 = 20 \text{ mEq of unmeasurable anions}$$

This value indicates there is an elevation of the unmeasurable anions in this patient.

The anion gap increases in metabolic acidosis resulting from an abnormal increase in organic acids. Examples are starvation, diabetic ketoacidosis, and lactic acidosis. The anion gap remains normal in metabolic acidosis owing to bicarbonate loss (for example in diarrhea or lower gastrointestinal fistulas) or administration of chloride-containing acids, such as ammonium chloride.

Other laboratory data

Other laboratory data also may provide clues to causes of acid-base disturbances. For instance, an elevated blood urea nitrogen would suggest renal failure and possible metabolic acidosis, while abnormal pulmonary function tests would suggest potential respiratory acid-base imbalances.

Arterial blood gases

As mentioned earlier, definitive diagnosis of acid-base imbalances depends upon arterial blood gas values. The values important in acid-base interpretation and the pH, PCO_2, and a measure of base (HCO_3 or base excess). Base excess is the preferred measure of base, because it measures both bicarbonate and other buffer anions of whole blood, such as those of hemoglobin and plasma proteins. Base excess reflects only metabolic activity. It is reported as base mEq/L above or below the normal range of buffer base (Shapiro 1973). Thus, a negative base excess actually means a base deficit. When evaluating a patient's blood gases, always compare the reported values to the normals for your institution. Also compare them to the actual or expected normal values for your patient, as indicated by previous measurements or pre-existing conditions such as chronic obstructive pulmonary disease.

pH   First evaluate the general acid-base status by examining the pH. The normal range is 7.35–7.45. If the value is lower than normal (below 7.35), an acidosis is present. If the value is elevated (above 7.45), an alkalosis is present. If the value is within the normal range, there are two possibilities. The patient could have a normal balance or an abnormal process which is compensated. Since you cannot tell which situation exists from examining the pH alone, just note at this point whether the value is normal and, if so, whether it falls more toward the acid side of the normal range or more toward the alkaline side.

PCO_2   Evaluate the respiratory parameter by examining the PCO_2. The normal range is 35–45 mm Hg. Decide whether the value is normal, elevated above 45 and therefore tending to make the blood acidic, or decreased below 35 and therefore tending to make the blood alkaline.

HCO_3 or base excess   Evaluate the renal parameter by examining the HCO_3 or base excess. Normal ranges are 23–28 mEq/L for HCO_3 and +2.5 to −2.5 for base excess. Decide whether the value is normal, elevated and therefore tending to make the blood alkaline, or decreased and therefore tending to make the blood acidic. (For the sake of simplicity, only one measure of base is given in the following examples.)

Next, compare the pH, PCO_2, and base value to each other. Since blood gas values can indicate a variety of disorders and stages of compensation, a given set of numbers may be compatible with more than one interpretation. Explain *each* value, considering *all* the possible interpretations.

After considering the possible interpretations of the values, choose the most probable one for your patient, based on the clues from the other patient data and the likelihood of a given combination of disorders. To clarify whether a set of values is due to a compensated or uncompensated disturbance, you may find it helpful to plot the values on an acid-base map, such as that shown in Figure 11-2.

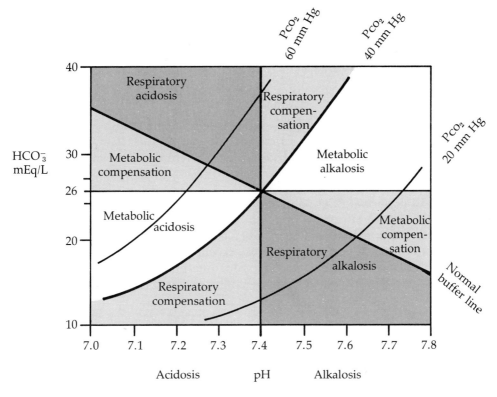

Figure 11-2.   Diagram of acid base relationships. (After Davenport, H., 1969. *The ABC of acid-base chemistry.* 5th ed. Chicago: University of Chicago Press. Used with permission of the publisher.)

To use the map, follow these steps:

1. You should know the patient's pH, PCO_2, and HCO_3^- for best results.

2. The pH values run horizontally. The HCO_3^- values run vertically. The PCO_2 values are shown in diagonally curved lines (isobars).

3. Plot the values on the appropriate scales. Usually, they will intersect either at the center of the diagram or in one of the eight surrounding areas. The exact center of the diagram represents a completely normal acid-base balance. Each of the eight areas represents a single uncompensated or compensated disturbance.

4. If the values do not fall within the same area, a mixed disturbance may be present.

Following are principles and examples illustrating interpretation of acid-base values. The various possibilities for interpretation are summarized in Table 11-5.

Abnormal pH and abnormal PCO_2 or HCO_3^-   If only the pH and one other value are abnormal, the blood gases indicate a single uncompensated disorder. You can identify the disorder by deciding which process the pH represents and which other value (the PCO_2 or HCO_3^-) is abnormal.

Example: pH 7.50, PCO_2 40 mm Hg, HCO_3^- 31 mEq/L

The pH tells you an alkalosis is present, because it is elevated. Since the PCO_2 is normal, a respiratory disorder cannot be the cause. The HCO_3^- is elevated, making the blood more alkaline. These values therefore indicate an uncompensated metabolic alkalosis.

Normal pH, abnormal PCO_2, and abnormal HCO_3^-   If the pH is normal but both the PCO_2 and HCO_3^- are not, the values indicate a compensated single disturbance. Determining whether the pH lies more toward the acid or alkaline end of the normal range will help you decide whether the imbalance is an acidosis or alkalosis. Double-checking your interpretation with the acid-base map is wise, to be sure that values you think are due to compensation actually are.

Example: pH 7.42, PCO_2 50 mm Hg, HCO_3^- 32 mEq/L

The pH is normal, but more toward the alkaline end of the range. The PCO_2 is elevated, tending to make the blood acidic. The HCO_3^- is elevated, tending to make the blood alkaline. The values represent a metabolic alkalosis compensated by increased CO_2 retention. Plotting the values on the acid-base map confirms this interpretation.

Abnormal pH, abnormal PCO_2, and abnormal HCO_3^-   If all three values are abnormal, they indicate either a single disorder with incomplete compensation

Table 11-5 Arterial blood gas interpretation

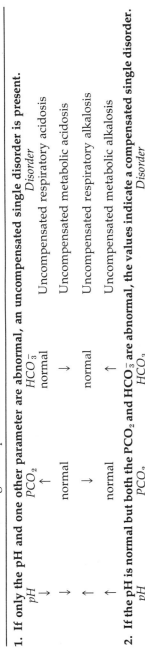

1. If only the pH and one other parameter are abnormal, an uncompensated single disorder is present.

pH	PCO_2	HCO_3^-	Disorder
↓	↑	normal	Uncompensated respiratory acidosis
↓	normal	↓	Uncompensated metabolic acidosis
↑	↓	normal	Uncompensated respiratory alkalosis
↑	normal	↑	Uncompensated metabolic alkalosis

2. If the pH is normal but both the PCO_2 and HCO_3^- are abnormal, the values indicate a compensated single disorder.

pH	PCO_2	HCO_3^-	Disorder
Acid normal	↑	↑	Compensated respiratory acidosis
Acid normal	↓	↓	Compensated metabolic acidosis
Alkaline normal	↓	↓	Compensated respiratory alkalosis
Alkaline normal	↑	↑	Compensated metabolic alkalosis

3. If the pH, PCO_2, and HCO_3^- all are abnormal, they indicate an inadequately compensated single disorder or a mixed disorder.

pH	PCO_2	HCO_3^-	Disorder
↓	↑	↑	Inadequately compensated respiratory acidosis
↓	↓	↓	Inadequately compensated metabolic acidosis
↑	↓	↓	Inadequately compensated respiratory alkalosis
↑	↑	↑	Inadequately compensated metabolic alkalosis
Very ↓	↑	Slightly ↑ or →	Mixed respiratory and metabolic acidosis
Very ↑	↓	Slightly ↑ or →	Mixed respiratory and metabolic alkalosis
Slightly ↑ or →	↑	↑	Mixed respiratory acidosis and metabolic alkalosis
Slightly ↑ or →	↓	→	Mixed respiratory alkalosis and metabolic acidosis

Key: ↑ denotes an increased value; ↓ denotes a decreased value.

or a mixed disorder. Plotting the values on the map, scanning the patient's history, noting other signs and symptoms, and considering the serum electrolytes will help you distinguish between these two possibilities.

Example: pH 7.09, PCO_2 69 mm Hg, HCO_3^- 22 mEq/L

In this example from McCurdy, the pH is very acidic. The PCO_2 is elevated and the HCO_3^- is slightly depressed. The pH and PCO_2 values indicate a respiratory acidosis, but the HCO_3^- is decreased when it should be either normal or increased if only a single disorder is present. The decreased HCO_3^- suggests an accompanying metabolic acidosis. Plotting the values on the map puts the pH and PCO_2 in the area for respiratory acidosis, but the HCO_3^- value does not fall in the same area. In fact, the combination of pH and HCO_3^- values falls in the area for metabolic acidosis. When you examine the serum electrolytes, they are as follows: Na^+ 135, K^+ 6.3, Cl^- 93, and CO_2 23. The sum of the bicarbonate and chloride values is 115. Subtracting this number from the sodium concentration, 136, gives an anion gap of 21. This increased anion gap confirms that a metabolic acidosis is indeed mixed with the respiratory acidosis.

Venous acid-base values   So far, we have been discussing arterial values. In some cases, an arterial blood sample may be unavailable. Shapiro states that peripheral venous blood is acceptable for acid-base measurement only if it is drawn without a tourniquet from a patient with good peripheral perfusion. Normally, the venous PCO_2 is slightly higher (40–50 venous versus 35–45 arterial), and the pH slightly lower (7.31–7.41 versus 7.35–7.45) than arterial blood. Bicarbonate and base excess values are about the same.

Treatment planning and implementation

Collaborate with the physician to relieve both the causes and the effects of acid-base disturbances.

Respiratory acidosis

If the patient has a compensated respiratory acidosis from chronic pulmonary disease and is asymptomatic, no treatment is necessary. Should the acidosis be acute, uncompensated, and/or symptomatic, treatment is aimed at removing the cause. Mechanical ventilation may be necessary to lower the PCO_2 and maintain ventilation. If so, it must be provided cautiously. Eccessive lowering of the PCO_2 can precipitate respiratory alkalosis. Also, if renal compensation is underway, a too rapid lowering of the PCO_2 (before the elevated HCO_3^- level has time to decrease) can precipitate metabolic alkalosis.

Bicarbonate administration may be indicated if the acidosis is severe. Any electrolyte imbalances present also may require treatment. For example, significant hyperkalemia may necessitate insulin and dextrose infusions, ion exchange resins, or dialysis.

Metabolic acidosis

Treatment of metabolic acidosis involves both therapy of the underlying disorder and bicarbonate replacement. Treating the underlying disorder involves such activities as insulin and glucose administration in diabetic ketoacidosis, improvement of oxygenation in lactic acidosis so that aerobic metabolism can resume, and so on. Bicarbonate replacement is calculated as follows:

1. The liters of extracellular and intracellular fluid containing bicarbonate are estimated by multiplying the body weight in kilograms times 0.4.
2. The bicarbonate replacement per liter is calculated by comparing the desired and actual bicarbonate levels, or by noting the base deficit.
3. The estimated total dose is obtained by multiplying the liters of fluid (from step 1) by the replacement per liter (from step 2).

For instance, for a 70 kg person with a base excess of -10:

$$70 \times 0.4 \times 10 = 280 \text{ mEq sodium bicarbonate}$$

Particular care must be taken to avoid rapid replacement of bicarbonate. As mentioned above, HCO_3^- ions do not equilibrate across the blood brain barrier as rapidly as CO_2. This fact may be responsible for a lag of variable length between the rapid onset of metabolic acidosis and the maximal development of hyperventilation, and another lag between the rapid administration of bicarbonate and the cessation of hyperventilation. If the blood pH is returned rapidly to normal, the patient will continue to hyperventilate (because it takes several hours for the bicarbonate to alter the CSF pH), and the patient may develop a respiratory alkalosis. Usually, about two thirds of the calculated dose is given in the first 24 hours, and the patient's response is checked before the physician decides whether further bicarbonate administration is necessary.

Respiratory alkalosis

Respiratory alkalosis is treated by reducing the patient's need to hyperventilate. For example, correction of an underlying hypoxia often will restore the respiratory pattern and therefore the PCO_2 to normal. If the patient is being mechanically ventilated, decreasing the rate or tidal volume or adding extra tubing (to increase deadspace) will cause the PCO_2 to rise. Should the hyperventilation result from emotional excitement, having the person breathe into a paper bag is a convenient way to restore normal PCO_2 and eliminate the frightening symptoms of numbness, tingling, lightheadedness, and so on. This intervention must be followed by counseling to help the person become aware of the role he plays in inducing symptoms and to relieve his emotional stress.

Metabolic alkalosis

Metabolic alkalosis is treated by removing the underlying cause and by replacing chloride. Examples of treating the underlying problem are relieving prolonged vomiting and replacing fluid and electrolytes lost through nasogastric suction. Depending upon the patient's electrolyte status, chloride may be supplied as sodium chloride, potassium chloride, or ammonium chloride. If symptoms of calcium deficiency are present due to the decrease in ionized calcium, calcium gluconate may be given intravenously.

Mixed disorders

Treatment of mixed disorders combines the principles governing the treatment of each individual disorder. For instance, to relieve a combined respiratory and metabolic acidosis due to severe hypoventilation, you must both improve ventilation (to relieve the respiratory acidosis) and oxygenation and circulation (to relieve the lactic acidosis). The combination of two acidoses or two alkaloses must be treated promptly and vigorously. They tend to block compensation for each other and therefore produce severe acid-base and electrolyte disturbances. The combination of an acidosis and an alkalosis is tolerated better by the body. They tend to have opposite effects on the bicarbonate/carbonic acid ratio and therefore produce a nearly normal pH.

General nursing care measures

In addition to the measures specific to the acid-base disturbance(s), provide the more general nursing care related to cerebral status changes; respiratory changes; and arrhythmias, angina, or shock. For instance, for the confused patient, provide a safe environment, orient him to reality, and reassure him that his confusion probably will disappear as the condition is treated. Place the hyperventilating patient in a position that does not compromise diaphragmatic excursion. Decrease angina by assisting the person with activities of daily living to reduce myocardial workload. For more ideas on how to help these patients, review other chapters related to these symptoms.

Outcome evaluation

Evaluate the patient's progress toward a healthy acid-base status. Outcome criteria by which you can judge the effectiveness of care are as follows:

- Level of consciousness restored to pre-imbalance state
- Respiratory rate and tidal volume within patient's normal limits (WNL)
- Cardiac rate and rhythm normal for patient

- Extremities warm and dry (and pink if the patient is Caucasian)
- Serum electrolytes WNL for patient
- Arterial blood gases WNL for patient

References

Guyton, A. 1976. *Textbook of medical physiology.* 5th ed. Philadelphia: W. B. Saunders Company.
Detailed presentation of principles of acid-base regulation.

McCurdy, D. 1972. Mixed metabolic and respiratory acid base disturbances. *Chest* 62(2):35S–44S.
Essential reading if you want to delve beyond the basic imbalances.

Oh, M. and Carroll, H. 1977. Current concepts: the anion gap. *N. Engl. J. Med.* 297:814–817.
Concept, abnormalities, and clinical application of the anion gap.

Reed, G., and Sheppard, V. 1977. *Regulation of fluid and electrolyte balance.* Philadelphia: W. B. Saunders Company.
Programmed instruction format facilitating comprehension of clinical physiology related to fluid, electrolyte, and acid-base imbalances.

Shapiro, B. 1973. *Clinical application of blood gases.* Chicago: Yearbook Medical Publishers, Inc.
Basic physiology, clinical interpretation, and clinical application of blood gases.

Supplemental Reading

Broughton, J. 1971. Understanding blood gases. Reprint No. 456. Ohio Medical Products.
Basic concepts; compensation versus correction of abnormalities.

Keyes, J. 1974. Blood gases and blood gas transport. *Heart Lung* 3:945–954.
Physiology of O_2 and CO_2 transport, including Bohr and Haldane effects.

Sharer, J. 1975. Reviewing acid-base balance. *A.J.N.* 75:980–984.
Brief review of control mechanisms and imbalances.

Weisberg, H. 1962. *Water, electrolyte, and acid-base balance.* 2nd ed. Baltimore:William & Wilkins Company.
Detailed information on normal and pathological physiology of water, electrolytes, and acid-base balance.

Chapter 12

Nutrition

In our concern about immediately life-threatening problems in the critically ill, it is easy to overlook nutritional needs. This is unfortunate, because malnutrition can produce a plethora of insidiously debilitating states, such as weakness, fatigue, and poor wound healing.

Outline

Assessment   History / Physical examination / Laboratory data

Nutritional planning and implementation   Total parenteral nutrition (TPN) / Initiating TPN therapy / Catheter insertion / Nutrients supplied via TPN / Importance of physical activity / Potential complications / Discontinuation of TPN

Outcome evaluation

Objectives

- Recognize conditions often present in the critically ill which increase calorie needs or limit nutrient utilization
- State the estimated amount of calories and nitrogen needed by an "average" critically ill patient to maintain positive nitrogen balance
- Recognize signs and symptoms of inadequate nutrition

- Perform a basic physical examination of the abdomen
- Recognize liver enlargement
- Define total parenteral nutrition (TPN)
- Assist the physician and patient during TPN catheterization
- Prevent or relieve complications of catheter insertion
- State the following characteristics of TPN solutions as a class: calorie sources, nitrogen sources, calorie/nitrogen ratio, glucose concentration, and osmolality
- Explain the importance of maintaining physical activity in the TPN patient
- Prevent or alleviate complications of TPN therapy
- Evaluate the patient's progress according to specified outcome criteria

Assessment

An evaluation of the patient's nutritional status attempts to determine whether the nutritional intake is sufficient for his or her needs. Any nutritional textbook can give you information on average daily needs for calories, protein, and so on, in the healthy adult. There is, however, a dearth of specific information on the nutritional needs of the critically ill. In addition, there is a lack of clinically feasible tests to determine nutritional status. As a result, clinical assessment of nutrition in the critically ill is largely empirical. Table 12-1 suggests a format for nutritional assessment by the critical care nurse.

History

A healthy adult needs approximately 1800 calories a day to maintain biochemical functions (Weimar 1978) plus an additional amount which varies according to physical activity. Nutritional assessment begins with a review of the patient's history for conditions which increase nutrient needs or interfere with nutrient intake and absorption.

Conditions which increase needs   The major conditions which increase needs for calories, protein, carbohydrates, and fats are pre-existing depletion, trauma, infection, and intense muscular activity.

When a person absorbs no food, initial energy needs can be met from glycogen stores or more commonly from gluconeogenesis from protein stores. The glycogen stores are exhausted within a few hours, while protein breakdown continues as the chief energy source for a few days. This protein breakdown causes a urinary nitrogen loss of 10–15 gm per day in addition to the normal loss which occurs because of obligatory protein turnover. After a few days, the energy source shifts to keto acids, which are derived from free fatty acids. This

Table 12-1.   Nutrition assessment format

1. History _____

2. Physical

   General appearance _____

   Weight _____ Change _____

   Mouth: Dentition _____

       Tongue _____

       Oral hygiene _____

       Gag reflex _____

       Swallow reflex _____

   Abdomen

       Inspection _____

       Auscultation _____

       _____

       Percussion and palpation

         Liver _____

         _____

         Spleen _____

         _____

         Tenderness _____ Rigidity _____ Free fluid _____

       Anus and rectum _____

3. Laboratory tests and diagnostic procedures

   _____

4. Other _____

shift spares some protein loss but does not stop it completely. Trauma or infection appears to accelerate protein catabolism. Calorie administration by itself will stop the increased catabolism in starving patients, but not in injured patients (University of California Hospitals, San Francisco [UCSF] 1976). Dudrick, Ruberg, Long, Allen, and Steiger (1972) estimate that the "average" depleted patient or patient with major complicated surgery needs 2500–4000 calories and 12–24 gm of nitrogen daily to maintain a positive nitrogen balance. If the patient has a fever, he will need approximately 600 calories more per degree Fahrenheit (UCSF 1976). Additional muscular activity, such as struggling during mechanical ventilation or shivering during hypothermia, will increase needs further.

Conditions which limit nutrient intake   Be alert for conditions which limit the patient's intake and absorption of nutrients. For instance, inadequate oral intake of nutrients will occur in anorexia, nausea, vomiting, coma, oral trauma, and endotracheal intubation. Expect limited nutrient absorption in such states as persistent diarrhea, inflammatory bowel lesions, intestinal fistulas, bowel resection, gastrointestinal obstruction, and paralytic ileus.

Patterns of eating and elimination   Include in your assessment the person's usual eating and elimination patterns. A knowledge of preferred foods, portion sizes, and meal frequency can be quite helpful in encouraging food intake in the anorexic patient. An awareness of normal bowel elimination patterns is essential in avoiding constipation, fecal impaction, or unnecessary use of laxatives, enemas, or suppositories.

Physical examination

Nutritional assessment continues with a physical examination of the patient's general appearance, mouth, abdomen, anus, and rectum.

General appearance   The patient's general appearance provides an overall view of the adequacy of nutrition. Look particularly at body mass, skin color, and mental status. Record the patient's weight, noting any change from his or her previous weight.

Mouth   Examine the mouth for adequacy of dentition, tongue movement, and oral hygiene. Also note whether the gag and swallow reflexes are intact.

Abdomen   Next, examine the patient's abdomen. As you do so, keep in mind the location of various abdominal organs (Figure 12-1). Instead of following the usual sequence of inspection, palpation, percussion, and auscultation, alter the order to inspection, auscultation, percussion, and palpation. Auscultation should precede percussion and palpation because the latter two can change the frequency of bowel sounds. Percussion should precede palpation because it usually is easier to identify the location of abdominal organs through percussion than through palpation. As you examine specific organs, you may find it helpful to alternate percussion and palpation. The following is a procedure for abdominal examination.

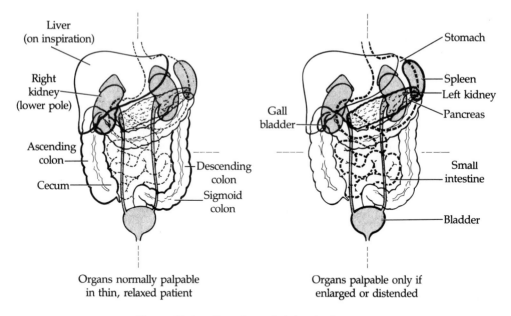

Organs normally palpable
in thin, relaxed patient

Organs palpable only if
enlarged or distended

Figure 12-1.   Location of abdominal organs.

1. First, inspect the abdomen, looking especially at its contour and symmetry. Also look for pulsations, scars, and distended superficial veins (seen in portal obstruction and venous thrombosis).

2. Next, auscultate the abdomen in all four quadrants. Listen for bowel sounds, bruits, and friction rubs. Normal bowel sounds are intermittent and vary in frequency, intensity, and pitch. Sounds that are intensified, weak, or absent, are abnormal. Loud gurgling sounds signify either increased intestinal motility, as in diarrhea or nervous tension, or early intestinal obstruction. Occasional, weak sounds suggest poor peristalsis. Absent sounds occur after handling of the bowel during surgery, during severe electrolyte disturbances, in peritonitis, and in advanced intestinal obstruction. Listen for 2–5 minutes in each quadrant before deciding that bowel sounds are absent (American Journal of Nursing 1974).

Bruits may be audible in patients with arteriosclerosis, hypertension, aortic aneurysms, masses compressing the aorta, and renal artery stenosis. Peritoneal friction rubs may be heard over the right lower costal margin, owing to hepatic tumors or abcesses, or over the left lower costal area, owing to splenic infarction.

3. Percuss the abdomen lightly. Normally, you will hear tympany over the stomach and intestine (therefore, over most of the abdomen). Tympany is a long, very hollow sound which indicates gas in an enclosed chamber. It resembles the sound you can hear by puffing out your cheek and percussing it. Over

organs, a short, high-pitched sound called dullness will be heard. (If you wish to review percussion technique and the characteristics of percussion notes, see Chapter 9.)

Estimate the size of the liver by percussing in the right midclavicular line down from lung resonance to dullness and up from abdominal tympany to dullness. It is important to note both the location of the borders and the distance between them. The upper border of the liver usually is at the fifth–seventh intercostal space. The normal distance between the upper and lower borders is 6–12 cm in the right midclavicular line and 4–8 cm in the midsternal line (Bates 1974). A normal-sized liver may be displaced downward, as in emphysema, or upward, as in ascites or abdominal tumors. As a result, a liver edge below the costal margin does not necessarily indicate liver enlargement.

Percuss the lower left anterior rib cage, listening for the change from lung resonance to the tympany of the gastric air bubble. This bubble may vary considerably in size. When quite large, it can alert you to gastric dilatation and the need for nasogastric decompression.

Nurses usually do not percuss the spleen, which appears as a small oval area of dullness from the ninth to eleventh ribs just posterior to the midaxillary line.

One of the most important findings you may detect on abdominal percussion is free fluid in the abdominal cavity. Two findings may point to free ascitic fluid: shifting dullness or a fluid wave. At least approximately 500 ml of fluid must be present for these signs to be positive (DeGowin and DeGowin 1976). To test for shifting dullness, first place the patient on his back and percuss each flank. If free fluid is present, you will hear tympany over the midabdomen and dullness in the flanks. Mark the points at which dullness appears. Next, turn the patient to one side and repeat the percussion. If ascitic fluid is present, gravity will cause it to collect in the dependent flank, and the level of dullness on that flank will be closer to the umbilicus. The upper flank, in contrast, now will sound tympanitic. Finally, turn the patient to the opposite side and repeat the procedure. By comparing the levels of dullness, you can estimate whether a small, moderate, or large amount of fluid is present.

When the patient has a large amount of ascites, you may detect a fluid wave (Figure 12-2). Have a second person place the ulnar surface of his hand along the midline of the abdomen and apply firm pressure. This pressure will minimize the possibility of a wave traveling through the abdominal wall itself. Place one of your hands along the patient's flank and sharply strike the opposite flank with your other hand. If you feel the wave with the palpating hand, free fluid is present.

4. Palpate the abdomen lightly (Figure 12-3). Place your hand on the abdomen with your forearm parallel to the floor at the level of the anterior abdominal wall. Put your fingers together and use the pads of your fingertips to feel for tenderness and resistance. Resistance may be voluntary, due to patient discomfort or apprehension, or involuntary, due to peritoneal irritation. If you encounter re-

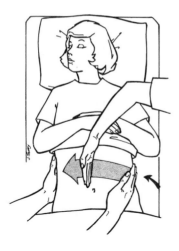

Figure 12-2. Percussion of fluid wave.

sistance, try to differentiate the type by ensuring that the patient is relaxed—
make sure he's positioned comfortably and your hands are warm; try to distract
him with conversation. You also can feel for the normal relaxation of the rectus
muscles on expiration (Bates 1974). Rigidity that continues in spite of these
maneuvers probably is involuntary.

Palpate areas of known tenderness last. If pain is present, check for rebound
tenderness, a reliable sign of peritoneal inflamation. Rebound tenderness is pain
which occurs after the release of pressure. To elicit this response, press firmly
over a quadrant of abdomen other than the tender one and release the pressure
suddenly. If the patient feels a sharp stab of pain over the suspected area (*not*
over the site on which you pressed), rebound tenderness is present (DeGowin
and DeGowin 1976). This test can provoke severe pain and muscle spasm, which
interfere with further examination. For this reason, it is wise to postpone it until
the end of the examination.

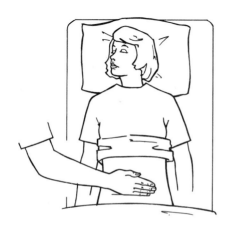

Figure 12-3. Light palpation.

After light palpation to identify resistance and tenderness, palpate more deeply for masses and abdominal organs. Refer back to Figure 12-1. Those which you normally may be able to feel in the thin, relaxed patient are the liver; the lower pole of the right kidney; ascending, descending, and sigmoid colon; cecum; and aorta. Unless they are enlarged or distended, you normally cannot feel the gallbladder, spleen, pancreas, stomach, small intestine, or bladder.

For deep palpation, ask the patient to breathe through his mouth. Place your hand as for light palpation. On each expiration, press slowly and firmly, each time increasing the depth of palpation until you have palpated as deeply as you can. During inspiration, maintain but do not increase the pressure. Instead, concentrate on feeling whether the organ is descending toward your fingers. Once you have located it, use your fingers to slide the abdominal wall back and forth over the organ to assess its shape, hardness, smoothness, and mobility.

To palpate the liver, stand on the patient's right side (Figure 12-4). Slide your left hand under and parallel to the eleventh and twelfth ribs. Place your right hand on the abdomen below the lower border of liver dullness, which you identified previously. Point your fingers toward the right costal border. Ask the patient to take a deep abdominal breath, blow it out, and take another deep breath. As the patient exhales, gently push your fingers inward and upward under the costal margin. You may be able to feel a firm ridge of pressure come down to meet your fingertips; this is the lower border of the liver. If you feel the edge, repeat the maneuver medially and laterally. Note the smoothness of the edge and any tenderness. Since the liver normally is not palpable, blunt percussion over the liver is an alternate method of detecting tenderness. To perform blunt percussion, place your left hand on the lower right lateral rib cage. Make a fist with your right hand and lightly strike your left hand.

The spleen usually is not palpable unless it is enlarged about three times (Bates 1974). To check for splenic enlargement, stand at the patient's right side (Figure 12-5). Reach over the patient and place your left hand under the left low back ribs. Place your right hand below the left costal margin on the anterior abdomen. Ask the patient to take a deep breath, lift with your left hand, and press inward with your right.

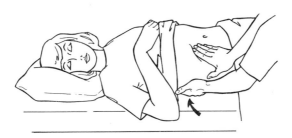

Figure 12-4. Palpation of liver.

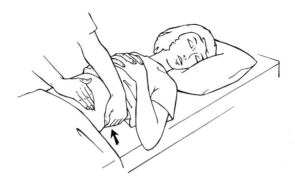

Figure 12-5.   Palpation of spleen.

Anus and rectum   Complete the physical examination of the gastrointestinal system by examining the anal area and rectum. Examine the anal area for hemorrhoids, fissures, rectal prolapse, or skin excoriation. Unless the date of the last bowel movement is known, ask the physician whether it is safe to perform a digital examination of the rectum. Early detection of fecal matter in the rectum can avoid the development of a fecal impaction, but it may be necessary to delay this examination if the patient's condition is unstable or might be adversely affected by rectal stimulation.

Other signs and symptoms   Conclude your nutritional assessment by scanning data from examination of the patient's other body systems. Signs of possible nutritional deficiencies include lethargy, fatigue, poor wound healing, poor resistance to infection, chronic weight loss, scaly skin, stomatitis, hair loss, and signs and symptoms of electrolyte depletion.

Laboratory data

Although there are no easily performed laboratory tests of nutrition per se, certain abnormal laboratory tests can be found in malnutrition. Among findings suggestive of nutritional deficiencies are a decreased hemoglobin level, diminished lymphocyte count, reduced serum albumin level, and abnormally low serum electrolyte concentrations.

Nutritional planning and implementation

Patients maintained solely on routine intravenous solutions receive highly inadequate nutrition. For example, a liter of 5% dextrose in water contains only approximately 200 calories. Ways to enhance the intake of adequate nutrients include such well known nursing measures as small, frequent feedings, selection of foods the patient enjoys, provision of a pleasant eating environment, and social interaction during meals. Dietary supplements may be prescribed for patients whose calorie needs cannot be met with the usual oral diet. Tube feedings may be indicated for patients with functioning gastrointestinal tracts who are unable to take food orally, such as those with esophageal lesions. When gastrointestinal intake and absorption is inadequate or may be dangerous, the physician may prescribe total parenteral nutrition. Among the patients who can benefit from this technique are those with gastrointestinal fistulas, bowel obstructions or resections, severe burns, and inflammatory bowel disorders. The nursing care of the person receiving total parenteral nutrition is complex. Because of the degree of nursing skill required, the remainder of this chapter is devoted to this nutritional technique.

Total parenteral nutrition (TPN)

Total parenteral nutrition (TPN), also known as central venous alimentation or hyperalimentation, is defined as the "delivery of hypertonic glucose, protein hydrolysates or crystalline amino acid solutions, and supplementary minerals and vitamins, into the superior vena cava in amounts greater than required for nutritional equilibrium" (Dudrick, Long, Steiger, and Rhoads 1970).

TPN does not reverse catabolism per se but instead reverses negative nitrogen balance by providing more nitrogen than the amount lost. TPN probably should be considered in any patient who has had no food for five days and who is unlikely to eat for another week (UCSF 1976).

Initiating TPN therapy

If the physician orders TPN, assist him or her to initiate the therapy. The following sections provide guidelines for this procedure.

Informed consent   First ascertain whether the patient has given informed consent. If not, assist the physician in explaining the purpose, benefits, and risks of TPN and obtaining the patient's informed consent.

Baseline laboratory values   Assure that baseline laboratory values are obtained. Because of the complexity of TPN therapy, numerous baseline studies should be done. Authors differ somewhat on which studies to do and how frequently. The following studies usually are obtained before TPN is instituted: serum electrolytes, serum osmolality, fasting blood sugar, complete blood count, blood urea nitrogen, and serum protein and lipid levels. In addition, weigh the patient and obtain a chest x-ray, ECG, and urinalysis.

Adequate hydration   Assure adequate hydration. If the above studies or clinical evaluation indicate suboptimal hydration, consult with the physician and administer whatever fluids he or she recommends. Adequate hydration prior to the institution of TPN is essential. Not only is it technically difficult to insert the catheter in a constricted vein, but inadequate hydration also increases the risk of hyperosmolar nonketotic coma.

Supplies   Gather the necessary supplies. Bring to the bedside the following supplies: skin preparation supplies (acetone, iodine, alcohol, razor); 1% xylocaine; sterile gowns, masks and gloves; cutdown tray; 8-inch intracatheter; 250 ml isotonic intravenous solution; intravenous administration tubing, and extension tubing.

Catheter insertion

Assist both the patient and physician during insertion. Assist the patient by explaining steps in the procedure, answering questions, and observing for signs of discomfort or other problems. Assist the physician by monitoring the patient's condition and by acting as the unsterile person. Before the procedure starts, connect the isotonic intravenous solution, administration tubing, and extension tubing. Flush air from the tubing and cover its free end sterilely until the catheter is inserted.

The goal of the insertion is to place the tip of the catheter in the superior vena cava. The preferred approach is via either subclavian vein. The subclavian vein has a greater blood volume than other veins, so the hypertonic TPN solution is diluted more rapidly. This approach also allows the patient to move his neck and arms freely after insertion and simplifies the application of an occlusive dressing. The external jugular vein may be used instead, but it is less desirable because it has a lesser volume, use of this site limits neck movement, and nearby hair makes it difficult to apply an occlusive dressing. The brachial and axillary veins are avoided. Their smallness limits blood flow between the catheter and the vessel wall. The concentrated solution and limited arm movement which occur with use of brachial or axillary veins both predispose to phlebitis.

Avoiding potential complications   There are numerous potential complications of catheter insertion, including injury to the vein, thrombosis, pneumothorax, arterial puncture, air embolism, arrhythmias, and cardiac tamponade. Since these are the same as with any central venous catheter, see Chapter 2 if you wish to review signs, symptoms, and treatments. To help avoid these complications, maximize venous distention by positioning the patient as follows. Place a towel roll along the spine so the shoulders drop posteriorly, turn the head to the side opposite the insertion site, and place the patient in Trendelenburg position if tolerated.

Preparing the insertion area   Assist the physician in shaving the skin over the clavicle, shoulder, neck, and upper chest; defat the skin with acetone; and cleanse it with iodine and alcohol. The physician then will drape the area (including the head) with sterile towels. The physician will infiltrate local anesthetic into the skin, subcutaneous tissues, and periosteum at the lower border of the middle of the clavicle (Dudrick, Long, Steiger, and Rhoads 1970). Tell the patient to anticipate temporary stinging as the area is infiltrated. Also, be sure the patient knows that he can request more anesthetic if he starts to feel pain during the procedure.

Catheter placement   The physician will use a 2-inch 14 gauge needle and 3 ml syringe to locate the vein by passing the needle through the skin, toward the suprasternal notch, and behind and below the clavicle (Dudrick, Long, Steiger, and Rhoads 1970). Once blood is obtained, the physician will have the patient hold his breath and bear down (Valsalva maneuver) while the physician holds the needle hub, disconnects the syringe, and passes an 8-inch 16 gauge catheter its full length into the vein. When blood appears, attach the catheter hub to an isotonic intravenous solution. Tell the patient he may breathe again, and flush the catheter. The physician will withdraw the needle and cover it with the needle guard to minimize the chance of shearing the catheter. The physician may suture the catheter in place and apply an antiseptic ointment. Finally, the physician will paint the skin with benzoin, apply a dressing, secure a loop of the tubing over the dressing to decrease traction on the catheter, and apply an occlusive dressing.

Starting the TPN solution   Obtain a stat chest x-ray to locate the catheter tip. It is important to verify catheter placement by x-ray because the catheter can curl up or travel up the internal jugular vein instead of going down the innominate vein into the superior vena cava. Once catheter placement is verified, discontinue the isotonic solution and begin the TPN solution.

Nutrients supplied via TPN

As mentioned earlier, when protein undergoes gluconeogenesis, tissue nitrogen is excreted. A negative nitrogen balance will continue even if exogenous nitrogen is supplied unless adequate calories also are supplied. When both adequate calories and nitrogen are provided, the calories will be used for energy and the nitrogen for protein synthesis.

Calories   Theoretically, calories could be supplied as fat, alcohol, or carbohydrates, but use of alcohol and fat is limited by practical considerations. Alcohol causes sedation and possible liver toxicity. Although fat contains more calories per gram than carbohydrate or protein, fat emulsions cannot be used for total caloric intake because the rate of utilization of fat is limited and because the body requires the intake of some carbohydrate and amino acids as well as fat.

Hypertonic glucose is used most frequently because it is inexpensive, available in several concentrations, and relatively safe (Freeman and MacLean 1971).

Nitrogen   Nitrogen (N) can be supplied as protein, protein hydrolysates, or amino acids. Although the body can use protein supplied in plasma, whole blood, or albumin, time and energy are required to convert it to forms suitable for protein synthesis. Crystalline amino acid solutions are expensive. For these reasons, nitrogen is usually supplied as protein hydrolysates. Hydrolysis of 76 gm protein provides 100 gm of protein hydrolysates (Deitel 1973). Since 16% of the weight of amino acids is nitrogen, 6.25 gm of protein supply 1 gm of nitrogen. Hydrolysates and amino acid solutions contain both essential and nonessential amino acids.

Ratio of calories to nitrogen   As mentioned previously, calories must be supplied so that the nitrogen will be used for protein synthesis. The ratio of calories to nitrogen necessary for protein synthesis is approximately 150–200 cal: 1 gm N. Usually, the protein hydrolysates or amino acids are added to a 25% dextrose solution. Depending upon its composition, the TPN solution's osmolality will be approximately 1200–2000 mOsm/kg. Since normal serum osmolality is about 290 mOsm/kg, these solutions are extremely hypertonic.

Electrolytes   A variety of electrolytes may be added to the solution. In the absence of definitive data on daily needs for some electrolytes, their supplementation must be determined empirically. In addition, supplementation is influenced by the multiplicity of factors affecting electrolyte needs in a given patient. Furthermore, minimal and optimal amounts of electrolyte intake may differ. For these reasons, the prescribed electrolyte supplementation may vary considerably from patient to patient and institution to institution. Since electrolyte compositions of the different commercial solutions also vary, the physician should specify the desired total concentration of each electrolyte per liter. The pharmacist will add to the commercial solution the amounts necessary to provide the desired concentration.

Sodium chloride usually is added for maintenance. Since potassium is excreted when muscle breaks down, patients in negative nitrogen balance often have a potassium deficit. If protein is supplied without potassium, these patients will be unable to synthesize protein. To enhance synthesis, at least 3.5 mEq of potassium and 4 mEq of phosphate should be provided for each gm of nitrogen (Giovanoni 1976). Calcium often must be provided; although intestinal loss ceases with hyperalimentation, urinary loss is exaggerated by immobilization. Magnesium deficit is common in starvation. Although magnesium is necessary for optimal functioning of enzyme systems, the amount that should be supplied has not been established definitely. Iron is supplied only if the patient is deficient; if so, it must be given intramuscularly rather than in the TPN solution.

Vitamins and trace elements   Data on the need for vitamins and trace elements (such as zinc and cobalt) is incomplete. Dudrick, Long, Steiger, and Rhoads (1970) recommend that the patient be given 10 ml of fat and water-soluble vitamins daily. If hyperalimentation exceeds one month, they also recommend administration of trace elements. Freeman and MacLean (1971) advocate administration of one unit of plasma or whole blood twice a week to supply essential fatty acids and trace elements. Vitamin B_{12}, Vitamin K, and folic acid are given intramuscularly.

Importance of physical activity

Promote optimal utilization of the calories and protein TPN provides by maintaining physical activity. If the patient can tolerate ambulation, encourage it. If not, provide activity through active or passive exercises. Exercise minimizes protein breakdown, helps to assure that weight is gained as lean muscle rather than adipose tissue, and lifts your patient's spirit as he sees his strength increasing. Explain the rationale for exercise's importance to him, and together set short-term goals by which he can judge his improvement.

Potential complications

Prevent and/or respond promptly to complications of TPN. As you would expect with so complex a therapy, the potential problems are numerous. They include allergy, infection, hyper- or hypoglycemia, fluid overload, protein overload, bleeding, metabolic acidosis, fatty acid deficiency, and electrolyte imbalances.

Allergy   Observe for allergy. Signs of allergy, a rare complication, are fever or shaking chill within the first 15–30 minutes of administration or allergic signs such as wheals or hives. These reactions are seen only with the protein hydrolysates, not with the crystalline amino acids. If they do occur, stop the TPN solution immediately and switch to 10% glucose temporarily while you notify the physician. The reactions usually disappear when the solution is discontinued, but if they are severe or persistent the physician may prescribe antihistamines (Freeman and MacLean 1971).

Infection   Guard against infection by following these guidelines:

1. Prevent infection through meticulous aseptic technique.

2. Use as few connections in the line as possible. Avoid "piggybacks" and stopcocks and tape all connections securely. (These measures will prevent both infection and air embolism.) Some physicians advocate the use of filters in the line. Others avoid them, because they may clog, or release a bolus of bacteria if they break; furthermore, they may stop bacteria but not their toxins.

3. Refrigerate solutions until 30 minutes before use, when you may allow them to warm naturally. Solutions usually are ordered daily from the pharmacy, which prepares them under a laminar-flow hood.

4. Do not hang solution that appears cloudy or has a precipitate. Do not save a discontinued bottle and rehang it later.

5. Minimize fibrin deposition along the catheter. Fibrin deposition is believed to provide a focus for infection and thrombosis. Do not administer blood through the line, or withdraw blood samples (unless checking for contamination of the catheter itself). Also, avoid using the line to measure central venous pressure.

6. Avoid administering drugs routinely via the line as they may precipitate. (Most physicians do not add antibiotics routinely to the TPN solution, either. Routine use can promote superinfections and some antibiotics may interact with chemicals in the fluid.)

7. Change the bottle, intravenous tubing, and filter (if you are using one) at least every 24 hours. Place the patient flat; if you do not, disconnecting the tubing may allow air to be sucked into the vein by negative thoracic pressure. Aseptically connect the new bottle to the new tubing and clear air from the line. Stop the flow in the old tubing. Then quickly and sterilely disconnect the old intravenous tubing from the extension tubing, which remains attached to the catheter hub underneath the dressing. Connect the new intravenous tubing to the extension tubing. Have the patient perform a Valsalva maneuver while you disconnect and reconnect the tubing to avoid a possible air embolism.

8. Change the dressing when soiled, and as specified by the physician (typically every other day). Since you will change the extension tubing at the same time, again place the patient flat. Wear a sterile mask and gloves. Remove the old dressing. Clean and examine the skin for erythema and any drainage. Examine the catheter to be sure it still is sutured in place and make sure the needle guard still is closed. Apply antiseptic ointment if recommended at your institution. Change the extension tubing. (You may find it helpful to grasp the catheter *hub* with a hemostat while you do this. Do *not* clamp the catheter itself; although you may prevent an air embolus, you may produce a catheter embolus!) Redress the site occlusively. Write the date on the dressing so other staff can remember when the next change is due. Chart the procedure and your observations, and alert the physician to any troublesome signs such as a loose suture.

9. Observe the patient closely for indications of bacterial or fungal infection. The most common bacterial contaminant is streptococcus. The catheter also may become contaminated with Candida, especially if the patient has been on TPN longer than 15 days (Freeman and MacLean 1971); is receiving protein hydrolysates; and is being medicated with broad spectrum antibiotics, immunosuppressives, or steroids (UCSF 1976). Because Candida sepsis may be asymptomatic in its early stages, Freeman and MacLean (1971) recommend routine weekly blood

and urine cultures for both bacteria and fungi. Redness, swelling, heat, or tenderness at the insertion site or along the catheter course; fever; or chills are signs of infection. If you suspect infection, alert the physician. Change and culture the bottle, tubing, and filter. The physician will draw blood cultures from both the catheter and a peripheral vein and try to identify possible foci of infection other than the catheter itself, such as a urinary tract, respiratory, or wound infection. If one is identified, the physician will treat that infection and leave the catheter in place. If no other source can be located, the doctor will remove and culture the catheter. TPN may be resumed at another site. Note that only the development of a new infection warrants catheter removal. The patient with an established infection may be started on TPN precisely to reverse the nutritional depletion that contributed to that infection.

Hyperglycemia   Be alert for hyperglycemia. The development of hyperglycemia is undesirable for a number of reasons. Excess glucose increases serum osmolality, causing a fluid shift from the intracellular to extracellular space. It also causes an osmotic diuresis, resulting in both extracellular and intracellular dehydration. The increased volume of plasma dilutes the serum sodium— producing hyponatremia—and also dilutes the serum bicarbonate—creating a hypertonic metabolic acidosis (Freeman and MacLean 1971).

Hyperglycemia can result from an excessive total load of glucose, too rapid an infusion rate, or diminished glucose tolerance. Prevent hyperglycemia by incorporating these measures into the patient's care:

1. During the intial stabilization period (4–7 days), increase the TPN rate gradually according to the physician's orders and the patient's tolerance. TPN increases the glucose, protein, osmolar, and volume loads on the patient. Most patients can increase their ability to cope with these loads if they are introduced slowly. One example of administration follows. On the first day, the physician may order administration of 1000 ml of TPN solution over 24 hours and the rest of the patient's fluid requirements as routine intravenous fluid. Each day, one liter of TPN solution may be added and one liter of other fluid deleted, until the total desired TPN solution is being administered.

2. Maintain the flow rate ordered by the physician. Most physicians specify that a constant flow rate be maintained over 24 hours to prevent deleterious swings in blood glucose and serum osmolality. Parsa, Thornton, and Ferrer (1972) adjust infusion rates according to the patient's blood glucose and whether the solution contains insulin. They recommend the following guidelines. If the solution contains insulin or if it does not but the blood glucose is below 150 mg%, give the solution at a constant rate. If the solution does not contain insulin and the blood glucose is above 150 mg%, use a slower rate during the night. They believe that persistent hyperglycemia *may* exhaust the beta cells and contribute to the later development of diabetes. Slowing the rate of course will lower the blood glucose level.

Use an infusion pump to maintain the flow of solution within 10% of the rate ordered by the physician (Ruberg 1974). Check the accuracy of the flow rate periodically. (If no pump is available, use a volume control chamber to limit the volume that could be infused accidentally.) Time-tape the bottle to indicate how much solution should be infused over a given period. This will provide a double check on pump accuracy.

Do *not* increase flow rate to "catch up" an infusion that is behind schedule.

3. Monitor blood glucose levels daily during stabilization and weekly thereafter. Anticipate that the blood glucose will rise. It should stabilize under 200 mg%.

4. Check urine sugar and ketones every 6 hours, using a double-voided specimen. Urinary sugar should be 1–2$^+$ and ketones should be negative or small. Due to variations in renal threshold for glucose, urine dextrose determinations do not indicate accurately blood glucose levels. If you and the physician anticipate or experience difficulty in stabilizing the patient on TPN, do not rely on urine glucose determinations. Instead, use reagent indicator strips to test the patient's blood glucose level.

5. Expect that diabetic patients or those with relative pancreatic insufficiency will need exogenous insulin. As a guideline, Dudrick, Ruberg, Long, Allen, and Steiger (1972) recommend adding to the TPN solution 5–25 units of insulin per 1000 calories of glucose.

6. Anticipate that patients who are on high dose steroids or undergoing increased stress (such as during surgery, the early postoperative period, or sepsis) will have a relative glucose intolerance. These patients will need insulin coverage when TPN is used. Freeman and MacLean (1971) recommend that TPN be interrupted during the operative and early postoperative period and 10% glucose given instead. At the University of California Hospitals in San Francisco, either the rate of 25% dextrose is reduced gradually over the 12–24 hours before surgery to approximately 40 ml/hr, or the rate first is slowed and the solution then changed to 10% dextrose. This latter practice both minimizes the hazards of glucose intolerance and prevents the inadvertent administration of a bolus of greatly hypertonic fluid during surgery.

7. Anticipate that patients with cardiac, renal, or hepatic disease will require adjustments in TPN volume or composition. For information on specific modifications, consult the Freeman and MacLean or Giovanoni references.

8. Monitor the patient for signs of hyperglycemia. Signs of hyperglycemia are: an increased urinary output, a urinary glucose level of 3–4$^+$ and/or ketone level greater than small; confusion, headache, lethargy, convulsions, or coma; nausea, vomiting, or diarrhea; dehydration; or a blood glucose level over 200 mg%. Notify the physician, who will order the infusion rate slowed or supplemental insulin administered.

If the above neurological signs and symptoms appear slowly (over days to weeks) and are accompanied by profound dehydration, a blood sugar over 600 mg%, and a serum osmolality over 330 mOsm/kg, the patient has developed a hyperosmolar hyperglycemic nonketotic state (HHNKS) (UCSF 1976). In this condition, an inadequate supply of insulin, probably due to pancreatic exhaustion, allows glucose to accumulate in the blood. Enough insulin is produced to prevent the use of fatty acids as an energy source, so ketones are *not* released. The syndrome thus differs from diabetic acidosis, in which diminished glucose utilization *does* provoke ketone production. Urinary glucose and ketone levels reflect this distinction. In diabetic acidosis, both glucose and ketone levels are high. In HHNKS, marked glycosuria occurs without ketonuria.

The mortality of the syndrome is high. A hyperosmolar hyperglycemic nonketotic state is best prevented by vigilant attention to the measures outlined above to prevent hyperglycemia. If HHNKS does occur, collaborate with the physician to treat it aggressively. The UCSF protocol recommends the following procedure:

1. Stop the TPN infusion.

2. Replace the fluid deficit with hypotonic fluids, as ordered by the physician. Half the needed volume should be replaced in the first 24 hours. If the patient is hypotensive or hyponatremic, normal saline is used; otherwise, 0.45% sodium chloride solution usually is used. When the blood sugar reaches 250 mg%, glucose solutions may be resumed.

3. Administer insulin as ordered by the physician. Doses depend upon hourly blood glucose and serum osmolality levels. Give the insulin intravenously and watch the patient closely because he may be more sensitive to insulin than the ketoacidotic patient.

4. Administer potassium according to the physician's orders. Patients with diabetic ketoacidosis develop a systemic acidosis which causes hyperkalemia. Those with HHNKS do not and may require earlier potassium replacement due to urinary losses. Doses depend on serum potassium determinations.

Hypoglycemia   Hypoglycemia also is a constant threat to patients on TPN. Signs and symptoms of hypoglycemia include profuse sweating, palpitations, convulsions, and/or coma, accompanied by a normal urine volume and negative urinary glucose level. Hypoglycemia can occur as a rebound phenomenon if the TPN solution is stopped suddenly, especially in patients receiving exogenous insulin. In this situation, the pancreas continues to produce high levels of insulin, causing blood glucose to drop precipitously. Prevent rebound hypoglycemia with these measures:

1. Use an infusion pump to maintain a constant flow rate.

2. Prevent kinking, clotting, and displacement of the catheter. If the flow slows, check for these causes. If they are absent, try changing the filter, if one is in use.

3. Avoid giving blood or other solutions through the catheter, because you will interrupt the flow of TPN solution.

4. If the patient is receiving insulin, give it intravenously rather than subcutaneously. By doing so, any accidental interruption in solution flow will be accompanied by an appropriate interruption in insulin administration.

5. If the patient is receiving exogenous insulin, maintain urine dextrose at 1–2+ (Parsa, Thornton, and Ferrer 1972).

6. If you are unable to use an infusion pump and there is an unplanned interruption in administration, restart the infusion within 2–4 hours; this may avoid a hypoglycemic reaction (Parsa, Thornton, and Ferrer 1972).

7. If abrupt changes in flow occur, notify the physician promptly so he/she can order appropriate changes in therapy.

8. When the physician orders the solution discontinued, taper it off gradually. Guidelines are presented later in this chapter.

Fluid overload   Observe for fluid overload. Weigh the patient daily under the same conditions and maintain strict intake and output records. Also consult with the physician about the expected rate of weight gain from tissue synthesis; the goal usually ranges up to 2½ pounds per week. More may be desirable, especially if the patient's hydration is very poor or fat stores are depleted severely. A gain in excess of the amount for a specific patient may represent fluid overload rather than increased lean body mass.

Patients without cardiac, renal, or hepatic disease usually can tolerate 3000–4000 ml fluid per day.

Protein overload   Watch for signs of protein overload. Monitor the BUN and creatinine daily until stable and then weekly. If signs of pre-renal azotemia appear, the physician may change from protein hydrolysates to amino acid solutions to lower the protein load on the kidneys.

Bleeding   Be alert for bleeding. Monitor CBC, prothrombin time, and platelet count weekly. Malnourished patients often have anemia and/or hypoproteinemia. Alert the physician if you suspect either condition, since administration of whole blood, plasma, or albumin may be needed. As TPN continues, improved protein synthesis may enable the patient to maintain hemoglobin and protein levels on his own (Dudrick, Long, Steiger, and Rhoads 1970).

Metabolic acidosis   Be alert for the signs of metabolic acidosis. They include restlessness, disorientation, coma, hyperventilation, hyperkalemia, arterial pH below 7.35, and serum bicarbonate below 23 mEq/L. Possible causes of metabolic acidosis in TPN patients include hyperglycemia, excessive additions of sodium chloride or potassium chloride to TPN solutions, or administration of crystalline amino acid solutions that contain cationic amino acids or that are derived from chloride or hydrochloride salts. If the problem results from excessive sodium or potassium chloride administration, the physician can substitute sodium or potassium bicarbonate, acetate, or phosphate for electrolyte replacement.

Fatty acid deficiency   Watch for fatty acid deficiency. Scaly skin, hair loss, poor skin turgor, poor wound healing, and decreased resistance to infections result from fatty acid deficiency. Such deficiency occurs because hypertonic dextrose provokes hyperinsulinemia, which in turn inhibits lipolysis, and because the TPN solution does not contain fatty acids. Alert the physician if you note these signs and administer fat emulsions as ordered. You may give fat emulsion safely via a peripheral vein because it is isotonic. For patients on TPN longer than one week, the UCSF protocol advocates the weekly administration of 2–3 bottles (1.0–1.5 L) of Cutter Laboratories' Intralipid 10%, which is a fat emulsion derived from soybeans. Do not add any drugs, electrolytes, or other nutrients to the bottle because you may disturb the emulsion's stability. For the first 30 minutes, give the solution at the rate of 1 ml/min while you observe for dyspnea, allergic reactions, vomiting, or chest pain. If no untoward reactions occur, you may increase the rate to the limit specified by the physician. Serum lipids will rise during the infusion but should return to normal within 4 hours after the infusion ends (UCSF 1976).

Electrolyte imbalances   Maintain electrolyte balance. Monitor serum electrolytes daily until stabilized and weekly thereafter. Watch for signs and symptoms of developing imbalances. Potential electrolyte imbalances during TPN include hypo/hypernatremia, hypokalemia, and hypophosphatemia.

Changes in weight, blood pressure, pulse volume, skin turgor, level of consciousness, and respiratory rate may indicate sodium imbalances, which are discussed in detail in Chapter 6. Hyponatremia is fairly common and may be due to true sodium loss or dilution of serum sodium by fluid shift from the intracellular to extracellular compartment. As mentioned above, sodium is added routinely to the solution to meet maintenance needs. Freeman and MacLean (1971) recommend no treatment for hyponatremia if the serum sodium concentration is above 130 mEq/L. If it is below that level, they advocate checking the blood glucose level: an elevated blood glucose associated with a diminished serum sodium implies a fluid shift into the extracellular space due to the osmotic pull of glucose. They recommend administration of insulin or potassium to increase cellular uptake of glucose, slowing the rate of TPN administration, or temporarily discontinuing the TPN and switching to 10% glucose. Patients with true sodium losses, of course, should be given additional sodium.

Hypernatremia may occur secondary to excessive osmotic diuresis. If the elevation in serum sodium is accompanied by lethargy, hyperventilation, or coma, suspect the occurrence of hyperosmolar hyperglycemic nonketotic diabetic acidosis (Freeman and MacLean 1971).

Weakness, cramps, nausea or vomiting, paresthesias, and ECG changes suggest hypokalemia, also discussed in Chapter 6. Potassium needs are increased during TPN, due to stress, osmotic diuresis, and increased protein synthesis. Dudrick, Long, Steiger, and Rhoads (1970) advocate a ratio in the TPN solution of 3.5 mEq potassium per gram of nitrogen to provide enough potassium for protein synthesis and a normal serum potassium level.

Lethargy, paresthesias, seizures, coma, and dysarthria are signs of hypophosphatemia. This condition can develop from the increased demand for phosphate for production of proteins, membrane phospholipids, deoxyribonucleic acid, and adenosine triphosphate (ATP), and from the increased need for buffering of acidic wastes produced by the accelerated metabolic rate. A diminished phosphate level can cause decreased levels of ATP and 2, 3 diphosphoglycerate in red cells (Travis et al 1971). Since these compounds bind to hemoglobin, their deficiencies are associated with a leftward shift of the oxyhemoglobin dissociation curve; that is, the red cells' affinity for oxygen is increased so less oxygen is available to the tissues. Hypophosphatemia also may produce a decreased ATP level in leukocytes, leading to a theoretical decrease in ability to combat infection (Craddock et al 1974). To prevent these problems, the physician often will order 10–15 mEq/L of phosphate added to the TPN solution. Since supplemental phosphate can cause a drop in serum calcium, calcium must be provided also. Add the calcium and phosphate to separate bottles because they precipitate when mixed together.

Discontinuation of TPN

The physician will discontinue TPN when the condition necessitating its use is alleviated and the patient shows progress toward adequate nutrition.

Parsa, Thornton, and Ferrer (1972) recommend varying the discontinuation technique according to whether the solution contains insulin. If it does, they advocate substituting 10% or 20% dextrose for the TPN solution and tapering the administration rate over 4–8 hours. If the solution does not contain insulin, they recommend decreasing the rate of TPN solution 5–10 drops per minute each hour until the rate is zero. Freeman and MacLean (1971) recommend a different discontinuation technique. When the patient is eating 1500 calories a day and receiving one bottle of TPN solution, they suggest substituting 10% glucose for the TPN solution for 4–6 hours at 50 ml/hour and then removing the catheter.

While returning to oral intake, the patient may have little appetite because of all the glucose being supplied intravenously. Slowing the rate and providing appetizing meals, perhaps with some pleasant social interaction, will help to stimulate his or her appetite.

Outcome evaluation

Evaluate the patient's progress toward adequate nutrition according to these outcome criteria:

- Weight gain within limits specified for the patient, usually 2½ pounds per week
- Increased muscle mass
- Improved wound healing
- Absent or diminishing signs of infection
- Hemoglobin, serum albumin, and lymphocyte levels WNL for patient
- Serum electrolytes WNL for patient

References

American Journal of Nursing Company. 1974. Patient assessment: examination of the abdomen. *A. J. N.* 74:1679–1702.
Programmed instruction on abdominal anatomy and assessment techniques.

Bates, B. 1974. *A guide to physical examination.* Philadelphia: J. B. Lippincott Company.
Abdominal anatomy, examination techniques, normal and abnormal findings contained in Chapter 9 along with numerous diagrams.

Craddock, P., Yawata, Y., Van Santen, L. et al. 1974. Acquired phagocyte dysfunction, a complication of hypophosphatemia of parenteral hyperalimentation. *N. Engl. J. Med.* 290:1403–1407.
Study of 18 hyperalimented dogs, showing a relationship between hypophosphatemia and decreased leukocyte ATP content.

Deitel, M. 1973. Intravenous hyperalimentation. *Can. Nurse* 69:38–42.
Technical aspects of nursing care.

DeGowin, E., and DeGowin, R. 1976. *Bedside diagnostic examination.* 3rd ed. New York: Macmillan Publishing Company.
A classic physical examination text with key signs and symptoms in boldface.

Dudrick, S., Long, J., Steiger, E., and Rhoads, J. 1970. Intravenous hyperalimentation. *Med. Clin. North Am.,* 54:577–589.
Catheter insertion technique, composition of solutions, and administration. Includes case studies.

Dudrick, S., Ruberg, R., Long, J., Allen, T., and Steiger, E. 1972. Uses, non-uses and abuses of intravenous hyperalimentation. In *Intravenous hyperalimentation,* eds. G. Cowan, Jr. and W. Scheetz. pp. 111–118. Philadelphia: Lea and Febiger.
Types of patients who can benefit, circumstances in which hyperalimentation should not be used, and common errors.

Freeman, J., and MacLean, L. 1971. Intravenous hyperalimentation: A review. *Can. J. Surg.* 14:180–192.
Indications and complications of hyperalimentation and adjustments in therapy for patients with heart failure, renal failure, and liver failure. Contains comprehensive review of physiology of solution components.

Giovanoni, R. 1976. The manufacturing pharmacy solutions and incompatibilities. In *Total parenteral nutrition*, ed. J. Fischer. Boston: Little, Brown and Company.
Detailed information on solutions. Remainder of text includes comprehensive treatment of principles; electrolyte supplementation; complications; nursing care; and adaptations for renal, cardiac, hepatic, gastrointestinal, burn, and pediatric patients.

Parsa, M., Thornton, B., and Ferrer, J. 1972. Central venous alimentation. *A. J. N.* 72:2042–2047.
Brief review of administration and complications.

Ruberg, R. 1974. Hospital practice of total parenteral nutrition. In *Symposium on total parenteral nutrition, Nashville, 1972*, eds. P. White and M. Nagy. pp. 349–355. Acton, Mass.: Publishing Science's Group.
Complications of TPN and guidelines for physicians and nurses.

Travis, S., Sugarman, H., Ruberg, R., et al. 1971. Alterations of red cell glycolytic intermediates and oxygen transport as a consequence of hypophosphatemia in patients receiving intravenous hyperalimentation. *N. Engl. J. Med.* 285:763–768.
Complex study of eight patients demonstrating that hypophosphatemia shifts the oxygen-hemoglobin dissociation curve to the left, causing increased red cell affinity for oxygen.

University of California (San Francisco) Hospitals. 1976. Protocol for total parenteral nutrition. Unpublished booklet. San Francisco: University of California.

Weiman, T. Nutritional requirements of the trauma patient. *Heart Lung* 7:278–285.
Review of nutritional needs; advantages and disadvantages of feeding tubes and gastrostomy tubes; full liquid, elemental, and low residue diets; and hyperalimentation.

Chapter 13

Communication

Communication is the dynamic, multisensory interaction by which a person shares thoughts and feelings with other people in his psychosocial environment. This chapter will not address psychiatric or communication disorders requiring specialized assessment and therapy; if you do encounter patients with such problems, seek consultation from and/or provide referral to appropriate professionals. Instead, this chapter will look at ways you can alleviate the impact of a critical illness on the psychosocial health of the previously well-adjusted person who is now stressed by a situational crisis.

Outline

Assessment   Process: history and physical examination / Content

Planning and implementation   Establishing a communication process / Fostering adaptation to the crisis / Maintaining your own emotional health

Outcome evaluation

Objectives

This chapter will help you to meet the following objectives.

- Assess your patient for communication input and output difficulties
- Identify your patient's expressed concerns, expectations of hospitalization, and significant others

- Determine the person's stage of adaptation to critical illness
- Plan and implement measures to improve communication with a patient who is (1) blind, (2) hemianopic, (3) deaf, or (4) unable to speak
- Plan and implement measures to support the person experiencing emotional shock or disorganization
- Foster movement into the stages of reorganization and resolution
- Maintain your own emotional health when working with the critically ill
- Evaluate the patient's progress toward satisfactory communication according to outcome criteria

Assessment

Communication consists of both process and content. Your goals in assessing your patient's communications therefore are two-fold: to identify how the patient communicates and what the patient communicates. A suggested format for assessment is shown in Table 13-1.

Table 13-1   Communication assessment format

Process

1. History _____

_____

2. Physical

Vision _____

Reading ability _____

Hearing _____

Tactile perception _____

Speech _____

Writing ability _____

Gesturing ability _____

3. Diagnostic procedures and laboratory tests _____

_____

4. Other relevant data _____

Content

1. History

    Ethnic background _____

    Religion _____

    Education _____

    Occupation _____

    Usual coping methods

       Pain _____

    _____

    _____

       Anger _____

       Substance abuse _____

       Emotional problems _____

    _____

    _____

2. Current information

    Expressed concerns _____

    _____

    _____

    Expectations of hospitalization _____

    _____

    _____

    Significant others _____

    _____

    _____

    Apparent stage of adaptation to illness _____

    _____

3. Diagnostic procedures _____

4. Other relevant data _____

    _____

Process: History and physical examination

In order to communicate, a person must have both motivation and means. Although severe communication difficulties should be evaluated by specialists, you can perform a brief, functional assessment of communicative processes which can be a guide in future interactions with your patient. Most times, attentive observation of the patient will suffice. Occasionally, you may want to supplement observation with questions to the patient or family, or simple tests.

Porch (1976) identifies three ways in which thoughts and feelings can reach the brain: visual, auditory, and tactile. Each input modality requires the person to receive the stimulus, perceive its characteristics, and then associate it with previously integrated stimuli. There also are three ways in which the brain can communicate messages: speech, gestures, and writing. Each output modality requires the person to conceptualize an idea, formulate it into neural stimuli, and express it through motor activity.

Visual input   You will recall that the retina perceives light rays in a reversed fashion; that is, rays from the right side of the visual field strike the left side of the retina. Nerve fibers from the retina form the optic nerve. The inner halves of the two optic nerves cross in the optic chiasm and rejoin the outer halves to form optic tracts (Figure 13-1). Because of this partial crossing, each optic tract con-

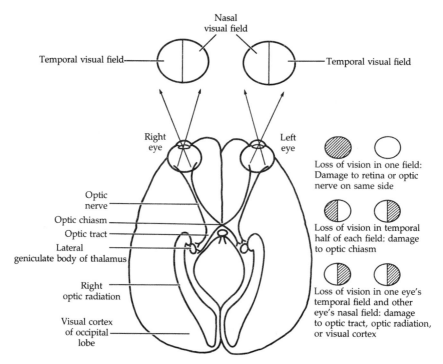

Figure 13-1.   Visual pathways.

tains fibers from the same half of each eye. For example, the right optic tract has fibers from the right half of each eye (which perceive rays from the left half of each visual field).

The tracts terminate in the thalamus (specifically, in the lateral geniculate bodies). From there, the optic radiations course to the visual portions of the occipital lobes.

Knowledge of this anatomy is important in understanding the various types of blindness. The patient who is blind in one eye but not the other has damage to the retina or optic nerve. Blindness in the temporal field of each eye (bitemporal hemianopia) results from a lesion involving the optic chiasm. The patient who is blind in the nasal field of one eye and temporal field of the other eye (homonymous hemianopia) is suffering from an injury to the optic tract, optic radiation, or visual cortex. For example, suppose your patient could not see anything in the temporal field of the right eye and the nasal field of the left eye. Light rays from these fields strike the left half of each retina. Because the partial crossing of the optic nerves occurs in the optic chiasm, impulses from the left half of each retina traverse the left optic tract, lateral geniculate body, and optic radiation to the visual cortex, any of which could be the site of the lesion.

When assessing visual input, note whether the patient has any visual deficits. These may be pre-existing (such as blindness, cataracts, or decreased visual acuity) or associated with the current illness (such as hemianopia, a vision loss in half of each eye's visual field, which often accompanies hemiplegia). Find out if the person reads Braille, uses glasses, or wears contact lenses. Also estimate the patient's reading level as a guide for future teaching techniques.

Auditory input   Auditory impulses are transmitted from the cochlea along the acoustic (eighth cranial) nerve to the brainstem. From there, they ascend to the thalamus and the auditory area in the temporal lobe. If the person fails to respond normally to sound, a conductive or sensorineural hearing loss may be present. A conductive loss results from conditions which block the transport of sound to the middle ear, such as impacted cerumen, middle ear infections, or a perforated eardrum. A sensorineural loss means that the inner ear is unable to transmit sound energy to the brain. An example of sensorineural hearing loss is streptomyocin ototoxicity. If the person has a hearing deficit, note whether he or she uses sign language, wears a hearing aid, or can read lips.

Tactile perception   Tactile perception, while a lesser form of stimuli input, nevertheless is important. The person with a tactile deficit may have difficulty sensing objects in contact with him. As a result, he may be unable to distinguish objects by touch, perceive pain, or sense others' emotions expressed through touch. In addition to assessing whether the person perceives tactile stimuli normally, ask whether he or she likes to be touched by others. Some people find it warm and comforting; others experience it as a territorial intrusion.

Expressive output   Output consists of speaking, writing, and/or gesturing. Output difficulties usually are thought of as resulting from motor disturbances such as paralysis, Parkinsonism, or cerebral palsy. Among the critically ill, however, probably the number one output problem is the intubated patient. One ventilator patient, a physician, later described his communication difficulties vividly:

> I was lying there on my back with the respirator humming away, when I suddenly felt a wave of nausea. I immediately knew I'd developed gastric distention and that I was vomiting and aspirating a lot of gastric fluid. Since I couldn't talk with the endotracheal tube, I frantically signaled the nurse and tried to communicate I was aspirating. She tried to reassure me that I wasn't, but there was no doubt. It felt like it was at least a gallon, and I felt like I was drowning. . . . I still feel that had I been successful in my desperate attempts to pull the bite block and the tube out so I could vomit over the side of the bed, I would've been able to prevent much of the damage. . . . I just lay there waiting for my aspiration pneumonia to develop—which is exactly what happened.
>
> (Chaney 1975)

Ventilator patients who are paralyzed with pancuronium bromide or curare are in double emotional jeopardy. In addition to the terror of not being able to speak which can afflict any ventilator patient, these patients suffer the additional terror of being unable to move. Worse, staff often ignore them or treat them as if they were comatose. These patients need exceptional emotional support from a caring, sensitive staff and family. They also may benefit from sedation to blunt their perception and combat the panic provoked by paralysis.

Aphasia   Aphasia is the loss of verbal comprehension and/or expression; Porch describes it as disturbed input, integration, and output. Aphasia often accompanies strokes or head trauma and also may occur with cerebral hemorrhage or embolism.

Comprehension of spoken or written speech is a function of Wernicke's speech area in the temporal lobe. To distinguish a hearing deficit from receptive aphasia, make a loud sound next to the ear—the aphasic will be startled, the deaf person will not. The ability to write or speak is controlled by Broca's speech area in the frontal lobe, which directs the motor cortex and extrapyramidal system to produce coordinated movements of the muscles of speech or writing. Broca's area is located in the dominant hemisphere, that is, in the left frontal lobe if the person is right-handed, and vice versa. Thus, a right-handed person who develops right-sided paralysis usually loses his speech also, because both are controlled by his left hemisphere. In contrast, a right-handed person who develops left-sided paralysis usually retains his speech, because the paralysis results from a lesion in his nondominant (right) hemisphere.

Content

The sections above have described nursing assessment of methods of communication. Equally important is assessment of the thoughts and feelings the patient communicates—in other words, the content of communication. A comprehensive, highly theoretical discussion of communication content is beyond the scope of this book. Instead, this chapter will focus on practical ways you can assess the content of your patient's communications and intervene to assist his adaptation to the crisis of critical illness.

An assessment of content should include both history and current information.

History   The patient's ethnic status, religion, education and occupation provide information about the patient's background. As such, they can provide clues to his values and beliefs. They also can help you in identifying possible problem areas, such as differing health beliefs between the patient's culture and your own. To avoid stereotyping your patient, be sure to validate any suppositions you are tempted to make solely on the basis of background information.

Asking the person how he usually copes with stressful situations can help you to interpret more accurately his current behavior under stress. It also allows you to identify and support successful coping strategies or suggest alternatives to ineffective ones. Because many people have difficulty expressing pain and anger, be sure to ask how the person usually copes with these feelings. Also ask specifically about the use of alcohol, tranquilizers, sleeping pills, and other mood-altering substances. The patient's replies not only may provide insight into his coping abilities but also may help you anticipate some physiologic problems, such as delirium tremens following the sudden withdrawal of alcohol or convulsions following abrupt cessation of barbiturate abuse.

Inquire, too, about a history of emotional problems, recent or significant lifestyle changes, and the quality of previous health care experiences. Knowledge of past emotional problems, particularly those severe enough to warrant treatment, can be important in prevention and early recognition of psychotic episodes. Descriptions of lifestyle changes can lead to fruitful information about patient and family role dislocations, frustrations, and emotional losses such as the death of a spouse. Descriptions of past health care experiences can help you determine whether there are primarily unpleasant memories, which tend to create a negative set toward hospital care, or mostly positive memories, which create a favorable basis on which to build trusting relationships with health care providers.

Current information   The next section of your assessment should elicit data about the person's current emotional state. There are four areas to assess: expressed concerns, expectations of hospitalization, significant others, and stage of adaptation (which will be discussed in detail in the following section).

1. *Expressed concerns.* A critical illness imposes not only physiologic crises for the patient but also emotional problems for the patient and family. A crisis is defined as the emotional disequilibrium which results from the sudden disruption of one's customary behaviors, beliefs, or values. Each person responds individually in a crisis; elements of a situation which are stressful for one person may not be for another. The patient's emotional crisis may be provoked by his unfamiliar environment, forced dependency, fear of pain, fear of disfigurement or death, or other factors. A family member's crisis may be precipitated by fear of the outcome of the patient's illness, worry about finances, changed roles within the family, an unresolved pre-admission argument with the patient, or perhaps conflict between wanting to be with both the patient in the critical care unit and small children at home.

You can begin to determine what emotional problems are troubling the person through sensitive listening and observation of affect and behavior. If the person can verbalize, ask what is troubling him/her. If the person is unable to verbalize, you may have to attempt to deduce his/her feelings from facial expressions or perhaps from "yes/no" answers to questions you frame. In either case, be sure to validate with the person your interpretations of his/her feelings. Evaluate the person's response for its appropriateness to reality by assessing content/affect and verbal/nonverbal congruence.

2. *Expectations of hospitalization.* By asking the patient and/or family what they think will happen during and after the hospitalization, you may be able to identify unrealistic expectations or areas of ignorance, denial, or misconception about the plan of therapy. It also is helpful to ask about the experiences of relatives or friends with similar disorders. It is not uncommon, for instance, to discover that your preoperative patient has a positive attitude because a co-worker or neighbor was helped by similar surgery, or alternatively fears the surgery because his acquaintance developed a complication and died.

3. *Significant others.* Significant others are those persons who play key roles in the patient's life. Most often, they are relatives, though they may include friends, lovers, employers, other patients, and members of the hospital staff. (Throughout this book, the term "significant others" is used interchangeably with "family." "Family" means not just blood relatives but all those who care about and nurture the patient.) Try to identify the nature of their relationships with the patient before illness and their current levels of involvement. There may, of course, be some whose significance lies in negative or unhealthy relationships with your patient, such as an overly critical or demanding spouse.

Although you may have little time to devote to the family during the initial critical period, some attention to their needs can ease their anguish, enhance their ability to nurture the patient, and establish the foundation for a trusting relationship with the staff. Either you or a colleague should find out whether they will be able to visit, need assistance with shelter or child care, or are worrying about financial matters. You then can refer them to appropriate resources. You might offer to call those people to whom the family turns for support—perhaps other family members or spiritual advisors. Lastly, try to identify the family's feelings—such as helplessness, fear, anger, grief, guilt—and evaluate their apparent coping levels. Especially during admission and other crisis periods, some family members may become acutely anxious, hysterical, or depressed. Sedatives and tranquilizers may be prescribed but often have the detrimental effect of blunting perception and impairing thought processes, resulting in a sense of unreality and repression of feelings. A more creative and therapeutic response is referral to a crisis-oriented psychological service, such as an in-hospital psychiatric nurse consultant to your critical care unit, a crisis hotline, or a community counseling service.

Stage of adaptation   Adaptation to a crisis evolves in four stages: shock, disorganization, reorganization, and resolution. Descriptions of the stages and appropriate nursing interventions are based partially on Kuenzi and Fenton (1975), Roberts (1976), Scalzi (1973), and Wooley (1972).

You can identify the patient's stage of adaptation by assessing his/her affect, verbal statements, behavior, sleeping pattern, and gastrointestinal function. The length of time since the onset of the crisis is also an important factor to assess.

1. *Shock.* The shock phase begins with the onset of the crisis and usually lasts 24–36 hours. In this phase the person is stunned by what has befallen him. He may describe himself as feeling numb or extremely calm. He may minimize the severity of what has happened, say he is in control of the situation, or ignore it completely. He may be inappropriately calm or cheerful, keep interactions on a superficial level, or try to focus conversations on you and your interests. He may attribute his hospital admission to a desire to placate others, such as his spouse or doctor. All of these behaviors are manifestations of the patient's attempt to protect himself by denying reality.

2. *Disorganization.* The stage of disorganization evolves when the person begins to realize what has occurred and its implications for his future. It usually starts within one to two days and lasts a variable period of time, typically two to four weeks. Behavior during this stage may be marked by anxiety, depression, or anger. The anxious person displays signs of emotional agitation, muscle tension, and autonomic nervous system hyperactivity, such as restlessness, fidgeting, shaking, anorexia, nausea, diarrhea, sweaty palms, dry mouth, tachycardia, flushing, clenched hands, or rigid posture. He often has difficulty sleeping, concentrating, or making decisions. He may talk almost continuously, failing to respond to cues which normally indicate a transition between topics or the end of a conversation; silence seems intolerable to him.

The person may also respond with rage at the unfairness of what has happened and his inability to control it. He may be demanding or antagonistic, making disparaging remarks about his care. Attempts to help him are greeted with active rejection or passive-aggressive responses such as "yes, but. . . ." The anger often is displaced onto safer or more available targets. Minor annoyances such as a late visitor may escalate into major confrontations, as the person deliberately provokes arguments in which he can release his anger.

Withdrawal and depression may characterize the person who is unable to express his anger and so turns it inward. The depressed person looks sad and may cry easily and uncontrollably. He may move slowly, sleep excessively, eat poorly, and allow his grooming to deteriorate. He may curl into a fetal position or slump apathetically in bed. Often, he will not initiate conversation and will ignore others' conversational attempts or respond only with monosyllables.

The period of disorganization is painful but necessary. After the impact of the event has fragmented the person's self image, he needs to express his anxiety, rage, or depression before he can begin rebuilding his life. Premature (though well intentioned) interference with these expressions can prolong the period of time the person remains in this stage.

3. *Reorganization.* The next two stages, reorganization and resolution, usually occur after hospital discharge. In the reorganization stage, the person actively begins to identify ways to rebuild his life. He may question old assumptions and seek suggestions and guidance from others who are more knowledgeable than he, for instance physical therapists or members of self-help groups such as ostomy or myocardial infarction clubs. He may try out new attitudes and behaviors. He may grieve for parts of his lifestyle he cannot reincorporate, perhaps crying or reminiscing about them. At times, he may question whether rebuilding his life really is worth the effort. These periods of despair may be interspersed with progressively longer bouts of renewed determination.

4. *Resolution.* Resolution is achieved when the person has established a realistic view of himself as a person with some limitations. In this stage, his activities are appropriate for his capabilities. When necessary, he seeks help in a matter of fact rather than self-pitying manner. He may even discover new strengths, such as greater compassion for others or a desire to help others facing the same crisis he has experienced.

5. *Overlap.* The patient may display different stages of adaptation to different problems in his life. For example, the myocardial infarction patient may be undergoing disorganization in relation to his job involvement while still denying the infarction's implications for his future sexual activity.

The above assessment will help you to identify whether the patient is able to communicate freely, how well he is coping psychologically with his illness, the degree of assistance he needs from you, and the ways you can help him most effectively.

Planning and implementation

Once you have assessed the patient, you are ready to plan and implement nursing measures to foster communication.

Establishing a communication process

It is essential to individualize assistance for the person with process difficulties, taking into account both his deficits and remaining abilities. In the following sections are some suggestions for ways to help your patient communicate more effectively.

Input problems   Follow these guidelines to improve patient input:

1. If not already done, have a specialist evaluate severe vision or hearing deficits.
2. Because the hemianopic person has only half a visual field, she may not see objects on her blind side, such as some of the food on her plate or obstacles in her pathway (Porch 1976). Teach her to compensate by turning her head to scan her environment. Always approach her from her sighted side.
3. Assist the blind patient by providing auditory and tactile cues for activity. Always identify yourself when you approach her. The patient may have preferred ways of orienting herself to a strange environment; ask her or her family how you best can help.
4. To communicate with the hearing-loss patient, capture her attention, speak directly to her, talk slowly, and augment your speech with gestures. If necessary, write messages or use sign language if you and the patient know it.

Output difficulties   A variety of methods can be used to communicate with the patient able to formulate thoughts but unable to speak. If the loss of speech can be anticipated (for example, laryngectomee or electively intubated patient), discuss with the patient in advance which method she prefers. Follow these guidelines to improve patient output:

1. Develop a set of cards, each of which contains a phrase the patient may want to use frequently. If you put them on a ring, you, the patient, or visitor easily can flip to the one she wants (Cruzic 1976). The cards could be personalized for each patient by including the names of her family, physician, and so on. The idea also could be adapted for the patient who does not speak English; a bilingual person could write on one side of the card a foreign language phrase and on the other side its English equivalent.
2. If the patient can write, use a magic slate or pencil and paper.

3. A less desirable alternative is to show the patient an alphabet and have her point to the letters of words she wants to express. The patient may become discouraged because this method is so laborious.

4. Sometimes a person is unable to speak, write, or point, for instance if she is paralyzed or intubated with both arms restrained. In this case, use a variation of the yes-and-no method, such as one eye blink for yes and two for no.

It is very important that you remain calm and patient when trying to "talk" to a person with a communication deficit. The patient will pick up readily on your frustration or impatience and may become anxious, confused, or discouraged. Conversely, you can provide a real incentive to communication with an empathic comment such as "This is hard work for us, but I'm glad we can communicate with each other."

Be sure to alert other staff and, if necessary, visitors to the patient's method of communication, as she will feel less confused and insecure if others use a consistent approach. This is especially important if the person will be outside the critical care unit, for instance in the x-ray department or operating room.

Finally, when you leave your patient, always check that her call bell is within reach. If she is conscious but unable to use the call bell and also unable to make any noise to summon help, she should not be left alone. Many intubated, paralyzed patients have described the stark terror and loneliness they experienced when they realized their inability to attract others' attention.

Fostering adaptation to the crisis

Once a communication process is underway, focus on ways to enhance the patient's and family's adaptation to the crisis of critical illness.

Shock phase   To assist the patient and family through the shock phase, follow these guidelines:

1. To intervene effectively in a crisis, you first must establish rapport with the person. Because your time is limited, quickly establish rapport by introducing yourself and engaging direct eye contact. Sitting down (if possible) implies you have time to listen to the person. Spontaneous touching also can be very effective in establishing warmth and caring.

2. Reduce depersonalization by greeting the patient before you check the equipment monitoring him. As Roberts (1976) points out, too often we are guilty of approaching the bedside, checking the cardiac monitor, intravenous fluid, and other pieces of equipment, and *then* acknowledging the person to whom they are attached.

3. Provide anticipatory guidance. Explain the stages of adaptation, and instill hope that the current stage will not last much longer and that resolution can be

achieved. Point out that the adaptive process is not smooth, instead being marked by plateaus, surges, and occasional temporary regression to an earlier stage. The person may be quite distressed by his emotional lability, particularly if he is a person who values self control and independence.

Expect that admission, transfer, and discharge will be crisis periods. Whenever possible, prepare the person for their eventuality and provide intensified support at those times.

The first time the family sees their loved one in the critical care unit is usually a time of extreme stress. Prepare them by describing in advance the appearance of the person and the critical care environment. Help them to see the patient as a person alive and still needing and loving them. Accompany them into the unit to demonstrate emotional support and to provide physical support and comfort in case they become faint or extremely upset.

The development of complications can be another emotional crisis period during which the patient or family may retreat to an earlier stage of adaptation in an attempt to protect themselves. If the patient's prognosis is poor, you can help him/her and the family begin to adapt to impending death. They may be relieved that the patient's suffering will end soon and may be comforted by their ability to face the end honestly and openly. Alternatively, they may react with rage, despair, or withdrawal. For ways to help the dying person and his family, consult the extensive literature on death and dying.

4. Help the patient learn the patient role. As Scalzi (1973) points out, the patient unintentionally may fail to report important bits of information or fail to comply with health recommendations because no one has explained their significance. The patient and family will look to you for cues to acceptable behavior.

5. Use consistent patient care assignments. It is very difficult to establish a therapeutic relationship when you care for a different patient each day and the patient is exposed to a different nurse each day. (Even with consistent planning, the patient will be cared for by several nurses in one week.) Primary nursing is one promising approach to providing a key person with whom the patient can build a therapeutic relationship. Another innovation some critical care units are trying is the 12-hour shift. Within each 24 hour period, the patient then has two rather than three nurses caring for him.

Disorganization phase   To assist the patient and family through the disorganization phase, follow these guidelines:

1. Provide repeated explanations about aspects of the critical care environment and the patient's illness. Solicit feedback so you can clarify any misconceptions which persist.

2. Help the person to identify the causes of his feelings. It is much more difficult to cope with free floating anxiety or anger than that which consciously has been associated with a specific event.

3. Allow the person to experience his feelings. Following this recommendation is hard; often we openly or subtly urge the patient to feel differently because of our own discomfort. It is particularly important that you allow him/her to experience denial. Because we tend to view denial negatively, we overlook its value as an appropriate, protective response to an inability to alter threatening circumstances. Short-term denial can contribute to the patient's physical and emotional survival, since it conserves energy by obviating the "fight or flight" response and ego disintegration.

4. If the patient's use of denial leads him to life-endangering behavior, some intervention will be necessary. A typical example is the myocardial infarction patient who repeatedly gets out of bed against orders. Often in this situation, you end up threatening the patient, to no avail, and then label him as "denying his illness." This label conveniently identifies the problem as the patient's. A more productive response is to examine the staff's role in the problem. For example, perhaps the assumption that patients benefit more from bedrest than from limited out of bed activity is unwarranted for this person, and the physician could modify activity restrictions. Alternatively, perhaps the person does not believe the staff when they say activity will harm him. This can be especially true if he has been up several times already without apparent physical harm. In this case, you might propose a compromise, such as calling you for assistance when he plans to get out of bed.

5. Support the person's sense of self-esteem. Avoid threats, confrontation, and criticism. Praise him for his attempts to adapt. If they are inappropriate, acknowledge his efforts and tactfully suggest more effective means.

6. For suggestions on ways to help the patient undergoing sensory disturbances or concerned about body image or sexuality, see Chapter 14.

Reorganization and resolution phases   You will usually not encounter these phases during the patient's short stay in the critical care unit. However, during the time you care for the patient you can facilitate post-discharge adaptation by laying the groundwork for these future phases:

1. Restore some control to the person by developing his care plan together. If joint development is inappropriate for the patient's condition, at least share the care plan with the patient and family. Emphasize ways they can promote the patient's recovery. When you make rounds or give bedside reports to other staff, include the patient and family in your conversation.

2. Begin a teaching and rehabilitation program. Cassem and Hackett (1973) contend that such a program for myocardial infarction patients should begin no later than the third coronary care unit day. This recommendation is based on the timing of psychiatric consultation requests and their observation that the most depressing factor for patients was the feeling of being "all washed up" that was

engendered by inactivity. Their suggestions for physical activity include passive range of motion exercises, use of chair rest and bedside commode, and early mobilization. They state that taking a detailed activity history, teaching the patient and family about the metabolic cost of various activities, and clarifying misconceptions about the future are helpful both to dispel depression and to ensure a safe recovery.

3. Encourage the patient to participate in performing his care, consistent with his physical capabilities and emotional state. If the person is in emotional shock or extremely disorganized, he may be very dependent and need specific directions or actual physical assistance with activities of daily living. As his emotional immobilization decreases and his physical condition allows, gently encourage him to resume self-care. Even such simple activities as washing his own body can restore some control and power to him.

4. Help the person to set short-term goals which are both meaningful to him and manageable. Call to his attention achievement of these goals or other manifestations of improvement such as a lowered medication dosage or less need for suctioning.

5. Assist him to make necessary and feasible changes in his lifestyle. Help him identify necessary changes and options for implementing them.

6. Provide clear discharge instructions to the patient and family well in advance of the actual discharge period, which often is too hectic to allow assimilation of information. Solicit feedback on their interpretation of the instructions. This is particularly important in light of the study by Cassem and Hackett (1973). The authors visited 24 families of myocardial infarction patients 6–12 months after discharge. They reported that all families had developed steady conflicts, 75% of which centered on instructions for convalescence. Be sure to find out whether the discharge instructions are feasible; if not, modify them (with the physician's knowledge) or refer the person to a social service agency, public health nurse, or other community support group.

Summary   In a crisis, a person may manifest behaviors, such as confusion, hysteria, or withdrawal, which do not help him cope effectively with the sources of disequilibrium. Such nonproductive activities drain the person's energy and hamper adaptation to the crisis. Your skills at crisis intervention can assist him to regain emotional equilibrium and energy to cope productively with reality.

Maintaining your own emotional health

The critically ill patient and his family undergo intense emotional stress. In order to help them cope effectively, you must be emotionally well nourished yourself. Unfortunately, many factors in the critical care environment mitigate against your maintaining enough emotional energy to spare some for the patient and family. Just as a patient can experience sensory overload, you can, too, from beeping monitors, hissing ventilators, fast-paced staff conversations, and incessantly ringing telephones. Even more draining can be the emotional overload which can result from daily exposure to a tense, pressured atmosphere in which you are expected to be highly observant and ready to respond instantly to a life or death crisis. You may feel anxiety, anger, or despair over the seeming futility of trying to save desperately ill patients or contend with staff or equipment shortages. You also may find yourself threatened by the air of competition which all too often characterizes the staff of a critical care unit. You may feel that you cannot seek support from your colleagues for fear of seeming unprofessional or weak. Sometimes it may seem as though these factors conspire to utilize so much of your emotional energy that you have none left over for important people in your personal life, much less your patient or his family.

Following are some suggestions which the author has found particularly useful for maintaining emotional health while nursing the critically ill.

Separation of professional and personal lives   Clearly separate your professional and personal lives. This can be hard to do, particularly if you work extra shifts or socialize only with other people who work in the same unit. A period of time each day or week unconnected with your nursing can refresh your spirit immensely.

Alternate demand periods   Within your professional practice, alternate periods of high and low emotional demands. If you are allowed to choose your patient assignments, occasionally choose "easy" patients instead of constantly taking the most difficult ones. If you find yourself frequently depressed and exhausted, consider temporarily transferring out of the unit to a less intense patient care environment. Some hospitals have exchange programs between nurses on the critical care unit and a related general ward. Short practice periods in the other's customary unit allows the general duty nurse to maintain her acute care skills and understanding of the patient's experience, while helping the critical care nurse to defuse her involvement, develop her communication and teaching skills, and maintain an awareness of the continuity of patient care beyond her unit.

Support person or group   Identify a support person or, better yet, a group with whom you can explore work-related emotional problems. A regular meeting with a skilled facilitator can provide a safe and supportive atmosphere for you and your co-workers to emotionally nurture each other by defusing some of the stress you feel, venting fears and frustrations, working out intrastaff conflicts, and recognizing each other for things well done. Cassem and Hackett (1975) identify the following steps as characteristic of successful support groups: 1) identification and acknowledgment of feelings; 2) sharing of feelings; and 3) examination of the details of a specific experience such as a cardiac arrest, with appropriate support, praise, and criticism. Through these steps, you and other group members can integrate an experience, gain a perspective on it, and apply what you have learned to future situations.

Coping with unsafe conditions   Band together with your colleagues to reduce stress resulting from unsafe working conditions. For instance, clear documentation of inadequate patient care due to staff shortages can have much more of an impact on hospital administration than generalized complaints or verbal blasts. If your attempts to alter conditions endangering patient care are ignored, consider contacting your local professional organization for assistance.

Outcome evaluation

Evaluate the patient's progress toward satisfactory communication and adaptation to illness. By discharge from the critical care unit, the patient ideally should meet these outcome criteria:

- If conscious but unable to speak, can communicate wants and feelings through an alternate communication process
- No longer exhibits manifestations of denial of illness
- If anxious, angry, or depressed, expresses: (1) awareness that such feelings are part of the normal process of adaptation; and (2) ability to cope with such feelings
- Is receiving preparatory assistance with reorganization and resolution through participation in a beginning teaching and rehabilitation program

References

Cassem, N., and Hackett, T. 1973. Psychological rehabilitation of myocardial infarction patients in the acute phase. *Heart Lung* 2:382–388.
Results of interviews with M. I. patients after discharge; recommendations for starting rehabilitation during acute stage to prevent psychological "crippling"; tables of metabolic expenditures for various types of activity.

——————— 1975. Stress on the nurse and therapist in the intensive care unit and the coronary care unit. *Heart Lung* 4:252–259.
Psychiatrists' use of support group to help coronary care unit nurses cope with work-related emotions.

Chaney, P., ed. 1975. Ordeal. *Nursing 75* 5(6):27–40.
Four first-hand accounts of reactions to hospitalization by a psychologist with cerebral palsy, a physician with multiple complications following liver surgery, a new mother with an atypical

stroke, and a nurse psychotherapist with mononucleosis. Highly recommended for insight into patient's perceptions of care.

Kuenzi, S., and Fenton, M. 1975. Crisis intervention in acute care areas. *A. J. N.* 75:830–834.
Applications of crisis theory to the critically ill and their families.

Porch, B. 1976. Communication. In *Rehabilitation: a manual for care of the disabled and elderly.* 2nd ed., eds. G. Hirschberg, L. Lewis, and P. Vaughan, pp. 100–139. Philadelphia: J. B. Lippincott Company.
Communication input, integration, and output; patient examination; causes and management of communication disorders.

Roberts, S. 1976. *Behavioral concepts and the critically ill patient.* Englewood Cliffs, New Jersey: Prentice-Hall.
Etiology and suggested interventions for powerlessness, loneliness, hopelessness, territorial intrusion, and other emotions afflicting the critically ill. Highly recommended.

Scalzi, C. 1973. Nursing management of behavioral responses following an acute myocardial infarction. *Heart Lung* 2:62–69.
Manifestations of and recommended nursing responses to anxiety, denial, depression, and aggressive sexual behavior.

Wooley, A. 1972. Excellence in nursing in the coronary care unit. *Heart Lung* 1:785–792.
Nursing implications of stages of adaptation of acute myocardial infarction patients.

Supplemental reading

Griffin, J. 1975. Family decision: a crucial factor in terminating life. *A.J.N.* 75:794–796.
Eloquent plea for allowing time for evolution of family's acceptance of discontinuing life support measures.

Kiely, W. 1973. Critical care psychiatric syndromes. *Heart Lung* 2:54–57.
Factors determining person's reaction to stress of critical illness.

Medearis, N. 1974. Training your staff effectively. *Nursing '74* 4(3):43–50.
Commonsense overview of principles of adult learning and ways to implement them in the critical care setting.

Murray, R., and Zentner, J. 1976. Guidelines for more effective health teaching. *Nursing '76* 5(2):44–63.
Tips on creating an effective learning environment and selecting goal-appropriate teaching strategies.

Reichle, M. 1973. Psychological aspects of the acutely stressed in an intensive care unit. In *Respiratory intensive care nursing*, ed. S. Bushnell, pp. 219–230. Boston: Little, Brown and Company.
Stresses on patients, families, and staff in critical care units.

Snyder, J., and Wilson, M. 1977. Elements of a psychological assessment. *A.J.N.* 77:235–239.
Suggestions for assessing psychological areas such as coping mechanisms, motivation, and support systems.

Tom, C. 1976. Nursing assessment of biological rhythms. *Nurs. Clin. North America* 11:621–631.
Assessment of objective and subjective data related to circadian rhythms.

Wacker, M. 1974. Analogy: weapon against denial. *A.J.N.* 74:71–73.
Use of analogy to minimize denial and serve as model for adjustment. Alternative to staff's direct confrontation of patient problem behavior.

Chapter 14

Activity

Rest in bed is anatomically, physically, and psychologically unsound. Look at a patient lying long in bed. What a pathetic picture he makes! The blood clotting in his veins, the lime draining from his bones, the scybala stacking up in his colon, the flesh rotting from his seat, the urine leaking from his distended bladder, and the spirit evaporating from his soul.

(Asher 1947)

Critically ill patients suffer severe restrictions in activity, and these restrictions can have far-reaching consequences. Your efforts during the acute period can influence not only your patients' survival but also their convalescence and eventual resumption of a satisfying lifestyle.

Outline

Assessment   History / Physical examination / Diagnostic procedures and laboratory tests

Planning and implementation   Fluid balance / Aeration / Nutrition / Communication / Activity / Stimulation

Outcome evaluation

Objectives

This chapter will assist you in meeting the following objectives.

- Identify the factors influencing the patient's activity level
- Plan and implement measures to prevent potential complications of bedrest

- Evaluate the effectiveness of preventative measures according to specified outcome criteria

Assessment

Any patient can suffer the detrimental effects of decreased activity. However, some patients need only minimal teaching and supervision while others need extensive assistance to avoid complications from decreased mobility.

To assess the type and amount of assistance your patient needs, you must obtain an activity history and perform a physical assessment of the patient. A recommended format for activity assessment is shown in Table 14-1.

Table 14-1   Activity assessment format

1. History

   Past activity level _____

   Current activity

   Prescribed (include estimated duration) _____

   _____

   _____

   Actual _____

2. Physical

   Perception of pressure: normal _____ absent _____ diminished _____

   If absent or diminished, specify how _____

   Skin integrity _____

   Activity impediments:

   Cast_____

   Diminished joint mobility _____

   Low tolerance for physical exertion_____

   Other (specify) _____

2. Diagnostic procedures and laboratory tests _____

4. Other relevant data _____

History

Begin your assessment by soliciting an activity history. Ask the person to describe his activities of daily living both before and after his illness. Include such activities as sleep, hygiene, physical exercise, and recreation. Often, asking the person to describe a typical day in his or her life will elicit revealing information about self-imposed activity restrictions.

Determine both the current activity level prescribed by the physician and the patient's actual activity level. Evaluating both aspects of current activity can help you identify the patient who is physically or emotionally unable to allow himself the degree of activity the physician approves, or, conversely, the patient who refuses to accept prescribed activity restrictions. Under the prescribed activity level, it is helpful to include a projection of the expected length of activity restriction.

Physical examination

Examine the patient physically to evaluate perception of pressure, skin integrity, and possible impediments to activity. Observe whether the patient appears to perceive sensations normally, by observing responses to diagnostic and therapeutic procedures and internal cues such as a full bladder. Note whether the person is confused, or receiving sedatives, tranquilizers, or other drugs which blunt perception. Determine whether the skin, especially that over bony prominences, appears intact and healthy. Note the presence of casts, pre-existing limitations of joint motion, or precarious intravenous lines. Assess whether the person is weak; becomes faint, dizzy, tachycardic, dyspneic, or diaphoretic on exertion; or seems extremely fatigued after activity.

Diagnostic procedures and laboratory tests

Under the category of diagnostic procedures and laboratory tests, make a note of formal range of motion evaluation by a physical therapist, electromyography, or other diagnostic data related to activity, if any has been obtained.

Planning and implementation

The activity assessment described above will help you plan and implement ways to prevent or combat the effects of restricted activity. These effects are numerous and can be grouped conveniently according to the six FANCAS categories: fluid balance, aeration, nutrition, communication, activity, and stimulation.

Fluid balance

Fluid balance is controlled by the cardiac, vascular and renal systems, each of which suffers when activity is restricted.

Cardiovascular effects   The cardiovascular system deteriorates rapidly on complete bedrest. The major manifestations of this deterioration are orthostatic hypotension, tachycardia, and accelerated thrombus formation.

Normally, neurovascular reflexes cause automatic blood pressure adjustment to changes in body position. Arteriolar and venous constriction, increased plasma catecholamine, tachycardia, decreased intrathoracic pressure, the pumping action of leg muscles, and venous valves all help to compensate for assumption of an upright posture (Weissler and Warren 1974). With prolonged bedrest, venous pooling results from loss of muscle tone. The nervous system also appears to habituate to the decreased pressure, lessened resistance, increased flow, and dilated vessels which characterize the supine position (Browse 1965). Because the person no longer can compensate quickly for position changes, sudden upright posture causes blood to pool in the muscles and abdomen, and the person faints. The abrupt drop in blood pressure due to the change of position is called orthostatic hypotension.

One study by Taylor, Henschel, Brozek, and Keys (1949) revealed that healthy young men developed orthostatic hypotension, tachycardia at work, and tachycardia at rest after 21 days of bedrest. Tachycardia at rest increased at the rate of one beat per minute every two days.

Cardiac workload increases on bedrest, not only because of tachycardia but also because of increased circulating blood volume. Chapman's study (1960) of healthy males on bedrest found a 41% increase in stroke volume and a 24% increase in cardiac output.

The diminished cardiac reserve which results from the increased workload significantly interferes with the patient's ability to perform muscular work. Taylor, Henschel, Brozek, and Keys reported that after three weeks, moderate work provoked tachycardia of 40 beats per minute over baseline values, and the ability to walk a 10% incline at 3.5 miles per hour decreased by 75%. These healthy men needed 5–10 weeks of physical conditioning before their cardiovascular functions returned to normal.

The strain on the heart is intensified during Valsalva maneuvers which bedfast patients may do as frequently as 10–20 times an hour while moving in bed or straining to move their bowels (Luckman and Sorensen 1974). Valsalva maneuvers increase intrathoracic pressure and decrease venous return; when intrathoracic pressure drops again, it is followed by a rebound increase in venous return.

The nursing profession has long been aware of the increased danger of thromboemboli on bedrest. Factors predisposing to thromboemboli include blood stasis, pressure on the veins, dehydration, and sudden bursts of activity.

(See Chapter 5 for information on vascular assessment and blood clotting, and Chapter 10 for a detailed discussion on pulmonary thromboembolism.)

To minimize cardiovascular deterioration, turn the patient frequently, implement a graded exercise and activity program, and prevent constipation. Detailed guidelines for these interventions are presented later in the chapter. Also teach the person to avoid Valsalva maneuvers by exhaling when he moves about in bed, exercises, or moves his bowels. Ambulate the person as soon as possible, but do it gradually. Accustom the person to having his or her head elevated first; then allow the person to dangle the legs over the side of the bed, and finally assist the patient to stand. This process of getting up slowly allows time for the neurovascular system to accommodate to the change in position so the person will not faint.

Renal function   The major renal problems associated with bedrest are stasis, infection, and stone formation.

Although the supine position does not significantly affect nephron function per se, the kidney must excrete a greater solute load than normal because of tissue breakdown and bone demineralization. Urinary stasis develops because the supine position inhibits both the flow of urine into the ureter and the expulsion of urine from the bladder. In the upright position, gravity helps urine to empty from the renal pelvis into the ureter. In the supine position, the beneficial effect of gravity is lost, and renal stones may develop because of urinary stasis in the renal pelvis.

Bedrest also can lead to bladder distention and stasis. Urination normally requires coordinated interaction among the detrusor muscle of the bladder and the internal and external urethral sphincters. An emptying reflex is triggered when the volume of the adult bladder approaches 400–500 ml, although a person can inhibit it for a while because the external sphincter is under voluntary control. In the upright position, when a person responds to the urge to empty the bladder, he relaxes the external sphincter. The detrusor muscle contracts reflexly, increasing bladder pressure and opening the internal sphincter so urine is released. In the supine position, however, it is harder to relax the external sphincter, so reflex emptying is more difficult to achieve. Sometimes the person can compensate with an increase in abdominal pressure. If the urge to void is ignored or not perceived, however, the bladder distends and urine eventually spills out due to the pressure of the excessive volume. Urinary incontinence contributes to skin breakdown and to patients' discouragement and anxiety. With repeated bladder distention, the urge to urinate becomes weaker, and back pressure may damage the kidneys. The stagnant urine also becomes more alkaline than normal, making the bladder more prone to infection and stone precipitation.

Several factors contribute to precipitation of urinary stones. The excretion of calcium, phosphates, and other minerals is increased due to protein breakdown and bone demineralization, so their concentration in urine is increased. Urine becomes alkaline because of infection and decreased production of acid metabolites owing to lessened muscular activity. Stones precipitate more easily in an alkaline solution. Renal stones occur in 15–30% of immobilized patients, usually developing after 14–21 days of immobilization (Luckman and Sorensen 1974).

To discourage stasis, infection, and stone precipitation, include these measures in your nursing care:

1. Diminish protein breakdown and bone demineralization with position changes, range of motion exercises and, if possible, weight bearing (by getting the patient up in a chair, standing at the bedside, or walking).

2. Encourage production of dilute, acid urine. Place the patient on intake and output. Give about 3000 ml fluid daily to maintain a dilute urine of approximately 1500 cc. Maintain physical activity and avoid urinary tract infections. Diet also can help to acidify the urine. Intake of high alkaline ash foods should be limited. These include dairy products, citrus fruits, and carbonated drinks. The ingestion of high acid ash foods should be encouraged. Common acid ash foods are meat, cereal, poultry, and fish. Use litmus paper to check urinary pH periodically. Urinary stones can be prevented by maintaining a urinary pH of 6.0 or less (Hirschberg, Lewis, and Vaughan 1976).

3. Facilitate bladder emptying. If the patient's condition precludes voluntary urination, provide for urinary drainage by using intermittent catheterization, a condom catheter for males or an indwelling catheter. Catheterization is at best a mixed blessing because of its potential as an infection route. Employ a closed urinary drainage system, and use a needle and syringe to withdraw urine specimens from the tubing without breaking the system.

For the person who can urinate voluntarily, periodically check for bladder distention. Try to encourage relaxation of the external sphincter by providing privacy when the person needs to void, using a commode chair, or letting the male patient stand. The two latter measures also contribute to improved drainage from the kidneys because of upright posture, and lessened nitrogen and mineral breakdown because of weight bearing activity. If the patient must remain in bed, promote urination by elevating the head of the bed, pouring warm water over the perineum, running water in a sink, or teaching the patient to empty the bladder manually if necessary.

Aeration

Among factors which compromise respiratory function in the bedridden patient are weakness, dehydration, obesity, body positions or incisions which restrict diaphragmatic or costal movement, and medications that depress respiration or the cough reflex. Lying down reduces vital capacity about 4% (300–400 ml), according to Browse (1965). In addition, because the patient is not engaging in activity, he takes fewer deep breaths, which normally re-expand collapsed alveoli. Atelectasis may develop and predispose the person to respiratory infections. The lack of frequent position changes makes drainage and expulsion of respiratory secretions more difficult. Hypoxia, respiratory acidosis, and even respiratory failure may develop if the patient is not mobilized. The venous stasis which occurs on bedrest predisposes to pulmonary emboli, particularly when the patient is remobilized after prolonged inactivity.

To avoid respiratory complications, follow the preventive measures given in the nursing care plans for atelectasis, respiratory failure, and pulmonary embolism (Chapter 10) and respiratory acidosis (Chapter 11).

Nutrition

Both the intake and elimination of food suffer in the bedridden patient. During the acute phase of illness, the patient often receives only parenteral fluids, which are notoriously inadequate as a source of nutrition (see Chapter 12). Even when an oral diet is resumed, meals may be uneaten because of fasting for laboratory tests, poor appetite, nausea, and diminished interest in self care. Compounding the problem is accelerated catabolism leading to protein breakdown and negative nitrogen balance. Measures to promote food intake are discussed in Chapter 12.

Normal elimination of bowel contents depends on involuntary visceral reflexes assisted by voluntary breath holding and contraction of abdominal muscles. The bedridden patient may be less aware of the defecation reflex, be too weak to use his abdominal muscles, or try to inhibit the reflex because of embarrassment over lack of privacy. Then, too, with a diminished or absent food intake the gastrocolic reflex may be provoked only infrequently or weakly.

Any nurse who ever has removed a fecal impaction knows how uncomfortable it can be for the patient and how time consuming and unpleasant for both parties. To prevent constipation and impactions, follow these guidelines:

1. If admission to the critical care unit was sudden and unexpected, the patient may develop constipation due to material present in his intestines at the time he fell ill. Hirschberg, Lewis, and Vaughan (1976) recommend that you digitally examine the rectum every 2–3 days during the acute care of a recently disabled person. It is advisable to check with the patient's physician before carrying out this recommendation, in case rectal stimulation is contraindicated.

2. Maintain an adequate fluid intake. According to Hirschberg, Lewis, and Vaughan, if the patient is producing 1500 ml of urine daily, he probably also is getting enough fluid for normal bowel activity.

3. Discuss the patient's usual bowel pattern with him or his family and try to duplicate it as closely as possible. If the patient is allowed to eat, high roughage foods and naturally laxative foods can be quite helpful. So can simple exercises to strengthen abdominal muscles such as contracting them several times an hour (while exhaling).

4. Straining with bowel movements should be avoided because it is a Valsalva maneuver which in susceptible patients can provoke hemorrhoids, rectal prolapse, bradycardia, heart block, myocardial infarction, or strokes. If the person is straining, teach him to exhale while tightening his abdominal muscles. Also ask the physician for an order for a stool softener (such as diocytl sodium sulfosuccinate 250 mg b.i.d.).

5. Occasional use of suppositories, laxatives, or enemas may be necessary, but avoid relying on them because they disrupt the normal bowel pattern.

6. Bedridden patients often view the bedpan as an invention of the devil, finding it uncomfortable, embarrassing, and tiring to use. Cassem and Hackett (1973) point out that using a bedpan requires as much energy as wheeling a 115 pound wheelbarrow, beating carpets, or swimming 20 yards a minute. Check with the physician about use of a commode instead; it requires less energy to use and more closely duplicates the American culture's usual position for bowel movements.

7. Try to provide as much privacy as possible. For example, your patient will appreciate your thoughtfulness in giving him a call bell to signal you when he is done rather than having you inquire brightly every few minutes "Are you done yet?" Another help is to attach a sign to the curtain or door saying "Please don't interrupt for a few minutes" to protect the patient against intrusion by doctors on rounds, x-ray or laboratory technicians, dietary or housekeeping personnel, and visitors. It is amazing how many people unwittingly can troop in during the "private, relaxed, unhurried" time the patient needs to move his bowels! Because patients may inhibit bowel activity due to embarrassment over expulsive smells and noises, it is helpful to provide air freshener and sound from a radio or television.

Communication

The patient on bedrest may be less motivated to communicate with others because of fatigue, anxiety, depression, or poor self-esteem; or less able to communicate because of coma, lethargy, confusion, or actual impediments such as an endotracheal tube. Dietrick, Whedon, and Shorr (1948) reported that during six weeks immobilization, each of their four healthy male subjects manifested signs of increased stress, anxiety, hostility, increased sexual tension, and violent emotional reactions whenever their positive personal relationships with physicians and nurses were threatened.

Please see Chapter 14 for ways to assist patients with communication of their needs, wishes, hopes, and fears.

Activity

Normal musculoskeletal function depends on both tonic activity and periodic increases in stress. Immobilization contributes to four undesirable musculoskeletal consequences. The first three—muscle weakening, restricted range of joint motion, and pressure ulcers—can develop rapidly. The fourth, osteoporosis, is a long-term complication of chronic bedrest.

Muscle weakening   When at complete rest, a muscle loses approximately 10–15% of its strength per week (Kottke 1965). In addition to causing generalized weakness and poor stamina, muscle disuse can result in reversible atrophy and also contribute to limitations of joint movement.

Restricted range of motion   Sometimes when you try to move a joint passively through its full range of motion, you will encounter resistance, with or without pain. Such resistance can result from a variety of causes, such as spasticity, scars, edema, arthritis, or disuse. Kottke (1971) states that gross evidence of restricted motion begins within about four days and develops progressively. When soft tissue structures around a joint shorten and the joint cannot be moved even when the person is anesthetized, a contracture exists. Contractures are extremely difficult to treat, often requiring prolonged physiotherapy or surgery.

Limitations of joint movement often reflect a patient's position in bed. Prolonged plantar flexion may lead to contractures of the gastrocnemius and soleus muscles and Achilles tendon (footdrop). These contractures seriously interfere with a person's ability to walk. Limited movement of the hip and knee joints makes walking difficult because balance is precarious when joints are out of alignment. Hip adductor tightness can make perineal care difficult and cause a scissors gait. Shoulder or hand contractures limit many activities of daily living and job skills. Restricted range of motion also may harm joints further by placing unusual stresses on them.

Pressure ulcers   Pressure ulcers are necrotic areas which develop from excessive pressure over prolonged periods. They commonly involve the skin and soft tissue but over time can extend through muscle and fascia into bone. There may be a significant amount of tissue necrosis before the overlying skin breaks down (Kosiak 1958). Hirschberg, Lewis, and Vaughan (1976) assert that a pressure ulcer can be caused by as little as one hour of pressure and immobility and frequently results from one interval of continuous pressure.

Pressure ulcers develop first as tender, reddened areas. As pressure continues, the skin becomes edematous and then necrotic. In the necrotic stage, the reddened tissue first becomes blue, and then becomes black and sloughs off.

Treatment of pressure ulcers is difficult. A variety of methods are used, mostly on an empirical basis. Among the treatment methods that have been advocated are applying granulated sugar or various ointments to the ulcer; exposing it to ultraviolet light; or placing the patient on flotation therapy.

Osteoporosis   Bone deposition depends on the interplay between osteoblastic and osteoclastic activity. Osteoblasts lay down the matrix in which bone salts precipitate. Osteoblastic activity is proportional to the bone's motion and weight bearing, so immobilization diminishes osteoblastic function. Osteoclasts are believed to secrete enzymes which absorb the matrix and bone salts. Osteoclastic activity continues unabated during immobilization. Since osteoclastic destruction exceeds osteoblastic deposition, the bone becomes depleted of matrix, calcium, phosphorous, and nitrogen. Osteoporosis thus represents decreased total volume of bone rather than changed composition of bone. The result is porous bone which is readily compressed or fractured. Osteoporosis takes weeks to develop and therefore is a problem more of the chronically ill person than of the acutely ill one. Prevention of osteoporosis cannot be achieved by passive range of motion exercises; it requires active exercises and weight bearing.

Minimizing complications   To minimize muscle weakening, restricted ranges of motion, pressure ulcers, and osteoporosis, utilize these measures:

1. The bed should have a firm mattress. Place a footboard at its end, preferably leaving space between it and the mattress for the patient's heels or toes.

2. Avoid excessive, prolonged pressure on bony prominences through frequent turning and judicious positioning. These nursing interventions are so crucial that they are described extensively in the following pages.

   If the person has diminished sensation or motor activity, turn him or her at least every two hours. If the patient is completely unable to sense pressure or shift body weight, turn him or her at least hourly. Each time you turn the person, leave him or her in a position which maintains functional alignment and minimizes pressure on bony prominences.

   With every position change, inspect the skin on which the patient was resting. Look for blanching, reactive hyperemia lasting more than five minutes, edema, tenderness or blisters. These are early signs of skin breakdown. It is imperative that the site be relieved of further pressure. Among the common ways to relieve pressure are foam pads, sheepskins, or an alternating pressure mattress. Most nurses already are familiar with these methods.

   An alternate method of relieving pressure depends upon pillows placed to suspend bony prominences above the bed. The following paragraphs describe in detail how to position patients. An asterisk (*) marks pillows placed to suspend bony prominences. These pillows may be deleted safely if the skin shows no signs of incipient breakdown and the period of bedrest is expected to be brief.

   A. *Supine position.* Align the head with the spine. Use one pillow or none at all; habitual use of more than one encourages the bedridden patient to develop a rounded back. *Place one pillow under the shoulder blades and one under the coccyx. Extend the legs and place the feet against the footboard. If there is no space between the mattress and footboard to suspend the heels, place a pillow lengthwise under each calf to prevent the heels from pressing on the bed. If the hip rotates outward, use a trochanter roll to keep it in correct position. Place a pillow between the legs if excessive hip adduction is a problem.

In this position, vary the position of upper extremities from time to time to maintain shoulder and elbow range of motion. Sometimes, extend the arms and place them close to the body. At other times, abduct the upper arms and flex the elbows; point the hands toward the head or the feet. If an upper extremity is paralyzed, support it on a pillow or in a sling across the chest to prevent subluxation of the shoulder. Keep the wrists extended, and use hand rolls to prevent flexion contractures.

The supine position causes knee strain and can contribute to back-knee deformity if the quadriceps, hamstrings, or gastrocnemius muscles are paralyzed. This disability occurs when posterior knee ligaments stretch, making the joint unstable so that it later is unable to bear weight properly. To prevent this deformity in the hemiplegic, place a small roll under the knee to flex the joint about 10°–20° (Hirschberg, Lewis, and Vaughan 1976). Check with the physician before doing this, since the risk of increased popliteal pressure from the roll may outweigh the benefit of knee flexion.

B. *Prone position.* The supine position encourages hip and knee flexion contractures, especially if the head or foot of the bed is elevated. To avoid these contractures, if the patient can tolerate it, place him prone at least twice a day for 30 minutes. The prone position also is helpful in draining posterior lung segments and relieving pressure on the back of the head, sacrum, and heels.

Place the patient so that his toes fit in the space between the mattress and footboard. (Alternatively, extend the hip with pillows above and below the knee so that normal ankle flexion may be maintained.) Turn the head laterally. *Place pillows above and below the knee and under the sternum. Abduct the arms, rotate them outward, and flex the elbows.

Because this position is difficult to achieve or contraindicated when patients have anterior incisions, chest tubes, or artificial ventilators, critically ill patients often are turned only three-quarters prone.

C. *Lateral position.* Turn the patient on his side and place the lower leg in a neutral position. *Place one pillow under the lateral chest, one under the hip, and one under the calf, to relieve pressure on the trochanter, femoral condyle, and malleolus. Support the entire upper leg on pillows. Move the upper hip slightly forward, flex the hip slightly, and flex the knee 90°. Use sandbags to support the feet at 90° flexion. Flex or extend the lower arm slightly. Flex the upper arm at the shoulder and elbow and support it on pillows. Place a small pillow under the head to align the head and spine.

Patients who are completely alert usually can change position at will, though they often need encouragement to turn and assistance so they do not entangle themselves in the various cables and tubes attached to them. Remind them to avoid Valsalva maneuvers.

3. Implement a graded exercise and activity program. Little has been written specifically about exercise suitable for patients in critical care units. The author has culled from physical therapy and nursing sources those exercise concepts adaptable to the critical care setting. The following recommendations are offered to conserve the patient's energy, maintain muscle strength and joint mobility, and prevent disabilities secondary to prolonged bedrest. (They are not intended as therapeutic measures for patients who already have musculoskeletal disabilities; consult a physical therapist for guidance in those circumstances.)

To implement a safe and effective exercise program, you should know the patient's estimated capacity for activity, the energy cost of various activities, and signs that the patient should decrease or discontinue an activity. Guidelines for implementing an exercise program follow. Since these are based on myocardial rehabilitation literature, you may need to adapt them to other types of patients. Furthermore, since guidelines by their very nature are general, a physician should evaluate any exercise program for a specific individual.

The American Heart Association has identified four functional classes of cardiac patients. Class I patients do not have any unusual tiredness, dyspnea, angina, or palpitations with ordinary physical activity. Class II patients are comfortable at rest but develop symptoms with ordinary physical activity. Class III patients are comfortable at rest but develop symptoms with less than ordinary activity. Class IV patients may have symptoms even at rest and these symptoms worsen with any physical activity. Most cardiac patients in critical care units fall into functional classes III or IV.

Numerous studies of energy metabolism have identified the metabolic cost of various activities. These costs are expressed in calories or metabolic units, which are not equivalent to each other. Trombly and Scott (1977) have generated several useful tables of metabolic costs of various activities and a table which specifies the maximal energy expenditures, both in calories and in METs, for each of the American Heart Association's functional classifications. Selected information from their work is presented in Table 14-2.

During the initial post-admission period, the patient's symptoms may worsen with any physical activity and may be present even at rest. Complete chair rest or bedrest is indicated. You should feed the patient and bathe him completely. An exercise program should not be started if any contraindications to activity are present (Table 14-3).

When the physician determines that the patient is stable and progressing satisfactorily, a graded exercise and activity program may be started. Initially, only low level energy expenditures are permissable. Provide passive range of motion exercises to all extremities five times each at least once a day. These exercises can be integrated pleasantly with daily patient care activities such as bathing, position changes, postural drainage, and chest physiotherapy. Remember to stabilize the body part proximal to the joint as you move the body part distal to it. (Also consider teaching family members to do some of these exercises. Performing the exercises may help them feel they are contributing

Table 14-2   Maximal energy expenditures for AHA functional classifications

Class	Limitation of physical activity	Comfortable at rest?	Responses to physical activity
I	None	Yes	No undue responses to ordinary activity
II	Slight	Yes	Fatigue, dyspnea, angina, palpitations with ordinary activity
III	Marked	Yes	Fatigue, dyspnea, angina, palpitations with less than ordinary activity
IV	Severe	Yes or No	Worsening of symptoms with any activity

their loved one's well being and reduce some of their anxiety and boredom with long periods of inactivity in waiting rooms.)

As soon as feasible, teach the alert patient active exercises. The key to maintaining muscle strength is not the number of repetitions of an exercise so much as it is the degree of muscle contraction achieved. Kottke (1965) states that a few strong contractions lasting just a few seconds each day can be sufficient to combat loss of muscle strength.

There are many variations of active exercises. Whichever you prefer, be sure to give your patient specific directions, and instruct him to avoid Valsalva maneuvers on exertion. Demonstrate the exercises and have him return the demonstration to obtain feedback on his learning.

The Cardiac Rehabilitation Program at Grady Memorial Hospital and the Emory University School of Medicine in Atlanta, Georgia, provides a detailed model of a graded activity program (Wenger 1973). This program is divided into four phases: coronary care unit, remainder of hospitalization, convalescence,

Maximum cal/min			
Continuous workload	*Intermittent workload*	*Maximal METS*	*Examples of energy expenditures*
4.0	6.0	6.5	Bowel movement—bedpan	4.7 cal
			Showering	4.2 cal
3.0	4.0	4.5	Dressing, bathing, shaving	3.8 cal
			Walking 2.5 mph	3.6 cal
			Bedside commode	3.6 cal
			Feeding	3.0 cal
2.0	3.0	3.0	Combing hair	2.5 cal
			Washing hands, face	2.5 cal
			Shaving	2.5 cal
			Dressing, undressing	2.3 cal
			Standing	2.0 cal
			Getting out of and into bed	1.65 METS
1.0	2.0	1.5	Eating—sitting	1.5 METS
			Sitting in bed	1.5 cal
			Lying in bed	1.4 cal
			Standing, relaxed	1.4 cal
			Sitting in chair	1.2 cal
			Conversation	1.2 cal
			Rest—supine	1.0 cal

Data from Trombly, C., and Scott, A. 1977. *Occupational therapy for physical dysfunction.* Baltimore: Williams and Wilkins Company.

and recovery and maintenance. The first two phases are subdivided into fourteen steps, progression through which is specified by the patient's primary physician. The exercise and activity program is integrated with a predetermined educational program designed to facilitate adaptation to an altered lifestyle. The activities for each step are delineated in Table 14-4.

According to this program, the first active exercises you would teach your patient are ankle plantar flexion and dorsiflexion. He may feed himself, if you elevate the head of the bed and support his trunk and arms with an over-the-bed table. (Using the table in this fashion diminishes gravity and thus lessens energy expenditure.) As the patient performs physical activity, observe his electrocardiographic pattern and periodically check his pulse rate, blood pressure, and symptoms. Signs that activity should be decreased or discontinued are increased ST segment deviation, significant arrhythmias, a heart rate above 120 beats per minute, a fall in systolic blood pressure more than 20 mm Hg, chest pain, or dyspnea (Wenger 1973).

Table 14-3   Contraindications to exercise

1. New or progressive angina pectoris
2. Impending or very recent myocardial infarction
3. Uncontrolled congestive heart failure
4. Uncontrolled hypertension
5. Arrhythmias
    a. Second and third degree A-V block
    b. Fixed rate pacemakers
    c. Ventricular tachycardia
    d. Uncontrolled atrial fibrillation
    e. Frequent premature ventricular contractions at rest which increase with exercise
6. Gross cardiac enlargement
7. Valvular disease—moderate to severe
8. Outflow tract obstructive disease
9. Recent pulmonary embolism
10. Uncontrolled diabetes mellitus
    Note: Use caution with certain drugs:
        Reserpine
        Propranolol
        Guanethidine
        Procainamide
        Ganglionic blocking agents

From: Wenger, N. 1973. *Rehabilitation after Myocardial infarction.* Dallas: American Heart Association. © Reprinted with permission, American Heart Association.

As the patient's condition and tolerance for activity improve, he may progress to washing his hands and face, brushing his teeth (in bed), and dangling his legs over the side of the bed once a day.

In the next activity step, the patient undertakes active assistive exercises, in which he moves the part as much as he can and you then help him to complete the motion. Wenger recommends these exercises, four times each: shoulder flexion; elbow flexion and extension; hip flexion, extension, and rotation; knee flexion and extension; and foot rotation. Concomitant with this exercise step, the patient may begin using a bedside commode, bathing himself completely, and sitting in a chair for short periods twice a day. (Be sure that the edge of the chair is several inches in back of the popliteal space to avoid deleterious pressure on the popliteal vessels.)

The patient next advances to resistive exercise, repeating the above exercises five times each with minimal resistance. He or she also stiffens all muscles three times; sits in a chair three times a day; changes his or her own gown; and engages in light crafts such as hand sewing, leather lacing, and copper tooling.

By this point, the patient usually is ready for transfer out of the coronary care unit. During the remainder of hospitalization, the person undertakes more difficult exercises and increasing self-care activities.

As mentioned above, the exercise and activity program is integrated with a predetermined educational program. The educational program is designed to

Table 14-4 14-step program inpatient rehabilitation after myocardial infarction*

	Exercise	Ward activity	Educational & craft activity
Step 1	Passive ROM to all extremities (5X ea), teach pt active plantar and dorsiflexion of ankles to do several times per day.	Feeding self sitting with bed rolled up to 45°, trunk and arms supported by over-bed table.	Initial interview and brief orientation to program.
Step 2	Repeat exercises of Step #1.	1. Feeding self. 2. Partial AM care (washing hands & face, brushing teeth) in bed. 3. Dangle legs on side of bed (1X).	Light recreational activity, such as reading.
Step 3	Active assistive exercise in shoulder flexion and elbow flexion and extension, hip flexion, extension and rotation, knee flexion and extension, rotate feet. (4X ea).	1. Begin sitting in chair for short periods as tolerated, 2X/day. 2. Bathing whole body. 3. Use of bedside commode.	More detailed explanation of program. Continue light recreation.
Step 4	Minimal resistance, lying in bed above ROM 5X ea. Stiffen all muscles to the count of 2 (3X).	1. Increase sitting 3X/day. 2. Change gown.	Begin explanation of what is an MI. Give pt pamphlets to read, begin craft activity: 1. Leather lacing. 2. Link belt. 3. Hand sewing, embroidery. 4. Copper tooling.
Step 5	Moderate resistance in bed at 45° above ROM exercises, hands on shoulders elbow circling (5X ea arm).	1. Sitting ad lib. 2. Sitting in chair at bedside for meals. 3. Dressing, shaving, combing hair—sitting down. 4. Walking in room 2X/day.	Continue education about healing of heart, reasons for early restriction in activity.

*The inpatient phase of the Myocardial Infarction Program at Grady Memorial Hospital and the Emory University School of Medicine. ROM, range of motion; 5Xea, five times each; MI, myocardial infarction; pt, patient; OT, occupational therapy.

Table 14-4 *(continued)*

	Exercise	Ward activity	Educational & craft activity
Step 6	1. Further resistive exercises sitting on side of bed, manual resistance of knee extension & flexion, (7X ea movement). 2. Walk distance to nearest bathroom and back, (note if patient needs assistance).	1. Walk to bathroom, ad lib if pt can tolerate. 2. Stand at sink to shave.	Continue craft activity or supply pt with another one. Pt may attend group meetings in a wheelchair for no more than 1 hour.
Step 7	1. Standing warm-up exercises: a. Arms in extension and shoulder abduction, rotate arms together in circles, (circumduction) 5X ea leg. b. Stand on toes, 10X. c. May substitute abduction 5X ea leg. 2. Walk length of ward hall (50 ft) and back to room at average pace.	1. Bathe in tub. 2. Walk to telephone or sit in waiting room (1X/day).	1. May walk to group meetings on the same floor.
Step 8	1. Warm-up exercises: a. Lateral side bending, 5X ea side. b. Trunk twisting, 5X ea side. 2. Walk 1½ lengths of hall, down 1 flight of stairs, take elevator up.	1. Walk to waiting room 2X/ day. 2. Stay sitting up most of the day.	Continue all previous craft and educational activities.
Step 9	1. Warm-up exercises: a. Lateral side bending, 10X ea side. b. Slight knee bends 10X with hands on hips. 2. In- crease walking distance, walk down 1 flight of stairs.	Continue above activities.	Discussion of work simplification techniques and pacing of activities.
Step 10	1. Warm-up exercises: a. Lateral side bending with 1 lb weight (10X). b. Standing—leg raising leaning against wall, 5X ea. 2. Walk 2 lengths of hall and downstairs, take elevator up.	Continue all of previous ward activities.	1. Pt may walk to OT Clinic & work on craft proj. for ½ hr. a. Copper tooling. b. Wood-working. c. Ce- ramics. d. Small weaving proj. e. Metal hammering. f. Mosaic tile. 2. Discussion of what exercises pt will do at home.

	Exercise	Ward activity	Educational & craft activity
Step 11	1. Warm-up exercises: a. Lateral side bending with 1 lb weight leaning against wall 10X ea side. b. Standing leg raising 5X ea. c. Trunk twisting with 1 lb weight 5X ea side. 2. Repeat part 2 of Step 10.	Continue all of previous ward activities.	Increase time in OT Clinic to 1 hour.
Step 12	1. Warm-up exercises: a. Lateral side bending with 2 lb weight 10X. b. Standing—leg raising leaning against wall, 10X ea. c. Trunk twisting with 2 lb weight, 10X. 2. Walk down 2 flights of stairs.	Continue all of previous ward activities.	Continue craft activity with increased resistance.
Step 13	Repeat all exercises of Step 12.	Continue all of previous ward activities.	Complete all projects.
Step 14	1. Warm-up exercises: a. Lateral side bending with 2 lb weight 10X ea side. b. Trunk twisting with 2 lb weight 10X ea side. c. Touch toes from sitting position, 10X. 2. Walk up flight of 10 stairs and down.	Continue all of previous ward activities.	Final instructions about home activities.

From: Wenger, N. 1973. *Rehabilitation after Myocardial infarction.* Dallas: American Heart Association. ©Reprinted with permission, American Heart Association.

facilitate adaptation to a healthier lifestyle and covers such topics as the anatomy and physiology of the heart, myocardial infarction, diet, discharge medications, activity after discharge, follow-up care, and community resources.

A progressive activity program such as this can promote venous flow, muscle strength, endurance, joint mobility, skin integrity, and other indices of physiological health. Equally important is its impact on the person's psyche. It counteracts the feelings of helplessness, hopelessness, and powerlessness which accompany critical illness, and, as the person sees concrete evidence of his returning strength, it promotes confidence and optimism for the future.

Stimulation

A frequent accompaniment to decreased mobility is impaired ability to perceive and respond to one's environment. Among the most common alterations are sensory disturbances, body image changes, and impaired expression of sexuality.

Sensory disturbances   The proportion of patients who suffer sensory disturbances in critical care units is uncertain. Some reports of postcardiotomy patients reveal the occurrence of sensory disturbances. Their frequent occurrence in other patients is supported by the author's experience in critical care units and in post-ICU and post-CCU interviews with patients. Many patients probably do not report sensory disturbances because they are not asked specifically about them or are afraid of appearing crazy.

Laboratory studies of sensory deprivation usually are not directly applicable to the critical care setting because of extreme experimental conditions such as gloves, opaque eyegoggles, and earplugs. Studies in more hospital-like environments are sparse. One study that does provide some insight is that reported by Downs (1974). Her subjects were 90 male and 90 female adults, 18–35 years old, who were believed healthy, had normal hearing and vision, and were not on drugs. She placed them on bedrest for 2¾ hours in a room which simulated a semiprivate hospital room. Her study was intended to measure the effects of personality and varied auditory input on cardiovascular function, motor activity, and time perception; data on abnormal sensory experiences was not solicited. A fascinating, incidental finding of her study was that at least 20% of her subjects suffered sensory distortions which they knew were neither real nor dreams. Among the distortions reported were cooking odors; ceiling lights about to fall down; sensations of floating above the bed; detachment of body parts; and changes in room temperature, light, and sound intensity. Subjects also reported being lonely, bored, unable to concentrate, and irritated by the aimless wandering of their minds. To emphasize, these experiences were suffered by normal healthy young adults after less than three hours bedrest!

Patients in critical care units are subjected to a distressing amalgam of unit noise: beeping sounds from cardiac monitors; whooshing sounds from ventilators; ear-piercing alarms; rattling trays; flushing toilets; snatches of conversation; and hospital pages. They are in unfamiliar beds in unfamiliar rooms which are lit constantly and may have no windows out of which they can look. They are connected by myriad tubes and wires to strange machines which watch them unceasingly. They have regressed to being bathed, fed, and toileted by strangers. They are deprived of undisturbed sleep for more than two or three hour stretches. Their minds may be clouded by their diseases, fluid and electrolyte imbalances, or drugs. As Smith (1973) writes, "The environment of a critical care unit possesses the unique ability to deprive a patient of meaningful sensory input while exposing him to a continual bombardment of unfamiliar stimuli causing potential sensory overload." All this is at a time when they are trying to cope with life-threatening illnesses which may have been thrust upon them with shocking suddenness. It is a wonder that all of them do not report sensory disturbances!

To help your patient maintain accurate sensory processing while on bedrest, use these measures:

1. Introduce yourself and briefly explain what you will be doing each time you care for a new, confused, or comatose patient. Touch the patient to express warmth and caring and to provide tactile stimulation.

2. Take a nursing history from the patient (and/or family). Ask him to describe his normal pattern of activities and how he reacts when it is disrupted significantly. Use this information to duplicate his normal patterns of eating, sleeping, bathing, toileting, etc., as closely as possible.

3. Orient the patient and his family to the unit. Explain the purpose of equipment used in his care and how to summon help. Describe visiting policies, eating facilities for visitors, the location of nearby telephones, and if necessary the locations of possible overnight accommodations.

4. Encourage his family and friends to visit. Suggest that they bring items which would be meaningful to him, for instance, snapshots or tape recordings of children too young to visit. Books, magazines, crossword puzzles, etc. can be tangible expressions of affection for him as well as welcome diversions.

5. Help the patient remain oriented to time. Place a calendar and clock in his room. Each day, mention the day of the week, any special characteristics of the day (such as holidays), and the weather. Try to perform activities at a consistent time each day.

6. Reduce unnecessary stimuli. Roberts (1976) suggests dimming overhead lights for those patients who do not need continuous observation, taping over flashing lights on cardiac or intravenous fluid monitors, and placing standby equipment out of the patient's immediate environment. Other ways to reduce disturbing stimuli are to mute the hospital paging system inside critical care units and to ensure that telephones are answered promptly. A telephone that

rings and rings can be a real annoyance for the patient—imagine how aggravating it must be to lie immobile when you have been socialized to answer the phone!

7. Enhance the meaningfulness of necessary stimuli. Identify the noises of the cardiac monitor, ventilators, and other equipment the patient and family may hear. Clearly define their relatedness to the patient. It is common for a patient after surgery to assume that all nearby noises relate to him, when in fact some of them emanate from equipment used for the patient in the next bed. Always explain to the patient the steps of procedures you plan to perform and the sensations he may experience during them.

8. If at all possible, provide several hours of uninterrupted sleep at night, in as dark and quiet an environment as possible. Help the patient relax and prepare himself for sleep by following as closely as possible his presleep activities, by massaging his back and neck if he wishes, and by medicating him if he wants pain relief or a sleeping pill. Roberts (1976) suggests using eyeshades and earplugs if he has difficulty screening out unavoidable environmental stimuli. While he is asleep, try to avoid disturbing him by limiting the entry of other personnel into the room, perhaps with a humorous sign such as "Caution: exhausted patient. May attack if provoked!" When you must check him, try to avoid touching him and rely instead on visual and auditory cues such as unlabored respirations, pink skin, and a satisfactory cardiac pattern on the oscilloscope.

9. Provide some visual interest in the unit. An increasing number of critical care units are being decorated in bright, cheerful colors. Old calendars and magazines are good sources of inexpensive yet interesting pictures.

10. Provide a pleasant auditory environment. Maintain a sensitive but cheerful attitude; humor can be an excellent antidote to the gloom engendered by confinement in a critical care unit. Discuss with the patient his hobbies, current news events, or other topics which may interest him.

11. Either involve your patient in conversations or hold them out of his hearing. It is dehumanizing to tend to a patient's physical needs while you ignore his spirit—particularly if you are chattering or joking with colleagues about personal matters. Avoid conversations just outside a patient's room; patients often decipher such snatches of conversation incorrectly as applying to them. Keep conversations at the nurses' station (especially at change of shift) quiet.

12. An excellent investment of unit funds might be a small tape recorder. Patients could use it to "talk" to far away loved ones or play messages from them. Family members could bring in recordings of favorite music to soothe patients. Nurses might experiment with it as a supplement to change of shift reports or a teaching tool.

13. Alert the patient to the possibility that he may experience unusual ideas or feelings because of his illness, drugs, or the unfamiliar environment. Tell him these imaginings are common and do not mean he is going crazy. Ask him to tell you or other staff if these experiences occur. Also be alert for nonverbal cues such as a confused or frightened expression, sniffing, unusual body movements, or inappropriate speech. If the patient appears to be having a sensory disturbance, ask him to describe it, reassure him it is temporary, reorient him to reality, and try to identify and remove the cause.

Body image changes   Decreased mobility often provokes an altered body image. Pitorak (1975) describes body image as ". . . the picture of one's own body developed in his mind. Yet it isn't just a picture of the body, of course; it's a whole personal range of activity and possibility, an outstanding impression, the sum of one's life experiences and future hopes. It may not even be accurate, but it's real to the holder." Body image may include objects the person uses frequently (such as eyeglasses, dentures, or canes). It is shaped by powerful cultural norms and may have irrational aspects. Particularly in the American culture, those who are not young, slim, strong, and whole may view their bodies and themselves negatively.

In the critically ill, changes in body image may result from actual external physical alterations (such as scars or amputations) or awareness of internal disorders (such as chronic renal failure). Decreased mobility can affect body image through sensory deprivation or the increased dependency and changes in status and power which accompany immobility.

Body image changes create a distortion of self that can be extremely anxiety-provoking. Among the factors influencing how the patient adapts to the change in body image are its visibility; changes it imposes on his lifestyle and favorite activities; self-strengths; sources of support; and reactions of those around him, whether loved ones, strangers, or professional staff.

Ways you can help the patient adapt to an altered body image are these:

1. Find out how the body image has changed. Asking the patient how he viewed his body before his illness and how he feels now may unleash a torrent of feelings and give you clues to ways you can assist him.

2. Listen supportively as he talks about and tries to work through his feelings. Also be alert for nonverbal cues such as a panicky or disgusted expression when he views a surgical wound.

3. Comment favorably upon those aspects of body image he values and still possesses.

4. Help the patient stay clean. A patient unable or too tired to care for himself can become very embarrassed and depressed about dirty hair, poor oral hygiene, or unpleasant body odors.

5. As soon as possible, encourage him to resume self-care. If he seems reluctant to care for an altered part himself, ask him to assist you (by holding tape, for instance) and demonstrate a matter-of-fact acceptance as you care for it, emphasizing positive aspects (for example, "The skin around your stoma's looking better—pink and healthy").

6. Consider asking the patient whether he would like someone who has coped with the same life experience to visit him and his family. Such a person can provide sensitivity, practical tips, and hope which excel even those offered by well-intentioned, knowledgeable staff.

Alterations in sexuality   Sexuality is an integral part of body image and is affected profoundly by decreased mobility. During the stage of fighting for survival, sexuality is low on the list of concerns of the patient, partner, and staff. After this initial period, however, it can become a primary (though often unexpressed) concern of the patient and/or partner. Because of their own discomfort with the topic, staff may assume with relief that if the person does not bring it up, he is not thinking about it. In fact, the person actually may be waiting for a cue that it is a permissible topic of discussion.

Counseling about resumption of sexual activity after hospital discharge can be started while the patient is still in the critical care unit. Such early counseling can contribute to a smoother, more rapid recovery by forestalling or alleviating concerns which plague the patient and partner. Among these concerns may be the possibility of harming the patient, changes in sexual interest, and worry about their ability to satisfy each other or have children. The partner in particular may feel resentful and guilty about finding the patient less attractive sexually, discovering the patient's sexual interest has waned, or having to assume a more active sexual role in their relationship.

Ways you can help the patient and/or partner include the following:

1. Develop an awareness of your own feelings and values about sex.

2. Indicate your willingness to discuss the topic, perhaps by asking whether the patient has thought about how his disability might temporarily or permanently affect his sexual relationships.

3. Learn about specific techniques which may apply to your patients; they vary with the disability. Couples may need to experiment with different times or positions for intercourse or alternate forms of pleasuring each other. You do not need to become an expert in order to share some basic knowledge which may help your patients. For instance, you can alert the male patient being discharged on antihypertensive medications that impotence may occur and point out that recent studies of female sexuality have shown that most women gain more pleasure from clitoral stimulation than from intercourse itself. (See the supplemental reading list for some sources of information about sexual functioning after various illnesses.)

4. If you feel too uncomfortable to explore the topic, refer the patient to other staff more comfortable with sexual counseling or to community groups such as a myocardial rehabilitation program or ostomy club for support in developing a satisfying sexual identity.

Outcome evaluation

Evaluate the effectiveness of your nursing care. This chapter has stressed nursing measures to prevent the hazards of decreased mobility. It is important also that you be able to spot developing problems early, call them to the physician's attention, and implement appropriate nursing care activities. Table 14-5 presents the signs and symptoms which should alert you to the possible ineffectiveness of preventive measures.

At the time of the patient's discharge from the critical care unit, the outcome criteria listed on the following page ideally should be met.

Table 14-5   Key signs and symptoms of physiologic complications of immobility

Signs and symptoms	*Possible cause*
When head or upper body elevated suddenly: pallor, fainting, weakness, clammy skin, tachycardia, hypotension	Orthostatic hypotension
Tender, inflamed veins	Venous thrombosis
Dyspnea, chest pain	Pulmonary embolus
Cold, painful, white, blue or mottled extremities, diminished pulses	Arterial embolus
Bone pain, easy fracturing	Osteoporosis
Resistance (with or without pain) to joint movement	Restricted range of joint motion
Abdominal distention, decreased appetite, headache, malaise, sacral pain, hard infrequent stools, straining, liquid stools	Constipation
Urinary frequency, urgency, burning; small amounts of cloudy, foul-smelling, alkaline urine; flank pain	Urinary tract infection
Flank pain, colicky abdominal pain, nausea and vomiting, hematuria, stones in urine	Kidney stone
Altered breath sounds, fever, productive cough	Respiratory infection
Skin blanching, erythema, edema, tenderness, or blisters, particularly over a bony prominence	Pressure ulcer

- Maintenance of consciousness, warm dry skin, and normal blood pressure when head is elevated suddenly
- Resting heart rate not exceeding admission heart rate plus 0.5 beat per minute per day of bedrest
- No redness, tenderness, or swelling over veins
- Urine 1500 ml/day, clear, acidic, with no stones and no foul odor
- Breath sounds clear bilaterally
- Arterial blood gas values within patient's normal limits (WNL)
- Weight WNL for patient
- Bowel movement of normal color and soft consistency at least twice a week
- No erythema, edema, tenderness, or pressure ulcers (over bony prominences in particular)
- Joints freely movable within range normal for patient
- If alert and physically able, patient correctly demonstrates appropriate exercises and states their purpose and frequency
- Patient states he is aware that possible sensory disturbances do not mean he is becoming crazy
- Patient may verbalize beginning awareness of changes in body image and sexuality and beginning ability to cope with them

References

Asher, R. 1947. The dangers of going to bed. *Brit. Med. J.* Dec 13, 1947:967–968.
Brief description of effects of immobility.

Browse, N. 1965. *Physiology and pathology of bedrest.* Springfield, Ill.: Charles C. Thomas Company.
Comprehensive presentation of pathophysiologic changes occurring during bedrest.

Cassem, N., and Hackett, T. 1973. Psychological rehabilitation of myocardial infarction patients in the acute phase. *Heart Lung* 2:382–388.
Rationale and recommendations for early mobilization; brief tables of metabolic costs of self-care, industrial, housework, and recreational activities.

Chapman, C. et al. 1960. Behavior of stroke volume at rest and during exercise in human beings. *J. Clin. Invest.* 39:1208–1213

Deitrick, J., Whedon, G., and Shorr, E. 1948. Effects of immobilization upon various metabolic and physiologic functions of normal men. *Am. J. Med.* 4:3–32.
Comprehensive four-month study of bedrest's physiological and psychological effects on four healthy men immobilized for six weeks.

Downs, F. 1974. Bedrest and sensory disturbances. *A. J. N.* 74:434–438.
Sensory distortions experienced by subjects on short period of bedrest for an unrelated experiment.

Hirschberg, G., Lewis, L., and Vaughn, P., eds. 1976. *Rehabilitation: a manual for care of the disabled and elderly.* 2nd ed. Philadelphia: J. B. Lippincott Company.
Comprehensive yet concise presentation of pathophysiology, rehabilitation concepts, and practices in hemiplegia, paraplegia, quadriplegia, chronic arthritis, amputations, communication deficits, and cardiorespiratory disorders. Highly recommended.

Kosiak, M. 1958. Evaluation of pressure as a factor in the production of ischial ulcers. *Arch. Phys. Med.* 39:623–629.
Pathophysiology of ischial decubiti, focusing particularly on interplay of degree and duration of pressure.

Kottke, F. 1965. Deterioration of the bedfast patient: causes and effects. *Public Health Reports* 80:437–447.
Etiology and pathophysiology of body systems changes induced by bedrest.

_____. 1971. Therapeutic exercise. In *Handbook of physical medicine and rehabilitation,* eds. F. Krusen, F. Kottke, and P. Ellwood, pp. 365–406. Philadelphia: J. B. Lippincott Company.
Physiology of connective tissue; mechanics of ambulation; detailed exercises to maintain range of motion, develop coordination, increase muscular strength, and improve endurance.

Luckman, J., and Sorensen, K. 1974. *Medical-surgical nursing: a psychophysiologic approach.* Philadelphia: W. B. Saunders Company.
Outstanding text containing a comprehensive chapter on the body's response to bedrest and immobility.

Olson, E., et al. 1967. The hazards of immobility. *A. J. N.* 67:781–796.
Effects of bedrest on various body systems; related nursing measures.

Pitorak, E. 1975. Rheumatoid arthritis: living with it more comfortably. *Nursing* 5(2):33–35.
Body image changes in the rheumatoid arthritic; factors influencing adaptation to changes in body image.

Roberts, S. 1976. *Behavioral concepts and the critically ill patient.* Englewood Cliffs, New Jersey: Prentice-Hall.
Numerous clinical examples illustrating application of theoretical constructs to behaviors of the critically ill. Particularly recommended chapters related to activity are those on body image and self concept, emotional-touch deprivation, sleep deprivation, and environmental overdose.

Smith, J. 1973. Adverse effects of critical care units. In *Critical Care Nursing,* eds. C. Hudak, B. Gallo, and T. Lohr, pp. 16–20. Philadelphia: J. B. Lippincott Company.
Sensory deprivation and overload, reality testing, and periodicity.

Taylor, H., Henschel, A., Brozek, J., and Keys, A. 1949. Effects of bedrest on cardiovascular function and work performance. *J. Appl. Physiol.* 2:223–239.
Study of healthy young men on 21 days of bedrest; revealed rapid development and persistence of orthostatic hypotension and tachycardia.

Trombly, C., and Scott, A. 1977. *Occupational therapy for physical dysfunction*. Baltimore: Williams and Wilkins Company.
Written by two professors of occupational therapy, this book contains many sections of interest to nurses: photographs of range of motion; activities appropriate for patients with arthritis, myocardial infarction, amputations, and other disorders; tables of expected activities for patients with spinal cord injuries at different levels; tables of metabolic costs of various activities.

Weissler, A., and Warren, J. 1974. Syncope and shock. In *The heart*. 3rd ed., eds. J. Hurst and R. Logue, pp. 570–585. New York: McGraw-Hill Books, Inc.
Pathogenesis of various syncope syndromes, including orthostatic hypotension.

Wenger, N. 1973. Rehabilitation after myocardial infarction. Dallas: American Heart Association.

———, Gilbert, C., and Skorapa, M. 1971. Cardiac conditioning after myocardial infarction: an early intervention program. *Cardiac Rehab* 2:17–19.
These sources present rationale, patient evaluation, contraindications, and step by step implementation of myocardial rehabilitation program at Grady Memorial Hospital and Emory University School of Medicine, Atlanta, Georgia.

Supplemental reading

Bierman, W., and Ralston, H. 1963. Respiratory and metabolic changes during passive and active movement of the lower extremities. *Arch. Phys. Med.* 44: 560–564.
Detailed discussion of respiratory changes and metabolic demands engendered by different types of exercise.

Crigler, L. 1974. Sexual concerns of the spinal cord-injured. *Nurs. Clin. North Am.* 9:703–717.
Neurophysiology of male and female sexual function; effects of spinal cord injury; specific counseling suggestions.

Drury, J. 1972. Handbook of range-of-motion exercises. *Nursing* 2(4):19–22.
Photographs of range-of-motion exercises for shoulder, elbow, hand, hip, knee, and foot.

Griffith, G. 1973. Sexuality and the cardiac patient. *Heart Lung* 2:70–73.
Review of studies on sexual activity and myocardial stress; ways to modify sexual activity to decrease stress; symptoms indicating excessive stress during sexual activities.

Hanlon, K. 1975. Maintaining sexuality after spinal cord injury. *Nursing* 5(5):58–62.
Anatomy and physiology of male sexual function; helpful ways to approach sexual counseling.

Kottke, F. 1971. Common cardiovascular problems in rehabilitation. In *Handbook of physical medicine and rehabilitation*, eds. F. Krusen, F. Kottke, and P. Ellwood, pp. 666–689. Philadelphia: W. B. Saunders Company.
Cardiac work at rest and during activity; peripheral vascular disease; lymphedema.

MacRae, I., and Henderson, G. 1975. Sexuality and irreversible health limitations. *Nurs. Clin. North Am.* 10:587–597.
Nursing assessment and interventions for patients with sexual disabilities due to paraplegia, arthritis, amputations, myocardial infarction, and emphysema.

Puksta, N. 1977. All about sex. . . after a coronary. *A. J. N.* 77:602–605.
Points to cover in assessment and teaching of myocardial infarction patients.

Stanford, D. 1977. All about sex. . . after middle age. *A. J. N.* 77:608–611.
Specific physiologic changes in sexual responses of older males and females.

Zelechowski, G. 1977. Helping your patient sleep: planning instead of pills. *Nursing* 7(5):63–65.
Measures to induce sleep; brief explanation of stages of sleep.

Chapter 15

Stimulation

In the FANCAS system, stimulation is defined as the process by which a person receives, interprets, and integrates impulses into a unified response (Swendsen 1975).

Outline

History

Physical examination Assessment of the level of consciousness / Examination of the cranium and neck / Assessment of the cranial nerves / Assessment of the sensorimotor function of the extremities / Examination of the vital signs

Diagnostic procedures Cerebrospinal fluid sampling / Electroencephalography / Pneumoencephalography and ventriculography / Cerebral arteriography / Computerized axial tomography

Objectives

- Assess the level ot consciousness.
- Identify the major structures contained in the anterior, middle and posterior fossae
- Define foramen magnum, dura mater, arachnoid, pia mater, falx cerebri, tentorium cerebelli, and cisterna magna
- Name the cerebral artery or arteries supplying the frontal lobe, parietal lobe, temporal lobe, occipital lobe, cerebellum, and brainstem

- Distinguish nasal mucus from a cerebrospinal fluid leak
- Examine the pupillary reflexes
- Briefly explain the tests for doll's eyes phenomenon and ice water caloric stimulation
- Assess the sensorimotor function of the extremities
- Recognize decorticate and decerebrate rigidity
- Differentiate between upper and lower motor neuron disease, specifying the kind of reflexes and paralysis seen with each
- Name the functions of the autonomic nervous system (ANS)
- Describe the origin, ganglionic characteristics and chemical mediators for the sympathetic and parasympathetic divisions of the ANS
- Recognize and state the significance of (1) post-hyperventilation apnea, (2) Cheyne-Stokes respiration, (3) prolonged hyperventilation, (4) apneustic respiration, and (5) ataxic breathing
- Describe the formation and circulation of cerebrospinal fluid
- Differentiate among lumbar, cisternal, and ventricular punctures in terms of indications, contraindications, and nursing care
- Provide the nursing care to patients undergoing (1) electroencephalography, (2) pneumoencephalography, (3) ventriculography, (4) cerebral arteriography, and (5) computerized axial tomography

Stimulation is mediated by the nervous system, a wondrously complex constellation of structures. These structures can be divided anatomically into those inside the skull and vertebral column—that is, the central nervous system consisting of the brain and spinal cord—and those outside the bony structures— that is, the peripheral nervous system consisting of the cranial, spinal, and autonomic nerves. The nervous system can be subdivided functionally into voluntary versus involuntary functions or sensory versus motor functions. Although these distinctions are helpful in developing a cognitive framework for understanding the nervous system, they blur in practical application to patient assessment. The assessment plan which follows is one of several ways to organize a practical, convenient assessment of a system which defies neat compartmentalization (Table 15-1).

History

The history of a patient with a neurological disorder often is quite extensive. When obtaining a history or reading the history recorded by the physician, remember to focus on information that is relevant to the person's present condition and has implications for his or her nursing care. Examples are a history of convulsions, language disturbances, paralysis, or Parkinson's disease. An im-

Table 15-1   Stimulation assessment format

1. History _____

2. Physical

   LOC _____

   Skull _____Neck _____

   Eyes: Corneal reflex _____

       Pupil size _____

       Reaction to light _____

   Extremities:

       Sensory function _____

       Voluntary motor function _____

       Reflex motor function

           DTRs _____

           Babinski _____

           Posturing _____

       Smoothness and coordination of movement _____

   _____

3. Diagnostic procedures and laboratory tests _____

   _____

4. Other relevant data _____

portant item to note is the length of the person's illness. If the illness is of recent onset, the patient and family may still be in the shock or disorganization phases of crisis (discussed in Chapter 13). On the other hand, if the illness has been prolonged, the person may have adapted to the chronic illness but need emotional support to cope with the discouragement caused by an acute exacerbation of the illness.

Physical examination

The key structures of the brain are shown in Figure 15-1.

The major divisions of the brain are classified according to embryological development as the forebrain, midbrain, and hindbrain (Jacob, Francone, and

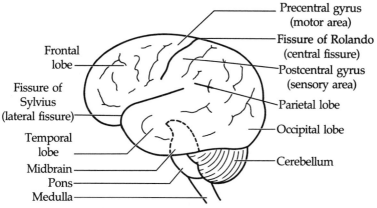

Figure 15-1.   Lateral view of brain.

Lossow 1978). The forebrain is composed of the cerebrum and diencephalon. The cerebrum consists of two identical cerebral hemispheres connected by the corpus callosum. Each hemisphere has four lobes: the frontal, parietal, temporal, and occipital. The diencephalon contains several structures around the third ventricle, the most important ones being the thalamus and hypothalamus. The next major part of the brain is the midbrain (mesencephalon), which connects the forebrain and hindbrain. The hindbrain consists of the cerebellum, pons, and medulla oblongata. The cerebellum sits below the occipital lobes and partially covers the brainstem. It, too, has two hemispheres connected to each other and the brainstem by tracts called cerebellar peduncles. Often, the midbrain, pons, and medulla collectively are called the brainstem. The brainstem thus extends from the diencephalon to the spinal cord. The functions of the various parts of the brain will be explained as the assessment plan progresses.

For easy reference, the functions of brain structures also are summarized in Table 15-2.

Assessment of the level of consciousness

Consciousness is mediated by the reticular activating system, which begins in the brainstem and ascends through the midbrain and thalamus to the cerebral cortex (Figure 15-2). The following description of this system is based on Guyton (1976).

The brain stem reticular formation receives input from collaterals of sensory neurons (from the cranial nerves or from ascending tracts between the spinal cord and thalamus or cerebellum) and motor neurons (descending from the cortex). It also receives stimuli from the hypothalamus, believed to contain indirect wake and sleep "centers." It integrates these stimuli and gives rise to the ascending reticular activating system, whose neurons project diffusely to the thalamus and hypothalamus. The brain stem reticular formation is believed to be responsible for general wakefulness; when it is stimulated, it causes diffuse

Table 15-2   Functions of brain structures

Structure	Functions
Cerebrum	Gray and white matter with sensory, motor, and integrative functions
A. Cerebral cortex	Outer layer consisting of gray matter
1) Frontal lobe	Complex intellectual functions such as memory, judgment, and problem solving; personality
Precentral gyrus	Primary motor area
2) Temporal lobe	Primary auditory area; taste, smell; comprehension of speech
3) Parietal lobe (specifically, postcentral gyrus)	Primary somatic sensory area
4) Occipital lobe	Primary visual area
B. Internal capsule	White matter; sensory and motor tracts, located between thalamus and basal ganglia
C. Basal ganglia	Gray matter deep in each hemisphere; coordination of muscular activity; automatic movements of expression
Diencephalon	Gray matter between cerebrum and midbrain; structures around third ventricle, particularly thalamus and hypothalamus
A. Thalamus	Gray matter located against lateral walls of third ventricle; reception of sensory impulses: participation in arousal mechanism; conscious awareness of crude sensations; relay of sensations to cortex for fine discrimination
B. Hypothalamus	Regulation of activity of autonomic nervous system; secretion of hormonal releasing factors, antidiuretic hormone and oxytocin; participation in arousal mechanism; control of appetite and body temperature
Brainstem	
A. Midbrain (mesencephalon)	White and gray matter connecting cerebrum and pons; contains nuclei of third cranial nerve (including the pupillary reflex center) and nuclei of fourth and part of fifth cranial nerves
B. Pons	White matter and nuclei of fifth to eighth cranial nerves; participation in regulation of respiration; projection tracts between brain and spinal cord
C. Medulla oblongata	Mostly white matter and nuclei of ninth to twelfth cranial nerves; cardiac, vasomotor, and respiratory reflex centers; also reflex centers for sneezing, coughing, vomiting, swallowing; projection tracts between brain and cord
D. Reticular activating system	Diffuse gray and white matter in brainstem core; relays impulses from cord and specialized sensory tracts to thalamus and then to cortex; portion rostral to midpons functions to arouse cerebral cortex and to maintain consciousness
Cerebellum	Coordination of muscular activity; maintenance of muscle tone, equilibrium, and posture

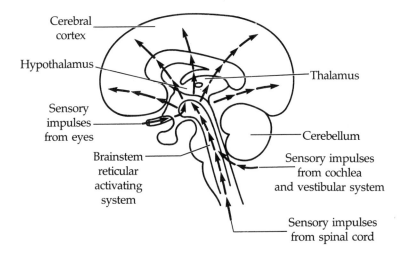

Figure 15-2. Reticular activating system.

activation of the entire brain. The thalamus has two functions in this system: it relays stimuli diffusely from the brain stem to the cortex and also selectively activates specific cortical areas. For full consciousness, the person must have both a functioning reticular activating system and relatively intact cerebral hemispheres (Plum and Posner 1972).

To assess the level of consciousness, ask the patient questions designed to test orientation to person, place, and time; insight; recent memory; and remote memory. For example, you might ask: "Who are you? Where are you? What month is this? Why are you here? What has happened to you in the last six hours? About how long ago did ____ (a remote event the patient is likely to know about) occur?" or similar questions.

Describe the level of consciousness in general terms only if they are known and agreed upon by all staff with whom you communicate. Jimm (1974) recommends the following descriptions:

Full consciousness: The person is alert and oriented to person, place, and time. He displays insight into his condition and recent and remote memory. He talks willingly, coherently, and clearly.

Early clouding of consciousness: The person appears alert and oriented at times but thinks slowly and displays lapses of memory and insight. He may ask repetitive questions whose answers he seemed to understand earlier.

Confusion or delirium: The person may be quiet and cooperative, or restless and irritable. He is not oriented to time or place, and may display delusions or hallucinations.

Stupor: The person is drowsy and hard to arouse, responding only if a stimulus is repeated. He responds purposefully to pressure and pain.

Coma: The person is unarousable, with no purposeful response to pressure or pain.

If such definitions are not commonly agreed upon, avoid using general terms. Instead, record the stimulus you used and response the patient exhibited, for example, "Patient responded to pressure on Achilles tendon by kicking nurse with other foot."

Examination of the cranium and neck

The skull is formed of many bones, the major ones of which are the frontal, parietal, temporal, occipital, and sphenoid bones and the cribiform plate. Disruption of these bones implies potential damage to the underlying structures.

The interior of the skull is divided into three areas. The anterior fossa contains the frontal lobes of the brain. The middle fossa contains the temporal, parietal, and occipital lobes. The posterior fossa contains the brainstem and cerebellum. At the base of the skull is an opening called the foramen magnum, through which the spinal cord emerges. Other openings in the skull provide passageways for the cranial nerves.

Between the skull and the brain, and between the vetebral column and spinal cord, are membranes called meninges. The outermost layer, the dura mater, is a tough membrane which adheres to the skull, though not to the vertebral column. The middle layer is the arachnoid. The innermost membrane, the pia mater, adheres to the brain and cord.

Folds of the dura support the brain. The midsagittal fold which divides the cerebral hemispheres is known as the falx cerebri. Its posterior portion swoops out laterally and anteriorly to form the tentorium cerebelli, which separates the middle from the posterior fossae, that is, the temporal and occipital lobes from the cerebellum and most of the brainstem. Structures contained in the anterior and middle cranial fossae thus are described as supratentorial, while those in the posterior fossa are infratentorial.

The spaces outside and between the meninges are named for their locations: between the skull and dura is the epidural space; between the dura and arachnoid is the subdural space; and between the arachnoid and the pia is the subarachnoid space. The larger subarachnoid spaces are called cisterns, the largest, the cisterna magna, being located between the foramen magnum and the first cervical vertebra.

The meninges provide spaces for the potential accumulation of blood and cerebrospinal fluid. Cerebrospinal fluid (CSF), which circulates in the subarachnoid space, will be discussed in detail later in the chapter. While inspecting and palpating the cranial bones, look for cerebrospinal fluid leaks, which usually appear as clear, colorless fluid oozing or dripping from the ear or nose or down the posterior pharynx. To differentiate the fluid from mucus, test it for glucose—CSF contains glucose, but mucus does not. The presence of blood in the fluid will invalidate this assessment tool, because blood contains glucose, too.

The arterial blood supply to the brain arises from the two internal carotid arteries anteriorly and the two vertebral arteries posteriorly (Figure 15-3). You

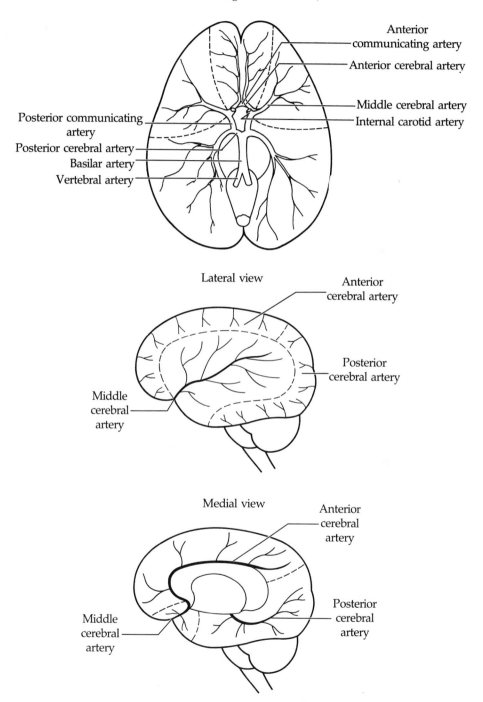

Figure 15-3. Major cerebral arteries and their areas of distribution.

may recall that the first three branches of the aorta are the brachiocephalic (which subdivides into the right common carotid and right subclavian arteries), the left common carotid, and the left subclavian arteries. The common carotid arteries give rise to the internal carotid arteries, which enter the skull through the cranial floor. The subclavian arteries give rise to the vertebral arteries, which travel up through the transverse processes of the cervical vertebrae and through the foramen magnum to unite into the basilar artery. The internal carotid arteries and basilar artery join at the base of the brain in the circle of Willis. The internal carotid arteries give rise to the anterior and middle cerebral arteries. The basilar artery gives rise to the posterior cerebral arteries. The circle of Willis provides for collateral circulation among all of these intracranial arteries so that even if one of the internal carotid or vertebral arteries becomes occluded, blood supply to the brain is maintained.

The anterior cerebral artery serves the anterior and middle portions of the brain tissue along the falx cerebri, that is, part of the frontal and parietal lobes. The middle cerebral artery nourishes the lateral part of the hemisphere, that is, portions of the frontal, parietal, and temporal lobes. The posterior cerebral artery serves the posterior surface of the hemisphere, that is, part of the temporal lobes and all of the occipital lobes. Branches of the vertebral and basilar arteries nourish the cerebellum and brainstem.

Branches of the cerebral arteries travel from the circle of Willis out over the surface of the cortex in the subarachnoid space. The meningeal arteries travel between the dura and skull. The veins draining the cortex travel mostly in the subarachnoid space. They empty into the superior sagittal sinus, inferior longitudinal sinus, and cavernous sinus, all of which eventually empty into the internal jugular vein and thus to the right atrium. Trauma to the cranium may lead to arterial or venous bleeding, depending upon the location of the injury.

While examining the skull, note also whether the person can touch his chin to his chest or whether nuchal rigidity (a sign of meningeal irritation) is present. (Do not flex the neck if trauma to the cervical spine is suspected.)

Assessment of the cranial nerves

Twelve pairs of cranial nerves emanate from the brain (Figure 15-4). The critical care nurse rarely performs a comprehensive evaluation of cranial nerves, instead focusing on those whose dysfunction may indicate life threats or seriously interfere with activities of daily living. The cranial nerves of primary importance to the critical care nurse thus are the optic (II), oculomotor (III), trigeminal (V), acoustic (VIII), glossopharyngeal (IX), and vagus (X). Several of these nerves have been mentioned in previous chapters: the optic and acoustic in Chapter 13 (Communication), the glossopharyngeal in Chapter 12 (Nutrition), and the vagus in Chapters 2 (Cardiac Assessment) and 3 (Arrhythmias and Conduction Defects). This chapter focuses on nursing examination of the patient's eyes. Such examination provides considerable information about the function of cranial nerves II, III, and V.

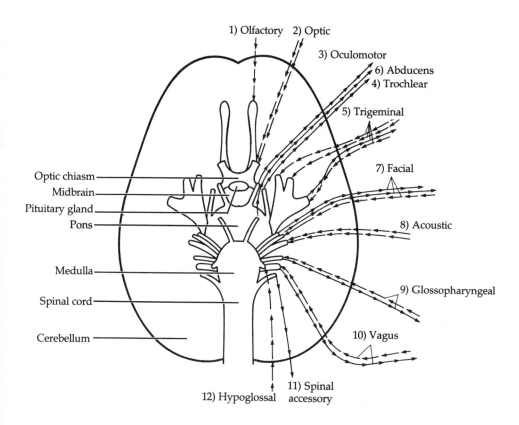

Nerve	Type	Major functions
1) Olfactory	Sensory	Smell
2) Optic	Sensory	Vision
3) Oculomotor	Motor	Eye movements (except those mediated by fourth and sixth cranial nerves), pupil size, and accommodation
4) Trochlear	Motor	Eye movements (superior oblique muscle)
5) Trigeminal	Sensorimotor	Sensations from face, cornea, teeth, tongue, nasal and oral mucosa; mastication
6) Abducens	Motor	Eye movements (lateral rectus muscle)
7) Facial	Sensorimotor	Taste from anterior two-thirds of tongue, facial expressions, salivation
8) Acoustic	Sensory	Hearing, equilibrium
9) Glossopharyngeal	Sensorimotor	Taste from posterior third of tongue, pharyngeal sensations, swallowing, salivation, reflex control of blood pressure, pulse, and respirations
10) Vagus	Sensorimotor	Sensation and movement of pharynx, larynx, thoracic and abdominal viscera
11) Spinal accessory	Motor	Movements of head, shoulders, pharynx, and larynx
12) Hypoglossal	Motor	Movements of tongue

Figure 15-4.   Cranial nerves.

When first examining a patient's eyes, note whether a corneal reflex is present. If the person does not blink spontaneously, test the reflex. With a fine wisp of cotton, approach the eye from the side. Avoid the eyelashes and touch the cornea lightly. Normally, this sensation is perceived by the trigeminal nerve and provokes intense blinking. If this reflex is absent, the cornea may become inflamed or ulcerated due to dryness, scratches, or particles which get in the eye. These conditions can deteriorate into inflammation of the iris and blindness. To prevent damage, lubricate the eye with artificial tears and cover with an eye shield. Periodically remove the shield, clean the eye area, and check for inflammation.

Next assess pupil size and response to light. Pupils should be equal in size, unless a congenital disparity exists or constricting or dilating eyedrops have been used in one eye. Anisocoria (unequal pupils) is probably unimportant unless other evidence of a third cranial nerve lesion exists, such as sluggish pupil constriction or diminished medial rectus function (inability to move the eye toward the nose). To enhance accuracy in communication, it is best to specify pupil size in millimeters (Figure 15-5) and also specify the degree of light in which you observed the eyes; for example, "dilated pupils" is less informative than "pupils 8 mm in brightly lit room."

Testing pupillary response to light involves testing both the optic and oculomotor nerves. The following testing procedure is recommended (*American Journal of Nursing* 1975). Darken the room if possible. If the patient is conscious, ask him to focus on a distant point. This will minimize the reflex constriction which occurs with focusing on a nearby point.

Place the edge of your hand along the patient's nose (to avoid the consensual response, explained below). Shine a bright light into one eye and observe the speed with which it constricts (direct light reflex). Repeat the procedure with the other eye. Each eye should constrict briskly. Next, remove your hand and shine the light so it strikes both eyes equally and simultaneously. Remove it and repeat. Each eye should constrict and dilate equally. Finally, put your hand on the patient's nose again. Shine the light in one eye and observe whether the other eye constricts; then test the other eye. When one eye is stimulated, the other should constrict (consensual light reflex). The reason this occurs is that one eye perceives the light and transmits impulses to the brain via the optic system; the brain, however, stimulates both oculomotor nerves.

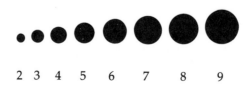

2   3   4   5   6   7   8   9

Figure 15-5.   Gauge of pupil size in millimeters.

A dilated, sluggish pupil is an ominous sign which can indicate impending herniation of the brainstem. Recall that a fold of dura, the tentorium, separates the cerebral hemispheres from the cerebellum. An opening in it, called the incisura or tentorial notch, allows the upper brainstem and its nerves and blood vessels to pass through. When supratentorial pressure increases, the structures near the notch become compressed. One of these structures is the third cranial (oculomotor) nerve. This nerve contains motor fibers (for eye movement) in the center and parasympathetic fibers (for pupillary constriction) on the outside. Compression of one oculomotor nerve causes loss of parasympathetic stimulation to the eye on the same side. Sympathetic stimulation continues unopposed, because the sympathetic fibers are not compressed. (The sympathetic pathway originates in the hypothalamus and courses through the brainstem to the upper three segments of the thoracic spinal cord where the sympathetic nerves to the eye originate.) The result is pupillary dilation and loss of the reflex response to light on the same side as the compression. If pressure is bilateral, both eyes will become dilated and sluggish. (For a complete discussion of abnormalities of pupil size and reflexes, see Plum and Posner.)

In addition to testing corneal and pupillary reflexes, you should understand the significance of two tests the physician may perform to evaluate oculocephalic reflexes. These tests are the doll's eyes phenomenon and caloric stimulation.

To test for the doll's eyes phenomenon, the physician holds the patient's eyelids open and rotates the head from side to side. In the normal (awake) patient, reflex eye movement cannot be elicited consistently because the patient can exert cortical control of eye movement. In the comatose patient, this maneuver sometimes will cause both eyes to move laterally in the direction opposite to the head rotation (Figure 15-6). This conjugate (parallel) lateral gaze is labelled a positive, normal, or intact doll's eyes response. To understand the significance

Head in neutral position	Head rotated to patient's left	
Eyes midline	Positive response: eyes move in relation to head	Negative response: eyes do not move in relation to head

Figure 15-6.   Doll's eyes phenomenon.

of this response, recall that the vestibular apparatus transmits information about head position along the acoustic nerve to the pons. The nerves controlling lateral gaze are the sixth cranial nerve from the pons and the third cranial nerve from the midbrain. A positive doll's eyes response indicates that information enters the lower pons, ascends to the upper pons and midbrain, and exits the appropriate cranial nerves, in other words, the brainstem is intact. A positive doll's eyes response thus means the coma-producing lesion is either supratentorial or metabolic. An absent (negative) doll's eyes reflex in a comatose patient usually indicates that the lesion is in the brainstem itself (Plum and Posner 1972). An exception is the negative doll's eyes response seen in sedative drug intoxication (the only metabolic encephalopathy in which negative doll's eyes is seen). This exception is important to remember, since drug-induced coma is very common. (The author is indebted to Dr. Roger Simon, Assistant Professor of Neurology at the University of California, San Francisco for a delightful way to remember the information about doll's eyes responses. He points out that expensive china dolls, such as his mother's, have eyes suspended on weights so that they move back and forth as the head is turned. Cheaper, "junky" dolls have painted-on eyes which remain fixed in the position of the head. Thus, eyes that remain fixed in midposition during head turning = junky doll = bad, while eyes that move from the midline during head rotation = expensive china doll = mother = good!)

Ice water stimulation (ice water calorics) is a maneuver that is physiologically identical to the doll's eyes maneuver but more powerful in inducing eye movements. The following descriptions are based on Plum and Posner (1972) and Carini and Owens (1974). After examining the ear for intactness of the tympanic membrane, the physician places the patient with the head elevated 30 degrees above the horizontal to provide maximal stimulation of the semicircular canal. He then uses a large syringe, filled with ice water, and a small catheter to slowly irrigate the canal until nystagmus or ocular deviation occurs (or 200 ml of water have been used). The response in the normal awake patient is nystagmus after 20–30 seconds, with slow movement toward the irrigated ear and rapid movement away. The slow phase of nystagmus indicates that impulses are being transmitted from the semicircular canal along the vestibular portion of the acoustic nerve to the pons; out along the sixth cranial nerve; and up into the midbrain and out along the third cranial nerve. The sixth nerve causes the eye closest (ipsilateral) to the irrigated ear to move laterally, while the third nerve causes the opposite (contralateral) eye to move medially. The mechanism for the quick phase of nystagmus is in the brainstem, but it is not well explained anatomically.

In the comatose patient, you may see the eyes move slowly toward the irrigated ear and remain there for 2–3 minutes; the fast return to midline (quick phase) has disappeared. This response indicates that the lesion is supratentorial or metabolic. If you see an extremely abnormal response, such as downward deviation and rotary jerking of one eye, the lesion is in the brainstem or cerebellum (the abnormal response will vary with the precise location of the lesion).

Assessment of the sensorimotor function of the extremities

The next step in assessment of stimulation is evaluation of limb sensation and movement. Interpretation of sensation and movement of the extremities requires not only comprehension of cranial function but also awareness of spinal cord function.

The vertebral column is made up of seven cervical, twelve thoracic, and five lumbar vertebrae plus the sacrum and coccyx. Central openings in the vertebrae form the spinal canal, which contains the spinal cord. The cord proper extends from the base of the brainstem through the foramen magnum to the second lumbar vertebra, from which a fibrous band attaches to the coccyx. Between the vertebrae and the spinal cord are the spinal meninges (dura, pia, and arachnoid). The cord is supplied by the anterior and posterior spinal arteries, which arise from the vertebral arteries at the foramen magnum, and by the lateral spinal arteries. Cerebrospinal fluid circulates between the arachnoid and the cord.

As a critical care nurse you usually will not perform a separate, systematic test of various sensations in all parts of the body. Instead, focus on the extremities, and integrate your assessment of sensation with your assessment of motor activity.

Sensory information reaches the spinal cord and brain from a variety of sources. Impulses pass from a sensory organ to a peripheral nerve, which carries sensory and motor fibers from a fairly wide area of the body. The peripheral nerves are regrouped closer to the spinal cord into nerve plexes (Figure 15-7) and then into thirty-one pairs of spinal nerves. The pairs of spinal nerves correspond to the thirty-one spinal segments (eight cervical, twelve thoracic, five lumbar, five sacral, and one coccygeal). Near the cord, the spinal nerves split into posterior and anterior roots (Figure 15-8). The roots connect with gray matter shaped like two pairs of horns within the spinal cord. The posterior (dorsal) root carries sensory fibers into the cord. The anterior (ventral) root carries motor fibers back out from the cord. Specific skin segments innervated by the sensory roots are called dermatomes. Dermatomes overlap each other considerably; a simplified diagram appears in Figure 15-9. Knowledge of dermatome innervation aids the physician in localizing a lesion causing a sensory abnormality.

Synapses within the cord enable sensory impulses to: (1) enter a spinal reflex arc back to the motor root; and/or (2) ascend the spinal cord to the cerebellum via the spinocerebellar tract; and/or (3) ascend the spinal cord to the cortex. To reach the cortex, impulses travel up spinal tracts to the thalamus and pass through the internal capsule to the sensory cortex, which is located behind the fissure of Sylvius in the parietal lobe. Different types of sensory information ascend different spinothalamic tracts (Figure 15-10). Only the most clinically important tracts are discussed here. Fibers carrying pain and temperature impulses enter the dorsal root and synapse with another neuron. This neuron crosses to the opposite side of the cord and ascends the lateral spinothalamic

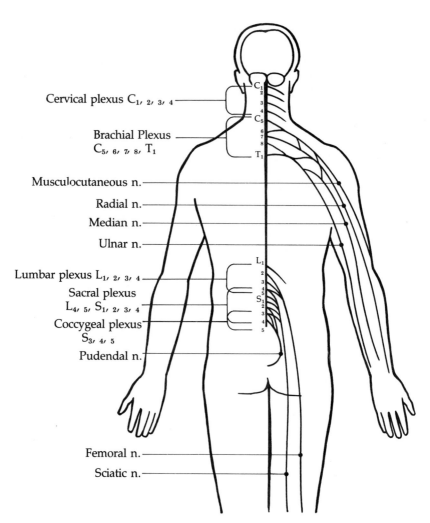

Cervical plexus C$_{1, 2, 3, 4}$

Brachial Plexus
C$_{5, 6, 7, 8}$, T$_1$

Musculocutaneous n.

Radial n.

Median n.

Ulnar n.

Lumbar plexus L$_{1, 2, 3, 4}$

Sacral plexus
L$_{4, 5}$, S$_{1, 2, 3, 4}$

Coccygeal plexus
S$_{3, 4, 5}$

Pudendal n.

Femoral n.

Sciatic n.

Figure 15-7. Spinal nerve plexes and major peripheral nerves arising from them.

tract to the thalamus. In the thalamus, the crude sensation is perceived and the neuron synapses with a third neuron. This third neuron travels through the internal capsule to the sensory cortex, where the stimulus is discriminated and localized. The loss of pain or temperature sensations on one side of the body may be due to damage to the sensory organs, peripheral nerves, spinal nerves, or dorsal roots on the same side, or (because pain and temperature fibers cross in the cord) damage to the lateral spinothalamic tract, thalamus, internal capsule, or sensory cortex on the opposite side of the body.

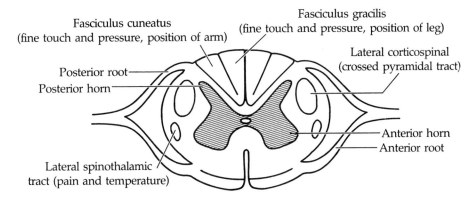

Figure 15-8.   Spinal cord in cross-section.

Fibers carrying fine touch and pressure impulses from the skin, and position and vibration impulses from muscles, tendons, and joints enter the cord and ascend uncrossed in the dorsal columns (posterior tract) to the medulla. (Impulses from the arm ascend in the column called the fasciculus cuneatus, those from the leg in the fasciculus gracilis). In the medulla, they synapse with another neuron. This neuron crosses within the medulla and ascends to the thalamus, which again perceives the general sensation. From the thalamus, a third neuron passes through the internal capsule to the sensory area in the parietal lobe.

Loss of fine touch, pressure, position, and vibration sensations on one side of the body can result from damage to the sensory organs, peripheral nerves, spinal nerves, dorsal roots, or dorsal columns on the same side of the body; damage to the medulla; or damage to the thalamus, internal capsule, or sensory cortex on the opposite side of the body.

Voluntary motor activity   Proceed with your examination by assessing the patient's motor function. Motor function can be classed conveniently into voluntary and involuntary activity.

Assess voluntary motor activity in the upper extremities by asking the patient to grip the second and third fingers of your hands. Note whether she is able to do so and compare the strength of her grip bilaterally. Alternatively, ask the patient to close her eyes and extend her arms for a few seconds. A drifting arm is an early sign of weakness. Assess voluntary motor activity in the legs by asking the patient to push her feet against your hands. (If the person does not respond to simple commands, test reflex motor activity with pressure or pain stimuli. Evaluation of reflex activity is discussed later in the chapter.)

Most voluntary activity originates in the primary motor cortex (precentral gyrus), which is a narrow strip in each frontal lobe, anterior to the fissure of Sylvius. Specific body parts are represented in a definite pattern, with the toes

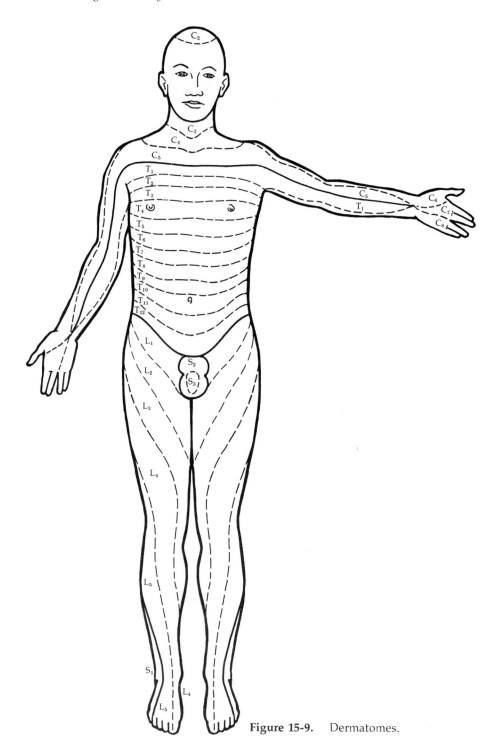

Figure 15-9.   Dermatomes.

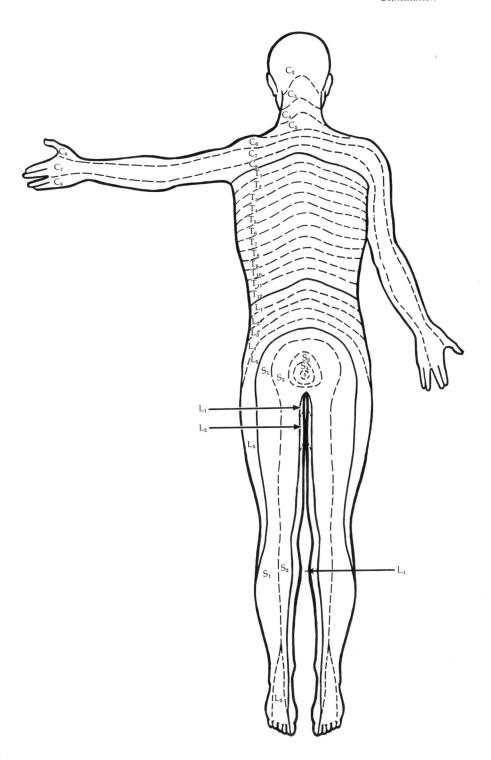

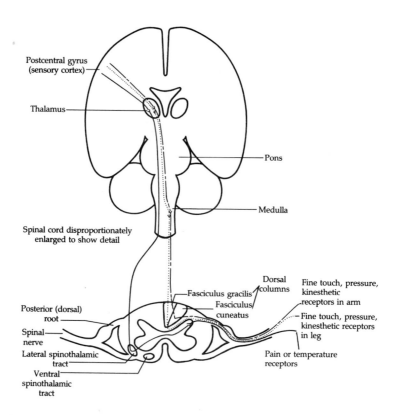

Postcentral gyrus
(sensory cortex)

Thalamus

Pons

Medulla

Spinal cord disproportionately
enlarged to show detail

Dorsal
columns

Fasciculus gracilis
Fasciculus
cuneatus

Fine touch, pressure,
kinesthetic
receptors in arm

Fine touch, pressure,
kinesthetic receptors
in leg

Posterior (dorsal)
root

Spinal
nerve

Lateral spinothalamic
tract

Ventral
spinothalamic
tract

Pain or temperature
receptors

Figure 15-10   Sensory (ascending) tracts for sensations from right side
of body.

closest to the top part of the hemisphere and the fingers closest to the fissure of
Sylvius (lateral fissure). Body parts are represented according to the discreteness
of their movement, for example, the hand is more highly represented than the
elbow.

From each motor cortex, fibers pass through the internal capsule on the same
side. (The capsules, which lie between the thalamus and basal ganglia, contain
both sensory and motor fibers.) The fibers continue to the medulla where they
are grouped to form the corticospinal (pyramidal) tracts (Figure 15-11). In the
medulla, most pyramidal fibers cross to the opposite side and continue down the
cord as the crossed pyramidal (lateral corticospinal) tract. Motor impulses leave
the cord via the anterior (ventral) horn and traverse spinal nerves, peripheral
nerves, and neuromuscular junctions before they reach the muscle itself.

Since the fibers cross in the medulla, voluntary movement initiated by the
motor cortex is manifested on the opposite side of the body. Thus, if your patient
has lost voluntary movement on one side of his body, it could result from
damage to the motor cortex, internal capsule, or medulla on the opposite side of

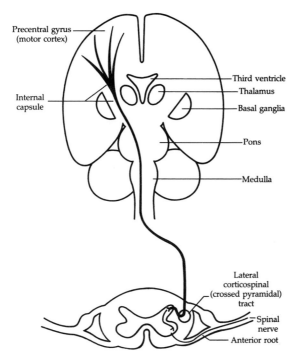

Precentral gyrus (motor cortex)

Internal capsule

Third ventricle
Thalamus
Basal ganglia

Pons

Medulla

Lateral corticospinal (crossed pyramidal) tract

Spinal nerve

Anterior root

Figure 15-11. Motor (descending) tracts for movement of right side of body.

the body; or the crossed pyramidal tract, ventral roots, spinal nerves, peripheral nerves, neuromuscular junctions, or muscles on the same side of the body.

Involuntary (reflex) motor activity   In addition to checking voluntary motor activity, it is important to evaluate involuntary (reflex) activity. Reflex activity can be classed into two broad types: autonomic and somatic. The autonomic nervous system will be discussed later in the chapter. Somatic reflexes are those mediated by the skeletal muscle cells. The cranial reflexes important for nurses to check have been discussed already and include pupillary, corneal, gag, and swallow reflexes. Spinal reflexes include deep and superficial reflexes. Deep reflexes usually are not tested by the critical care nurse; the physician tests them by briskly striking a partially stretched tendon or bony prominence with a reflex hammer and evaluating the resulting muscular contraction. Examples are the biceps and patellar reflexes.

The scale on which deep tendon reflexes are graded is as follows: 0^+ denotes no response; 1^+ denotes a reflex weaker than average; 2^+ denotes an average reflex; 3^+ denotes a reflex stronger than average; and 4^+ denotes a hyperactive reflex. A value of 1^+, 2^+, or 3^+ may be a normal reflex for the patient. An intact deep tendon reflex requires a healthy peripheral sensory nerve, spinal nerve, dorsal root, cord synapse, motor root, motor nerve, neuromuscular junction, and muscle. Reflex activity does not depend upon pyramidal or extrapyramidal tracts or the cerebellum, but they may influence the intensity and smoothness of a reflex.

Superficial reflexes are tested by stroking the skin. One superficial reflex you may have observed in males is the cremasteric reflex: stroking the inner thigh skin (such as when you manipulate a urinary catheter) causes testicular elevation on the same side. Critical care nurses evaluate superficial reflexes when they use light pressure to evoke a withdrawal response in a patient who does not respond to simple commands or check the plantar reflex for the Babinski sign.

To evaluate the plantar reflex, use a fairly sharp object such as a pen. Start at the outer edge of the heel. Stroke up the outer side of the sole and across the ball of the foot. Normally, the person will plantar flex the big toe. The abnormal response of dorsiflexing the big toe (and sometimes flaring the other toes) is called a positive Babinski sign and indicates damage to the pyramidal tract (Figure 15-12).

As mentioned earlier, if the person does not display voluntary motor activity, pressure or pain should be used to elicit reflex activity. Avoid pinching the patient as repeated pinching will bruise the patient. Instead, try light pressure by stroking the extremity; if no response, try deep pressure by pressing intensely on the sides of the fingertips or toes, the Achilles tendon, the supraorbital ridge, the trapezius muscle, or the sternum. Note the specific patient response and evaluate it as appropriate, inappropriate, or absent. Appropriate responses include pushing your hand away or withdrawing from the stimulus. They indicate that sensory function is intact and motor function from the cortex to the muscle is present to some degree. Inappropriate responses include unilateral or bilateral decorticate or decerebrate postures (Figure 15-13). The following information on these postures is from Plum and Posner (1972). If the patient's

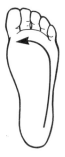 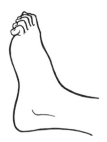 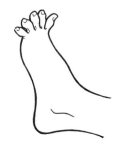

Stroke up sole of foot and across ball   Normal response—plantar flexion of all toes   Abnormal response—dorsiflexion of big toe with or without fanning of other toes.

Figure 15-12.   Babinski sign.

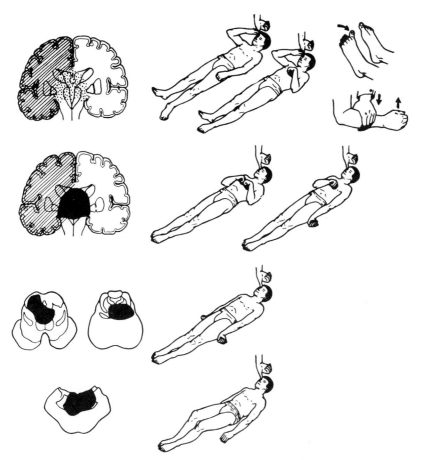

Figure 15-13.   Motor responses to noxious stimulation in patients with acute cerebral dysfunction. **Top line:** internal capsular or cerebral hemispheric lesions interrupting corticospinal pathways. The contralateral side shows hemiparesis or a decorticate response, and positive Babinski sign. The ipsilateral side shows appropriate response to stimuli but resistance to passive movement. **Second line:** deep hemispheric lesions starting to press on upper brainstem. The contralateral side displays the decorticate or decerebrate response, while the ipsilateral side is decorticate or appropriate response. **Third line:** an infarct destroying entire brainstem above the middle of the pons, or massive cerebral hemorrhages destroying or compressing the lower thalamus and midbrain. Both sides display decerebrate posturing. **Fourth line:** extensive damage to the brainstem down to or across the pons at the trigeminal level. The upper limbs show decerebrate signs, while the lower limbs remain flaccid or display a weak flexor response. (From Plum, F., and Posner, J., 1972. *The Diagnosis of Stupor and Coma.* 2nd ed. Philadelphia: F. A. Davis Company. Used with permission of the author and publisher.)

response is to bring his arm next to his body; flex his fingers, wrist, and arm; and extend his leg, rotate it internally, and plantar flex his foot, he is exhibiting decorticate posturing. This response is typical of the interruption of corticospinal pathways produced by a lesion in the motor cortex or internal capsule. If the patient's response is to rigidly extend his arms and legs, bring his arms close to his body and hyperpronate them, plantar flex his feet, and sometimes to arch his back (opisthotonus), he is displaying decerebrate posturing. This sign indicates a more life-threatening situation than decorticate posturing. It indicates a cerebral lesion which is compressing or destroying the lower thalamus and midbrain, or all the brainstem above the middle of the pons. Decerebrate changes in the arms with flaccidity or weak flexor responses in the legs are primitive reactions seen in patients with extensive brainstem damage.

There are some important points to remember about decorticate and decerebrate postures. The above descriptions are of full-blown responses; often, you will see only fragments of a posture, such as flexion of one arm. These fragments are important to note and report to the physician, as they are early indicators of abnormal responses. The postures may occur with or without your stimulation, and may be intermittent or continuous.

Motor neuron disease   Disorders causing loss of voluntary or reflex movement commonly are described as upper motor neuron or lower motor neuron disease. As mentioned earlier, peripheral nerves can carry motor and sensory fibers. The motor fibers eventually subdivide so that one motor fiber serves one muscle fiber. This last motor neuron innervating a muscle fiber is called the final common pathway because all motor impulses must pass through it to the muscle fiber.

Motor neurons serving the final common pathway are of two types. Those between the cerebral cortex and the motor nuclei of the brainstem or spinal cord are called upper motor neurons. Those between the motor nuclei of the brainstem (for cranial nerves) or the anterior horn cell in the spinal cord (for spinal nerves) and the muscle are called lower motor neurons.

Upper motor neuron disease produces hyperactive reflex activity· while the reflex arc remains intact, cortical inhibition is lost. Although reflex activity is retained, voluntary motor function is lost (spastic paralysis). An example of upper motor neuron disease is hemiparesis following a cerebrovascular accident. Lower motor neuron disease produces hypoactive reflexes, loss of voluntary movement, and muscle atrophy (flaccid paralysis). An example is anterior poliomyelitis.

Extrapyramidal system   During your assessment of motor activity, observe whether movements are smooth and coordinated. Background muscle tone, automatic movements (such as those which maintain posture), equilibrium, smoothness, and coordination of muscular activity are controlled by the extrapyramidal system. This system consists of the cerebellum, basal ganglia (gray matter in the cerebrum), and extrapyramidal pathways in the spinal cord.

The cerebellum, located below the occipital lobes of the cerebrum, consists of two hemispheres. Tracts (peduncles) connect the hemispheres to each other and to the brainstem. The cerebellum receives input from the motor cortex, brain stem, and peripheral areas. It modifies motor activity in numerous ways, which can be grouped into regulation of muscle tone, coordination of muscle movements, and maintenance of equilibrium.

The basal ganglia are bodies of gray matter found beneath each cerebral hemisphere. They control habitual acts and help adjust muscle tone.

Impulses from the cerebellum and basal ganglia are transmitted to the muscles via extrapyramidal pathways in the spinal cord. Thus, loss of smoothness and coordination can result from damage to the cerebellum, basal ganglia, and/or extrapyramidal pathways in the cord.

Patterns of pathology   So far, correlation of signs and symptoms and sites of dysfunction has been presented beginning with the symptom and then identifying possible sites. As you have seen, most symptoms can be due to lesions in a variety of sites. The differential diagnosis of pathology requires extensive education and experience in neurology, and is based upon the level and extent of symptomatology and a knowledge of the patterns of findings produced by lesions in different sites. Some patterns of pathology which you may observe are presented in Table 15-3. It is useful to acquaint yourself with them, both to understand how a neurologist identifies the site of a lesion and to predict a patient's deficits from a medical diagnosis so you can better plan nursing care.

Examination of the vital signs

Vital signs can provide valuable clues to nervous system function but must be interpreted with caution due to the multiplicity of factors which influence them. It is also important to remember that changes in level of consciousness are earlier, more sensitive indicators of central nervous system dysfunction than are vital sign changes.

Autonomic nervous system   Although vital signs can be affected by the voluntary nervous system, they are controlled primarily by the involuntary or autonomic nervous system (ANS). This complex system is responsible for unconscious control of involuntary muscles and most glands. It therefore regulates vital signs, fluid intake and output, appetite, gastrointestinal activity, carbohydrate and fat metabolism, sleep, and sexual functioning. Its effects are widespread because they are exerted both by nerves and by chemical mediators.

Overall control of the ANS resides in the hypothalamus. From the hypothalamus, neurons descend through the brainstem and spinal cord and end in three groups. One group of neurons is clustered in the brainstem (around the nuclei of the third cranial nerve in the midbrain and the seventh, ninth, and tenth cranial nerves in the medulla). Another group of neurons is located in the cord around the thoracic and upper lumbar vertebrae, and the last group is

Table 15-3   Patterns of Pathology

Type of loss	Location of lesion
Sensory	
1. Decrease or loss of all sensation in area served by peripheral nerve	Peripheral nerve
2. Decrease or loss of all sensation in dermatome	Sensory (dorsal) root
3. Decrease or loss of pain and temperature sensation on one side of body	Lateral spinothalamic tract on opposite side of body
4. Decrease or loss of fine touch discrimination, vibration awareness, awareness of limb position	Dorsal column (fasciculus gracilis or cuneatus) on same side of body
5. Decrease or absence of all sensation on one whole side of body	Thalamus on opposite side of body
6. Retention of crude sensation with loss of fine discrimination on one whole side of body	Sensory cortex on opposite side of body
Motor	
1. Loss of reflex activity with retention of voluntary activity	Sensory neuron on same side of body
2. Loss of voluntary activity below level of lesion with retention of reflex activity (spastic paralysis)	Corticospinal (pyramidal) tract (upper motor neuron); side of body depends on level of lesion
3. Loss of voluntary and reflex activity below level of lesion (flaccid paralysis)	Lower motor neuron on same side of body
4. Decrease or loss of fine sensation and voluntary movement on entire side of body, with retention of crude sensation and reflex activity	Internal capsule
5. Decrease of muscle tone; inability to synchronize movements, gauge distance and speed, alternate movements quickly; intention tremor; poor equilibrium; voluntary and reflex motor activity present	Cerebellum
6. Rigidity, resting tremor, involuntary movements such as in Huntington's chorea; voluntary and reflex motor activity present	Extrapyramidal system

centered around the sacral portion of the cord (Figure 15-14). The thoracolumbar group gives rise to the sympathetic division of the ANS, and the cranial and sacral groups form the parasympathetic division.

Neurons from the thoracic and lumbar area leave the cord through its anterior roots and form an interconnected chain of ganglia on either side of the vertebral column and along its complete length. Since these sympathetic ganglia are close to the cord, fibers between the cord and the ganglia (preganglionic fibers) are short, while those between the ganglia and effector organs (postganglionic fibers) are long. The primary chemical mediator exerted by sympathetic

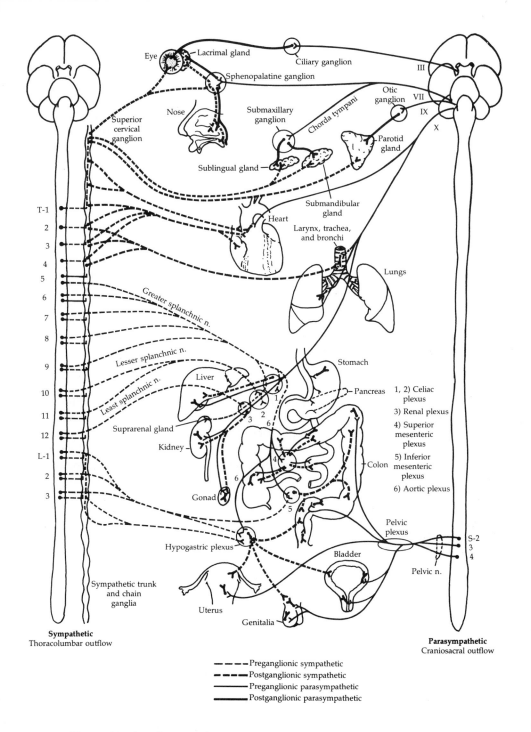

Figure 15-14. Autonomic nervous system. (From Jacob, S., and Francone, C., 1965. *Structure and Function in Man.* Philadelphia: W. B. Saunders Company. Used with permission of the author and publisher.)

fibers is noradrenalin; drugs that mimic its effects are called adrenergic or sympathomimetic agents.

In contrast to the sympathetic system, neurons from the cranial and sacral parts of the ANS form parasympathetic ganglia near the effector organs. Their preganglionic fibers thus are long and their postganglionic fibers short. The parasympathetic fibers secrete acetylcholine, and drugs mimicking its effects are known as cholinergic agents.

The distribution of fibers to effector organs does not necessarily follow the distribution of spinal nerves and is determined partially by the embryonic origin of the organ. Most muscles and glands are innervated by both sympathetic and parasympathetic fibers; their effects are antagonistic but balanced.

Changes in temperature   Although temperature is regulated by the hypothalamus, changes in temperature more often reflect infection in other body sites than hypothalamic dysfunction. Metabolic coma, exposure to extreme cold, and hypothalamic disorders may produce a temperature drop (Plum and Posner 1972), while a rise may occur with cerebrospinal fluid infection, blood in the CSF, dehydration, or exposure to extreme heat.

Changes in blood pressure   Blood pressure is influenced by the vasomotor center in the lower pons and upper medulla. This center exerts its effects on blood vessels through the sympathetic vasoconstrictor system, which contains fibers to all blood vessels except capillaries. The lateral portions of the vasomotor center excite the sympathetic vasoconstrictor fibers, while the medial portion inhibits them. The vasomotor center responds to a variety of stimuli, including input from the cerebral cortex, hypothalamus, and reticular substance of the pons, midbrain, and diencephalon; central and peripheral chemoreceptors which sense changes in CO_2 concentration of the CSF and arterial blood; and peripheral baroreceptors which sense changes in blood pressure. Because of the influence of peripheral reflexes and other factors, the cardiovascular system is able to function even without central nervous system regulation. Blood pressure changes do occur with posterior fossa lesions, hypertensive encephalopathy, and following subarachnoid hemorrhage, but otherwise appear inconsistently or not at all. As a result, blood pressure changes are not very useful as indicators of neurological status.

Pulse rate and volume changes   As with blood pressure, the pulse rate and volume are under both peripheral and central control. The pulse is influenced by the vasomotor center in the lower pons and upper medulla. The lateral portions send excitatory impulses via the sympathetic nerves to the heart, thus increasing pulse rate and myocardial contractility. The medial portion sends inhibitory impulses to the heart via the vagus nerves (part of the parasympathetic system), thus slowing the heart rate. Arrhythmias may occur due to pressure on the vasomotor center or, more commonly, blood gas alterations which accompany brain disorders.

Respiratory changes   Respiration is influenced by many levels of the brain and cannot occur without central nervous system regulation of skeletal muscles (Plum and Posner 1972). Since respiration also is influenced by metabolic factors, they must be ruled out before one assumes a neurological basis for abnormal respiration.

The respiratory center in the medulla and pons consists of three areas: the rhythmicity center in the medulla and the apneustic and pneumotaxic centers in the pons (Guyton 1976). The medullary center sets the basic respiratory rhythm of a short inspiration and longer expiration. Without input from additional areas, however, its activity is weak and uncoordinated. The apneustic and pneumotaxic centers in the pons are not required for the basic rhythm of respiration but do function to make it smoother and stronger. Influences from stretch receptors in the lung, peripheral and central chemoreceptors, the spinal cord, midbrain, and cerebral cortex also modify respiratory rate, depth, and pattern.

As explained in Chapter 9, the most potent stimulus to respiration is the CO_2 concentration or pH of cerebrospinal fluid bathing the respiratory center. The CSF in turn is influenced by changes in CO_2 concentration or pH in arterial blood. Increased CO_2 concentration (decreased pH) causes the rate and depth of respirations to increase (hyperventilation), while decreased CO_2 concentration (increased pH) causes the respiratory rate and depth to decrease. Plum and Posner (1972) state that when hyperventilation reduces arterial CO_2 tension below its normal resting level, the stimulus that causes rhythmic breathing appears to arise from the forebrain. In other words, rhythmic breathing due to normal variation in CO_2 appears to originate in the respiratory center, while that following hyperventilation appears to originate in the forebrain.

Respiratory patterns thus can be used as a reliable guide to the level of neurological involvement once metabolic causes (such as diabetic ketoacidosis) have been ruled out. Following are the most common respiratory changes in neurological patients, based on Plum and Posner's descriptions (Figure 15-15).

After taking five or six deep breaths, the normal person experiences either no apnea or apnea of less than 10 seconds; presumably, the lowered arterial CO_2 tension produced by this hyperventilation has been followed by a forebrain stimulus to respiration. If breathing ceases for more than 12 seconds after this maneuver (post-hyperventilation apnea), the forebrain response is lacking and the person will resume breathing only when the accumulating CO_2 in the blood again stimulates the respiratory center. Post-hyperventilation apnea indicates a diffuse process affecting both cerebral hemispheres, such as metabolic disease, dementia, or hypertensive encephalopathy.

Smoothly alternating hyperpnea and apnea is known as Cheyne-Stokes respiration. It results from the combination of an increased respiratory center response to CO_2 stimulation (which produces the hyperpnea) and a decreased forebrain response to lowered CO_2 (which produces the apnea). The neurological cause usually is bilateral lesions deep in the cerebral hemispheres and basal ganglia that also damage the internal capsules. (Cheyne-Stokes respiration in cardiac failure probably results from prolonged circulation time between the

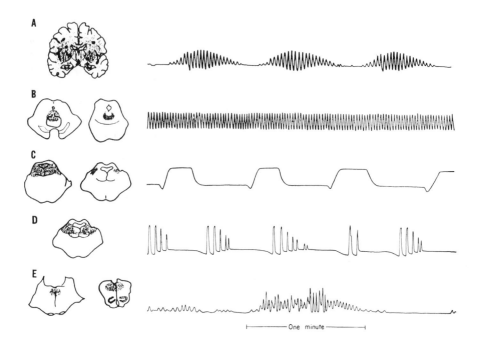

Figure 15-15. Abnormal respiratory patterns associated with pathologic lesions (shaded areas) at various levels of the brain. Tracings by
chest-abdomen pneumograph, inspiration reads up. **A,** Cheyne-Stokes
respiration; **B,** central neurogenic hyperventilation; **C,** apneusis; **D,** cluster breathing; **E,** ataxic breathing. (From Plum, F., and Posner, J., 1972.
The Diagnosis of Stupor and Coma. 2nd ed. Philadelphia: F. A. Davis Company. Used with permission of the publisher.)

lungs and brain. This delay allows large changes in blood gas concentration to
occur before the respiratory center detects and reacts to them.)

A pattern of prolonged, rapid hyperpnea occurs in some patients with lesions in the low midbrain and upper pons, and many patients in whom cerebral
hemorrhage has caused herniation through the tentorial notch and resulting
midbrain compression. Plum and Posner called this pattern central neurogenic
hyperventilation. Recently, however, the genesis of this pattern in neurological
patients has been disputed. It is possible that the pattern arises from hypoxia
associated with the neurological disorders rather than a central neurogenic
mechanism per se (Shapiro 1975). Hyperpnea is also seen in pulmonary edema,
heart failure, and hepatic coma.

Brief (2–3 second) pauses at the end of inspiration characterize apneustic
breathing. Expiratory pauses and other irregularities may be present as well.
This pattern indicates extensive pontine lesions.

Varying groups of breaths with irregular in-between pauses (cluster breathing) typify lesions in the lower pons or upper medulla.

Totally irregular respiration indicates damage to the respiratory center in the medulla, such as that produced by cerebellar, pontine, or medullary hemorrhage. Called ataxic breathing, this type consists of random shallow and deep breaths with irregular apneic pauses. It indicates disrupted coordination between inspiratory and expiratory neurons in the medulla. With respiratory center damage, the patient is more susceptible to depressant drugs and less susceptible to usual chemical stimulation than normal, so that respiratory depressants or sleep may produce apnea. (Interestingly, the center frequently responds to cortical control, so the patient can continue breathing by conscious effort.) This type of breathing necessitates mechanical ventilation.

Diagnostic procedures

Numerous diagnostic procedures are available to aid the physician and you in assessing the location and extent of neurological damage and the prognosis for recovery. The ones reviewed here are those done most commonly on the critically ill: cerebrospinal fluid sampling, electroencephalography, pneumoencephalography, ventriculography, cerebral arteriography, and computerized axial tomography. Intracranial pressure monitoring is discussed in the next chapter.

Cerebrospinal fluid sampling

Cerebrospinal fluid (CSF) is secreted from blood primarily by the choroid plexus. The plexus consists of tufts of capillaries and epithelium lining the brain's ventricular system. The ventricular system is composed of two lateral ventricles, a central third ventricle, a fourth ventricle located between the brainstem and cerebellum, and interconnecting canals (Figure 15-16).

One lateral ventricle sits in each cerebral hemisphere and consists of an anterior horn in the frontal lobe, a body in the parietal lobe, a posterior horn in the occipital lobe, and an inferior horn in the temporal lobe (Carini and Owens 1974). From each lateral ventricle, CSF passes through a foramen of Monroe into the third ventricle and then through the aqueduct of Sylvius into the fourth ventricle. It then passes through openings in the fourth ventricle into the subarachnoid space. After flowing over the brain and down around the spinal cord, it is drained from the subarachnoid space through the arachnoid villi, which project into the superior sagittal sinus, the large superficial midline sinus of the dura mater.

CSF functions to cushion and nourish the brain. It is formed and absorbed constantly, at the rate of 400–500 ml in 24 hours; at a given moment, about 140 ml is circulating. It is clear, colorless, and odorless, and normally contains no red cells and few white cells. Glucose content varies with the serum glucose level, averaging about 60% of the serum glucose. The normal value is approximately 50–75 mg/100 ml. Protein concentration varies with the sampling site, normally measuring 5–15 mg/100 ml in the ventricles, 15–25 mg in the cisterna magna,

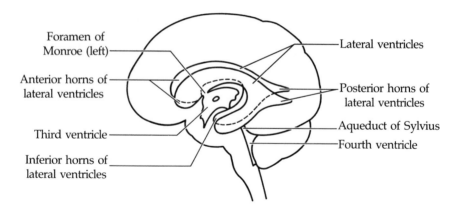

Foramen of
Monroe (left)

Anterior horns of
lateral ventricles

Third ventricle

Inferior horns of
lateral ventricles

Lateral ventricles

Posterior horns of
lateral ventricles

Aqueduct of Sylvius

Fourth ventricle

Figure 15-16.   Ventricular system (left lateral view).

and 15–45 mg in the spinal canal (Brunner and Suddarth 1975). Normal specific gravity is 1.007. Opening pressure varies with position, up to 200 mm H_2O recumbent and up to 300 mm H_2O sitting.

Samples of CSF can be obtained from the lumbar subarachnoid space of the spinal canal, the cisterna magna (the large subarachnoid space below the occipital bone), and the lateral ventricles. For sampling at any site, the patient and/or family should be prepared psychologically with a description of the benefits and risks, steps in the procedure, and normal sensations. An informed consent should be signed and the patient sedated if necessary. Lumbar and cisternal punctures may be done in the critical care unit; ventricular punctures usually are performed in surgery or in some cases on the unit. The following descriptions of the various procedures are based on Blount, Kinney, and Donohoe (1974), Brunner and Suddarth (1975), Carini and Owens (1974), and Kinney, Blount, and Donohoe (1974).

A lumbar puncture, the most common, may be done to measure CSF pressure, sample CSF, remove CSF to lower intracranial pressure, or inject contrast media or medications. Contraindications to a lumbar puncture are inflammation at the proposed injection site, a subarachnoid block, or greatly increased intracranial pressure; in the latter case, removal of CSF from the spinal canal could precipitate brain herniation. To assist with a lumbar puncture, explain to the patient that the procedure will last only a few minutes and usually is not painful; that the doctor will give him a local anesthetic to reduce the feeling of pressure from the needle insertion; that he will lie on his side and should stay very still; and that he may experience short pains in his legs or pelvis if the needle brushes nerves to those areas. Bring to the bedside a lumbar puncture tray, local anesthetic, sterile gloves, and a bandaid. Place the patient on his side with his back at the edge of the bed and his spine curved, or have him sit up and bend over a bedside table. You may need to hold a restless patient. The physician will clean the skin, and infiltrate it with a local anesthetic. He then will insert the needle and stylet at the level of the iliac crests. Insertion of the needle at this level places its tip in the spinal canal below the termination of the cord. After removing the stylet, the physician will connect the manometer, measure opening pressure, drain off fluid into laboratory tubes, measure closing pressure, remove the needle, and cover the puncture site with a small bandage. During the procedure, reassure the patient, remind him not to move, and observe for a change in the level of consciousness, which may signify herniation. After the procedure, observe for changes in the level of consciousness or vital signs, meningeal irritation, and edema or hematoma at the puncture site. Headache is common and may be eased by having the patient remain prone for 1–6 hours, increased fluid intake, and analgesics. Transient back and leg pain may result from nerve root irritation.

A puncture of the cisterna magna may be done if a lumbar puncture is contraindicated or a subarachnoid block is present. Contraindications to a cisternal puncture are posterior fossa pathology or greatly increased intracranial pressure. To assist with a cisternal puncture, explain the procedure to the patient. Shave the nape of the neck and place the patient on his side with his back at the edge of the bed and a sandbag under his head. Bend his head slightly forward and hold it firmly. The physician will clean and anesthetize the skin, and insert the needle below the occipital bone in the midline. The test proceeds as does a lumbar puncture and observations are the same (with the exception of back and leg pain, which do not occur with a cisternal puncture). Headache usually does not follow a cisternal puncture.

A ventricular puncture is done if lumbar and cisternal ones are contraindicated, ventriculography is planned, or ventricular drainage is necessary for increased intracranial pressure. It cannot be used to visualize the cranial subarachnoid space. This procedure is not done in the critical care unit except for emergency ventricular drainage through a previously established burr hole. To assist with emergency drainage, place the patient on his side opposite the lateral ventricle to be tapped and hold his head. The physician will prepare the skin, insert the needle into the ventricle and proceed as above. (The patient without a previous burr hole is taken to the operating room. After the site is shaved, the physician cleans and anesthetizes the skin. He then incises the scalp, makes a burr hole through the skull, incises the dura, and inserts the needle into the ventricle.) Nursing care following a ventricular puncture consists of 10–15 degree elevation of the head; bedrest for 24 hours; neurologic checks every 30–60 minutes until stable; and maintenance of a dry, sterile dressing over the sutured skin incisions. The patient should be watched closely, as he may develop an anaphylactic reaction to the contrast media; headache; respiratory distress; convulsions; or increasing intracranial pressure.

Electroencephalography

In this procedure, the electrical activity of the brain is recorded from scalp electrodes. The electroencephalogram (EEG) is used to diagnose disorders which cause changes in electrical patterns, such as epilepsy, tumors, and brain death.

Other than an explanation to the patient, no particular preparation is necessary. The patient will be taken to a soundproofed, electrically-shielded room or, if he is too sick to be moved, the EEG will be recorded at the bedside. Electrodes are applied with paste or needles to the scalp over the various lobes and the tracing is recorded while the patient remains relaxed and still to avoid creating electrical artifacts. The EEG may take up to 2 hours and will be interrupted periodically so the patient can change position. Alert the patient in advance that he will be asked to hyperventilate for a short time to provoke any abnormal discharge; he can anticipate transient lightheadedness or dizziness during this hyperventilation.

An EEG is not painful and does not produce any post-procedure complications.

Pneumoencephalography and ventriculography

These diagnostic tests are performed outside the critical care unit, usually in the neuroradiology department. Both pneumonencephalography and ventriculography involve removal of cerebrospinal fluid and injection of air to visualize the ventricular system. When a lumbar or cisternal puncture is used, the procedure is called pneumoencephalography; when a ventricular puncture is used, the procedure is called ventriculography. Both procedures allow the physician to evaluate the patency of the ventricular system, localize intracranial masses, and detect cerebral atrophy. In addition, pneumoencephalography allows visualization of the intracranial subarachnoid space. When the physician suspects greatly increased intracranial pressure or a lesion in the posterior fossa, the procedure of choice for CSF sampling is ventriculography. The reason is greater danger of brain herniation through the tentorial notch or foramen magnum when pressure is released from below the brain by lumbar or cisternal puncture.

Prior to the procedure, collaborate with the physician to explain to the patient and/or family its benefits and risks and secure written consent. Also teach the patient what to expect before, during, and after the procedure. The patient should anticipate a sedative the night before the procedure, unless one is contraindicated (for example by fluctuating levels of consciousness). He should also expect no food or water for eight hours before the procedure; shaving of the entry site; and premedication (if used in your institution). Before premedicating him, remember to assess and record his vital signs, level of consciousness, pupillary activity, and extremity sensorimotor function.

As part of your pre-procedure teaching, inform the patient of the procedural details pertinent to your institution. Usually, he will be taken to the neuroradiology department and restrained in a special chair with x-ray plates directly in front of his face. He will be draped and given local or general anesthesia. If a local anesthetic is planned, be sure to prepare him for the likelihood of headache, nausea, and vomiting during the procedure. These reactions are more severe with pneumoencephalography.

The physician will make the appropriate puncture (see section on CSF sampling for details). In a ventriculogram, he gradually will remove up to 50 ml of CSF and replace it with air or oxygen. In a pneumoencephalogram (PEG), he will inject a small amount of air or oxygen before removing any CSF, to visualize the third and fourth ventricles; after obtaining an x-ray of them, he gradually will remove up to 30 ml of CSF and replace it with air or oxygen. During the removal and injection period, assisting staff will provide emotional support and monitor the patient closely for the anticipated effects mentioned above and for signs of increased intracranial pressure.

The needle will be removed and x-ray studies will be done with the patient's head tilted in various positions. He will be returned to his room unless immediate surgery is indicated.

Post-procedure, keep him in bed for 24 hours (flat for a PEG and with head elevated 15° for a ventriculogram) and assist him in turning side to side every two hours. Perform a neurological assessment every 30 minutes to 4 hours, depending upon the patient's stability. Watch for sustained severe headache, convulsions, shock, and other signs of increased intracranial pressure or meningitis. Treat minor problems (such as nausea and vomiting) symptomatically, according to the physician's orders. Encourage an oral or intravenous fluid intake of 2500–3500 ml unless a high fluid intake is contraindicated by increased intracranial pressure or co-existing problems such as congestive heart failure. The patient usually can increase activity on the second day, though he may continue feeling tired, headachy, and irritable for several days.

For a first-hand account of the sensations involved in pneumoencephalography, see the article by Blackwell (1975).

Cerebral Arteriography

In this diagnostic maneuver, contrast media is injected into the cerebral circulation to visualize the arteries and veins. It is used to detect aneurysms, occlusions, hematomas, tumors, and other lesions sizable enough to destroy cerebral vessels.

Before the procedure, assist the physician in explaining its benefits and risks and secure informed consent. Particularly prepare the patient for the sequence of steps and the intense burning sensation he may experience when dye is injected. This sensation is normal and lasts for 20–30 seconds.

Pre-procedure preparation usually includes a sedative the night before, nothing by mouth for 8 hours before the procedure, and shaving of the proposed injection site. Just before the patient leaves the unit, you should record a current neurological assessment and *then* premedicate him.

The patient will be taken to the neuroradiology department and placed on a movable x-ray table. Depending upon the anticipated site of pathology, the physician will plan to inject the carotid artery (to visualize the anterior, middle, and posterior cerebral arteries) or the vertebral artery (to visualize it and the basilar artery). The carotid and vertebral arteries can be punctured directly or reached by a catheter advanced from other arteries, such as the femoral or brachial (Donohoe, Blount, and Kinney 1974). The physician will prepare the skin, inject local anesthesia, make a percutaneous entry into the vessel, introduce and advance a catheter under fluoroscopic examination, and inject radiopaque dye while repeated x-rays are taken. During this time, the patient will be monitored closely for an anaphylactic reaction and signs of increased intracranial pressure.

After the procedure is completed, he will be returned to his room. Perform neurologic checks every 30 minutes to 4 hours, depending upon his stability. Also follow the measures outlined in the section on cardiac catheterization (Chapter 2) for potential complications after catheterization. Patients usually recover from this procedure without severe reactions, in a few hours.

To experience cerebral arteriography vicariously, see Blackwell's article or talk with patients who have undergone the procedure. Seeking this information will sensitize you to the concerns of patients and help increase your ability to alleviate their worries.

Computerized axial tomography

Computerized axial tomography (CAT scanning) is a neurodiagnostic procedure that utilizes a computer to analyze x-ray data. Although a beam of x-ray photons is used, the data is recorded numerically rather than in a conventional x-ray.

Patient preparation for a CAT scan should include a brief description of the equipment and procedure. The patient must hold very still approximately 4 minutes for each scan, as even small movements induce artifact. If the patient is unable to hold still, sedation may be necessary. The scan is safe and painless; the only unpleasant sensation the person might experience is a brief burning sensation if contrast media are used.

The following information on CAT scans is derived from Ambrose (1973). The reference line for the planes of scanning is the orbitomeatal line, the line between the outer angle of the eye and the external auditory meatus. When the patient goes for a CAT scan, this line is marked on his face with a grease pencil. A strip of tape is placed on the side of his face in front of his ear, and the levels to be scanned are marked on it for reference in aligning the beam. The patient lies on a stretcher and his head is positioned within the section of the scanner containing the x-ray tube. The x-ray tube rotates 180° around the head, transmitting an x-ray beam (a scan) across the head in 1° steps. (Some newer scanners use several beams and rotate the tube several degrees in each step.)

During each scan, the two 13 mm slices of brain tissue on either side of the beam are examined. In most cases, three scans (six pictures) are sufficient. Both the level and angle of the scans can be varied and recorded so that lesions can be localized exactly.

On the opposite side of the head from the beam is a crystal detector which reads the transmission. The readings form the basis of complex equations which the computer solves and transforms into absorption coefficients indicating the density of predetermined small volumes of brain tissue.

The data from the scan is available in three forms: a computer printout, cathode tube or television tube display, and a photograph of the display. The computer printout consists of numbers indicating the absorption values on an arbitrary scale, usually 1000 units. (Water is given a value of 0, bone +500, and air −500. The density values of intracranial structures have been identified; for example, CSF is 0–10 units).

The computer constructs a picture based on the density values and displays it on a screen. The picture varies in light intensity from white (high density structures) to black (low density structures). The picture shows structures as if you were looking from above at a transverse slice of the brain. Major anatomical structures are identified by size, shape, and location. Easily identified structures are white matter, gray matter, Sylvian fissures, fissure of Rolando, lateral ventricles, third ventricle, choroid plexuses, and calcified pineal body. For detailed study, areas of display can be enlarged.

Abnormalities are detected by deviations from normal density and sometimes also by displacement of normal structures. To be located, a lesion's density must differ from that of surrounding normal tissue. Lesions which are less dense than normal (therefore appearing as low numbers on the printout or black areas on the picture) are areas of tissue necrosis (malignant tumors and infarctions), edema, degenerative changes, cysts, and hemorrhages which have not yet clotted. Lesions causing increased density include blood clots and calcium deposits in tumors. Radiopaque contrast media can be injected intravenously to increase the density of vascular structures and enhance the detection of abnormal densities.

CAT scanning equipment is very expensive and therefore its current availability is limited. In institutions which have scanners, the CAT scan has markedly reduced the incidence of pneumoencephalography. PEGs are still useful for diagnosing abnormalities in the basal cisterns and posterior fossa. These areas are hard to see on CAT scans because of computer artifact resulting from the sudden large density contrast between air-filled sinuses and bony structures. While CAT scans have reduced the use of cerebral arteriography for tumor screening, the cerebral arteriogram is more precise than the scan for visualizing vascular anatomy and abnormalities such as aneurysms or occlusions. The CAT scan can show hemorrhage in the hemispheres, ventricles, cerebellum, or brainstem; such hemorrhage cannot be detected by other procedures.

No special physiologic care is necessary after a scan, other than observing for a possible allergic reaction to the contrast media.

References

Ambrose, J. 1973. Computerized transverse axial scanning (tomography): Part 2. Clinical application. *Brit. J. Radiol.* 46:1023–1047.

Lucid explanation of underlying principles and clinical applications. Numerous normal and abnormal scans (computer printouts and photographs) with autopsy specimens.

American Journal of Nursing. 1975. Patient assessment: neurological examination. Part I: cranial nerves 75:9 (P.I. 1–24):
Programmed instruction on basic anatomy, physiology, and assessment techniques.

Blackwell, C. 1975. PEG and angiography: a patient's sensations. *A.J.N.* 75:264–266.
Personal account of sensations experienced by nurse who underwent pneumoencephalography and carotid arteriography; contains specific advice on patient teaching.

Blount, M., Kinney, A., and Donohoe, K. 1974. Obtaining and analyzing cerebrospinal fluid. *Nurs. Clin. North Am.* 9:593–609.
Techniques, nursing care, and interpretation of abnormal findings.

Brunner, L., and Suddarth, D. 1975. *Textbook of medical-surgical nursing.* 3rd ed. Philadelphia: J. B. Lippincott Company.
Review of basic neuroanatomy and diagnostic procedures contained in Chapter 35, "Patients with Neurologic and Neurosurgical Problems."

Carini, E., and Owens, G. 1974. *Neurological and neurosurgical nursing.* 6th ed. St. Louis: C. V. Mosby Company.
Basic nursing text which includes anatomy and physiology of nervous system, diagnostic procedures, medical therapies, medications, and symptoms and nursing care for a wide variety of neurological disorders.

Donohoe, K., Blount, M., and Kinney, A. 1974. Cerebral circulation and cerebral angiography. *Nurs. Clin. North Am.* 9:623–631.
Description of cerebral blood flow, indications, technique, and nursing care related to cerebral angiography.

Guyton, A. 1976. *Textbook of medical physiology.* 5th ed. Philadelphia: W. B. Saunders Company.
Comprehensive reference text on normal anatomy and physiology.

Jacob, S., Francone, C., and Lossow, W. 1978. *Structure and function in man,* 4th ed. Philadelphia: W. B. Saunders Company.
Normal anatomy and physiology text less detailed than Guyton.

Jimm, L. 1974. Nursing assessment of patients for increased intracranial pressure. *J. Neurosurg. Nursing* 6 (July 1974): 27–38.
Well-written article that integrates assessment techniques, findings, and related anatomy and physiology.

Kinney, A., Blount, M., and Donohoe, K. 1974. Cerebrospinal fluid circulation and encephalography. *Nurs. Clin. North Am.* 9:611–621.
CSF dynamics, pneumoencephalography, and ventriculography.

Plum, F., and Posner, J. 1972. *The diagnosis of stupor and coma.* 2nd ed. Philadelphia: F. A. Davis Company.
Medical text on differential diagnosis of conditions producing stupor and coma. Diagnostic procedures are integrated with relevant anatomy and physiology and illustrated with clinical examples.

Shapiro, H. 1975. Intracranial hypertension: therapeutic and anesthetic considerations. *Anesthesiology:* 43:445–471.
Pathophysiology, manifestations, and treatment of increased intracranial pressure.

Swendsen, L. 1975. *FANCAS: a framework for nursing assessment.* University of California School of Nursing, San Francisco.
Definitions and examples of FANCAS categories.

Supplemental Reading

American Association of Neurosurgical Nurses. 1977. *Core curriculum for neurosurgical nursing.* Baltimore: American Association of Neurosurgical Nurses.
Behavioral objectives, detailed outline format covering functional neuroanatomy and physiology, patient assessment, nursing care in numerous pathological states. Highly recommended.

Goodman, M. and Aung, H. 1978. Cerebral death: theological, judicial, and medical aspects. *Heart Lung* 7:477–483.
Fascinating review of religious, legal, and medical perspectives on assessment of cerebral death.

Mandrillo, M. 1974. Brain scanning. *Nurs. Clin. North. Am.* 9:633–640.
Brief description of technique, interpretation, and implications for nursing care.

Chapter 16

Increased Intracranial Pressure

The concept of increased intracranial pressure is one that underlies a spectrum of acute disorders affecting stimulation (the ability to perceive and to respond to one's environment). Increased intracranial pressure can be anticipated in such diverse neurological conditions as cerebral edema, subarachnoid hemorrhage, and post-craniotomy.

It is a misconception that increased intracranial pressure always is harmful to the patient. As Mitchell and Mauss (1976) point out, many everyday activities such as isometric exercise, sexual intercourse, and straining at bowel movements can cause spikes of pressure far above normal levels. Moreover, benign intracranial hypertension (caused by jugular venous or vena caval obstruction) can cause extremely high intracranial pressures which nevertheless are well tolerated by many of these patients.

While these examples are enlightening, it is imperative to realize that for patients in critical care units, acute increases of intracranial pressure (especially focal increases) can be lethal. This chapter focuses on ways you can anticipate, prevent, and ameliorate detrimental increases in intracranial pressure (ICP).

Outline

Assessment   Risk conditions / Signs and symptoms / Measuring intracranial pressure

Planning and implementing care   Oxygenation and ventilation / Prevention of obstructions to venous outflow / Prevention of increases in intrathoracic pressure / Minimizing arterial hypo- and hypertension / Prevention of infection / Signs of impending herniation / Neurogenic pulmonary edema / Implementing medical therapy

Outcome evaluation

Objectives

- Recognize patients at risk of increased ICP
- Briefly describe why the classic generalized signs are unreliable indicators of increased ICP
- Name three types of intracranial pressure monitoring, and give one advantage and one disadvantage of each
- Assist with insertion of a ventricular catheter or subarachnoid screw
- State the normal range of intracranial pressure in mm Hg and cm H_2O
- Define cerebral perfusion pressure and explain how to estimate it
- State the normal response when intracranial compliance is tested and the significance of an abnormal response
- Plan and implement nursing care for patients with increased ICP
- Differentiate among the pathophysiology of central (transtentorial) herniation, uncal herniation, and herniation through the foramen magnum
- Briefly describe the signs of each stage of: a) central herniation; and b) uncal herniation
- Identify the physiologic mechanism by which hyperventilation may avert imminent herniation
- Evaluate the patient's progress according to specified outcome criteria

Assessment

The intracranial contents consist of brain tissue and extracellular fluid (subdivided into blood, cerebrospinal fluid, and interstitial fluid). Since the amount of interstitial fluid is negligible, for practical purposes the intracranial volume (ICV) equals the sum of brain volume (BV), cerebrospinal fluid volume (CSFV), and cerebral blood volume (CBV), that is, $ICV = BV + CSFV + CBV$. The volume within each intracranial compartment exerts pressure. Since the easiest pressure to measure is that of CSF, it is the pressure commonly referred to as *intracranial pressure*.

When the volume of one compartment increases, the total pressure will increase also unless there is a reciprocal change in another compartment. Fortunately, although the skull is a nondistensible structure, it has openings for the spinal cord, cranial nerves, and blood vessels. Through these openings, cranial contents can escape, thus lowering intracranial pressure. The major pressure buffer is CSF, for two reasons: 1) the dura covering the spinal cord is loosely attached and can expand readily to accommodate CSF leaving the cranial subarachnoid space; 2) CSF absorption by the arachnoid villi is partially dependent on CSF pressure. The ability of CSF to buffer pressure changes is compromised when an expanding mass blocks subarachnoid pathways or when CSF absorption is diminished.

Risk conditions

Be alert for patients with actual or potential increases in intracranial pressure. Conditions increasing the patient's risk include mass lesions such as cranial tumors, hematomas, and arteriovenous malformations; brain swelling due to cerebral vascular congestion or edema, such as in thrombosis, embolism, and infection; obstructive hydrocephalus; and hypertensive encephalopathy.

Signs and symptoms

Maintain a high index of suspicion for signs and symptoms of increased ICP. The classic generalized signs and symptoms are a nonspecific headache; blurred or double vision; personality changes; decreased level of consciousness; papilledema (due to pressure transmission via CSF in the subarachnoid space around the optic nerve); occasionally nausea and vomiting; and bradycardia and systemic hypertension (Cushing response). When decompensation occurs, the pulse becomes irregular and tachycardic, and the pulse pressure narrows. See Chapter 15 for a discussion of various respiratory patterns which may be seen.

These classic signs and symptoms are notoriously unreliable indicators of the onset and degree of increased ICP. Because they are nonspecific, a condition other than increased ICP may provoke them. Even in increased ICP, they appear only after pathologic changes have occurred and poorly reflect the degree of pressure elevation, since they are influenced by the rapidity with which pressure increases. Thus, a slow-growing tumor can produce a severe rise in ICP with minimal or absent signs and symptoms. Finally, even if the classic manifestations are present, they may be transient. For these reasons, patients likely to suffer acutely increased ICP ideally should have the benefit of direct monitoring of CSF pressure. Such monitoring does not, however, eliminate the need for astute bedside physical assessment.

Measuring intracranial pressure

The following sections describe techniques of intracranial pressure monitoring.

Types of pressure monitoring   Although CSF pressure can be evaluated by lumbar punctures, such readings are isolated and inaccurate in the presence of subarachnoid block. More importantly, lumbar punctures present a danger of herniation in those patients who most need pressure evaluation. In contrast, an intracranial transducer, ventricular catheter, or subarachnoid screw can monitor intracranial pressure accurately and continuously, without danger of herniation through the foramen magnum. The three cranial areas monitored most frequently are the epidural space, the subarachnoid space, and the lateral ventricle.

Epidural monitoring is done with an intracranial transducer, or an intracranial balloon connected to an external transducer. The dura is not opened, so there is less danger of cranial infection than with other methods. The internal transducer reduces the danger further, but it is affected by heat and cannot be recalibrated. Epidural monitoring does not allow for CSF drainage or testing of intracranial compliance.

The ventricular catheter is inserted under local anesthesia, through a drill hole in the skull and a puncture of the dura, into the frontal or occipital horn of the lateral ventricle in the nondominant hemisphere. Advantages include the abilities to drain CSF, recalibrate the transducer, test compliance, and instill contrast media for visualization of the size and patency of the ventricular system. Disadvantages include the technical difficulty of insertion in the presence of marked cerebral edema and the potentials for infection, CSF loss, and blockage of the catheter by blood clots.

The subarachnoid screw is a small hollow screw whose tip sits in the cranial subarachnoid space. Advantages include ease of insertion, ability to recalibrate the transducer as necessary, and potential for draining CSF. Disadvantages are possible infection, CSF loss, inability to instill contrast media, and possible blockage of the screw by brain tissue.

Since the ventricular catheter and the subarachnoid screw are used more frequently, the remainder of this chapter is devoted to the care of patients being monitored by these methods.

Insertion of the ventricular catheter or subarachnoid screw   To prepare the patient and family for insertion, explain that monitoring is a temporary measure to enable the nurses and doctors to detect the onset of increased intracranial pressure and intervene early to prevent or ameliorate its detrimental effects. Explain that the scalp will be numbed with local anesthesia and that the insertion itself will be painless. Briefly explain the set-up and monitor, so that the family will not be horrified by the tubes and wires connected to their loved one's brain.

Gather the equipment necessary for the monitoring: the catheter or screw; an insertion tray containing a syringe and needle for anesthesia, scalpel, drill, sutures, and dressing supplies; skin preparation solution; local anesthetic; sterile gloves; monitor; transducer; high-pressure tubing; two 3-way stopcocks; one 2-way stopcock; stopcock porthole cap; a 10 ml syringe; a small syringe; bag of IV flush solution; IV tubing; IV pole; and carpenter's level.

Assemble the equipment sterilely before the catheter or screw is inserted.

Set up the flush system by connecting the flush solution, IV tubing, and a 3-way stopcock. This set-up will serve as your fluid source but should not be attached to the monitoring system because of the danger of inadvertently administering a large amount of fluid into the ventricle or subarachnoid space. Fill one 10 ml syringe with fluid and a small syringe with the amount of fluid specified by the physician for flushing the catheter or screw (usually 0.1 ml).

To set up the monitoring system, follow this procedure. Refer to Figure 16-1 as you read this procedure.

1. Place a three-way stopcock on the straight transducer arm, and a two-way stopcock on the angled transducer arm.
2. Connect the large syringe with flush solution to the side port of the three-way stopcock on the straight transducer arm.
3. Turn the three-way stopcock attached to the straight arm so that the open end port is shut off.

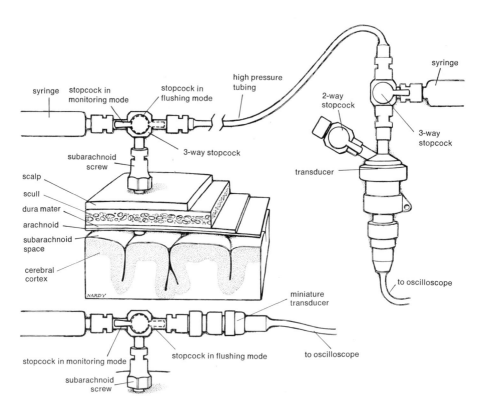

Figure 16-1. Intracranial pressure monitoring with a subarachnoid screw. (From Johnson, M., and Quinn, J., 1977. The subarachnoid screw. © March 1977, The American Journal of Nursing Company. Reproduced with permission of artist Neil O. Hardy and publisher, from the *American Journal of Nursing* 77:3.)

4. Turn the two-way stopcock on the angled arm so that fluid can flow out its open end port.

5. Flush the transducer and two-way stopcock. When you see fluid coming out the open port of the two-way stopcock, continue flushing slowly. Apply a porthole cap to the two-way stopcock, turn that stopcock off to the transducer, and turn the three-way stopcock off to the transducer. Then release the pressure you have been exerting on the plunger of the syringe. (If you released the pressure first and then closed off the ports, you might suck small air bubbles back into the ports. By continuing to flush as you close off stopcock ports, you avoid this possibility.)

6. Connect high pressure tubing to the open end port of the three-way stopcock.

7. Connect another three-way stopcock to the free end of the high pressure tubing. Turn its handle so that the side port is closed.

8. Flush the tubing and open end port of this three-way stopcock. When fluid drips out the open port, continue flushing as you close it off with the second syringe (containing more flush solution).

9. Turn the handle on this three-way stopcock so fluid drips out its side port. Cap the side port. Leave this stopcock so that the side port is open to the transducer. (After the catheter or screw is inserted, it will be connected to this side stopcock port.)

10. Then turn the handle on the three-way stopcock attached to the transducer so that the transducer is open to the high pressure tubing.

11. Mount the transducer on an IV pole so it is level with the reference point of the catheter or screw specified by the physician.

12. Connect the transducer to the oscilloscope and turn it on. Calibrate the transducer according to the manufacturer's directions.

Assist the physician in inserting the catheter or screw. The physician will shave, clean, and infiltrate the insertion site with a local anesthetic. He then will incise the scalp, drill a hole, puncture the dura, and insert the catheter or screw. Remove the cap covering the stopcock side port and connect the catheter or screw. At this point, you should see a waveform on the oscilloscope. The physician will suture the incision and apply a sterile dressing.

Nursing care responsibilities   The following sections describe nursing responsibilities related to intracranial pressure monitoring.

Obtain accurate pressure measurements. Follow these steps each time you measure the pressure:

1. Place the patient in the baseline position, as you will get false pressure changes if the level of the head has changed in relation to the transducer. Use

the carpenter's level to verify that the transducer is level with the catheter or screw. (Some units are using miniature transducers attached directly to the sensing device and taped to the head to preclude measurement error from failure to level the transducer.)

2. Observe the waveform of the oscilloscope to verify patency of the line. If it appears flattened (dampened), consult the physician. Many physicians do not want the patency of the system disturbed. If the physician does want you to flush the system, proceed as he or she recommends. One flushing method follows. Fill a syringe only with the amount of flush solution specified by the physician. Connect it to the three-way stopcock attached to the catheter or screw. Turn the stopcock so it is off to the transducer, that is, so the syringe and catheter or screw are connected. *Slowly* flush the catheter or screw. (Do not aspirate first, as you would with a line for monitoring vascular pressure. Aspiration may suck brain tissue into the screw.) Turn the stopcock so the catheter or screw and transducer are reconnected. Again observe the waveform. If it remains dampened, notify the physician.

3. Do not measure the pressure when the patient is moving, coughing, sneezing, using abdominal muscles to inspire, or has his head turned, since these actions will cause temporary increases in intracranial pressure.

4. Balance and calibrate the transducer as frequently as the manufacturer recommends.

Analyze the pressures critically. Remember that the trend is more significant than an isolated reading. Compare the readings to the patient's norm rather than an arbitrary standard; the patient with chronically increased intracranial pressure will have a higher "normal" value than the patient being monitored to detect the onset of increased pressure. Reported normal ranges are 4–15 mm Hg or 50–200 mm H_2O (Hanlon 1976). Following are guidelines for pressure analysis:

1. You may see frequent pressure changes with a given patient. Pressures normally fluctuate with cardiac pulsations (transmitted to the CSF through the choroid plexus) and changes in the thoracic and abdominal pressures (transmitted to the CSF through the vena cava and the jugular veins).

2. You also may see spontaneous abnormal variations in pressure called pressure waves (Figure 16-2). Lundberg (1960) has described three types of abnormal pressure waves. B waves are sharp, rhythmic waves with a saw tooth appearance. They occur every 30 seconds to 2 minutes and raise intracranial pressure up to 50 mm Hg. C waves are smaller rhythmic waves which occur every 4–8 minutes and raise intracranial pressure as much as 20 mm Hg. B and C waves coincide with rhythmic respiratory variations in blood pressure, but their significance is unclear. Most important are A waves, commonly called plateau waves.

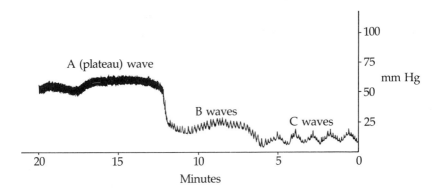

Figure 16-2. Intracranial pressure waves. Composite diagram of A (plateau) waves, B waves, and C waves. See text for discussion.

These waves raise intracranial pressure 50–100 mm Hg and last for 5–20 minutes (Mauss and Mitchell 1976). These sustained pressure elevations occur on an already elevated mean intracranial pressure baseline exceeding 20 mm Hg. Plateau waves are believed to be significant because they may reduce cerebral perfusion pressure and contribute to brain cell hypoxia. Supporting this assumption is Lundberg's observation that transient displays of the classic signs of increased pressure most often occurred at the peak of plateau waves. Of particular importance to nursing is his observation that above a baseline pressure of 20 mm Hg, transient pressure rises may summate into plateau waves.

3. In addition to evaluating absolute pressure values, note the amplitude of the recording. As mentioned above, changes in cardiac pulsations are transmitted to the CSF through the choroid plexus. Normally, as cranial blood pressure rises and falls, blood and CSF escape and return through patent outflow channels in the foraminae at the base of the skull. These compensatory mechanisms keep intracranial pressure relatively constant, so the cardiac pulse produces only slight variations between the high and low values on ICP recordings. As ICP increases, the outflow of CSF and blood is reduced. Since less compensation for pressure changes occurs, they are reflected more distinctly in ICP recordings as a widened amplitude. When ICP becomes great enough to interfere severely with blood outflow, pulsations from the choroid plexus diminish, the amplitude of the recording decreases, and death ensues (Hanlon 1976).

4. Also monitor cerebral perfusion pressure, which is the difference between cerebral arterial and venous blood pressures. Cerebral arterial pressure approximates mean systemic arterial pressure, and cerebral venous pressure approximates intracranial pressure when ICP is elevated. To estimate cerebral perfusion pressure, first note the systolic and diastolic systemic blood pressures, preferably from an arterial monitoring line. Subtract the diastolic from the systolic, take

one-third the difference, and add it to the diastolic pressure to get the mean systemic arterial pressure. From the mean systemic arterial pressure, subtract the intracranial pressure to get the approximate cerebral perfusion pressure (CPP). Normal CPP is 80–90 mm Hg (Hanlon 1976). CPP can be reduced by either a drop in arterial pressure or a rise in intracranial pressure. As intracranial pressure increases and cerebral blood flow slows, compensatory cerebral vaso-dilatation occurs (autoregulation). Although this compensation increases blood flow, it also increases ICP; the net result is a decrease in cerebral perfusion pressure. At a CPP of 40 mm Hg, cerebral perfusion fails, and cerebral hypoxia ensues.

5. Test cranial compensation if ordered by the physician. The compensatory mechanism can be elevated with ventricular monitoring systems by introducing a known amount of fluid into the ventricle and noting the compliance (change in volume per unit of pressure change). The volume/pressure relationship can be illustrated by a curve such as that in Figure 16-3. The exact configuration varies from individual to individual. The normal relationship is depicted by the lower part of the curve—a small increase in pressure causes only a small increase in volume. If the patient's ICP is relatively normal, instilling a small amount of fluid causes only slight increases in ICP and amplitude. If the ICP is increased signifi-cantly (upper portion of the curve), the pressure will rise dramatically and the amplitude will increase considerably. The point at which this occurs also varies among individuals.

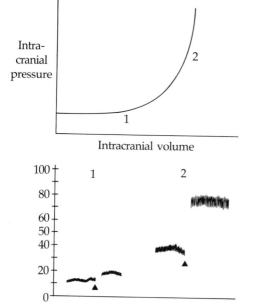

Figure 16-3   Diagram representing rela-tionship of theoretical volume/pressure curve (upper figure) and compliance test (lower figure) for two hypothetical pa-tients. Patient 1, on lower part of volume/pressure curve, has normal baseline pressure and normal response to instillation of 2 ml of fluid (marked by ▲). Patient 2, on upper part of volume/pressure curve, has elevated baseline pressure and abnormal compliance test: pressure sharply increases and amplitude of recording increases.

Anticipate and prevent complications of monitoring. Implement the following measures for patients on ICP monitoring:

1. Observe the waveforms periodically to detect *obstruction* in the line. If the form appears dampened, check for kinks in the tubing and flush the system if ordered by the physician.

2. Avoid *infection* by scrupulous aseptic technique. Breaks in technique are particularly likely when you are setting up the system and when you are preparing to flush the system. Remember that filling the syringe from a separate IV bag and transferring it to the stopcock means you are using an open system. (If your unit recommends connecting the IV bag so that you have a closed system and less chance of infection, be *absolutely sure* you keep the stopcock to the bag closed when you are not filling the syringe. You can kill the patient by accidentally leaving the stopcock open and infusing fluid into the ventricle or subarachnoid space.) Change the flush solution and tubing every 24 hours. Draw off 2 ml of CSF daily for culture and sensitivity determination.

3. Observe the system for *CSF leaks*, which are dangerous because they allow a pathway for infection and because they lower the pressure in the system and allow brain tissue to be sucked against or into the catheter or screw. If you see fluid on the stopcocks or tubing, tighten or replace them. If you are unable to stop the leak, turn the stopcock attached to the catheter or screw off to the direction of the leak, cover the leak with a sterile towel, and notify the physician (Johnson and Quinn 1977).

Planning and implementing care

Many maneuvers that nurses commonly use in caring for critically ill patients may have deleterious effects on patients already suffering from increased ICP. To understand why, it is helpful to review intracranial dynamics briefly.

Oxygenation and ventilation

Cerebral blood flow varies in response to metabolic changes, specifically the arterial partial pressures of CO_2 (P_aCO_2) and O_2 (P_aO_2) and the level of lactic acid. Within the normal range of P_aCO_2 (35–45 mm Hg), changes in CO_2 level exert more effect on CSF than do changes in O_2 level (Shapiro 1975). The oxygen level exerts its greatest power when P_aO_2 drops below normal. P_aCO_2 and cerebral blood flow vary directly. As P_aCO_2 increases, cerebral vessels dilate; since their resistance decreases, cerebral perfusion pressure and blood flow increase. The relationship between P_aO_2 and cerebral blood flow is inverse—as P_aO_2 drops, cerebral vessels dilate and CBF increases. Lactic acid accumulation also causes vasodilatation.

When intracranial pressure rises, venous outflow and therefore cerebral blood flow decrease. As a result, more CO_2 accumulates in cerebral vessels, and less oxygen than normal is available to the cells. The CO_2 excess and oxygen deficit both cause vasodilatation, which reduces resistance and increases cerebral blood flow toward normal (metabolic autoregulation). Unfortunately, the increased blood flow tends to increase intracranial pressure even more. The following sections describe ways of maintaining oxygenation and ventilation to lessen this vicious cycle.

Airway patency   Establish and maintain a patent airway. When positioning a patient to maintain airway patency or for intubation, remember that a stiff neck may indicate cerebellar tonsillar herniation (Shapiro 1975). Forceful neck flexion in this situation can compress the vital centers in the medulla and kill the patient.

Hypoxemia and/or hypercapnia   Avoid hypoxemia and/or hypercapnia, either of which can cause vasodilatation with a resultant further increase in ICP. Particularly important measures are close monitoring of arterial blood gases, preoxygenating before suctioning, and limiting suction to 10–15 seconds in the apneic patient to minimize CO_2 accumulation. For other measures to maintain oxygenation and ventilation, see Chapter 10.

Prevention of obstructions to venous outflow

Try to prevent obstructions to venous outflow from the brain. Such obstructions not only increase pressure in the capillary bed (predisposing toward cerebral swelling) but also diminish absorption of CSF. Since CSF is absorbed by the arachnoid villi into the sagittal sinus and then into the jugular veins, pressure resulting from compression of the jugular veins will be transmitted back into the brain. A continuing rise in pressure may precipitate reduction in one of the other volumes. Blood volume may decrease, causing ischemia, or brain tissue may herniate.

Unless specifically ordered by the physician, do not place the patient with increased ICP flat or in Trendelenburg's position. Instead, keep the head of the bed elevated to increase the pressure gradient between the brain and heart. Although 30° is a common elevation, the degree of elevation often must be individualized. Position the head and neck midline to avoid jugular venous compression. Recent research indicates that extreme hip flexion also elevates ICP and should be avoided. For example, if you must catheterize a female with increased ICP, flex the legs as little as possible.

Prevention of increases in intrathoracic pressure

Prevent avoidable increases in intrathoracic pressure. If the physician plans to insert a jugular venous catheter, you must modify your usual preparation of the patient. Avoid placing him in Trendelenburg position and having him execute a Valsalva maneuver, as you do with other patients to minimize the danger of air embolism due to negative intrathoracic pressure. Instead, the physician should prevent air being sucked into the catheter during insertion by maintaining suction on the catheter with a syringe.

Take actions to avoid other Valsalva maneuvers. For example, teach the patient to exhale when moving his bowels; assist him to turn; and keep fecal contents soft through diet, fluid intake, and/or stool softeners. While a Valsalva maneuver alone may not be sufficient to cause a plateau wave, its combination with other pressure-increasing actions can cause a sustained increase in intracranial pressure.

Minimizing arterial hypo- or hypertension

Minimize bursts of arterial hypertension or hypotension. Both systemic arterial pressure and intracranial pressure strongly influence cerebral perfusion. Cerebral perfusion pressure (CPP) equals mean systemic arterial pressure (MSAP) minus ICP, that is, $CPP = MSAP - ICP$. Within a MSAP of 50–150 mm Hg, the diameter of cerebral blood vessels (and therefore their resistance) alters automatically to maintain a constant perfusion pressure. This type of automatic regulation is known as pressure autoregulation and is essential in avoiding drastic changes in CBF. Given a normal ICP (4–15 mm Hg), pressure autoregulation will maintain CPP at about 80–90 mm Hg (Hanlon 1976).

Autoregulation is believed to fail when ICP exceeds approximately 33 mm Hg (Reivich 1968), mean systemic arterial pressure falls below 50 mm Hg, or CPP drops below 40 mm Hg (Hanlon 1976). When autoregulation fails, cerebral blood flow no longer alters appropriately with pressure or metabolic needs; instead, cerebral blood flow fluctuates directly with systemic blood pressure. Increases in mean SAP pound more blood into cerebral vessels, further elevating ICP and worsening cerebral edema. Conversely, decreases in mean SAP worsen cerebral ischemia. In this situation, even the brain's desperate needs for oxygen and removal of CO_2 and lactic acid cannot provoke improved cerebral blood flow.

Many nursing care activities cause an arousal response accompanied by increased systemic blood pressure. Among the stimuli that can provoke this arousal response are an endotracheal tube, suctioning, chest physiotherapy, and pain. Use blood pressure and intracranial pressure monitors to evaluate your patient's response to these circumstances and adapt your care accordingly. For instance, try timing suctioning or chest PT for intervals of peak sedation; check with the physician about using topical anesthesia if suctioning provokes hypertensive episodes; use muscle relaxants as ordered by the physician if repeated explanations are ineffective in calming the patient fighting an endotracheal tube and if your evaluation reveals he is not hypoxic. Decrease the occurrence of painful stimuli or any other nonspecific stimuli which provoke the hypertensive response in your particular patient.

Also try to reduce the risk of small pressure increases summating into plateau waves. If you must do two activities, each of which causes a pressure increase, time your care judiciously so that pressure can diminish after the first activity before you institute the second.

Prevention of infection

Infection can be catastrophic in patients on ICP monitoring. Meticulous sterile technique and prompt antibiotic therapy if signs of infection appear may protect the patient against meningitis or fullblown sepsis. Because sepsis can lead to increased cardiac output and vasodilatation, it can contribute to a dangerous rise in intracranial pressure. Since early septic shock is "warm shock" and so insidious, see Chapter 5 if you wish to review signs, symptoms, prevention, and treatment.

Signs of impending herniation

Observe closely for signs of impending herniation. There are two main routes of herniation: through the tentorial notch and through the foramen magnum.

You will recall that the tentorium cerebelli separates supratentorial and infratentorial structures and contains an opening, the tentorial notch or incisura, through which the midbrain passes. There are two clinically important types of supratentorial herniation: central and uncal. The following descriptions are taken from Plum and Posner (1972).

Central herniation   In central (transtentorial) herniation, an expanding lesion forces the hemispheres and basal nuclei downward through the tentorial notch, progressively compressing the diencephalon, midbrain, and pons. Displacement of branches of the basilar artery causes ischemia and severe brainstem deterioration. Central herniation also can block the aqueduct of Sylvius, between the third and fourth ventricles. This blockage, which cannot be diagnosed clinically, robs the brain of its ability to displace fluid from the ventricular system to compensate for increased brain volume and causes a severe rise in supratentorial pressure. However, impaired CSF circulation probably is less instrumental in causing herniation than the factor initially causing the increase in intracranial pressure.

Central herniation generally causes ischemia to advance in a rostral-caudal (head-tail) direction. Plum and Posner describe manifestations typical of four stages of progression: early diencephalic, late diencephalic, midbrain-upper pontine, and lower pontine-upper medullary. These changes are shown in Figure 16-4.

The earliest sign in the diencephalic stage is diminished alertness characterized by difficulty in concentration, memory lapses, lethargy, and stupor.

Pupils are small (2–3 mm). Although on superficial examination they may appear not to react to light, a closer look reveals that they react rapidly but only within a small range of contraction. The doll's eyes reflex is present. The ice water caloric test provokes normal slow movement but diminished or absent fast movement. Respirations may be a relatively normal pattern interspersed with yawns, sighs and pauses, or Cheyne-Stokes breathing. Motor responses to a painful stimulus are appropriate in the early diencephalic stage but progress to decorticate posturing in the late diencephalic stage.

In the midbrain-upper pontine stage, pupils become somewhat dilated (3–5 mm) and fixed to light. The doll's eyes response disappears and the ice water caloric response becomes harder to provoke. Respirations may change from Cheyne-Stokes to sustained hyperventilation. (This hyperventilation used to be called central neurogenic hyperventilation [CNH]. Current thinking attributes the tachypnea to hypoxia rather than a central neurogenic mechanism [Shapiro 1975]). Decerebrate posturing occurs in response to painful stimuli or spontaneously.

In the lower pontine-upper medullary stage, the pupils remain fixed in midposition. Both the doll's eyes and ice water caloric responses are absent. Respirations become more or less regular but shallow. The patient remains flaccid except sometimes for nonpurposeful flickers of movement in response to painful stimuli.

In the terminal medullary stage, medullary ischemia causes ataxic respirations, varying pulse rates, hypotension, dilated pupils, and respiratory arrest.

The authors point out two exceptions to the generalization of rostral-caudal progression in untreated supratentorial lesions: acute cerebral hemorrhage, and lumbar punctures in patients with impending herniation. In both cases, sudden medullary failure may occur. In acute cerebral hemorrhage, structures around the fourth ventricle are compressed by hemorrhage into the ventricular system. In the second case, the extraction of spinal fluid apparently removes support from the brain, allowing it to herniate into the foramen magnum.

Uncal herniation   The uncus, a medial portion of the temporal lobe, overhangs the edge of the tentorial notch. Expanding lesions in the temporal lobe or lateral middle fossa can force the uncus over the edge of the incisura. This uncal herniation compresses the midbrain (which passes through the notch) up against the opposite edge of the tentorial opening. The oculomotor nerve and posterior cerebral artery are adjacent to the uncus. Uncal herniation often traps them against the opposite incisural edge too. Compression of the oculomotor nerve is discussed below. Posterior cerebral artery compromise can provoke occipital ischemia, edema and infarction. Uncal herniation also can compromise CSF circulation by compressing the aqueduct of Sylvius, with the results indicated above under central herniation.

The type of herniation does not correlate consistently with the site of lesion. Uncal herniation is more common than central herniation in neurological

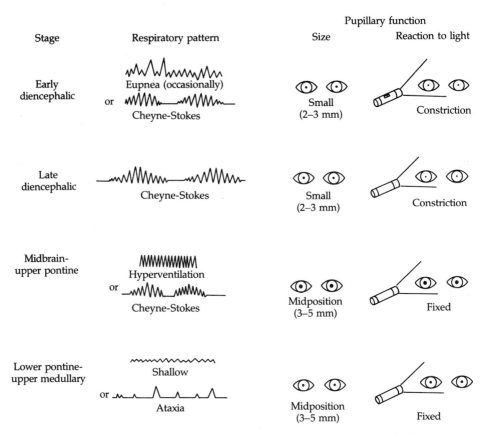

Stage	Respiratory pattern	Pupillary function	
		Size	Reaction to light
Early diencephalic	Eupnea (occasionally) or Cheyne-Stokes	Small (2–3 mm)	Constriction
Late diencephalic	Cheyne-Stokes	Small (2–3 mm)	Constriction
Midbrain-upper pontine	Hyperventilation or Cheyne-Stokes	Midposition (3–5 mm)	Fixed
Lower pontine-upper medullary	Shallow or Ataxia	Midposition (3–5 mm)	Fixed

Figure 16-4. Central syndrome signs. (From McNealy, D., and Plum, F., 1962. Brainstem dysfunction with supratentorial mass lesions. *Ar-*

emergencies such as rapid expansion of a cerebral hematoma. Central herniation is more common in subacute and chronic disorders and is harder to recognize.

Because of the anatomical location of the uncus, uncal herniation produces early stages that are different from central herniation: the third nerve stage and the midbrain-upper pontine stage (Figure 16-5). The earliest consistent sign is not the level of consciousness (which may vary from diminished alertness to coma) but rather a unilaterally dilating pupil.

Compression of the third cranial nerve first affects the pupillary parasympathetic fibers which make up the outer portion of the nerve, causing a unilaterally dilated pupil on the affected side. When you flash a light in that eye, the pupil will react sluggishly or not at all, although the other eye will respond consensually. Similarly, a light flashed in the nonaffected eye will provoke a normal direct reflex in it but a sluggish or absent consensual response in the affected eye. This pupillary abnormality may be the only sign of early uncal

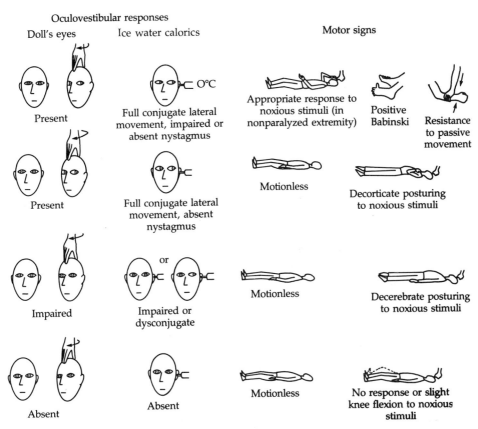

Oculovestibular responses

Doll's eyes — Ice water calorics

Motor signs

Present — Full conjugate lateral movement, impaired or absent nystagmus — Appropriate response to noxious stimuli (in nonparalyzed extremity) — Positive Babinski — Resistance to passive movement

Present — Full conjugate lateral movement, absent nystagmus — Motionless — Decorticate posturing to noxious stimuli

Impaired — or — Impaired or dysconjugate — Motionless — Decerebrate posturing to noxious stimuli

Absent — Absent — Motionless — No response or slight knee flexion to noxious stimuli

chives of Neurology 7:10–32. Copyright © 1962, American Medical Association. Used with permission of the author and publisher.)

herniation. Increasing pressure next affects the fibers in the center of the third cranial nerve which control oculomotor-mediated eye movement. As a result, diplopia and ptosis appear, and the eye (when resting) looks downward and outward due to the unopposed action of the sixth cranial nerve.

Uncal herniation is particularly dangerous because it tends to progress rapidly to produce irreversible midbrain-upper pontine damage. Within a few hours, the patient may be comatose. In this stage, pressure on midbrain corticospinal and other tracts results in hemiparesis, bilateral plantar flexion, and decerebrate posturing to noxious stimuli. The opposite pupil may dilate and be fixed to light; eventually both pupils dilate to 5–6 mm and become fixed to light. Doll's eye and ice water responses are abnormal and the respiratory pattern becomes Cheyne-Stokes or sustained hyperventilation. After this stage, the uncal syndrome progresses in the same fashion as the lower pontine–upper medullary stage of central herniation.

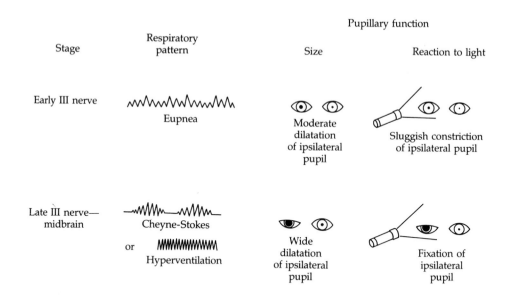

Figure 16-5.   Uncal syndrome signs. (From McNealy, D., and Plum, F., 1962. Brainstem dysfunction with supratentorial mass lesions. *Archives of*

Herniation through the foramen magnum   If cranial pressure becomes extremely high rapidly, the medulla and cerebellum may herniate through the foramen magnum at the base of the skull. This herniation is a catastrophe, as it compresses the vasomotor and respiratory centers in the medulla and the vertebral-basilar artery system which nourishes the brainstem. This type of herniation is pathologically distinct but not clinically distinct. Manifestations are those of rostral-caudal transtentorial herniation, as described above. The patient dies from cardiorespiratory arrest.

Nursing implications   The above descriptions of downward brain herniation accentuate the importance of conscientious physical examinations by nurses and prompt reactions at the *first* signs of possible impending herniation. Alert the physician if you observe any signs of possible incipient herniation, even if they are transient or equivocal.

For the patient on continuous intracranial pressure monitoring, notify the physician promptly if there is a consistent rise in ICP, plateau waves, or widening of the pulse pressure, so that CSF drainage, mannitol administration, or other therapy can be instituted. A change in the recording from a consistently high ICP and wide amplitude to a high ICP and narrow amplitude implies failure of the compensatory mechanism and impending death (Hanlon 1976).

Should you suspect imminent herniation, immediately summon medical assistance. Meanwhile, hyperventilate the patient to reduce the PCO_2. This action will constrict the cerebral vessels, temporarily decrease intracranial pressure

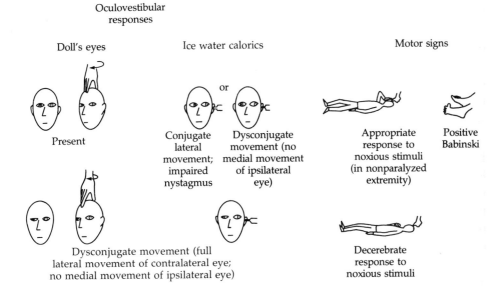

Oculovestibular responses

Doll's eyes

Present

Dysconjugate movement (full lateral movement of contralateral eye; no medial movement of ipsilateral eye)

Ice water calorics

Conjugate lateral movement; impaired nystagmus

Dysconjugate movement (no medial movement of ipsilateral eye)

Motor signs

Appropriate response to noxious stimuli (in nonparalyzed extremity)

Positive Babinski

Decerebrate response to noxious stimuli

Neurology 7:10–32. Copyright © 1962, American Medical Association. Used with permission of the author and publisher.)

and may avert herniation long enough for more definitive medical therapy to be instituted.

Neurogenic pulmonary edema

Be alert for the development of neurogenic pulmonary edema. The literature contains many conflicting reports on the relationship between neurologic disease and pulmonary edema. A recent review of sixty-three reports concluded that the proposed mechanisms remain speculative and require further investigation (Rossi and Graf 1976). For a review of signs, symptoms, and treatment of pulmonary edema see Chapter 10.

Neurogenic pulmonary edema usually is refractory to diuretics and cardiotonics unless ICP is reduced. Until then, ventilation with positive end-expiratory pressure (PEEP) is useful in maintaining oxygenation. Because PEEP increases intrathoracic pressure, however, its use is not without danger. Extreme elevation of the head of the bed is recommended to minimize its effect on intracranial pressure. Other problems associated with PEEP are discussed in Chapter 10.

Implementing medical therapy

An important aspect of nursing the patient with increased ICP is implementing the plan of medical therapy. Definitive therapy, of course, varies with the cause.

Hypertonic agents are used to reduce cerebral edema. Hypertonic agents are only temporary measures which bide time for more definitive treatment. Commonly used agents include mannitol (the drug of choice), urea, and glucose. When hypertonic agents are used, be alert for the development of congestive heart failure. Also watch for increasing cerebral edema which may occur when these drugs pass through the disrupted blood-brain barrier and raise brain osmolality. To reduce the risk of ICP rebound, only a portion of the volume lost during diuresis should be replaced. Mannitol is always administered intravenously through a filter because it crystallizes; failure to use a filter can cause microemboli to be introduced into the patient's bloodstream (Saper and Yosselson 1975).

Continuous hyperventilation may be tried if drug therapy is ineffective. Lowering the P_aCO_2 normally constricts the cerebral vasculature and therefore lowers ICP and improves compliance. Unfortunately, this effect depends upon retained CO_2 responsiveness, which often is lost if extensive tissue is diseased or the brain has suffered an anoxic insult. Moreover, CSF pH and cerebral blood flow return to normal after several days of hypocapnia in normal man (Severinghaus 1965). If the same occurs with the increased ICP patient, continuous hyperventilation loses its effectiveness, and intermittent hyperventilation also may no longer be effective in reducing acute increases in ICP.

Treatment of lesions in the posterior fossa may include ventricular drainage to reduce supratentorial pressure. It is important to remember, however, that the lesion still can press on the brainstem and precipitate cardiopulmonary arrest.

Outcome evaluation

Evaluate the patient's progress according to these outcome criteria:

- Return to premorbid level of consciousness
- Pupils of equal size which accommodate briskly to light
- Blood pressure, pulse, respirations, and temperature within normal limits (WNL) for the patient
- Appropriate motor responses to stimuli

References

Hanlon, K. 1976. Description and uses of intracranial pressure monitoring. *Heart Lung* 5:277–282.
Brief descriptions of types and uses of monitoring; clear illustrations of recordings showing normal and abnormal compliance tests and pressure waves.

Johnson, M., and Quinn, J. 1977. The subarachnoid screw. *A. J. N.* 77:448–450.
Description and nursing care related to use of the screw in intracranial pressure monitoring.

Luckmann, J. and Sorensen, K. 1974. *Medical-surgical nursing.* Philadelphia: W. B. Saunders Company.
Comprehensive text covering care of a wide variety of patients. Highly recommended.

Lundberg, N. 1960. Continuous recording and control of ventricular fluid pressure in neurosurgical practice. *Acta Psychiat. Neural. Scand.* 36:7 (Supplement 149).
Original description of ventricular pressure waves in patients with expanding brain lesions.

Mauss, N., and Mitchell, P. 1976. Increased intracranial pressure: an update. *Heart Lung* 5:919–926.
Review of recent research on ventricular pressure: relationships to vital sign changes, suggestions for nursing care.

Mitchell, P., and Mauss, N. 1976. Intracranial pressure: fact and fancy. *Nursing* 6(6):53–57.
Misconceptions about intracranial pressure and implications for nursing care.

Plum, F., and Posner, J. 1972. *Diagnosis of stupor and coma.* 2nd ed. Philadelphia: F. A. Davis Company.
Supratentorial, subtentorial, and metabolic diseases causing coma; pathophysiology of signs and symptoms; psychogenic unresponsiveness; brain death. Concepts are explained clearly and comprehensively, and illustrated with numerous clinical examples. Highly recommended.

Reivich, M. 1968. Regulation of cerebral circulation. *Clin. Neurosurg.* 16:378–418.
Techniques used to measure cerebral blood flow; cerebral perfusion pressure; factors controlling cerebrovascular tone.

Rossi, N., and Graf, C. 1976. Physiological and pathological effects of neurologic disturbances and increased intracranial pressure on the lung. A review. *Surg. Neurol.* 5:366–372.
Review of sixty-three articles relating to neurogenic pulmonary edema.

Saper, J., and Yosselson, S. 1975. Raised intracranial pressure: diagnosis and management. *Postgraduate Medicine* 57(4):89–94.
Brief presentation of signs, symptoms, and therapy.

Severinghaus, J. 1965. Role of cerebrospinal fluid pH in normalization of cerebral blood flow in chronic hypocapnia. *Acta Neurol. Scand.* Suppl. 14:116–120.
Interrelationships of chronic low pCO_2 CSF pH, and cerebral blood flow.

Shapiro, H. 1975. Intracranial hypertension: therapeutic and anesthetic considerations. *Anesthesiology* 43:445–471.
Pathophysiology, manifestations and treatment; effects of anesthetics on intracranial pressure; review of 149 references.

Chapter 17

Using FANCAS in a Service Setting

Throughout this book, the components of FANCAS have been isolated for analysis and description. A patient, of course, cannot be compartmentalized so neatly. His very nature mandates a holistic approach to his care, one which interweaves consideration of his physiological, psychological, social, and spiritual attributes.

Preceding chapters have discussed in detail not only the *what's* of patient care but also the *how to's* and *why's*. Such detail is appropriate for educational purposes. In the setting of a busy critical care service, however, such detail is inappropriate if not impossible to include on a patient's care plan. This chapter will present one feasible method of care planning in a critical care setting and illustrate its application with hypothetical clinical examples.

Figure 17-1 presents data obtained during a critical care nurse's assessment of Karen J. on the day before her cardiac surgery. (The assessment form presents a suggested order in which to assess items. If she preferred, the nurse could have done a head to toe assessment and then grouped the data under the relevant categories.)

Care planning theory

A patient assessment is of little benefit to the bedside nurse unless its data is used to formulate a plan of care. A particularly logical system of care-planning has been developed by Mayers (1972). She recommends that an individual patient care plan contain four sections: overall planning information; medications, treatments and diagnostic tests; a checklist of standard or frequently ordered care; and unusual problems.

Overall planning information

The overall planning information section includes identifying information (such as name and hospital number), diagnosis, physician's expectations regarding

Figure 17-1   Critical care nursing assessment guide

Name **Karen J.** Age **48** Sex **F** Hospital # **000000**

Date **9/24/77** Assessor **Nancy Holloway, RN**

Chief Complaint **"short of breath, very tired, weight loss x 1½ yrs"**

Medical Diagnosis **severe mitral regurgitation, significant mitral stenosis;**

for valve replacement 9/25

Allergies **eggs**

Fluid Balance

Cardiac

1. History **Rheumatic fever, age 12**

   P.A.T. after catheterization 3 weeks ago—converted p̄ treatment

   c̄ Quinidine. Has been on Lanoxin, Hydrodiuril, KCl—last doses 9/23

2. Physical

   A. Inspection/palpation

      PMI **5th ICS at anterior axillary line**

      Precordial movements **apical thrill**

   B. Auscultation

      Heart sounds

      S$_1$ **nl**   S$_2$ **opening snap**

      S$_3$ **none**   S$_4$ **none**

      Murmurs **holosystolic III/VI apex → axilla**

      diastolic IV/VI axilla → apex

      rubs **none**

3. Diagnostic procedures and laboratory tests

   Cardiac pressures RA **2** RV **40/4** LA **19**

   (continued)

Material in this chapter is based on Mayers. A systematic approach to the nursing care plan, 1972. Courtesy of Appleton-Century-Crofts, Publishing Division of Prentice-Hall.

Fig. 17-1 *(continued)*

LV **120/8** PA **40/16** Aorta **120/70** PCWP **22**

CVP **16**

ECG **NSR at 72, ST depression "consistent with digitalis intoxication"**

Chest X-ray **results not yet reported**

Cardiac cath **3 weeks ago. Cardiac output and index nl; LV function**
good. Mitral valve gradient 16, area 0.9 cm²

Enzymes **SGOT 23, LDH 212, CPK 8**

Other

4. Other relevant data **none**

Vascular

1. History **neg**

2. Physical

A. Inspection/Palpation

Skin color **pale** temperature **warm**

trophic changes **neg**

vascular lesions **neg**

tenderness **neg** Homan's sign **neg**

edema **neg**

Neck veins **distended at 90°**

HJR **neg**

Arterial pulses

carotid **2⁺ =** brachial **2⁺ =** radial **2⁺ =**

femoral **2⁺ =** popliteal **2⁺ =**

dorsalis pedis **2⁺ =** posterior tibial **2⁺ =**

(continued)

B. Auscultation

Bruits ___neg___

BP ___120/70—bilateral brachial___

pulse pressure ___50___ mean arterial pressure ___67___

3. Diagnostic procedures and laboratory tests

CBC RBC ___4,200,000___ Hgb ___14.5___ Hct ___38%___

Reticulocytes ___NA___ WBC ___8600___

Differential ___nl___

Clotting time ___NA___ PT ___12.9 (control 13.0)___

PTT ___47 (control 45.5)___

4. Other relevant data ___none___

Renal

1. History ___neg___

2. Physical ___neg___

3. Diagnostic procedures and laboratory tests

Urine volume ___24 hour unknown. Urinalysis sample 200 ml; voids___

___7–8 x/day s̄ difficulty___

sp.g. ___1.020___ osmolality ___NA___

urinalysis: color ___straw___ clarity ___clear___

pH ___6___ cells ___few white___

crystals ___0___ casts ___0___

bacteria ___0___

BUN ___7___ Creatinine ___0.8___

Creatinine clearance ___NA___ Hgb ___see above___

Hct ___see above___

Other _____

4. Other relevant data ___none___

(continued)

Fig. 17-1   *(continued)*

Fluid and electrolyte balance

1. History   anorexia x 1½ yrs, diuretics x 1 yr.
2. Physical

     Weight   46.5 kg   Estimated Normal Body Water   60%

     Intake and output (24 hr)   no definite data; pt describes as "average"

     Skin turgor   nl   Mucous membranes   hydrated

     Pulse rate and volume   72, normal   BP   120/70

     Other

3. Diagnostic procedures and laboratory tests

     Osmolality: serum   NA   urine   NA

     Electrolytes: serum Na^+ 136 K^+ 3.2

                 Cl^- 98 Ca^+ NA Mg^{++} NA

                 urine: Na^+ NA K^+ NA Cl^- NA

     Other

4. Other relevant data   none

Temperature   98.6° F

Aeration

1. History   DOE, PND, orthopnea x 1½ years; smoking history neg
2. Physical

     A. Inspection

          Thoracic shape   symmetrical, AP< lateral diameter

          Respirations: Rate   16   Rhythm   eupnea

          Chest expansion   equal bilaterally

(continued)

B. Palpation

    Trachea   <u>midline</u>

    Tactile fremitus   <u>nl</u>

C. Percussion   <u>nl</u>

D. Auscultation

    Breath sounds   <u>nl</u>

    Adventitious sounds: <u>few rales at bases; clear with coughing</u>

    Voice and whispered sounds   <u>nl</u>

E. Extrathoracic signs

    Cyanosis <u>neg</u> Clubbing <u>neg</u>

    Use of accessory muscles <u>neg</u>

    Other _____

3. Diagnostic procedures and laboratory tests

    Pulmonary function tests <u>not done</u>

      Inspiratory force _____ Compliance _____

      FEV_1 _____ TV _____ RV _____

      FRC _____ TLC _____ VC _____

      VD/VT Ratio _____

      Other _____

    Arterial blood gases <u>not done</u>

      F_IO_2 _____ PO_2 _____ PCO_2 _____

      A-a gradient _____ Shunt _____

    Chest X-ray <u>results not available</u>

    Other <u>NA</u>

Acid-base balance

1. History   <u>anorexia x 1½ yr; diuretics x 1 yr</u>

2. Physical   <u>neg</u>

(continued)

Fig. 17-1   *(continued)*

3. Diagnostic procedures and laboratory tests

Serum electrolytes Na^+ __136__ K^+ __3.2__ Cl^- __98__

CO $_2$ __NA__   Anion gap   __NA__

Arterial blood gases   pH __NA__   PCO $_2$ __NA__   HCO $_3$ __NA__

4. Other   __NA__

Nutrition

1. History   anorexia, fatigue x 1½ yrs. Usual elimination pattern
1/day-nl. color and consistency.

2. Physical _____

General appearance   thin, frail, pale

Weight   __46.5 kg__   Change?   loss of 13 kg in last 1½ yr

Mouth: Dention   upper and lower dentures

Tongue   nl appearance and movement

Gag reflex   intact

Swallow reflex   intact

Abdomen

Inspection   nl appearance

Auscultation   nl bowel sounds in all 4 quadrants; no bruits or rubs

Percussion and palpation

Tenderness   neg   Rigidity   neg

Liver   upper border 6th ICS, lower at costal margin; not tender

Spleen   5 cm oval 9th–11th ribs at MAL; not palpable

Rectum and anus $\bar{0}$ hemorrhoids

(continued)

3. Diagnostic procedures and laboratory tests

 Blood glucose 96

4. Other relevant data   none

Communication

Process

1. History   congenital deafness and slurred speech

2. Physical

 Vision nl

 Reading ability   college level

 Hearing   deafness–greater in R ear

 Tactile perception   nl

 Speech   slurred, hesitant

 Writing ability   nl

 Gesturing ability   nl

3. Diagnostic procedures and laboratory tests

4. Other relevant data   none

Content

1. History

 Ethnic background   Caucasian

 Religion   Baptist "but not strong faith"

 Education   2 yr RN–did not complete

 Occupation   homemaker

(continued)

Fig. 17-1   *(continued)*

Usual coping methods

Pain   withdraws physically and emotionally; has tears in eyes; doesn't like to ask for pain medication because of seeming weak and babyish

Anger   withdraws until cooled off

Substance abuse   none

Emotion problems   neg except for "hard time adjusting" when illness caused her to lose scholarship and drop out of school 2 years ago

2. Current information

Expressed concerns   will be embarrassed without dentures; husband will be shocked and upset when sees her post-op; won't know when daughter's baby born

Expectations of hospitalization   expects dangerous surgery, painful, unpleasant post-op period; worried about competence of staff, esp. supervision of students and new nurses; anticipates difficulty making needs understood

Significant others   husband Raymond and daughter Melissa. Raymond works in construction 8 AM–6 PM; off only on day of surgery. Melissa expecting baby any day. Neither present for any teaching–home is 3 hr drive from hospital

Apparent stage of adaptation to illness   disorganization–anxiety

3. Diagnostic procedures   none

4. Other relevant data   none

(continued)

Activity

1. History

Past activity level <u>sedentary x 1½ yrs due to fatigue and dyspnea;</u>
<u>played tennis and other active sports before that.</u>
<u>Sleeps 8 hrs a night (10 PM–6 AM) plus 3 naps per</u>
<u>day; bathes in evening; likes to read and sew.</u>

Current activity level

Prescribed (include estimated duration)

<u>complete bedrest; probably up in chair on 2nd p.o. day and</u>
<u>ambulating with assistance on 5th p.o. day</u>

Actual <u>bedrest, moving about freely</u>

2. Physical

Perception of pressure __✓__ normal ____ absent ____ diminished ___

If absent or diminished, specify how _____

_____

Skin integrity <u>no signs of breakdown</u>

Activity impediments ____ cast ____ diminished joint mobility _____

__✓__ low tolerance for physical exertion

____ other (specify) _____

3. Diagnostic procedures and laboratory tests

<u>__NA__</u>

4. Other relevant data <u>none</u>

Stimulation

1. History <u>neg</u>

2. Physical

LOC <u>alert and oriented</u>

(continued)

Fig. 17-1   *(continued)*

Cranium intact   Neck   flexible

Eyes: Corneal reflex   nl

Pupil size 3 mm, equal

Reaction to light   brisk and equal

Extremities:

Sensation   nl

Voluntary movement   moves all extremities freely

Reflex movement DTRs 2$^+$ and equal bilaterally; Babinski nl

bilaterally

Smoothness and coordination of movement   nl

3. Diagnostic procedures and laboratory tests

4. Other relevant data   none

Abbreviations: nl = normal; neg = negative; NA = not available.

convalescence, nursing's criteria for discharge, home care coordination activities, and other relevant data.

To determine priorities and plan care effectively, a nurse needs to know not only the patient's diagnosis, but whether his/her course is likely to be typical or complicated, how long he/she probably will be under care, and whether he/she will be able to return to his/her premorbid lifestyle. This information can be summarized under the section on physician's expectations for recovery.

The section on nursing criteria for discharge specifies patient-centered expected outcomes that are reasonable for the patient to achieve by discharge. They are used as the criteria against which to evaluate the effectiveness of the overall plan of care and to decide whether to discharge the patient from nursing responsibility.

The home care coordination section includes space for referrals to a discharge coordinator or home care agencies. The section for other relevant data provides a place to record miscellaneous information, such as unusual visiting schedules.

Medications, treatments, and diagnostic tests

The next major section of the care plan is an up to date abstract of the physician's orders for care. Because this section is so familiar to nurses, it will not be discussed further.

Checklist of standard and frequently ordered care

The checklist of standard and frequently ordered care provides a concise, efficient way to indicate standard elements of the patient's care. Included in this section are nursing routines, such as tracheostomy care; standard care plans; diet; activity level; hygienic activities; and vital sign checks. Also included is space for recording miscellaneous patient preferences, such as "wants to be called by nickname, Sunny."

Standard care plans delineate the usual problems which can be predicted from a patient's condition and those nursing activities likely to lead to successful resolution of the problems. They are written in advance and should be readily accessible to the nursing staff. They need not be rewritten for each patient but instead can be listed by title in this portion of the care plan. Standard care plans are appropriate for patients whose problems and progress fall within expected norms.

According to Mayers, standard care plans can be written for diagnoses, situations, or general physiological states. An intensive care unit, for example, might have standard care plans on pulmonary edema, postoperative ambulation, and sleep deprivation. Problems may be actual (one the patient definitely will have) or potential (one the patient is highly likely to develop). For instance, for patients with chest tubes, discomfort is an actual problem, while infection at the insertion site is a potential problem.

A standard care plan (SCP) should have four columns for usual problems, expected outcomes, deadlines, and nursing actions. Usual problems are those which occur frequently in groups of patients with similar disorders. They should include a brief statement of causation. For example, a standard care plan for pulmonary edema might include as a usual problem "dyspnea due to fluid-filled alveoli."

Expected outcomes are short-term objectives which must be achieved before the overall discharge criteria can be met. They should be specific measurable patient behaviors, that is, statements of what you can observe with your senses. For instance, suppose you were writing a standard care plan for congestive heart failure (CHF) and had identified as a usual problem "potential post-discharge recurrence of CHF due to failure to take medications." A statement such as "understands medications" would not be an acceptable expected outcome. Because it does not specify what you would observe the patient doing, it is too subject to varying interpretations by different members of the nursing staff. Acceptable expected outcomes might be 1) "correctly states name, purpose, and dosage schedule for each discharge medication''; and 2) ''states ability to pay for maintenance medications or has been referred to Social Service for financial assistance.''

Deadlines fall into two categories: estimated time limits for meeting expected outcomes, and intervals for documenting the patient's progress towards expected outcomes. In the case that an ultimate deadline cannot be predicted, only documentation intervals may be included.

Nursing actions are activities designed to facilitate the patient's achievement of the expected outcomes. They specify what is to be done, under what circumstances, and how frequently. An example might be ''Perform passive range of motion exercises for the paralyzed extremity five times every four hours while awake.''

Usual problems, expected outcomes, deadlines, and nursing actions can be derived from the staff's experience, a review of patient charts and/or a review of nursing literature. Nursing care for many critical care disorders has already been presented in this book and could be abstracted readily to Mayers' format. For other disorders not specifically addressed in this book, the core concepts can be used as ''building blocks'' in the development of a standard care plan.

Unusual problems

The last section of the individual care plan pertains to unusual problems, that is, those which are unique or require special attention. They may be unanticipated problems or anticipated ones with which the patient is not coping satisfactorily. Frequently, you may determine from your assessment that the patient does not have any unusual problems. In that case, you would note that decision in this section of the care plan. You would also specify a date for reassessment of the validity of your determination. If you did identify unusual problems, you would state for each one your judgment of its cause; expected outcomes; deadlines; and nursing actions.

This brief explanation will orient you to the system used in the care plan presented in this chapter. Readers who are interested in adapting this system in their practice settings should consult Mayers' book for greater detail.

Care planning application: Karen J.

After assessing the patient and recording the data, the nurse's next step is to develop a plan of care. Although not a part of Mayers' system, the FANCAS assessment format leads logically into the steps of identifying patient problems. The nurse begins with the standard care plan for mitral valve replacement (Figure 17-2) developed by the (hypothetical) nursing staff of the intensive care unit. After identifying actual and potential usual problems, the staff had written possible causes, expected outcomes, deadlines, and nursing orders. This care plan represented a consensus of the staff's judgments about nursing care and was supported by documentation in the nursing and medical literature. Because

Figure 17-2 Standard care plan

Overall planning information

Identifying information _____

Physician's expectations regarding treatment

regimen or course of convalescence:

( ) Typical or routine

( ) Atypical or complicated

If atypical or complicated, in what way? _____

Diagnosis __Mitral valve replacement standard care plan__

___(MVR SCP)—Intensive care unit phase___

Nursing's criteria for discharge (overall expected outcomes)

1. Vital signs within normal limits (WNL) for patient

2. Urinary output above 30 ml/hr with specific gravity WNL for patient

3. Arterial blood gas values WNL for patient after extubation

4. Arterial line discontinued

5. Peripheral pulses, limb temperature, and limb color WNL for patient

6. Level of consciousness WNL for patient

7. Medical/surgical problems (for example, arrhythmias) controlled by medical therapeutic plan

8. Patient and/or family demonstrate awareness of therapeutic plan and ability to cooperate with it

(continued)

Fig. 17-2 (continued)

Home care coordination activities

Usual problems	Expected outcomes	Deadlines	Nursing orders
Fluid balance			
1. Potential arrhythmias due to hypoxia; electrolyte imbalances; acid-base imbalances; medications; catecholamine stimulation; surgical trauma to circumflex coronary artery or conduction system; hypertension or hypotension; Valsalva maneuvers	1. Normal sinus rhythm (ideal) or spontaneous or artificial rhythm with regular ventricular rate between 60 and 100 beats per minute	Discharge (✓↑q↑8 hrs) 4th po↑ day (✓q 8 hrs)	1. Place on continuous ECG monitor on admission to ICU
			2. Run rhythm strip and mount it in chart with analysis every 4 hrs and prn for serious arrhythmia
	2. If premature beats present: 10 or fewer APBs or JPBs per minute; 4 or fewer VPBs per minute; no VPBs that are multifocal, more than 3 consecutive, or encroaching on T waves		3. Obtain 12-lead ECG↑ daily and prn for serious arrhythmia
2. Potential cardiac failure*			4. Check chart for medical orders re treatment of: arrhythmias, electrolyte imbalances, acid-base imbalances, hypo- or hypertension
3. Potential cardiac tamponade*	3. BP ± 20 mm Hg of patient's normal BP↑		
4. Potential shock*	4. Adequate peripheral perfusion as manifested by: absence of angina; mental state WNL for patient; urinary output WNL for patient; warm dry skin; peripheral pulse volume WNL for patient		5. Check BP and peripheral perfusion every 1–4 hrs
5. Potential fluid overload*			6. Reduce catecholamine stimulation by minimizing patient anxiety and pain and treating hypotensive episodes promptly
6. Potential hypokalemia*			7. Reduce Valsalva maneuvers by: (after extubation) reminding patient to exhale when moving about in bed; controlling pain; administering stool softeners when ordered by MD↑
7. Potential acute renal failure*			

Usual problems	Expected outcomes	Deadlines	Nursing orders
8. Potential infection due to contamination of indwelling arterial, venous, and urinary catheters; surgical incisions; artificial airway; atelectasis	1. Temperature WNL for patient 2. No purulent drainage, erythema, edema, or unusual tenderness at sites of indwelling catheters 3. Incisions healing without purulent drainage, skin breakdown or wound dehiscence 4. No purulent respiratory secretions		1. Check temperature every 4 hours 2. Check indwelling catheter and incision sites every shift 3. Use meticulous sterile technique with catheter care, wound care, and suctioning 4. Discontinue catheters per MD orders as soon as BP stable; patient taking fluids orally; and patient alert enough to use urinal or bedpan 5. Inform MD of temperature spikes; obain blood cultures and catheter cultures as ordered 6. Check chart for orders for antipyretics and/or antibiotics
Aeration 9. Potential acute respiratory failure* 10. Potential atelectasis* 11. Potential pulmonary edema* 12. Potential pulmonary embolus*			

(continued)

Fig. 17-2 *(continued)*

Usual problems	Expected outcomes	Deadlines	Nursing orders
Nutrition			
13. Potential acute gastric dilatation or paralytic ileus due to anesthesia	1. Undistended abdomen 2. Bowel sounds WNL for patient on auscultation and percussion 3. Abdominal x-rays show no abnormal accumulation of air or fluid in stomach or bowel	3rd po day ($\sqrt{}$ q 8 hrs)	1. Insert and/or connect nasogastric tube to suction per MD order 2. Auscultate abdomen to detect absence of bowel sounds 3. Palpate and percuss abdomen and measure abdominal girth to detect distention 4. Give nothing by mouth until MD orders
14. Potential ulceration due to stress: steroid drugs; GI† tract ischemia	1. NG† drainage pH above 3 2. No blood in NG drainage or stool 3. Hematocrit WNL for patient	Discharge ($\sqrt{}$ q 8 hrs)	1. Check NG drainage acidity q 8 hrs 2. Administer antacids per MD orders to keep pH of NG drainage above 3 3. Check NG drainage and stool for blood
Communication			
15. Anxiety due to fear of pain, complications, death; separation from loved ones; unfamiliar environment; dependency; inability to control environment	1. Relaxed facial expression 2. Relaxed body posture 3. Discusses questions and worries with staff 4. BP, pulse, and respirations WNL for patient	($\sqrt{}$ q 8 hrs)	1. Implement Preoperative Cardiac Surgery Teaching Program in conjunction with nursing staff on preoperative unit 2. Nurse who will receive patient postoperatively: visit patient on day before surgery; assess understanding of preop teaching program and appropriateness of taking patient and family to visit ICU† 3. Assess need for analgesics by noting groaning, frowning, unexplained restlessness, unwillingness to move.

Usual problems	Expected outcomes	Deadlines	Nursing orders
			Control pain by giving analgesics before patient requests
			4. When stripping chest tubes, turning patient, or performing other painful procedures, alert patient to likelihood of pain, premedicate if necessary, and provide reassurance and encouragement
			5. Splint incision with pillow or sheet during movement, coughing, and chest physiotherapy
			6. Assist patient to cope with fears of dependency and loss of control by acknowledging their presence, involving patient in individualizing plan of care as necessary, emphasizing ways patient can contribute to recovery, allowing patient to make choices about timing of care, and encouraging patient to perform self-care when appropriate to physical status
			7. Assign same staff to care for patient whenever feasible
			8. Explain bedside activities and likely patient sensations, even if patient appears unconscious
			9. Encourage visits and phone calls from loved ones
			10. If severe anxiety persists despite nursing measures, consult MD re sedation

(continued)

Fig. 17-2 *(continued)*

Usual problems	Expected outcomes	Deadlines	Nursing orders
Activity			
16. Decreased mobility*			
Stimulation			
17. Potential decreased perception and interpretation of stimuli due to sleep deprivation; medications; post-cardiotomy or ICU psychosis; cerebral hypoxia or emboli	1. Alert and oriented to person, place, time, recent and remote memory	Discharge (√ q 8 hrs)	1. As soon as patient returns to unit, begin orienting to reality 2. Assess level of consciousness every hr until stable 3. Make environment meaningful by explaining objects and noises; remind patient if discussed during preop teaching 4. Schedule care to allow as much undisturbed sleep as possible

*Due to the large number of problems identified in this care plan, only selected representative problems have been fully illustrated with possible causes, expected outcomes, deadlines, and nursing orders. The starred problems are discussed in other chapters and the reader can easily derive causes, outcomes, deadlines, and orders for these problems if desired.

†Abbreviations: WNL, within normal limits; APB, atrial premature beat; JPB, junctional premature beat; VPB, ventricular premature beat; MD, doctor of medicine; po, postoperative; BP, blood pressure; NG nasogastric; ICU, intensive care unit; re, regarding; ECG, electrocardiogram; prn, as necessary; q, every; √, document summary evaluation in patient's chart, GI, gastrointestinal.

this plan had been developed prior to Karen's expected ICU admission, the nurse does not need to rewrite an extensive care plan. Instead, she needs only to alert the staff to review the data gathered in her assessment; to review the SCP; and to individualize the patient's care plan (see Figure 17-3) if any unusual problems may develop. The following paragraphs describe the nurse's thinking as she reviews and analyzes the data under each FANCAS section:

1. Fluid balance.
Cardiac   Her left atrial, pulmonary capillary wedge, and right-sided pressures are elevated, but these elevations are typical for her disorders. The apical thrill, murmurs, increased mitral valve gradient and decreased valve area are all typical, too. Potential atrial arrhythmias are usual problems with mitral stenosis and regurgitation, due to volume overload of the atria or hypoxia secondary to pulmonary congestion. Her cardiac strengths are her normal rhythm, left ventricular and aortic pressures, left ventricular function, cardiac output, cardiac index, and serum enzymes. Our standard care plan on mitral valve replacement is appropriate for her.
Vascular   Her vascular status doesn't pose any problems. The only pathologic finding is the jugular venous distention, but that's just another sign of her right-sided failure.
Renal   Everything's normal here.
Fluid and electrolytes   Her serum potassium's low—that might have potentiated her digitalis toxicity. It's not clear why her potassium level's low—she was on a potassium-wasting diuretic, but also on an oral potassium supplement. Maybe she didn't take the supplement regularly—it does taste awful. This needs to be explored if she'll be discharged on digitalis.

2. Aeration. Her dyspnea on exertion and paroxysmal nocturnal dyspnea are signs of her mitral valve disease and should be relieved by her surgery. Her lungs are clear now, and she'll need the usual post-op chest care to keep them that way. No unusual problems here.

3. Nutrition. She says she's not been hungry for a long time and often is too tired to fix nourishing meals; this is borne out by her chronic weight loss. She'll be N.P.O. during the operative period; since she's already depleted of nutrients, poor wound healing and resistance to infection are possibilities. This is an unusual problem.

4. Communication. There are a lot of problem signals here:
Worry about cost of hospitalization   She says their insurance won't cover the bill. The Social Service Department might be able to help with this.
Worry about her husband and daughter   She's really upset about not being with her daughter during labor. She also seems concerned her husband will lose his job if he takes time off, yet angry that he's not here when she needs him. She also said she's afraid he'll be shocked and upset when he first sees her after the operation. This amount of anxiety about her family is unusual.
Communication barriers   She has trouble both hearing and speaking, and is worried that staff will ignore her or not understand what she needs. Also, she'll

Figure 17-3 Individual nursing care plan

Overall planning information

Physician's expectations regarding treatment regimen
of course of convalescence:

(√) typical or routine

( ) atypical or complicated

If atypical or complicated, in what way? _____

_____

_____

Nursing's criteria for discharge (overall expected outcomes) _____

As specified in mitral valve replacement SCP

Home care coordination activities   Referral to Social Service 9/24

Other relevant data   husband Raymond, grown daughter Melissa

Identifying information:

Karen J.   #000000

48 year old female

Dr. Sabatier

Diagnosis: severe mitral regurgitation, significant mitral
stenosis. For mitral valve replacement 9/25

Medications, treatments and diagnostic tests

Date	Medications	Date	Treatments	Date	Diagnostic tests
9/24	Allergic to penicillin Check chart for post-op orders				

Checklist of standard and frequently ordered care

Nursing routines

✔ Mitral valve replacement
✔ Hemodynamic monitoring lines
✔ Urinary catheter
✔ Artificial airway
✔ Mechanical ventilation
✔ Chest drainage
✔ Range of motion exercises

Activity:
    bed rest

Hygiene:
    bed bath

Diet:
    N.P.O.

Frequently ordered items

  Oral temperature
✔ Rectal temperature
✔ Pulse, respirations
✔ Blood pressure
✔ Intake and output
✔ Specific gravity

Patient preferences, miscellaneous information:

Prefers bath in evening. Usually sleeps 10 PM—6AM and naps 3 x day.

Wants to be called by first name.

(continued)

Fig. 17-3 *(continued)*

Unusual problems

✔ Fluid balance   Aeration   ✔ Nutrition   ✔ Communication   Activity   Stimulation

Date	Unusual problem	Expected outcomes	Deadlines	Nursing actions
9/24	Possible recurrence of digitalis intoxication after discharge due to failure to take prescribed K⁺ supplement	(none possible to define yet)	3 days after transfer to general unit	Gather more information about cause of hypokalemia and knowledge re: relationship between K⁺ and digitalis
9/24	Potential poor wound healing or wound infection due to inadequate nutrition (also see mitral valve replacement SCP, problem 8: infection)	1. See SCP 2. Eats all food on tray 3. Gains weight at rate specified by MD	7 days po (✔ daily)	1. See SCP 2. Replace dentures after extubation 3. As soon as bowel sounds return, check with MD about high calorie diet and desired rate of weight gain 4. Send consult to dietitian to plan hospital meals around favorite foods, and (before hospital discharge) to help her plan nutritious meals needing minimal preparation at home 5. During meals, encourage eating; help if too tired 6. Save items uneaten at meals (if appetizing) and offer as snacks 7. Weigh q.o.d.
9/24	Difficulty communicating due to: a) congenital deafness R > L b) slurred speech	1. Able to indicate needs 2. No tense expression, frowning or other signs of frustration	24 hr po (✔ daily thereafter)	1. Look directly at her 2. Enunciate clearly and slowly 3. Direct speech more toward her left ear

Date	Unusual problem	Expected outcomes	Deadlines	Nursing actions
	c) tendency to withdraw emotionally when upset or in pain d) postoperative intubation	3. No periods of emotional withdrawal longer than 30 minutes		4. Use gestures to supplement speech 5. While intubated, use personalized communication cards on ring (already prepared for her at unit secretary's desk) 6. After extubation, listen to speech patiently and attentively; watch gestures 7. After extubation, use Magic Slate if speech unintelligible 8. Watch for withdrawn expression or tears in eyes 9. Offer pain medication according to your judgment in addition to her requests 10. If withdrawn, gently ask why. If no reply, allow short period of withdrawal (her usual pattern) and ask again
9/24	Anxiety due to: a) worry over husband and daughter b) expectation of painful and unpleasant postoperative period c) fears about staff competence d) also see mitral valve replacement SCP, problem 15: anxiety	1. See SCP	24 hr po (✔ daily thereafter)	1. See SCP 2. Allow husband to visit whenever able to come 3. Before husband's first visit, explain wife's and unit's appearance 4. Accompany husband on first visit 5. Encourage husband to verbalize reactions after visit and clarify misconceptions

(continued)

Fig. 17-3 *(continued)*

Date	Unusual problem	Expected outcomes	Deadlines	Nursing actions
				6. Notify patient promptly of baby's birth when daughter or husband calls
				7. If possible, do not assign students or new nurses to care for her. If unavoidable, provide supervision and discuss their uncertainties re: knowledge or skill away from bedside

be intubated for several hours postoperatively. She may have unusual trouble getting adequate pain relief and emotional support because of her tendency to withdraw, too. These difficulties make communication an unusual problem for her.

Anxiety about staff competence She's knowledgeable about technical details of care, and is apprehensive about a painful, unpleasant postoperative period. She's also concerned about poor care from inexperienced staff. This degree of anxiety about staff competence is unusual.

5. Activity. She is sedentary because of her fatigue and is on bed rest. She really sleeps a lot now. Although she'll be sedated from the anesthetic and analgesics, her decreased mobility will probably not be much of a problem, since she is moving about in bed freely now and the surgeon anticipates getting her out of bed within three days after the surgery. This decrease in mobility represents a usual problem.

6. Stimulation. Everything looks good here except her speech difficulty, which has already been considered.

After identifying the patient's problems and differentiating the usual, unusual, and possible problems, the nurse wrote the care plan in Figure 17-3. The FANCAS checklist under the unusual problems section provides a quick indicator that the patient's problems have been assessed systematically. It is not part of Mayers' original system.

This plan of care clearly indicates much of the care anticipated for Karen the next day. It will, of course, be updated when her postoperative orders arrive in the unit and as changes in her condition necessitate. Left in the cardiac surgical unit the evening before surgery, it can alert the nurses to Karen's unusual problems in advance of her actual admission. It thus can reduce the staff's anxiety about their unknown patient and ensure that attention is paid early to her unusual problems.

Because it will accompany her upon discharge from the critical care unit, it also can facilitate continuity of care. It shows which of Karen's unusual problems received early care-planning attention, which ones are receiving continued nursing intervention, and which ones still need to be explored. A care plan such as this is invaluable in facilitating the provision of personalized nursing care, both during the crucial early postoperative days and beyond the critical care experience.

References

Mayers, M. 1972. *A systematic approach to the nursing care plan.* New York: Appleton-Century-Crofts.

Application of systematic problem solving to nursing practice; care-plan components; care-planning in hospitals, institutions, community agencies, and nursing education; numerous case studies demonstrating use of care plans.

APPENDIX

FANCAS:
An Educational Framework

In 1975, the author used FANCAS as the conceptual framework for planning a critical care educational program offered by the Department of Nursing Service at the University of California, San Francisco. The course consisted of 480 hours of didactic and clinical learning related to adult and pediatric patients with cardiovascular, respiratory, neurological, renal, and endocrine disorders. This appendix will describe the mechanics of establishing such a program and include examples from the UCSF Core Critical Care Course. The author's intent is to encourage and assist other critical care educators to establish similar programs.

Assessment of the need for and feasibility of a critical care educational program

Determining need for a course

To assess the need for such a program, look at such factors as your community's pool of experienced critical care nurses, critical care educational programs offered by nearby colleges or schools of nursing, your critical care patient load, the quality of nursing care in your critical care units, your institution's policies regarding staffing of critical care units, and your success in recruiting and retaining critical care nurses.

In early 1975, it was obvious that a program to prepare registered nurses for critical care nursing was needed at our institution. Although San Francisco is a mecca for registered nurses, competition for experienced critical care nurses was keen among the city's numerous critical care units. Many nurses were interested in entering the field, but most schools of nursing did not equip their students with the necessary knowledges and skills for safe, effective critical care practice. Inexperienced nurses required extensive orientation, which often was truncated because of the pressing need for nurses to provide patient care. Furthermore, at the UCSF campus alone, there were four critical care units, with another scheduled to open in the near future. The four units had a total of 11,668 patient days during fiscal year 1974.

A limited number of critical care courses and workshops were available locally, but they were an expensive, inefficient way to educate nursing staff. We were unable to meet our desired nurse/patient staffing patterns without frequent pleas to already overworked nurses to work extra shifts. Overtime costs were prohibitive and morale suffered as nurses struggled to maintain quality patient care. We believed that a comprehensive educational program could benefit both our nursing staff and their critically ill patients.

Identifying the goal

The overall course goal should be identified clearly. After considerable discussion, we defined our overall goal as the education of registered nurses without previous critical care experience to function as beginning practitioners in our critical care units.

Examining the feasibility of meeting the goal

Feasibility assessment necessitates projection of preparation and teaching time necessary, course enrollment, educational resources, and financial expenses and resources. Both the planning and teaching of course content are very time-consuming. We estimated 5.5 months of full-time preparation for the course. In fact, it took approximately 2.5 months more to plan objectives, class content, clinical experiences, and evaluation methods. We also estimated that three months of classes and clinical experience would be necessary to prepare a registered nurse for beginning practice in our critical care units, which are quite sophisticated. We identified a capacity to educate twenty students in the course.

Our educational resources were substantial. Within the Department's Division of Staff Development, there was a masters-prepared instructor with expertise in coronary and cardiac surgical nursing. This instructor was relieved of all other responsibilities to become the course coordinator and primary instructor.

A senior staff nurse who was also a pediatric nurse practitioner and experienced critical care nurse was appointed for three months to co-coordinate the course, particularly its pediatric aspects.

Faculty for the course included nursing staff in the various units, and members of the Schools of Nursing and Medicine. Our students had access to the University Library, books in the Staff Development Department, School of Nursing Learning Resource Center, and University Museum of Anatomy. Clinical resources included a 4-bed Coronary Care Unit, 12-bed Intensive Care Unit, 22-bed Neonatal Intensive Care Unit, 4-bed Pediatric Special Care Unit, 24-bed Pediatric Surgical Ward, 27-bed Neurosurgery Ward, Cardiac Catheterization Laboratory, and operating rooms.

Financial expenses include the salaries of staff and students as well as expenses for books, films, and other educational aids. Financial resource options may be departmental allocation, fees from students, or perhaps a grant from the Department of Health, Education, and Welfare or other funding agency.

Our total program costs, almost $90,000, were met by a departmental allocation. The bulk of this expense was salaries. Because our goal was to improve patient care in our units, we opted not to enroll any nurses not employed by our hospital. Although we considered an enrollment fee, we rejected it as prohibitive for students; based on a comparison with already available shorter courses, we estimated $1500 as a comparable fee for our course. Instead of charging a fee, we asked each student to make a moral commitment to work at our hospital for a year after completing the course. We did not apply for a funding grant from an outside agency because of time constraints.

Planning the program

Planning is *the* crucial step in successful implementation of a program like this. Involved in course planning are the steps of obtaining input from key people, selecting a conceptual framework, developing behavioral objectives, planning class and clinical content, scheduling learning experiences, planning evaluation methodology, deciding upon course credit, deciding how to best utilize course graduates, and defining the criteria and process of student selection.

Obtaining input from key people

No matter how elegant, an educational design will fail unless it is supported by the people whom it will affect most. We found it helpful to establish two planning committees. The first, responsible for organizational planning, consisted of the Director of Nursing, Assistant Director for Fiscal Affairs, Assistant Director for Staff Development, Administrative Supervisor for CCU and ICU, and the course coordinator.

The second committee, called the Liaison Committee, consisted of the course coordinator and the head nurse of each clinical unit involved in the program. This committee's purposes were to provide input into the selection of candidates, help develop course content, and plan and facilitate clinical supervision of the learners. The committee met two hours a week. To facilitate planning within a limited time period, the program coordinator developed proposals which then were reviewed by the committee for completeness and feasibility. The head nurses were enthusiastic about the course's purposes and design, and contributed many helpful suggestions for refining the course's objectives, organization, content, and evaluation methods.

The committee developed an explicit statement of the responsibilities of the course coordinator for the didactic portion of the course, and the head nurses for the clinical portion of the course. By allowing each person to be clear about the responsibilities she was assuming, this statement helped to facilitate clear communication and smooth implementation of the program.

Selecting a conceptual framework for the course objectives and content

It is essential to establish a conceptual framework before defining objectives and selecting content. Without a framework, you easily can become muddled about what to include, and either cover unnecessary material or overlook important concepts. For example, you might focus all of your objectives and classes on physiological areas of critical care, overlooking the often-neglected psychological aspects.

The framework we selected integrated the concepts of nursing process, core knowledges and skills in critical care nursing, and FANCAS. The same framework upon which this book is based, it is discussed in Chapter 1.

Developing student behavioral objectives for each class and each clinical experience

Student behavioral objectives were defined for each class and each clinical experience. In addition to enhancing course planning and student learning, these student behavioral objectives were particularly useful in alerting guest lecturers and staff nurse preceptors to the ways they could assist students.

It is important to set realistic post-course expectations of students. Unless students have a prolonged period of time for learning, it is unlikely that they will be fully competent practitioners upon completion of the program. We encouraged the head nurses to plan additional practice in the individual unit to help our graduates adapt their core knowledges and skills to that particular unit.

Planning class and clinical content

Content development was a mammoth task. We found it helpful to use planning sheets, which contained five columns for class objectives, content, teacher activity, learner activity, and learning aids. These sheets oriented the teachers and learners to each class' purpose and the activities designed to meet it. They also reminded the teachers of nitty-gritty details such as arranging for necessary audiovisual aids or for patients to examine. An example of a planning sheet is shown in Table A-1.

The course coordinator also developed guidelines for the students to use in choosing clinical activities. These guidelines were based on the course objectives, course content, and suggestions from head nurses for good learning experiences in their clinical environments. An example is shown in Table A-2.

Table A-1 Clinical experience: physical assessment, weeks 2–6

Objectives	Content	Teacher activity	Learner activity	Learning aids

1. Given critically ill patients the nurse will perform physical assessments according to criteria established in the physical assessment class	As in physical assessment class	1. Select in advance patients for examination
		
		2. Observe learner's demonstration; correct techniques and interpretation of findings as necessary
			1. Examine at least 1 critical patient in each category:
			  a. neonate
			  b. older pediatric
			  c. adult
			
			2. Orally differentiate normal from abnormal findings
				Patients:
				  Neonate, older pediatric, adult

2. Given physical assessments performed by herself or others, the nurse will differentiate normal from abnormal findings				

Table A-2 Clinical experience: cardiac medical patients

A. *Recommended Types of Patients* (in preferred order):

1. Acute myocardial infarction

2. Pacemaker

3. Hemodynamic problem requiring pulmonary arterial line

4. Atrial arrhythmia

5. Angina

B. *Skills to Practice*

1. 12-lead ECG

2. Arrhythmia interpretation

3. CVP, PA, arterial lines

4. Pacemaker care

5. Assistance with pericardiocentesis

6. Working with monitors

7. Assistance with cardioversion

8. Defibrillation

Developing a workable class and clinical schedule

The class and clinical schedule must be planned meticulously, to ensure that content is presented in class before the nurse is expected to apply it in the clinical setting.

We opted to intersperse didactic and clinical experiences. This approach reinforced class material by providing prompt opportunities for clinical application and minimized the "information overload" on students. It was also dictated by the units' capacity for student experiences. Because UCSF is a teaching institution, our facilities were already being used by nursing students, medical students, nursing staff orientees, and many other learners. Most units could accomodate only 1–2 additional learners at any given time.

With experience, we settled on a mix of centralized and decentralized scheduling for clinical experiences. The coordinator developed a master schedule indicating which students would rotate into which units each week. Within that overall schedule, learners negotiated with the head nurse for specific times open for learning experiences. We deliberately avoided confining clinical experience within a Monday–Friday 9 A.M. to 5 P.M. time frame, which was already overloaded with learners and which did not necessarily coincide with useful patient care experiences, such as preoperative teaching sessions.

Our final course schedule consisted of 125 hours of didactic instruction on anatomy, physiology, assessment, pathophysiology, treatment, and nursing skills for common critical conditions. It also included 150 hours of supervised patient care and 205 hours of goal-directed independent study. Students participated in the course full-time for 12 weeks.

One initially perplexing problem was how many hours to allot to each segment of class and clinical. The breakdown we chose is shown in Table A-3. The course was planned so that the first six weeks were spent in class, on assessment rounds, in skills laboratories, and in observations of diagnostic and surgical procedures. Each of the remaining six weeks was planned for 24 hours of clinical experience and 16 hours of class, conference and independent study. The delay in introducing students to bedside care was intended to reduce their reality shock by equipping them with basic knowledges and skills, before exposing them to an environment in which a nurse often is evaluated initially on the sophistication of her knowledge and her rapid performance of technical skills. Unfortunately, for some students the early weeks were marked by increasing anxiety about their ability to care for patients. Perhaps this difficulty might have been avoided by earlier exposure to bedside care.

Planning must allow for library and study time. It is unreasonable to expect a learner to attend 40 hours of class or clinical a week and still prepare for classes, assignments, and tests. We found that the learners were so stimulated that they read voraciously, shortchanging themselves on sleep and activities with families and friends. In retrospect, our schedule did not allot enough time for study.

Table A-3   Allotment of class and clinical hours

Topic	Hours
Introduction	4
Normal anatomy and physiology	12
Physical assessment class	8
Physical assessment rounds	8
Diagnostic procedures	8
Observations of cardiac catheterization and neurodiagnostic procedures	8
Neonatal intensive care	10
ECG interpretation	20
Cardiovascular disorders and nursing care	8
Aeration disorders and nursing care	12
Neurological disorders and nursing care	3
Fluid, electrolyte, and endocrine disorders and nursing care	4
Renal disorders and nursing care	3
Communication with the critically ill	3
Gastrointestinal disorders and nursing care	3
Activity restrictions	3
Examinations	6
Observation of surgery	8
Bedside patient care:	
Coronary care unit	24
Intensive care unit	24
Intensive care nursery	24
Pediatric special care unit	24
Neurosurgical unit	24
Pediatric surgery unit	24

Planning evaluation methodology

It is important to plan evaluation methods before implementing the program so that necessary data can be collected at appropriate times. If you want to do a before and after comparison, for example, you must collect your "before" data in advance of program implementation.

You can determine what to evaluate by asking yourself what you want to know about various aspects of the program. Both ongoing and retrospective evaluations are helpful. Ongoing evaluation is invaluable in detecting problem areas during the program. Evaluation at the end of the program and several months later can help you determine whether you met your goals. In our case, we decided we wanted to know: a) how well the students learned the didactic material; b) how well they functioned in various clinical settings; c) whether the units provided an atmosphere conducive to learning; d) what the students and head nurses perceived as strengths and weaknesses of the program; e) what percentage of learners passed the course; and f) what percentage fulfilled the one-year post-course work commitment. We considered doing before and after comparisons of turnover rate, absenteeism, and quality of patient care but decided they were affected by so many variables it would be almost impossible to attribute any change to this specific program.

The methods we used to collect data varied. The methods used to evaluate students' theoretical learning were multiple choice examinations, a written case study and care plan, and a short class for unit staff on a topic chosen by the student. Evaluation of the student's clinical performance consisted of two parts. Each week, the staff nurse who precepted the learner rated the student on general clinical behaviors (Table A-4). The preceptor then discussed the evaluation with the learner to help her identify areas needing improvement. The second part of the clinical evaluation was a technical skills checklist (Table A-5) which the learner was expected to complete over several weeks. By the end of the course, the student was expected to achieve a satisfactory rating in all categories on both the general and technical clinical evaluations. To enhance student learning and observer objectivity, criteria for skill evaluation were developed and shared with students and preceptors (Table A-6). Items on both the general and technical evaluations were rated on a satisfactory or "needs improvement" basis; that is, either the learner did perform the behavior according to the criteria or she did not.

Criteria for "passing" levels on each evaluation method and the percentage contribution of each toward the final grade were clearly specified at the start of the course (Table A-7).

During the course, the students evaluated the clinical learning environment weekly, so that the environment could be improved while the course was still in progress. They used a form (Table A-8) designed by the head nurses and course coordinator to identify possible problem areas.

When the course was over, it was evaluated by the students (Table A-9) and by the head nurses (Table A-10). The results were summarized by the coordinator for feedback to the head nurses and Director of Nursing, and for improvement of the program should it be offered again.

The results of our evaluations will be discussed later.

Table A-4   Critical care course: clinical performance evaluation

Part I: General

Learner's name _____ Date _____

Unit _____ Type of patient (s) _____

Evaluator's name _____

Directions to learner: Obtain one evaluation at end of each clinical week and return to the course coordinator.

Directions to evaluator: Rate the learner's performance according to your observations as follows:

1. Not observed

2. Needs improvement

3. Satisfactory

Item	*Rating*
A. Assessment	
1. Performs physical assessment before caring for patient	_____
2. Recognizes changes in patient's condition	_____
3. Repeats physical assessment as indicated by changes in patient's condition	_____
4. Interprets assessment findings in relation to each other and underlying pathophysiology	_____
B. Planning	
1. Consults resource material and people when needed	_____
2. When asked, is able to state:	
a. patient's actual problems	_____
b. patient's potential problems	_____
c. pathophysiology of problems	_____
d. goals of care	_____

(continued)

Table A-4   *(continued)*

e. methods of care	_____

C. Implementation

    1. Responds appropriately to patient emergencies:

a. cardiac arrest	_____
b. acute respiratory distress	_____
c. shock	_____
d. hemorrhage	_____
e. other (please specify)	_____

    2. Responds appropriately to other changes in patient condition _____

    3. Demonstrates prevention of common problems by including in care:

a. measures to prevent sensory deprivation/overload	_____
b. safe electrical environment	_____
c. optimum positioning	_____
d. range of motion exercises	_____
e. patient participation in activities of daily living (when appropriate)	_____

    4. Communicates with patient and family in ways that explain care, allay anxiety, and recognize patient's individuality _____

    5. Utilizes opportunities for teaching patient, family, and/or staff _____

D. Evaluation

1. Evaluates effects of nursing actions	_____
2. Revises care plan according to evaluation	_____

Deciding upon credit for the course

Upon successful completion of our course, each student received a written certificate describing course content and attesting to her performance. Current alternatives to such certification might include community college or university

Table A-5   Critical care course: clinical performance evaluation

Part II: Technical

Learner's name _____

Directions to learner: Submit this form to the course coordinator at the end of the course, at which time you must have a rating of three in each category in each skill.

Directions to evaluator:

a. Demonstration—enter unit's initials if you have demonstrated to student

b. Return demonstration—Rate the student's performance according to your observations:

1. Not observed

2. Needs improvement

3. Satisfactory

Write the rating and your unit's initials. For criteria for rating, see the Critical Care Syllabus on your unit.

Skill	*Demonstration*	*Return Demonstration*
A. Demonstrates beginning proficiency in special assessment techniques.		
1. Cardiac monitor a. Electrodes and settings		
b. Response to arrhythmias		
2. 12-lead ECG		
3. CVP line		
4. PA line		
5. Arterial line		
6. Umbilical line		
7. LAP line		
8. Automatic blood pressure machine		

(continued)

Table A-5 *(continued)*

9. Chest drainage
10. NG drainage
11. Urinary drainage
12. Heart auscultation
13. Lung auscultation
14. Neuro signs
15. ABG interpretation
16. Electrolyte interpretation
B. Demonstrates beginning skill in performing or assisting with specialized treatment techniques.
1. Intubation
2. Extubation
3. ET suctioning
4. NT suctioning
5. Mechanical ventilation
6. CPAP
7. Chest PT
8. Hand ventilation
9. Pacemaker
10. Cardioversion/defibrillation
11. Gavage
12. Hyperalimentation
13. IV Drugs (preparation and monitoring of infusions)

credit, or continuing education credits from a state Board of Nursing or the American Association of Critical Care Nurses.

Deciding how to best utilize staff after course completion

We decided to place most course graduates in a critical care float pool. This placement provided educated staff to assist the regular nursing staff during peak

Table A-6 Example of criteria for clinical performance evaluation

Part II: Technical

Assessment skills

1. Cardiac monitoring
   A. Electrodes and settings
      1. Orients patient to purpose and technique of monitoring
      2. Applies leads in specified positions for unit
      3. Sets rate alarms
      4. Adjusts monitor controls to obtain clear pattern
      5. Demonstrates ability to trigger printout from: (a) bedside; and (b) central monitor
   B. Response to arrhythmias
      1. Evaluates patient
      2. Documents arrhythmia
      3. Interprets by self or obtains assistance in interpreting
      4. For ventricular standstill, begins CPR
      5. For ventricular tachycardia with hemodynamic decompensation or for ventricular fibrillation, defibrillates by self or obtains assistance in defibrillating
2. 12-lead ECG:
   A. Explains procedure to patient
   B. Applies leads in standard positions
   C. Records clear example of approximately 6 complexes per lead
   D. Labels leads, and labels ECG with name, time and date
3. Hemodynamic monitoring lines
   A. Assembles equipment in proper order
   B. Obtains accurate readings
   C. Interprets significance of readings

(continued)

Table A-6 *(continued)*

   D. Provides routine care (see Standard Care Plan on Hemodynamic Monitoring Lines)

   E. In addition for lines requiring transducers:

      1. Uses closed, continuous flush system as first choice; closed intermittent system as second choice; open flush system as last choice

      2. Follows specified steps in balancing and calibrating, including:

         a. Selects correct calibration number for arterial or venous use

         b. Opens system to air when calibrating

---

census periods, staff illnesses, and so on. It also gave the graduates a chance for additional clinical practice in a variety of settings. As vacancies occurred in unit staffs, they were filled from this pool by mutual agreement among the graduate, head nurse, and nursing administration.

Selection of students

The criteria and process for selection of students should be based on the course goals. Defining the criteria and process in advance of student selection allows you to be objective and impartial.

Table A-7 Evaluation

Method	Percent of grade	Criteria for credit
1. 4 written quizzes	20	70% of items on each quiz correct
2. 1 written final exam	15	70% of items correct
3. 6 general clinical evaluations	30	By end of course, rating of 3 on all items
4. 1 skill sheet	10	By end of course, rating of 3 on all items
5. 1 written case study	15	Assessments, care plans, and follow-up evaluation meet criteria specified on assignment sheet
6. 1 class for unit staff	10	Brief written evaluation by clinical preceptor

Table A-8   Critical care nursing course: student evaluation of clinical experience

Date _____   Unit _____

Please comment on these areas. Be specific. Feel free to add other comments.

1. Staff acceptance of you as an R.N. student.

2. Staff assistance and support of you

3. Opportunity to function independently, consistent with your level of expertise

4. Consistency between patient care taught in class and that given on unit

5. Consistency of teaching among staff

6. Accessibility of data relevant to patient care

7. Completeness and currentness of nursing care plans on Kardexes

8. Suggestions for improving clinical experience on this unit

---

   In committee meetings, we decided that the successful and satisfied critical care nurses we already knew possessed the following characteristics: intelligence; retentive memory for details; facility for independent, rapid and accurate decision-making; tolerance for high stress; physical stamina; conscientiousness; ability to remain patient-focused; and skill at determining priorities and organizing patient care activities. Although direct measurement of such characteristics was beyond our ability, we identified the following criteria for student selection:

- Registered nurse with no previous critical care experience
- Minimum of 6 months' staff nurse experience
- Demonstrated ability to provide quality patient care
- Personal motivation to master course content

Table A-9   Critical care course evaluation

1. What did you like most about the course?

2. What did you like least? How could these things be changed?

3. What topics should be added to/deleted from the course? Why?

4. Should the timing of any of the classes be changed? How?

5. Did you get what you wanted in taking the course? If not, what needs were you unable to meet?

6. Have your views of critical care nursing changed during the course? If so, how?

7. Did you have satisfactory role models in class? Clinical?

8. Should any of the evaluation methods be changed? If so, how?

9. Please evaluate the following by circling your response:

Length of total class segment	too short	about right	too long
Length of clinical segment	too short	about right	too long
Number of classes per day	too few	about right	too many
Independent study time	not enough	about right	too much

10. Would you recommend splitting this course into an adult course and a pediatric course? Why?

(continued)

11. Any further comments or recommendations about *class* segment of course:

12. Any further comments or recommendations about *clinical* segment of course:

13. Please comment on the course coordinator's effectiveness as a teacher:

   Presentation of content:

   Stimulation of you to learn:

   Supportiveness:

   Openness to constructive criticism:

   Other:

Table A-10   Core critical care course head nurse evaluation

1. What problems did you encounter during the course that you think have not been resolved? How could they be avoided/solved for the next course?

2. Did you think students had learned an adequate amount of theory before they came to your unit, so that they could take advantage of available clinical experiences? If not, what topics should be included next time?

3. What other comments or suggestions do you have in relation to the educational aspects of the program?

- Commitment to work in our critical care units for one year after completing the course
- Acceptance of the policies regarding floating and rotations of shifts and weekends which would apply after course completion

Approximately 4 months before the start of the course, we advertised it and the criteria for selection in our in-house nursing newsletter. The nurses who were interested met as a group with the course coordinator and the Assistant Director for Fiscal Affairs to learn about the selection process, course objectives, and other details. To assist potential applicants in assessing their aptitude for critical care nursing, we devised a questionnaire (Table A-12). The Assistant Director and the coordinator then interviewed the applicants and met individually with head nurses to evaluate the candidate's suitability for the course. These meetings focused on the candidate's demonstrated quality of patient care, decision-making ability, and skill at organizing patient care. Seventeen nurses were accepted out of 19 who applied from our hospital. (The remainder were selected by the coordinator and the Assistant Director from applicants for staff nurse positions at UCSF.) Beginning the selection process this far in advance allowed us to recruit and orient staff to replace those entering the program. Thus, disruption on the units from which students came was held to a minimum.

Responsibilities

It is essential to clearly define the responsibilities of the course coordinator, instructors and students. Advance clarification of responsibilities, rewards, and sanctions avoids many potential misunderstandings. We chose a learning contract, developed by the coordinator with student input, as the vehicle for clarification of the coordinator's and students' responsibilities. Each student received a copy of the contract which she and the coordinator signed. The learning contract is shown in Table A-12.

Clinical preceptor and student responsibilities during clinical experiences are shown in Table A-13.

Implementing the program

Implementation of an educational program as large as this requires a full-time coordinator to keep things running smoothly on a day to day basis. Even with such a coordinator, implementation may seem chaotic on some days.

"Shakedown" problems

No program runs smoothly the first time it is presented. Preparing yourself psychologically for the likelihood of unanticipated problems makes it easier to cope when you discover that vital piece of information you overlooked!

Table A-11 Core critical care course applicant self-assessment

This sheet is intended to help you think about a "match" between your preferences and the environments of Critical Care Units. Unless you prefer not to, please complete and return to the Assistant Director for Fiscal Affairs prior to your interview. During your interview, you and she will have an opportunity to discuss your self-assessment.

1. What is your philosophy of nursing?

2. Why do you want to work in Critical Care?

3. What are your strengths in caring for patients?

4. What are your areas that need strengthening in caring for patients?

5. What aspects of nursing do you enjoy most?

6. What aspects of nursing do you enjoy least?

7. Describe your preferred method of making (or obtaining) decisions about patient care.

8. What are your feelings about working with dying patients?

(continued)

Table A-11   *(continued)*

9. Describe your ability to learn:

   (a) basic sciences
   (b) behavioral sciences
   (c) technical skills

10. Describe the characteristics of your preferred work environment.

11. How much difficulty do you have adapting your body rhythms to working various shifts?

Table A-12   Core critical care course learning contract

Course coordinator

The course coordinator agrees to do the following:

A. In relation to students:

  1. Share with the students the learning philosophy underlying the course.

  2. Make explicit statements about the course's

    • structure

    • objectives

    • content

    • evaluation criteria and evaluation methods

  3. Provide a variety of learning experiences in the area of critical care.

  4. Elicit from the students frequent feedback about the appropriateness of course structure and content.

(continued)

5. Consider students' recommendations in revising the current and/or future course.

6. Orally share with students her decisions about their recommendations.

7. Provide oral or written positive reinforcement and constructive evaluation of students' learning progress.

8. Upon completion of the course:

   a. Place in each student's employee folder a statement reflecting course attendance and evaluation performance.

   b. Recommend to the Director of Nursing job placement for students.

      1. Students who fulfill the contract and meet the learning objectives will be recommended for placement in a critical care float pool, except for nurses from the 6th and 8th floors, who will return to those floors.

      2. Students who fulfill the contract but do not meet the objectives may be recommended for additional learning experiences before placement in the pool or for placement in non-critical areas.

B. In relation to instructors:

   1. Share the learning philosophy underlying the course.

   2. Establish (with input from the instructor) the objectives and content for a specific class.

   3. Assist the instructor in gearing the presentation to the level of a beginning critical care nurse.

   4. After presentation, share feedback from students about its appropriateness in meeting the class objectives, its organization, its suitability for beginners in critical care nursing, and suggestions (if any) for improving future presentations of the subject.

   5. Write a letter to the instructor thanking him or her for teaching the class.

   6. Send a copy of the letter to the instructor's immediate supervisor and the employee's folder (if applicable).

Table A-12   *(continued)*

Students

The Students agree to:

1. Share with the coordinator oral or written feedback about:

    a. The appropriateness of course objectives for their learning needs

    b. Workload

    c. Frustrations

    d. Suggestions for improving current or future courses

2. Attend all classes.

3. Arrive for class at the time it is scheduled to begin.

4. Notify the secretary in the Nursing Office and the secretary in Staff Development in advance of unavoidable absences.

5. Correctly answer formal and informal questions about material assigned for study prior to class.

6. Participate in demonstrations in class.

7. Orally contribute relevant comments to class.

8. Provide oral feedback to individual instructors during class about clarity of presentation and need for further explanation of concepts.

9. After class, provide the coordinator with written or oral feedback about:

    A. Whether the material was presented:

        1. according to the objectives and content listed in the class outline

        2. in an organized fashion

        3. at the level of the learner (beginning level in critical care).

    B. Suggestions for improving future presentations of the subject.

10. Meet criteria for all required clinical experiences.

11. Complete all required evaluation tools by specified dates.

12. Notify course coordinator if considering withdrawal from course.

(continued)

If the coordinator or student thinks the above agreements are being breached, he/she should promptly discuss the problem with the person not fulfilling the agreements. If this discussion does not resolve the problem, the following options are available:

A. For nonfulfillment by any party:

　1. Re-negotiation of the contract

B. For nonfulfillment by student:

　1. Transfer of student out of course and/or critical care float pool

　2. Termination of employment (for probationary employees)

C. For nonfulfillment by course coordinator:

　1. Submission of written statement agreed upon by student group that describes the counterproductive/ineffective behavior of the coordinator. The statement should be directed to the Coordinator of Staff Development.

I understand and agree to this contract:

Name ＿＿＿＿＿＿＿＿＿＿＿＿＿＿＿＿＿ Date ＿＿＿＿＿＿＿＿＿＿＿＿＿

Name ＿＿＿＿＿＿＿＿＿＿＿＿＿＿＿＿＿ Date ＿＿＿＿＿＿＿＿＿＿＿＿＿

Table A-13　Preceptor and student responsibilities for clinical experience

Learner	*Preceptor*
1. Select one patient from each category.	1. Serve as a resource in patient selection.
2. Arrange time with head nurse.	2. Coordinate student time on unit.
3. Do assessment.	3. Serve as a resource in assessment.
4. Read about pathology, care techniques, and drugs unfamiliar to you.	4. Serve as a resource in pathology, drugs, and care.
5. Write individualized care plan.	5. Discuss care plan with student.
6. Provide direct care.	6. Provide supervision as needed.
7. Attend pertinent patient conferences (optional).	7. Inform student of conferences.
8. Complete self-evaluation.	8. Complete student evaluation.
9. Complete evaluation of experience on unit.	9. Use feedback from students to improve clinical experience for next group.

One early crisis in our program was our students' sudden demand for a limited number of library references also used by other library patrons. The course reading load was heavy and students panicked when they could not obtain materials. Much to the coordinator's dismay, she discovered that requests for reserve status of reading materials should have been submitted six weeks earlier. This problem necessitated emergency revision of the reading list, diversion of some of our funds for duplication of dozens of articles, and establishment of a mini-library.

A crisis in the clinical segment developed when the census of one unit fell to zero for two weeks (even though it had been jammed for previous months!). Clinical assignments had to be revised and arrangements made for alternate clinical experiences.

Emotional support to the students

Students take an emotional risk when they enroll in a program like this. They essentially abandon their successfully established roles as competent practitioners in their home units to embark on an uncertain path in another branch of nursing. In addition, the content of such a course can be threatening. Our course was intellectually rigorous and we found some students needed assistance in reestablishing effective study habits, writing papers, and handling test anxiety.

Students also needed some assistance in differentiating themselves from the staff nurse role in the critical care units, so that they could leave the units without guilt when scheduled for classes, library time, etc. The potential conflict between the nurse's learning needs and the patient's care needs was minimized because the students were not counted as unit staff. They were on full salary as learners and their timesheets were maintained separately from unit staff.

One delightful by-product of the course was the friendships formed during it. The coordinator encouraged students to vent their frustrations and anxieties, and they quickly established supportive bonds with each other and with her. A welcoming party at the coordinator's home the day before the course helped to alleviate anxiety, too, by giving everyone an opportunity to meet informally in a social setting before tackling the course.

Evaluating the program

A thorough evaluation can indicate whether goals were met and can suggest areas for revision if the course is to be repeated. Our evaluations produced numerous insights, among which were the following.

1. Students liked most: the theoretical presentations, assessment rounds, observations of diagnostic tests and surgeries, availability of study time, variety of lecturers, and open atmosphere for questions and feelings.

2. They liked least: weekly unit rotations, problems with clinical scheduling, and the unwelcoming attitude of some staff nurses.

3. A few students reported becoming disillusioned with critical care nursing as they saw it practiced; however, others reported using negative role models as learning experiences. One student suggested using the time set aside for discussion of experiences to redefine their expectations and goals instead of dwelling on disappointment.

4. Most students thought the amount of clinical hours was about right. The group was split between thinking the total number of class hours was about right or not enough.

5. All but one learner completed and passed the course, in spite of its intellectual and emotional rigor. The nurse who did not complete the course had a passing grade at the time she withdrew.

6. 84% of the course graduates completed the one-year work commitment. Forty-seven percent were still employed at our institution two years after the course ended.

Summary

The Core Critical Care Course educated registered nurses without previous critical care experience to function as beginning practitioners in our critical care settings. Based within a Staff Development Division of Nursing Service, it was an exciting, innovative approach to providing competent and compassionate nurses to care for desperately ill patients.

Index